Interventional Radiology in Trauma Management

Jaime Tisnado, MD
Professor
Radiology and Surgery, Cardiovascular and Interventional Radiology
MCV Hospitals/VCU Medical Center
Richmond, Virginia

Rao R. Ivatury, MD
Emeritus Professor of Surgery
Immediate Past Chair
Division of Trauma, Critical Care, and Emergency Surgery
MCV Hospitals/VCU Medical Center
Richmond, Virginia

Thieme
New York • Stuttgart • Delhi • Rio de Janeiro

Executive Editor: Timothy Y. Hiscock
Managing Editor: Elizabeth Palumbo
Director, Editorial Services: Mary Jo Casey
Production Editor: Sean Woznicki
International Production Director: Andreas Schabert
Vice President, Editorial and E-Product Development: Vera Spillner
International Marketing Director: Fiona Henderson
International Sales Director: Louisa Turrell
Director of Sales, North America: Mike Roseman
Senior Vice President and Chief Operating Officer: Sarah Vanderbilt
President: Brian D. Scanlan

Library of Congress Cataloging-in-Publication Data

Interventional radiology in trauma management / [edited by]
    Jaime Tisnado, Rao R. Ivatury.
        p. ; cm.
    Includes bibliographical references and index.
    ISBN 978-1-60406-311-0 (hardcover) --
ISBN 978-1-60406-734-7 (eISBN)
    I. Tisnado, Jaime, editor of compilation. II. Ivatury, Rao R., editor of
compilation.
    [DNLM: 1. Wounds and Injuries--surgery. 2. Radiography,
Interventional--methods. 3. Wounds and Injuries--diagnosis.
WO 700]
RD33.55
617'.0757--
dc23   2013039569

© 2016 Thieme Medical Publishers, Inc.

Thieme Publishers New York
333 Seventh Avenue, New York, NY 10001 USA
+1 800 782 3488, customerservice@thieme.com

Thieme Publishers Stuttgart
Rüdigerstrasse 14, 70469 Stuttgart, Germany
+49 [0]711 8931 421, customerservice@thieme.de

Thieme Publishers Delhi
A-12, Second Floor, Sector-2, Noida-201301
Uttar Pradesh, India
+91 120 45 566 00, customerservice@thieme.in

Thieme Publishers Rio de Janeiro, Thieme Publicações Ltda.
Edifício Rodolpho de Paoli, 25º andar
Av. Nilo Peçanha, 50 – Sala 2508,
Rio de Janeiro 20020-906 Brasil
+55 21 3172-2297 / +55 21 3172-1896

Cover design: Thieme Publishing Group
Typesetting by Thomson Digital, India

Printed in China by Everbest Printing Co.   5 4 3 2 1

ISBN 978-1-60406-311-0

Also available as an e-book:
eISBN 978-1-60406-734-7

Important note: Medicine is an ever-changing science undergoing continual development. Research and clinical experience are continually expanding our knowledge, in particular our knowledge of proper treatment and drug therapy. Insofar as this book mentions any dosage or application, readers may rest assured that the authors, editors, and publishers have made every effort to ensure that such references are in accordance with **the state of knowledge at the time of production of the book.**

Nevertheless, this does not involve, imply, or express any guarantee or responsibility on the part of the publishers in respect to any dosage instructions and forms of applications stated in the book. **Every user is requested to examine carefully** the manufacturers' leaflets accompanying each drug and to check, if necessary in consultation with a physician or specialist, whether the dosage schedules mentioned therein or the contraindications stated by the manufacturers differ from the statements made in the present book. Such examination is particularly important with drugs that are either rarely used or have been newly released on the market. Every dosage schedule or every form of application used is entirely at the user's own risk and responsibility. The authors and publishers request every user to report to the publishers any discrepancies or inaccuracies noticed. If errors in this work are found after publication, errata will be posted at www.thieme.com on the product description page.

Some of the product names, patents, and registered designs referred to in this book are in fact registered trademarks or proprietary names even though specific reference to this fact is not always made in the text. Therefore, the appearance of a name without designation as proprietary is not to be construed as a representation by the publisher that it is in the public domain.

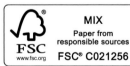

To Samantha, Melissa, Jamie for their love, support and encouragement and for being three great human beings.

Jaime Tisnado, MD

To My family: Leela, Gautam, Arun and the next generation: Mia, Nalin, Om Roshan, Veehan and Rohan for their unselfish love.

Rao R. Ivatury, MD

Contents

Foreword

I cannot think of a team better qualified than that of Jaime Tisnado and Rao R. Ivatury, internationally recognized experts in interventional radiology (IR) and trauma surgery respectively, to write and edit a comprehensive, single-volume text like the one you are holding that addresses the pivotal role of interventional radiology in the care of the trauma patient. However, this book is not limited to the description of interventional techniques but recognizes the importance of a team approach in the care of the trauma patient undergoing interventional procedures. To this end, the initial chapters focus on the critical roles of IR nurses, physician extenders, and radiology technicians in preparing for the procedure, assisting in its performance, and monitoring the critically ill patient before, during and following the intervention.

Equally important, the editors and authors underscore the significance of diagnostic imaging prior to the trauma patient's arrival to the IR suite as evidenced by chapters focusing on imaging of thoracic, abdominal, and peripheral vascular trauma. These chapters authored by well-known trauma radiologists provide in-depth, multimodality-based discussions regarding the diagnosis and characterization of a wide variety of injuries and are complemented by high-quality images. These chapters are particularly important as they demonstrate the manner in which the appropriate application of rapidly evolving technology plays an integral role in therapeutic decision making and provides information vital to planning interventional procedures. Particularly in the arena of CT, it may also permit the diagnosis of complex and at times clinically occult injuries in a rapid, non-invasive fashion.

In addition, by drawing on the clinical expertise of trauma surgeons and emergency medicine physicians, Drs. Tisnado and Ivatury have included chapters addressing trauma mechanisms and resuscitation of trauma patients —critical information for anyone involved in performing interventional procedures in the setting of trauma.

Utilizing these chapters to provide vital background information, the editors next focus on the performance of state-of-the-art interventional techniques used not only in the diagnosis but also in the treatment of trauma affecting virtually every major organ. This section of the book begins by addressing the most common angiographic procedures performed in the evaluation of trauma patients and then describes therapeutic interventional techniques such as embolotherapy, stenting, and balloon occlusion. In this way, the book reflects the *evolution of interventional radiology from a specialty that in its infancy was purely diagnostic to one that is now not only diagnostic but also therapeutic in many instances.*

Importantly, this book focuses on not only procedures used to diagnose and treat abdominal solid organ and peripheral vascular injuries but also techniques used to diagnose and treat head, neck, and spine trauma as well as trauma involving the heart and urinary tract. Also, the editors created sections dedicated to the discussion of filters, the performance of interventions in the pediatric trauma patient, and the role of interventional radiology in the management of iatrogenic trauma. Appropriately the editors conclude the book by looking to future developments and research in the exciting area of interventional radiology in trauma.

In summary, *Interventional Radiology in Trauma Management* will no doubt serve as an indispensable resource to radiologists, trauma surgeons, emergency medicine physicians, technicians, nurses and all others involved in the care of the trauma patients undergoing interventional radiology procedures.

Ann S. Fulcher, MD
Chairman and Professor of Radiology
Virginia Commonwealth University
Richmond, Virginia

Preface

Current therapy of trauma has evolved with developments in all fields: medicine, surgery, and radiology. With a wide spectrum of available techniques from minimally invasive to maximally intrusive, the focus is on minimizing blood loss, while striving to restore anatomic and physiologic function as rapidly as possible after injury. Surgical procedures still are the solution for the hemodynamically abnormal patients. For the vast majority of the remaining, however, treatment paradigms have shifted now to achieving these goals with as little as possible of the two inevitable consequences of operative trauma: tissue destruction and blood loss. The results of these newer concepts have been nothing short of spectacular: witness the control of injured subclavian artery or thoracic aorta without the mutilation of chest; arrest of major hepatic hemorrhage without incising the abdomen. The scope and the need for this relatively newer field, interventional radiology is expanding exponentially each day. The result: a new specialty of trauma management in its own right.

The editors of the current work have had the good fortune of decades of experience in these two fields, interventional radiology and surgery. As we began to collaborate in multiple challenges on a daily basis, it became apparent to us that the rapidly accumulating knowledge in this area is fragmented at best and incomplete at worst. The need for a single volume summarizing the state of the art was clear. Further, in keeping with the multi-dimensional approach to the current therapy of trauma, this book aims to bring forth the surgical and the I-R perspectives side by side whenever relevant.

The authors have been chosen for their special expertise and interest in the surgical and interventional aspects of trauma and all of them have given their time and talent with enthusiasm and energy. Our sincere appreciation goes out to them. We owe our administrative assistant, Mrs. Margie Smith an enormous debt of gratitude for her energy and commitment to this endeavour. This work would not have seen completion without the expert counseling of Mr. Owen Zurhellen and the skillful editing of Mrs. Elizabeth Palumbo from Thieme Publishers and we are grateful.

Acknowledgements

In the challenging management of complex trauma, the art and science of interventional radiology requires the expertise and commitment of many : administrators, radiologists, surgeons, anesthesiologists, intensivists, technologists, critical care nurses, "runners" to maintain a constant supply of life-sustaining fluids and equipment ….. just to name a few.

They convert the chaos of the I-R suite into an orchestrated concert culminating in yet another "save". These professionals deserve our eternal gratitude and acclaim, so they may take a bow and get back to their business of saving lives. We dedicate this book to these unsung heroes.

List of Contributors

Michel B. Aboutanos, MD, MPH
Associate Professor
Division of Trauma/Critical Care Surgery
MCV Hospitals/VCU Medical Center
Richmond, Virginia

John Henry Adamski II, MD, MSC, MPH, FACS
Medical Director
Trauma and Acute Care Surgery
Northeast Georgia Medical Center
Gainesville, Georgia

Marco A. Amendola, MD, FACR
Director of Medical Imaging
Innovative Cancer Institute
Voluntary Professor of Radiology
University of Miami
School of Medicine
220 Veleros Court
Coral Gables, Florida

Chad G. Ball, MD
Associate Professor of Surgery and Oncology
University of Calgary
Foothills Medical Center
Calgary, Alberta, Canada

Tiago Bilhim, MD, PhD, EBIR
Interventional Radiology
Saint Louis Hospital
Radiology Department
Faculdade de Ciencias Medicas
Universidade Nova de Lisboa
Lisbon, Portugal

Andre Biuckians, MD, MPH
Surgeon
Vascular Surgery Associates, LLC
Bel Air, Maryland

Megan L. Brenner, MD, MS, RPVI, FACS
Assistant Professor of Surgery
Trauma/Surgical Critical Care
R. Adams Cowley Shock Trauma Center
University of Maryland
Baltimore, Maryland

L. D. Britt, MD, MPH
Henry Ford Professor
Edward J. Brickhouse Chairman
EVMS Medical Group
EVMS Surgery
Norfolk, Virginia

Charles A. Bruno, Jr., DO
PGY-5 R1, Radiology, Interventional/Radiation Oncology
Hahnemann University Hospital/Drexel Medical
Philadelphia, Pennsylvania

Kim M. Caban, MD
Assistant Professor
University of Miami School of Medicine
Miami, Florida

Christine Craft, RN
Clinical Nurse II
MCV Hospitals
VCU Medical Center
Richmond, Virginia

Christopher J. Dente, MD
Associate Professor of Surgery
Emory University
Associate Medical Director
Marcus Trauma Center
Grady Memorial Hospital
Atlanta, Georgia

Thérèse M. Duane, MD
Associate Professor of Surgery
Division of Trauma/Critical Care Surgery
MCV Hospitals/VCU Medical Center
Richmond, Virginia

Marisa Duarte, MD
Interventional Radiology
Saint Louis Hospital
Lisbon, Portugal

Charles A. Ehlenberger, MD
Assistant Professor
Radiology Department
Vascular Interventional
MCV Hospitals
VCU Medical Center
Richmond, Virginia

Timothy C. Fabian, MD, FACS
Harwell Wilson Professor and Chairman
Department of Surgery
University of Tennessee Health Science Center
Memphis, Tennessee

David V. Feliciano, MD, FACS
Battersby Professor and Chief
Division of General Surgery
Attending Surgeon
Indiana University and IUH Methodist Hospitals
Indiana University Medical Center
Indianapolis, Indiana

Michelle Ferrari
[Deceased]

Mark Foley, MB, BCh, BAO
Fellow
University of Miami
Jackson Memorial Hospital
Miami, Florida

Sasikhan Geibprasert, MD
Toronto Western Hospital
University of Toronto
Division of Neuroradiology
Toronto, Ontario, Canada

Shima Goswami, MD
Instructor in Radiology
Newark Beth Israel Medical Center
Newark, New Jersey

James M. Haan, MD, FACS
Clincal Professor of Surgery
Kansas University School of Medicine
Medical Director, Trauma Survices
Via Christi Health
Wichita, Kansas

Robert A. Halvorsen, MD
Professor of Radiology/Director of Quality Assurance
MCV Hospitals/VCU Medical Center
Richmond, Virginia

Eric K. Hoffer, MD
Associate Professor of Radiology
Geisel School of Medicine
Dartmouth-Hitchcock Medical Center
Lebanon, New Hampshire

Rao R. Ivatury, MD
Emeritus Professor of Surgery
Immediate Past Chair
Division of Trauma, Critical Care, and Emergency Surgery
MCV Hospitals/VCU Medical Center
Richmond, Virginia

Paul R. Jolles, MD
Associate Professor, Radiology
MCV Hospitals/VCU Medical Center
Richmond, Virginia

Riyad Karmy-Jones, MD
Trauma and Thoracic/Vascular Surgery
Medical Director of Trauma
Legacy Emanuel Medical Center
Portland, Oregon

Timo Krings, MD, PhD, FRCP(C)
Professor of Radiology
Program Director – Neuroradiology
University of Toronto
Toronto Western Hospital
Toronto, Ontario, Canada

Daniel J. Komorowski, MD
Interventional Radiologist
MCV Hospitals/VCU Medical Center
Richmond, Virginia

Mark M. Levy, MD
Associate Professor
Virginia Commonwealth University Health System
Richmond, Virginia

Soroosh Mahboubi, MD
Pediatric Radiologist; Assistant
The Children's Hospital of Philadelphia
Philadelphia, Pennsylvania

Ajai K. Malhotra, MBBS (MD), MS, DNB, FRCS, FACS
Professor and Vice Chair
Division of Trauma/CC and Emergency Surgery
Associate Medical Director
Level-I Trauma Center, VCUHS
Richmond, Virginia

Timothy P. Maroney, MD
Professor of Radiology, Interventional/Radiation Oncology
Hahnemann University Hospital/Drexel Medical
Philadelphia, Pennsylvania

Julie Anne Mayglothling, MD
Assistant Professor
Department of Emergency Medicine
Department of Surgery
MCV Hospitals/VCU Medical Center
Richmond, Virginia

Gordon K. McLean, MD
Chief, Interventional Radiology
St. Clair Hospital
Pittsburgh, Pennsylvania

Felipe Munera, MD
Professor of Radiology
Medical Director Radiology Services
University of Miami Hospital
Jackson Memorial Hospital/Ryder Trauma Center/
   University of Miami Hospital
University of Miami Miller School of Medicine
Miami, Florida

Emanuele Orrù, MD
University of Padua – Radiology Institute
Policlinico Universitario
Istituto di Radiologia, Via Giustiniani 2
Padua, Italy

Mark S. Parker, MD
Associate Professor
Director, Medical Student Electives, Diagnostic Radiology
   (M-IV Program)
MCV Hospitals/VCU Medical Center
Richmond, Virginia

João Pisco, MD, PhD
Interventional Radiology
Saint Louis Hospital
Lisbon, Portugal

Uma R. Prasad, MD
Associate Professor
Department of Radiology
MCV Hospitals/VCU Medical Center
Richmond, Virginia

Carol Provost, RT (R) (CV), CIRCC
Rad Tech Billing Specialist
Department of Radiology
MCV Hospitals/VCU Medical Center
Richmond, Virginia

Marcus H.T. Reinges, MD
Professor
Department of Neurosurgery
RWTHAchen University
Aachen
Germany
Department of Neurosurgery
Justus-Liebig-Unversity Giessen
Giessen, Germany

Michael J. Rohrer, MD, FACS
Professor of Surgery
Chief, Division of Vascular and Endovascular Surgery
University of Tennessee Health Science Center
Memphis, Tennessee

Thomas M. Scalea, MD, FACS, FCCM
Physician-in-Chief, R. Adams Cowley Shock Trauma Center
Francis X. Kelly/MBNA Professor of Trauma Surgery
Director, Program in Trauma
University of Maryland School of Medicine/University of
   MD Medical Center
Baltimore, Maryland

Malcolm K. Sydnor, MD
Director, Vascular and Interventional Radiology
Associate Director, Residency Education
MCV Hospitals/VCU Medical Center
Richmond, Virginia

Jamie Tisnado, MD
Fellowship/Instructor
Radiology
Cornell University
Ithaca, New York

Jaime Tisnado, MD
Professor
Radiology and Surgery, Cardiovascular and Interventional
   Radiology
MCV Hospitals/VCU Medical Center
Richmond, Virginia

Jinxing Yu, MD
Associate Professor
Director, Oncologic Imaging
MCV Hospitals/VCU Medical Center
Richmond, Virginia

Wen-Yuan Zhao
Associate Professor
Shanghai Hospital
Second Military Medical University
Department of Neurosurgery
Shanghai, The People's Republic of China

1 Historical Aspects of Interventional Radiology

Jaime Tisnado and Rao R. Ivatury

In 1964 Charles Dotter was the first physician to treat peripheral artery disease with a catheter to open the blocked artery. Dotter came to be known as the "Father of Interventional Radiology" for pioneering this technique and was nominated for the Nobel Prize in Physiology or Medicine in 1978. Alexander Margulis coined the term "interventional" to describe the new, minimally invasive techniques that were to subsequently develop after Dotter's medical innovation. These radiologists—minimally invasive technologists—pioneered a new medical specialty with the invention of angioplasty and the catheter-delivered stent. Subsequent advances in angioplasty led to the development of endovascular stents to keep the dilated vessels open. In 1969, Dotter conceived the idea of expandable stents with an intra-arterial coil spring. The first stents developed by Dotter and Andrew Craig were made of nitinol. Stents soon expanded to other types such as the self-expandable Z stent, the self-expandable mesh stent, the knitted tantalum stent, and the balloon-expandable stent. Angioplasty and stenting soon found a venerable place in the modern management of cardiology.

Soon, interventional techniques were finding other applications. Selective infusion of vasopressors, selective arterial embolization to control hemorrhage, and transhepatic variceal embolization became life-saving, minimally invasive procedures that became commonplace in clinical practice. In the span of a few years, the interventional techniques expanded to other systems such as the biliary and urinary ducts. The field of interventional oncology was pioneered by other legendary pioneers such as White and Wallace.[1,2] The articles by Rosch et al.[1] and the 2000 RSNA Annual Oration in Diagnostic Radiology on "the future of interventional radiology" are mandatory for the student of history of I-R.

Many, many patients are now routinely saved by the interventional radiologist both in trauma and nontrauma situations. The following is a modified list of important milestones in the development of this constantly expanding, increasingly versatile specialty, adapted from the Society of Interventional Radiology website.[3]

1.1 Milestones in Interventional Radiology

1964 Angioplasty
1966 Embolization therapy to treat tumors and spinal cord vascular malformations by blocking the blood flow

1967 Closure of the patent ductus arteriosis, a heart defect in newborns of a vascular opening between the pulmonary artery and the aorta
1967 Selective vasoconstriction infusions for hemorrhage, now commonly used for bleeding ulcers, gastrointestinal (GI) bleeding, and arterial bleeding
1969 The catheter-delivered stenting technique
1970s Percutaneous removal of common bile duct stones
1970s Development of occlusive coils
1972 Selective arterial embolization for GI bleeding, which was adapted to treat massive bleeding in other arteries in the body and to block blood supply to tumors
1973 Embolization for pelvic trauma
1974 Selective arterial thrombolysis for arterial occlusions, now used to treat blood clots, stroke, deep vein thrombosis, etc.
1974 Transhepatic embolization for variceal bleeding
1980 Development of special tools and devices for biliary manipulation
1980s Biliary stents to allow bile to flow from the liver, saving patients from biliary bypass surgery
1981 Embolization technique for spleen trauma
1982 Transjugular intrahepatic portosystemic shunt (TIPS) to improve blood flow in damaged livers from conditions such as cirrhosis and hepatitis C
1982 Dilators for interventional urology; percutaneous removal of kidney stones
1983 The balloon-expandable stent (peripheral)
1990s Radiofrequency ablation for soft tissue tumors (i.e., bone, breast, kidney, lung, and liver cancer)
1991 Abdominal aortic stent grafts
1994 The balloon-expandable coronary stent
1999 Percutaneous delivery of pancreatic islet cells to the liver for transplantation to treat diabetes

References

[1] Rösch J, Keller FS, Kaufman JA. The birth, early years, and future of interventional radiology. J Vasc Interv Radiol 2003; 14: 841–853
[2] Becker GJ. Interventional radiology 2000 and beyond: back from the brink. The 1999 Charles T. Dotter Lecture. J Vasc Interv Radiol 1999; 10: 681–687
[3] Society of Interventional Radiology. The History of Interventional Radiology. Available at: http://www.sirweb.org/about-us/historyIR.shtml. Accessed May 14, 2012

2 Mechanism of Injury in Trauma

Thérèse M. Duane and Ajai K. Malhotra

The care of the acutely injured patient is linked closely between all members of the trauma team and the radiology and interventional radiology (IR) sections. Surgeons and physicians depend on radiographic studies to determine the extent of injury and need for intervention, either surgery or IR. Continued improvements in imaging capabilities are significantly benefiting the field of trauma.

Over the last few decades more-sophisticated imaging methods have been developed that are more sensitive and efficient, making it easier to diagnose injuries. Multidetector computed tomography (MDCT), for example, has become much more exact, allowing finer slices and three-dimensional (3D) reconstructions. MDCT also has become much faster procedure, allowing for the rapid identification of life-threatening injuries. A recent study that compared MDCT to conventional imaging demonstrated that it took significantly less time to diagnose and manage injuries in the MDCT group.[1]

Since the 1960s, radiology has advanced from providing a simple means of diagnosis to actual interventions and treatments. The benefits of IR management for acutely injured patients vary based on the specific type of injury. Certain injuries lend themselves to IR methods more than others. To appreciate the contributions of these imaging modalities it is important to have a clear understanding of the basic mechanisms of trauma. In this chapter we describe the various types of trauma—blunt, penetrating, and iatrogenic—as well as the damage to soft tissue, organs, vasculature, and bone caused by trauma.

2.1 Penetrating Trauma

2.1.1 Low-Velocity Weapons

Low-velocity penetrating trauma caused by knives or impalement have a pathway of destruction directly correlated with the pathway of the penetrating instrument. There is no associated tissue damage from a blast effect. Therefore, identification of the pathway of the weapon (whether a knife, an ice pick, or other) is often enough to allow for injury identification. For those patients in whom the offending instrument was removed, the main goal of the trauma team is to determine the depth and trajectory of the weapon. In the event the weapon or instrument remains in place, plain radiographs can usually identify the extent of the penetration. Furthermore, injury patterns with serrated instruments will differ from smooth instruments, leaving characteristic scrape marks particularly on the skin.[2]

Low-velocity penetrating trauma caused by guns, handguns, and "cheap" pistols ("Saturday special") can result in many different soft tissue injuries. Penetration of parenchyma can result in localized hemorrhage within an organ or a body cavity. For example, injuries to the thoracic cavity can result in a simple pneumothorax or a more complex hemopneumothorax.

The "cardiac box," defined both anteriorly and posteriorly by the clavicles superiorly, the midclavicular lines laterally, and the costal margins inferiorly, can easily be damaged by low-velocity weapons. Therefore, the cardiac box must always be evaluated closely and rapidly to avoid missing the potential consequences of cardiac tamponade.

Vascular injuries from low-velocity weapons are often small, yet lethal. Even small lacerations to vessels such as the femoral artery can result in exsanguination with amazing rapidity and alacrity. Occasionally, these injuries will undergo spasm or tamponade, providing time to gain control of the bleeding and repair the injury. When the instrument is serrated, the injury is often more difficult to repair because of the need to debride the vessel wall; clean edges are needed to perform an anastomosis. If there is a larger injury caused by a serrated blade, the vessels are less likely to constrict, retract, and temporarily stop the bleeding, thus promoting exsanguination and death.[3]

Bone fractures are less common with low-velocity weapons, but still can occur. More often, there is also penetration into the soft tissues or joint spaces resulting in open wounds. These wounds are far less extensive than those associated with blunt force trauma, described later in this chapter.

2.1.2 High-Velocity Weapons

Unlike low-velocity gunshot injuries, high-velocity gunshot wounds (GSW), caused either by a small- or large-caliber gun, pose a greater challenge in the identification of the bullet's pathway. Because of differences in tissue resistance, bullets rarely follow a straight line through the body. The variability of the trajectory presents a quandary for trauma and vascular surgeons. Therefore, a direct visual inspection via exploration in the operating room is the preferred diagnostic method, particularly in the unstable patient with a GSW to the torso.[4]

Vascular injuries associated with high-velocity weapons are associated with much more tissue destruction than with low-velocity penetrating trauma. Depending on the trajectory of the bullet, there may be direct damage resulting in a large defect (permanent cavity) and hemorrhage, or there may be a local blast effect (temporary cavity) resulting in acute thrombosis of a vessel.

In addition to the repair of the hole in the vessel, the intima extending proximally and distally away from the site of injury should also be evaluated because it is impossible to discern the extent of an injury by visual inspection of the adventitia. Resection of the vessel with primary anastomosis, bypass, or even temporary shunting depending on the patient's overall condition may be necessary.[5] There also tends to be more associated soft tissue injury, which may provide a tamponade effect, allowing time for vascular control, both proximal and distal.

Bones are more easily fractured by this mechanism of injury. These fractures are considered open, requiring emergent treatment to decrease infection risks. During the initial evaluation, it is extremely important to assess the vasculature to determine concomitant injuries that may need to be addressed first. When multiple injuries are identified, a coordinated approach is required to ensure an appropriate prioritization of injuries. Such an approach is often successful in saving lives and salvaging limbs and organs.[6]

2.2 Shotgun Blasts

A shotgun blast results in a combination of injuries that are both penetrating and blunt. The depth of penetration is dependent on the distance of the weapon from the patient. Numerous pellets may penetrate anywhere from superficial soft tissue to deeper organs and vessels. The pellets may also spray widely, so care must be taken to look thoroughly for possible injuries within and across the entire body.

A shotgun blast can cause significant damage to solid organs—disrupting parenchyma and causing hemorrhage. The pellets can also produce small holes throughout the gastrointestinal tract with subtle perforations that may be difficult to identify on an exploratory laparotomy. Vessels can receive direct penetration of pellets as well as thrombosis from the blast effect.

Fractures associated with this type of penetrating trauma are usually considered open fractures because of the extensive surrounding soft tissue damage. Early aggressive irrigation and debridement is important to minimize infection risk. These patients often require multiple episodes of operative debridement and skin grafting, and are expected to have a protracted hospital course.[7]

2.3 Blunt Trauma

In civilian practice, the majority of trauma is from blunt force. Unlike penetrating trauma, where the area of injury is usually localized to the area of penetration, blunt trauma can often result in injuries remote from the site of impact to the body. In general, there are two types of force that produce injuries to the body: rapid acceleration/deceleration and compression.

2.3.1 Acceleration/Deceleration

This force is also described as a "shear" and occurs when the body is rapidly accelerated, followed by a rapid deceleration. A head-on motor vehicle collision, when the vehicle comes to a very rapid stop, or a fall from a height where the human body is suddenly stopped as it hits the ground, are examples of rapid deceleration. Other examples of this are when a slow-moving or stationary vehicle is hit by a fast-moving vehicle, and the first vehicle, in turn, hits a stationary object such as an embankment. At the time of the first impact, the occupants of the stationary/slow-moving vehicle will undergo rapid acceleration, and when the vehicle hits the embankment and comes to a sudden stop, the occupants will undergo rapid deceleration. The same is observed when a pedestrian is struck by a motor vehicle and thrown in the air—rapid acceleration—and then hits the ground—rapid deceleration. Rapid acceleration/deceleration of the whole body can lead to many severe injuries anywhere in the body: head, neck, chest, abdomen, extremity. These injuries often occur where the anatomy and degree of fixation of an organ is altered, for example, at the fissure of the ligamentum teres in the liver, or the ligamentum arteriosum in the thoracic aorta.

2.3.2 Compression

Compression occurs usually at the site of impact of the body with another blunt object such as the steering column in a motor vehicle. It is similar to hitting a tissue or an organ with a hammer. The tissue or organ is compressed to a much smaller volume than usual, which leads to injuries to those tissues or organs.

A related force is "overpressure": Instead of a solid organ, a body cavity or a hollow or tubular organ is compressed by trauma, resulting in increased pressure within the cavity or lumen of the organ. If the pressure exceeds the tensile strength of the wall of the cavity or organ, then a rupture or explosion may occur. For example, after a direct blow to the lower abdomen when the urinary bladder is full of urine, the urinary bladder will rupture. A sudden blunt force to the entire abdomen results in a rupture of the diaphragm. Similarly, a rupture of the aortic valve (aortic insufficiency) or ascending aorta full of blood results in death from exsanguination.

2.3.3 Motor Vehicle Collisions

Motor vehicle collisions are the leading cause of trauma deaths and the second leading cause (after firearms) of nonfatal injuries.[8] There are five main forms of motor vehicle collisions: frontal, lateral, rear, rotational, and rollover. Each type has a specific injury pattern.[9] In reality, however, two or more forms are usually combined. The frontal impact is illustrative of how blunt force trauma can impact each of the major body regions. When a moving vehicle comes to an abrupt stop, the occupant's body continues to move forward due to inertia. In case of the driver, the first impact is usually around the knees as these hit the bottom of the dashboard. This direct impact can result in musculoskeletal extremity injuries. As the force transfers to the pelvis, it can lead to pelvic fractures. As the body continues to move forward, the next impact is to the torso as the torso hits the steering column. This leads to injuries to the thoracic skeleton, the abdominal and thoracic organs, and the thoracic and lumbar spine. Finally, the head is thrown forward and can strike the windshield, resulting in intracranial injuries or injury to the cervical spine.

Furthermore, depending on the height of the driver, the top of the steering wheel can impact the anterior neck resulting in injuries to the soft tissue of the neck, the aerodigestive tract, and the carotid and vertebral arteries. The exact pattern of injuries will depend on multiple factors, the most important of which are the speed of the vehicle at the time of the impact and the use of restraint devices such as seatbelts, airbags, etc.

Other factors that influence the injury pattern are the age, size, and the exact orientation of the victim at the time of impact. Although the injury pattern may be different for other forms of motor vehicle collisions, remember that a collision can lead to significant injuries in the entire body. A systemic approach to evaluating the entire body: head, neck, thorax, abdomen, pelvis, spine, and extremities is necessary to identify all injuries, and more importantly, to rule out injuries.

2.3.4 Falls

Falls are responsible for ~ 8% of trauma deaths. Furthermore, falls account for 33% of injury-related hospitalizations and 25% of injury-related visits to the emergency department. Falls are responsible for significant injury in the extreme age groups: the young and the old.[8,10] However, the pattern of injuries is quite different in the young and the elderly. In the former (< 5 years), the injuries from falls are usually minor and do not require much workup or hospital care.[11,12] Whereas in the elderly, falls are significant causes of morbidity and mortality. The elderly are less steady on their feet, have osteoporotic bones prone to fractures, and sometimes are on antithrombotic agents such as Plavix (clopidogrel bisulfate; Bristol-Myers Squibb Co., New York, NY), aspirin, or warfarin so even a minor fall can lead to a life-threatening intracranial bleed or other conditions.[13,14] These factors need to be addressed when planning a diagnostic workup and therapeutic options.

Falls from heights are extreme examples of a deceleration injury and usually occur in young adults from work or recreational activities. The injury patterns after falls from significant height are related to the orientation of the body at the time of ground impact. If the victim lands on their feet, the forces are transferred up the axial skeleton. Beginning with the heels (calcaneal fractures), up the lower extremity (tibial plateau and/or femoral fractures), through the pelvis (acetabular or posterior pelvic or other pelvic fractures), and up the spine (compression fractures of the vertebral bodies), vertebrae, anywhere in the spinal column.

2.3.5 Auto–Pedestrian Accidents

Pedestrians hit by motor vehicles (automobiles, trucks, busses) receive extreme energy transfers to their bodies. Even at a lower speed, a motor vehicle has substantial momentum based on its combination of mass and velocity. This high-energy transfer often results in multisystem injuries. The typical injury pattern involves a victim being hit in the lower extremities by the bumper, resulting in fractures of the lower extremities. Following this, the victim may be thrown in the air, and as the vehicle continues to move, the victim lands on the hood or windshield, resulting in torso injuries (skeletal and soft tissue). Finally, the victim falls off the hood onto the pavement, often landing on the head, which leads to intracranial injuries.[15] An extremely high index of suspicion, therefore, should be maintained for major multisystem injuries in any victim being struck by a motor vehicle.

2.4 Iatrogenic Injuries

Iatrogenic injuries may occur as a result of diagnostic, interventional, or surgical procedures. Iatrogenic trauma as a result of IR procedures is discussed in Chapter 25.

2.5 Conclusion

Detailed knowledge of the mechanisms of trauma injury is extremely useful for the trauma team in determining the types of injury a victim may have sustained. With this information, the trauma team can establish what diagnostic workup must be done, in what time frame, and what therapeutic options are available.[16]

References

[1] Wurmb T, Balling H, Fruhwald P, et al.. Polytrauma management in a period of change: Time analysis of new strategies for emergency room treatment. Unfallchirurg 2009; 112: 390–399

[2] Pollak S. [Pattern of findings in injuries caused by "survival knives"] Arch Kriminol 1989; 183: 11–20

[3] Sauvageau A, Trépanier JS, Racette S. Delayed deaths after vascular traumatism: two cases. J Clin Forensic Med 2006; 13: 344–348

[4] Eastern Association for the Surgery of Trauma (EAST) Guidelines. Penetrating Abdominal Trauma, Selective Nonoperative Management. Available a http.www.east.org. Accessed Oct. 30, 2014

[5] Subramanian A, Vercruysse G, Dente C, Wyrzykowski A, King E, Feliciano DV. A decade's experience with temporary intravascular shunts at a civilian level I trauma center. J Trauma 2008; 65: 316–324, discussion 324–326

[6] Ashworth EM, Dalsing MC, Glover JL, Reilly MK. Lower extremity vascular trauma: a comprehensive, aggressive approach. J Trauma 1988; 28: 329–336

[7] Bartlett CS, Helfet DL, Hausman MR, Strauss E. Ballistics and gunshot wounds: effects on musculoskeletal tissues. J Am Acad Orthop Surg 2000; 8: 21–36

[8] Fingerhut LA, Warner M Injury Chartbook. Health, United States, 1996–97. Hyattsville, MD: National Center for Health Statistics, 1997

[9] Siegel JH, Loo G, Dischinger PC et al. Factors influencing the patterns of injuries and outcomes in car versus car crashes compared to sport utility, van, or pick-up truck versus car crashes: Crash Injury Research Engineering Network Study. J Trauma 2001; 51: 975–990

[10] Rice DP, MacKenzie EJ, et al. Cost of Injury in the United States. San Francisco, CA: Institute of Health and Aging, University of California and the Injury Prevention Center, The Johns Hopkins University, 1989

[11] Scheidt PC, Harel Y, Trumble AC, Jones DH, Overpeck MD, Bijur PE. The epidemiology of nonfatal injuries among US children and youth. Am J Public Health 1995; 85: 932–938

[12] Rivara FP, Alexander B, Johnston B, Soderberg R. Population-based study of fall injuries in children and adolescents resulting in hospitalization or death. Pediatrics 1993; 92: 61–63

[13] Tinetti ME, Speechley M, Ginter SF. Risk factors for falls among elderly persons living in the community. N Engl J Med 1988; 319: 1701–1707

[14] Sorock GS. Falls among the elderly: epidemiology and prevention. Am J Prev Med 1988: 282–288

[15] Demetriades D, Murray J, Martin M et al. Pedestrians injured by automobiles: relationship of age to injury type and severity. J Am Coll Surg 2004; 199: 382–387

[16] Ruchholtz S, Nast-Kolb D, Waydhas C, Schweiberer L. [The injury pattern in polytrauma. Value of information regarding accident process in clinical acute management] Unfallchirurg 1996; 99: 633–641German

3 Resuscitation of the Traumatized Patient

Julie Anne Mayglothling, Michel B. Aboutanos, and Rao R. Ivatury

Trauma deaths show a trimodal distribution, with 50% of patients dying immediately at the scene from traumatic brain injury or exsanguination, 30% dying within several hours of reaching the hospital owing to hemorrhagic shock, and the remaining 20% dying within the coming days to weeks from multiorgan failure and sepsis (▶ Fig. 3.1).[1] Although immediate deaths are targeted by preventative measures, initial resuscitative and surgical techniques target both the second and third causes of trauma mortality. Failure to resuscitate optimally in the prehospital setting, the emergency department, and the intensive care unit can contribute to worsening hemorrhage, shock, and ultimately increased mortality.

In 1963, R. Adams Cowley described the "golden hour" as it relates to the predictive outcome of the traumatized patient whose increased oxygen demands needs to be met in an expeditious manner. Failure to meet the consumptive demands of the tissues with adequate oxygen delivery leads to accumulation of tissue oxygen debt. The ensuing inflammatory cascade at the cellular level results in endothelial damage, end organ dysfunction, and eventually death.

Resuscitation involves restoration of adequate tissue perfusion to meet the consumptive demands of the body. The ultimate goal of resuscitation is the prevention of an uncompensated anaerobic state and the reversal of metabolic hypoxia. To achieve such a goal, timely intervention with a goal-directed and targeted resuscitative strategy has been shown to improve outcome and decrease mortality.[2] Such concepts and goals are dependent on a multidisciplinary approach to the resuscitative management of the injured patient along with the critical use of clinical, as well as technological advances. These advances have expanded beyond monitoring capabilities to include therapeutic interventions that are currently vital to the management of the traumatized patient. These range from the use of ultrasonography (US) for difficult vascular access to critical hemorrhage control by interventional radiology (IR) in every body cavity from the embolization of a bleeding abdominal or pelvic organ to the endovascular control of an aortic injury.

In this chapter, we will review the current and evolving concepts in the resuscitation of the injured patient and the ongoing controversies about the ideal ways to restore physiologic function.

3.1 Shock and Oxygen Debt

Shock is defined as circulatory insufficiency that creates an imbalance between tissue oxygen supply and oxygen demand. Oxygen delivery (DO_2) is the product of the arterial oxygen content (CaO_2) and the cardiac output (CO). Systemic oxygen consumption (VO_2) comprises a delicate balance between supply and demand. In a normal physiologic state, the tissues consume ~ 25% of the oxygen delivered and venous blood returning to the right heart is therefore 75% saturated (mixed venous oxygen saturation in the pulmonary artery [Sm_{VO2}]). When the oxygen supply is insufficient to meet the demand of the tissues, the first compensatory mechanism is an increase in CO, thereby delivering more oxygen to the tissues. If this mechanism is insufficient to meet the demands of the tissues, then the amount of oxygen extracted from the hemoglobin by the tissues increases, which in turn causes the Sm_{VO2} to decrease. When these compensatory mechanisms fail to meet the demands of the tissues, the imbalance between oxygen supply and demand causes an oxygen debt, forcing the tissues to undergo anaerobic metabolism and the formation of lactate.

This oxygen debt, in addition to causing lactate formation and subsequent lactic acidosis, also causes activation of both coagulation and inflammatory cascades.[3] If uncorrected, this hypoperfusion has been implicated in ischemic cellular injury and cell death, which leads to systemic inflammatory response syndrome and irreversible multiple organ dysfunction syndrome (MODS). This response appears to be strongly related to both the severity and duration of shock,[4] which emphasizes the importance of early and adequate resuscitation.

Not all hemorrhage produces hemorrhagic shock, and patients may have ongoing hemorrhage with blood loss up to 30% of the circulating blood volume without manifesting low blood pressure (▶ Table 3.1). The importance of early recognition and reversal of this shock is paramount in trauma resuscitation.

3.2 End Points of Resuscitation

Control of hemorrhage is the first priority in patients with traumatic hemorrhagic shock, but concomitant fluid resuscitation with blood and crystalloids is also important to maintain end-organ perfusion. Historically, the resuscitation of the injured patient was based on normalization of heart rate and blood pressure, although these parameters have been shown to be sorely inadequate to assess oxygen delivery. Patients who manifest persistently abnormal vital signs despite fluid administration are clearly in a state of uncompensated shock and need further resuscitative efforts.[5,6] However, up to 85% of patients

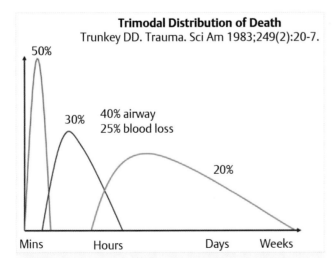

Fig. 3.1 The trimodal distribution of trauma deaths. (Used with permission from Trunkey DD, Trauma. Sci Am 1983;249(2):20–27)

Table 3.1 Classification system for hemorrhage

Parameter	Class I	Class II	Class III	Class IV
Blood loss (mL)	< 750 mL	750–1000	1500–2000	> 2000
Blood loss (%)	< 15%	15–30%	30–40%	> 40%
Pulse	< 100	> 100	> 120	> 140
Blood pressure	Normal	Narrowed pulse pressure	Decreased SBp < 90	Profoundly decreased
Respiratory rate	Normal	Slightly increased	Moderate tachypnea	Marked tachypnea
Central nervous system symptoms	Normal	Anxious	Confused	Lethargic

who normalize these parameters may still have evidence of ongoing hypoperfusion, leaving them in a state of "compensated shock."[7] Failure to recognize this inadequate tissue perfusion can worsen the systemic inflammatory response and increase multiorgan failure and subsequent death. In recent years, other resuscitative end points have been noted to more accurately reflect adequacy of oxygen delivery or the state of cellular dysoxia. These parameters include both global markers of resuscitation (lactate, base deficit, mixed venous oxygen saturation) and regional end points that look at specific organ-system perfusion (gastric tonometry, sublingual capnography, and near-infrared spectroscopy).

3.3 Lactate and Base Deficit

It is clearly recognized that elevated lactate and base deficit levels after trauma reflect impaired tissue perfusion and predict worse outcomes. The time to normalization of lactate levels has also been associated with outcome, with those patients able to normalize lactate levels within 24 hours showing improved mortality. In one study, patients who were unable to normalize lactate levels within 48 to 72 hours had a 100% mortality rate. This study confirmed that time to lactate clearance was an independent predictor of survival.[8] A more recent study showed 67% mortality for those patients who did not clear serum lactate within 48 hours.[9]

The Eastern Association for the Surgery of Trauma (EAST) attempted to develop evidence-based management guidelines for clinical practice on end points of resuscitation. They suggested a level I recommendation (the highest) that initial base deficit, lactate or gastric pHi from tonometry can be used to stratify patients with regard to the need for ongoing fluid resuscitation.[10] Although these studies clearly document that lactate is associated with adverse outcome in trauma, no prospective studies have investigated if standardized methods for trauma resuscitation would improve lactate clearance times.[11]

The use of mixed venous oxygenation saturation (SvO$_2$) levels reflects the adequacy of oxygen delivery to tissues in relation to global tissue oxygen demands. Gattinoni et al resuscitated a group of critically ill patients to a normal cardiac index (CI; 2.5–3.5 L/min/m^2), supranormal CI (≥ 4.5 L/min/m^2) or normal SvO$_2$ (≥ 70%). There were no differences in mortality or multiple organ dysfunction (MODS).[12] There are few specific data on the use of SvO$_2$ in trauma patients, but this parameter is used periodically as a marker of resuscitation.

Regional markers of resuscitation and tissue oxygenation, such as gastric tonometry, sublingual capnography, and near-infrared spectroscopy show promise in detecting early signs of organ hypoperfusion, mainly in the gastrointestinal system and skin. However, finding consistent, cost-effective ways to measure these continues to be a challenge and these tools are not widely used currently.

3.4 Fluid Resuscitation

Acute hemorrhage is the predominant cause of acute intravascular volume loss requiring aggressive resuscitation. The goal of restoring normal intravascular volume and normal arterial blood pressure with either isotonic crystalloid or colloid solution has been a mainstay of treatment of injured patients for decades. The aim of this fluid administration is to reestablish intravascular volume and maintain adequate perfusion pressure, thereby restoring oxygen delivery and ensuring perfusion to vital organs. The original studies that established the value of fluid resuscitation involved controlled hemorrhage models with fixed amounts of blood loss.[13] The limitation of this model is that it may not accurately represent the reality of traumatic bleeding which is an uncontrolled state. During the Vietnam war, more-aggressive crystalloid resuscitation became popular due to research that demonstrated that large volume isotonic crystalloid improved survival.[13] The recommendations for early and aggressive crystalloid administration persisted for decades and are now part of the Advanced Trauma Life Support course, which recommends 2 L of crystalloid therapy, followed by blood transfusion for patients that are persistently hypotensive.[14] Although it was once widely believed that early aggressive fluid resuscitation is beneficial, clinical studies have failed to provide conclusive evidence supporting this tenet, and this long-standing theory is being questioned. It is now recognized that resuscitation fluids are not completely innocuous and they may potentiate the cellular injury caused by hemorrhagic shock.[15]

3.5 Isotonic Crystalloid Solution

Isotonic crystalloid solutions, normal saline (NS), and lactated Ringer's solution (LR) have been the preferred resuscitation fluid in the United States for many years. Crystalloids are hypo-oncotic, and therefore, cause a substantial amount of the crystalloid to shift into the extravascular space. At best, 30% of the fluid remains intravascular. This is the physiological basis for the 3:1 ratio for isotonic crystalloid volume replacement: For every amount of blood lost, three times that amount of isotonic crystalloid is required to restore intravascular volume. The choice of NS versus LR solution has been controversial. There is no clear evidence that either of these solutions is superior to the other and they both have drawbacks. Infusion of either crystalloid causes significant immune activation and induction of cellular injury, LR increases cytokine release and may increase lactic acidosis when given in large quantities, and NS causes worsening acidosis secondary to hyperchloremia.[15] It appears as though the critically ill patients who develop late complications of increased inflammatory response have undergone severe hemorrhagic shock and massive fluid resuscitation.

3.6 Colloid Resuscitation

Although more expensive, colloids (dextran 70, hydroxyethyl starches, modified gelatins, albumin, or plasma protein fraction), theoretically make more sense in resuscitation. Colloids have larger molecular weight particles that should keep the solution in the intravascular space more than crystalloids, resulting in a more effective expansion of circulating blood volume. In addition, they promote less of an inflammatory process than isotonic crystalloid. Various colloid solutions have been compared with each other, as well as to isotonic crystalloid solutions. Multiple meta-analyses, as well as a Cochrane review, failed to show any evidence of improved outcome with the use of colloids; one study showed an increased risk of death in those patients who received albumin.[16,17] The largest randomized controlled trial of albumin versus saline, the SAFE trial (Saline versus Albumin Evaluation) enrolled over 700 patients requiring intravascular fluid resuscitation. Albumin was found to be no better than saline overall for resuscitation. However, it found increased mortality in trauma patients, especially those with traumatic brain injury.[18] For these reasons, as well as cost consideration, crystalloids tend to be the preferred fluid used for initial trauma resuscitation.

3.7 Hypertonic Saline

In 1980, Velasco et al showed that a small volume of hypertonic saline (HTS) was as effective as large-volume crystalloids in providing intravascular volume expansion during hemorrhagic shock.[19] Hypertonic saline has several theoretical and practical advantages over traditional isotonic crystalloids in both civilian and military trauma patients, so there has been great debate about its use. Theoretically, HTS has benefits with regard to hemodynamics, immune modulation, and intracranial pressure reduction. From a hemodynamic standpoint, the use of low-volume HTS, as opposed to higher volumes of isotonic crystalloids, avoids the overaggressive fluid administration that may increase blood loss through clot destabilization and hemodilution of clotting factors. The increased osmolarity of hypertonic saline allows the use of a much lower volume to achieve the same degree of plasma expansion. Similar to isotonic saline, HTS distributes into the extracellular space; however, HTS may initially draw fluid from the interstitial and intracellular compartments to the intravascular compartment, restoring mean arterial pressure with smaller fluid volumes.[20] From an immune perspective, the hyperinflammatory properties of isotonic saline are well established.[21] In contrast, both animal and human models demonstrate that HTS limits proinflammatory response of circulating inflammatory cells while enhancing T-cell function.[22,23] Because of its logistic advantages and immunologic benefits, HTS with or without dextran, seems to possess all the qualities of an ideal resuscitative fluid. Given both of the above mechanisms, HTS has the potential to influence both early and late mortality after traumatic injury (second and third peaks on mortality curves). The final theoretical benefit of HTS is in traumatic brain injury. The combination of increased osmotic pressure, which increases cerebral perfusion, along with decrease in ICP, should minimize the progression of secondary brain injury.

There have been several randomized controlled trials that have evaluated the use of hypertonic saline (7.5% normal saline with or without 6% dextran 70) for resuscitation of the hypovolemic trauma patient with mixed results.[24–34] Several of these studies evaluated survival as an end point; however, few were powered to show a difference in survival between treatment groups. A Cochrane Review concluded that there is no evidence that hypertonic crystalloids are better than isotonic crystalloids for fluid resuscitation in trauma.[33] In addition, a large, prospective, multicenter randomized trial by the Resuscitation Outcomes Consortium (ROC) evaluating the use of HTS in patients with traumatic hypovolemic shock was unable to demonstrate any improvement in mortality or subsequent organ failure. The study was stopped early due to futility.[34] Despite the theoretical advantages to the use of HTS over isotonic crystalloid, the clinical outcomes have not shown a benefit in trauma resuscitation and its use continues to be debated.

3.8 Blood Products

For trauma patients who demonstrate end-organ hypoperfusion despite crystalloid administration, either through hemodynamic instability or other end points of resuscitation, transfusion of blood products is warranted. Although this tenet sounds straightforward, the timing and extent of blood product transfusion in trauma resuscitation remains a subject of controversy. Fresh, warm whole blood most effectively restores red cell mass, plasma volume, clotting factors, and platelets. However, given shortages of blood products and current blood banking principles, the use of whole blood transfusions is frequently not realistic. The use of component product transfusion is the mainstay of transfusion practice, effectively utilizing a scare resource while matching the components transfused to the specific needs of the patient.

In the setting of trauma resuscitation, indications for blood component therapy can be divided into two main categories: (1) enhancement of oxygen carrying capacity by increasing RBC mass intravascular volume, and (2) replacement of coagulation components due to loss, dysfunction, or consumption.

Patients who remain hemodynamically unstable despite the infusion of 2 L of crystalloid necessitate immediate PRBC transfusion. Hypotension in the setting of trauma should be assumed to be secondary to acute blood loss until proven otherwise. Typed and cross-matched packed RBC should be transfused packed red blood cells regardless of serum hemoglobin levels. In the setting of active hemorrhage, hemoglobin and hematocrit values do not represent the extent of blood loss, and further transfusions are given based upon the patient's injuries and response to the initial transfusion. However, in the absence of ongoing blood loss or hemorrhagic shock, there is no benefit of a "liberal" transfusion threshold in hemodynamically stable trauma patients.[35] In a prospective study of over 15,000 trauma patients, blood transfusion was shown to be an independent predictor of mortality, intensive care unit (ICU) admission, ICU length of stay (LOS), and hospital LOS. Those patients who received blood transfusion in the first 24 hours were more than three times as likely to die.[36,37]

The use of fresh frozen plasma (FFP) in trauma resuscitation is also controversial; recommendations are changing as the understanding of traumatic coagulopathy is evolving. Most serum measurements of coagulation do not represent what is happening real time to the hemorrhaging trauma patient. Transfusion of plasma and cryoprecipitate has historically been based on clinical signs of coagulopathy. A further discussion of coagulopathy and use of clotting factors is in the Hemostatic Resuscitation section.

Transfusion of any blood products carries with it multiple risks, including an increased risk of infection, multi-organ failure (MOF), acute lung injury (ALI), and mortality for every unit of component administered. Practitioners must have a clear understanding of these risks to use blood component therapy safely and effectively.

3.9 Damage Control Resuscitation

Military conflicts frequently give rise to changes in trauma care; therefore, much of the treatment of civilian trauma patients is derived from military experience. War provides a concentrated population of patients in traumatic shock in whom re-evaluation of current practices and trials of new paradigms are initiated. Recent conflicts in Iraq and Afghanistan have given unprecedented opportunities to study patients with traumatic shock and have changed the way severely injured patients are resuscitated and surgically treated. The data from military operations have spurred evaluation of these concepts in civilian trauma centers as well.

The concept of damage control with regard to trauma care was initially described in the early 1990s with with the use of damage-control laparotomy. In contrast to definitive laparotomy, this surgical approach to severely injured patients involves initial control of life-threatening hemorrhage and contamination, followed by intraperitoneal packing and rapid closure with planned re-exploration at a later time once the patient is hemodynamically stabilized.[38] This approach has been shown to lead to improved outcomes for abdominal trauma[39]; its application has now been extended to include thoracic surgery and early orthopedic care. Damage-control resuscitation (DCR) is a treatment strategy for patients in severe hemorrhagic shock that targets the conditions that exacerbate hemorrhage, namely the three components of the lethal triad of hypothermia, coagulopathy, and acidosis. It includes the following:

- Hypotensive resuscitation
- Hemostatic resuscitation
- Prevention and treatment of acidosis and hypothermia
- The use of fresh, whole blood when available
- The use of factor VIIa for ongoing bleeding
- The above resuscitative efforts in combination with rapid surgical control of bleeding

3.10 Hypotensive Resuscitation

Since the 1950s, the traditional concept of resuscitation of the injured trauma patient has promoted aggressive fluid administration aimed at restoring intravascular volume. Although there is data to support this approach after hemorrhage is controlled, growing evidence over the past two decades indicates this approach may be harmful if applied prior to achieving adequate hemostasis. This practice, although widely implemented, may exacerbate bleeding by increasing hydrostatic pressure on established blood clots, diluting coagulation factors, and contributing to hypothermia. Hypotensive resuscitation, or permissive hypotension, is a strategy that aims to achieve the minimal perfusion pressure needed to maintain tissue oxygenation, while accepting lower than normal blood pressures until surgical control of hemorrhage can be achieved. This concept of limiting fluid resuscitation is not new. During World War I, surgeons called for the limited use of fluids and blood during hemorrhage, stating that "Injection of a fluid that will increase blood pressure has dangers in marked degree because the blood pressure has been too low and the flow too scant to overcome the obstacle offered by a clot. If the pressure is raised before the surgeon is ready to check any bleeding that may take place, blood that is sorely needed may be lost."[40] Subsequent recommendations promoted more liberal use of crystalloid and the concept of hypotensive resuscitation remained relatively dormant for the next 50 years.

There is extensive support for low-volume resuscitation in animal models. Studies consistently demonstrate that using lower than normal blood pressures as a guide to fluid resuscitation reduces the risk of death, regardless of the degree of hemorrhage.[41] The data in humans are less consistent. A major study supporting the concept of hypotensive resuscitation demonstrated that delaying resuscitation until bleeding was controlled improved overall survival in patients with penetrating torso injuries.[42] Patients randomized to the delayed fluid resuscitation group received an average of 375 mL of crystalloid compared with 2.5 L in the standard resuscitation group. In this study, prehospital times were short and patients were mostly young, so extrapolation to other populations or mechanisms of injury may not be appropriate. Two other smaller studies did not show a benefit of delayed fluid resuscitation, but both studies had considerable methodological shortcomings that may limit their conclusions.[43,44]

Despite the lack of conclusive evidence for hypotensive resuscitation, recommendations support the use of judicious fluid replacement in all trauma patients, but particularly in penetrating trauma with a surgically controllable source of bleeding. There needs to be a balance between the risk of worsening coagulopathy and bleeding against maintaining adequate end organ perfusion. For those patients with head injury, hypotensive resuscitation is not recommended due to the risk of secondary injury from hypoperfusion of the brain.[45]

3.11 Hemostatic Resuscitation

The acute coagulopathy of trauma has been rigorously studied since 2003, when Brohi et al first described the prevalence of coagulopathy and its profound impact in trauma. Brohi reported that the incidence of coagulopathy on presentation was close to 25% and increased with increasing severity of illness. In addition, for a given degree of injury, patients with coagulopathy were more likely to die than those without it. Shock appears to be the prime driver of early coagulopathy, and there is a dose-dependent association between degree of tissue hypoperfusion and admission markers of coagulopathy.[3]

Multiple mechanisms of traumatic coagulopathy have been hypothesized, including tissue trauma, hypoperfusion, acidosis, hemodilution, hypothermia, and inflammation.[46] Although the pathophysiology of traumatic coagulopathy is highly complex and not yet fully understood, the rapid identification and treatment of coagulopathy associated with major injury is now appreciated as central to improving outcome. This growing understanding of coagulopathy has encouraged the early and aggressive administration of clotting factors with transfusion of fresh frozen plasma (FFP), platelets, cryoprecipitate, as well as the use of recombinant factor VIIa.

Transfusion thresholds in the setting of acute trauma are not well established and coagulation parameters, such as prothrombin time (PT), international normalized ratio (INR) and partial prothrombin time (PTT) may not promptly and adequately represent the extent of coagulopathy. This complex and dynamic condition makes the recommendation of when and how much of these products to administer controversial. Until more definitive recommendations are put forth, most transfusion of clotting factors is based on a combination of clinical evidence of coagulopathy and abnormal laboratory parameters demonstrating disordered coagulation.

Massive transfusion (transfusion of ≥ 10 units of packed red blood cells [PRBCs] in a 24-h period) occurs in up to 8% of military patients and 3% of civilian trauma patients.[47] With the increased understanding of traumatic coagulopathy, recent recommendations from both the military and many civilian centers support transfusion of FFP and PRBCs in a 1:1 ratio for those patients who receive massive transfusion.[48–53] Previous ratios had ranged from 1:4 to 1:10 FFP:PRBC. These recent recommendations are still debated because many of these studies are retrospective and some of the military data are confounded by the use of whole blood and recombinant factor VIIa.[48,53] Although the optimal ratio of FFP:PRBC is still debated, it is likely that a transfusion ratio that mimics the replacement of whole blood, as close to 1:1 FFP:PRBC, is optimal. Regardless of the ratio of FFP:PRBC administered, it appears as though the implementation of any massive transfusion protocol decreases the overall consumption of blood products and reduces mortality of bleeding trauma patients.[53]

Platelet transfusion in patients requiring massive transfusion is also controversial. Quantitative platelet counts rarely represent platelet function, and laboratory values of platelet function, such as platelet mapping and thromboelastography, are infrequently used in the acute trauma setting. The effect of high platelet to PRBC and FFP ratio in patients receiving massive transfusion has only been studied in two retrospective studies that demonstrate improved survival with a 1:1:1 ratio.[50,51] This practice theoretically makes sense because it mimics the replacement of whole blood, but the practice is based on limited evidence. More studies need to be done before a definitive recommendation on platelet transfusion is made.

3.12 Whole Blood Transfusion

Over the past 40 years, transfusion in the developed world has evolved from the use of whole blood to largely component therapy. After the development of fractionation in the 1940s, component therapy has predominated as the primary transfusion approach, primarily due to concerns of resource utilization and safety. There are little data that compare component therapy with whole blood in rapidly bleeding trauma patients, and it is unclear if our current reliance on component therapy is clinically equivalent to the use of whole blood.[54] There are some recent retrospective data from military conflicts that suggest transfusion of whole blood is superior to component therapy in the massively transfused patient,[55,56,57] but strong prospective studies are lacking to make a recommendation for its use in the general trauma population. In addition, the military has a prescreened, pretyped population of donors that can be called upon as clinical needs arise, which is not representative of the civilian population.

3.13 Recombinant Factor VIIa

Recombinant factor VIIa is approved for use in patients with hemophilia and inhibitory antibodies, but its use in trauma and intracranial hemorrhage has also been studied.[58,59,60,61] Factor VIIa promotes coagulation both physiologically, through activation of both the intrinsic and extrinsic coagulation pathways, and pharmacologically, by acting directly on platelets causing a thrombin burst. Factor VIIa is known to rapidly correct PT and INR, as well as improve thromboelastograms; however, how this translates to clinical outcomes is unclear. Two multicenter, randomized, controlled trials demonstrated significant reductions in blood transfusion requirements in patients with blunt trauma, but no improvement in mortality.[58,59] The CONTROL trial, a phase III trial evaluating the role of factor VIIa in patients with traumatic hemorrhage, was stopped early because at the interim analysis, it was unlikely a benefit would be found given the preliminary results.[62] The role of factor VIIa and its cost effectiveness is still debatable: The current use of hemostatic resuscitation with high ratios of FFP:PRBC may make it difficult to show a mortality benefit with factor VII.

3.14 Hypothermia and Acidosis

Trauma patients are predisposed to hypothermia because of exposure by removal of clothing and opening of body cavities, and the administration of cold intravenous fluids and blood products. In addition, they have a decreased ability to maintain normothermia because of hemorrhage, anesthetic agents, and alcohol or drug intoxication. Consequently, hypothermia is common, and the degree of hypothermia correlates with the Injury Severity Score (ISS) and Trauma Score.[63] There is some evidence to support that hypothermia is an independent predictor of mortality after trauma.[64] The detrimental effects of hypothermia on coagulation, platelet function, and metabolism are well recognized, so its prevention and treatment are of high importance. Prevention of hypothermia is easier than reversal, and the importance of mitigating heat loss is a high priority. Recommendations to prevent hypothermia include increasing the ambient temperature in the resuscitation unit and operating room, and using reflective coverings on the patients, as well as warmed intravenous fluids.[65,66]

Therapeutic hypothermia has been well tested and supported for nontraumatic cardiac arrest and some hemorrhagic models.[67,68] This technique has not been adequately tested in trauma patients, mainly due to the concern for worsening coagulopathy, increased incidence of sepsis, and the metabolic consequences of rewarming and reperfusion. Therefore, at the current time, induced hypothermia remains a theoretical intervention that still warrants further study.[69]

Metabolic acidosis is the predominant defect resulting from persistent hypoperfusion and can arise from multiple etiologies in trauma, including lactate from hypoperfusion and resuscitation with crystalloid causing hyperchloremia and hypothermia.[70] Acidosis at or below pH 7.2 is associated with decreased contractility and cardiac output, vasodilation, hypotension, bradycardia, increased dysrhythmia, and decreased blood flow to the liver and kidneys.[71] In addition, acidosis can act synergistically with hypothermia to further worsen coagulopathy. Although correction of metabolic acidosis requires restoration of organ perfusion, acidosis may persist while ongoing attempts at resuscitation are underway. The traditional treatment for severe acidosis in critical illness is sodium bicarbonate, but there is little rationale for its use or evidence of its effectiveness in general or in the trauma population.[72] Administration of sodium bicarbonate produces carbon dioxide, which can require large increases in minute ventilation to clear, and can cause decreases in serum calcium levels, which has adverse effects on cardiac and vascular contractility.[73] This has led to a search for adjunctive pharmacologic treatments for acidosis, such as hydroxymethyl aminomethane (THAM), but the role of these agents in trauma resuscitation has yet to be elucidated.

3.15 Conclusion

The ideal resuscitation strategy for multiply injured patients remains a topic of ongoing debate. At present, no consensus has been reached on the ideal type and amount of fluid for early resuscitation and on the threshold for blood-product transfusion. Ongoing support for the deleterious effects of high-volume crystalloid administration encourages the judicious use of crystalloid and the early use of blood products to improve oxygen delivery, target coagulopathy, and minimize complications. Patients who receive a massive transfusion likely benefit from either transfusion of whole blood or component therapy that mimics whole blood content. Research is ongoing to further evaluate and support these recommendations.

References

[1] Committee on Trauma Research. Injury in America, a continuing public health problem. Washington, DC: National Academy Press; 1985:65–80

[2] Rivers E, Nguyen B, Havstad S et al. Early Goal-Directed Therapy Collaborative Group. Early goal-directed therapy in the treatment of severe sepsis and septic shock. N Engl J Med 2001; 345: 1368–1377

[3] Brohi K, Singh J, Heron M, Coats T. Acute traumatic coagulopathy. J Trauma 2003; 54: 1127–1130

[4] Rixen D, Siegel JH. Bench-to-bedside review: oxygen debt and its metabolic correlates as quantifiers of the severity of hemorrhagic and post-traumatic shock. Crit Care 2005; 9: 441–453

[5] Porter JM, Ivatury RR. In search of the optimal end points of resuscitation in trauma patients: a review. J Trauma 1998; 44: 908–914

[6] Scalea TM, Maltz S, Yelon J , et al. Resuscitation of multiple trauma and head injury: role of crystalloid fluids and isotopes. Crit Care Med 1994; 22: 1610–1615

[7] Abou-Khalil B, Scalea TM, Trooskin SZ, Henry SM, Hitchcock R. Hemodynamic responses to shock in young trauma patients: need for invasive monitoring. Crit Care Med 1994; 22: 633–639

[8] McNelis J, Marini CP, Jurkiewicz A et al. Prolonged lactate clearance is associated with increased mortality in the surgical intensive care unit. Am J Surg 2001; 182: 481–485

[9] Husain FA, Martin MJ, Mullenix PS, Steele SR, Elliott DC. Serum lactate and base deficit as predictors of mortality and morbidity. Am J Surg 2003; 185: 485–491

[10] Tisherman SA, Barie P, Bokhari F et al. Clinical practice guideline: endpoints of resuscitation. J Trauma 2004; 57: 898–912

[11] Napolitano LM. Resuscitation endpoints in trauma. Transfusion Alternatives in Transfusion Medicine. 2005; 6: 6–14

[12] Gattinoni L, Brazzi L, Pelosi P et al. A trial of goal-oriented hemodynamic therapy in critically ill patients. SvO2 Collaborative Group. N Engl J Med 1995; 333: 1025–1032

[13] Shires T, Coln D, Carrico J, Lightfoot S. Fluid therapy in hemorrhagic shock. Arch Surg 1964; 88: 688–693

[14] American College of Surgeons Committee on Trauma. Advance Trauma Life Support for Doctors Manual. Chicago, IL: American College of Surgeons; 1997:97–107

[15] Alam HB, Rhee P. New developments in fluid resuscitation. Surg Clin North Am 2007; 87: 55–72, vi

[16] Alderson P, Schierhout G, Roberts I, Bunn F. Colloids versus crystalloids for fluid resuscitation in critically ill patients. Cochrane Database Syst Rev 2000: CD000567

[17] Cochrane Injuries Group Albumin Reviewers. Human albumin administration in critically ill patients: systematic review of randomised controlled trials. BMJ 1998; 317: 235–240

[18] Finfer S, Bellomo R, Boyce N, French J, Myburgh J, Norton R SAFE Study Investigators. A comparison of albumin and saline for fluid resuscitation in the intensive care unit. N Engl J Med 2004; 350: 2247–2256

[19] Velasco IT, Pontieri V, Rocha e Silva M, Lopes OU. Hyperosmotic NaCl and severe hemorrhagic shock. Am J Physiol 1980; 239: H664–H673

[20] Järvelä K, Koskinen M, Kaukinen S, Kööbi T. Effects of hypertonic saline (7.5%) on extracellular fluid volumes compared with normal saline (0.9%) and 6% hydroxyethyl starch after aortocoronary bypass graft surgery. J Cardiothorac Vasc Anesth 2001; 15: 210–215

[21] Rhee P, Burris D, Kaufmann C et al. Lactated Ringer's solution resuscitation causes neutrophil activation after hemorrhagic shock. J Trauma 1998; 44: 313–319

[22] Bulger EM, Jurkovich GJ, Nathens AB et al. Hypertonic resuscitation of hypovolemic shock after blunt trauma: a randomized controlled trial. Arch Surg 2008; 143: 139–148, discussion 149

[23] Rizoli SB, Rhind SG, Shek PN et al. The immunomodulatory effects of hypertonic saline resuscitation in patients sustaining traumatic hemorrhagic shock: a randomized, controlled, double-blinded trial. Ann Surg 2006; 243: 47–57

[24] Mattox KL, Maningas PA, Moore EE et al. Prehospital hypertonic saline/dextran infusion for post-traumatic hypotension. The U.S.A. Multicenter Trial. Ann Surg 1991; 213: 482–491

[25] Holcroft JW, Vassar MJ, Turner JE, Derlet RW, Kramer GC. 3% NaCl and 7.5% NaCl/dextran 70 in the resuscitation of severely injured patients. Ann Surg 1987; 206: 279–288

[26] Vassar MJ, Fischer RP, O'Brien PE et al. The Multicenter Group for the Study of Hypertonic Saline in Trauma Patients. A multicenter trial for resuscitation of injured patients with 7.5% sodium chloride. The effect of added dextran 70. Arch Surg 1993; 128: 1003–1011, discussion 1011–1013

[27] Vassar MJ, Perry CA, Gannaway WL, Holcroft JW. 7.5% sodium chloride/dextran for resuscitation of trauma patients undergoing helicopter transport. Arch Surg 1991; 126: 1065–1072

[28] Vassar MJ, Perry CA, Holcroft JW. Prehospital resuscitation of hypotensive trauma patients with 7.5% NaCl versus 7.5% NaCl with added dextran: a controlled trial. J Trauma 1993; 34: 622–632, discussion 632–633

[29] Maningas PA, Mattox KL, Pepe PE, Jones RL, Feliciano DV, Burch JM. Hypertonic saline-dextran solutions for the prehospital management of traumatic hypotension. Am J Surg 1989; 157: 528–533, discussion 533–534

[30] Younes RN, Aun F, Accioly CQ, Casale LP, Szajnbok I, Birolini D. Hypertonic solutions in the treatment of hypovolemic shock: a prospective, randomized study in patients admitted to the emergency room. Surgery 1992; 111: 380–385

[31] Younes RN, Aun F, Ching CT et al. Prognostic factors to predict outcome following the administration of hypertonic/hyperoncotic solution in hypovolemic patients. Shock 1997; 7: 79–83

[32] Cooper DJ, Myles PS, McDermott FT et al. HTS Study Investigators. Prehospital hypertonic saline resuscitation of patients with hypotension and severe traumatic brain injury: a randomized controlled trial. JAMA 2004; 291: 1350–1357

[33] Bunn F, Roberts I, Tasker R, Akpa E. Hypertonic versus near isotonic crystalloid for fluid resuscitation in critically ill patients. Cochrane Database Syst Rev 2004; 3: CD002045

[34] Bulger EM, May S, Kerby JD et al. ROC investigators. Out-of-hospital hypertonic resuscitation after traumatic hypovolemic shock: a randomized, placebo controlled trial. Ann Surg 2011; 253: 431–441

[35] McIntyre L, Hebert PC, Wells G et al. Canadian Critical Care Trials Group. Is a restrictive transfusion strategy safe for resuscitated and critically ill trauma patients? J Trauma 2004; 57: 563–568, discussion 568

[36] Malone DL, Dunne J, Tracy JK, Putnam AT, Scalea TM, Napolitano LM. Blood transfusion, independent of shock severity, is associated with worse outcome in trauma. J Trauma 2003; 54: 898–905, discussion 905–907

[37] Carlson AP, Schermer CR, Lu SW. Retrospective evaluation of anemia and transfusion in traumatic brain injury. J Trauma 2006; 61: 567–571

[38] Rotondo MF, Schwab CW, McGonigal MD et al. 'Damage control': an approach for improved survival in exsanguinating penetrating abdominal injury. J Trauma 1993; 35: 375–382, discussion 382–383

[39] Moore EE. Thomas G. Orr Memorial Lecture. Staged laparotomy for the hypothermia, acidosis, and coagulopathy syndrome. Am J Surg 1996; 172: 405–410

[40] Cannon WB, Frasor J, Cowell EM. The preventive treatment of wound shock. JAMA 1918; 70: 618–621

[41] Mapstone J, Roberts I, Evans P. Fluid resuscitation strategies: a systematic review of animal trials. J Trauma 2003; 55: 571–589

[42] Bickell WH, Wall MJ, Pepe PE et al. Immediate versus delayed fluid resuscitation for hypotensive patients with penetrating torso injuries. N Engl J Med 1994; 331: 1105–1109

[43] Dutton RP, Mackenzie CF, Scalea TM. Hypotensive resuscitation during active hemorrhage: impact on in-hospital mortality. J Trauma 2002; 52: 1141–1146

[44] Turner J, Nicholl J, Webber L, Cox H, Dixon S, Yates D. A randomised controlled trial of prehospital intravenous fluid replacement therapy in serious trauma. Health Technol Assess 2000; 4: 1–57

[45] Stahel PF, Smith WR, Moore EE. Hypoxia and hypotension, the "lethal duo" in traumatic brain injury: implications for prehospital care. Intensive Care Med 2008; 34: 402–404

[46] Hess JR, Brohi K, Dutton RP et al. The coagulopathy of trauma: a review of mechanisms. J Trauma 2008; 65: 748–754

[47] Como JJ, Dutton RP, Scalea TM, Edelman BB, Hess JR. Blood transfusion rates in the care of acute trauma. Transfusion 2004; 44: 809–813

[48] Borgman MA, Spinella PC, Perkins JG et al. The ratio of blood products transfused affects mortality in patients receiving massive transfusions at a combat support hospital. J Trauma 2007; 63: 805–813

[49] Duchesne JC, Hunt JP, Wahl G et al. Review of current blood transfusions strategies in a mature level I trauma center: were we wrong for the last 60 years? J Trauma 2008; 65: 272–276, discussion 276–278

[50] Gunter OL, Au BK, Isbell JM, Mowery NT, Young PP, Cotton BA. Optimizing outcomes in damage control resuscitation: identifying blood product ratios associated with improved survival. J Trauma 2008; 65: 527–534

[51] Holcomb JB, Wade CE, Michalek JE et al. Increased plasma and platelet to red blood cell ratios improves outcome in 466 massively transfused civilian trauma patients. Ann Surg 2008; 248: 447–458

[52] Zink KA, Sambasivan CN, Holcomb JB, Chisholm G, Schreiber MA. A high ratio of plasma and platelets to packed red blood cells in the first 6 hours of massive transfusion improves outcomes in a large multicenter study. Am J Surg 2009; 197: 565–570, discussion 570

[53] Riskin DJ, Tsai TC, Riskin L et al. Massive transfusion protocols: the role of aggressive resuscitation versus product ratio in mortality reduction. J Am Coll Surg 2009; 209: 198–205

[54] Holcomb JB, Spinella PC. Optimal use of blood in trauma patients. Biologicals 2010; 38: 72–77

[55] Kauvar KS, Holcomb JB, Norris GC et al. Fresh whole blood in massive transfusion. J Trauma 2006; 61: 181–184

[56] Repine TB, Perkins JG, Kauvar DS, Blackborne L. The use of fresh whole blood in massive transfusion. J Trauma 2006; 60 Suppl: S59–S69

[57] Spinella PC, Perkins JP, Grathwohl KG et al. The risks associated with freash whole blood and RBC transfusions in a combat support hospital. Crit Care Med 2007; 35: S340–S345

[58] Boffard KD, Riou B, Warren B et al. NovoSeven Trauma Study Group. Recombinant factor VIIa as adjunctive therapy for bleeding control in severely injured trauma patients: two parallel randomized, placebo-controlled, double-blind clinical trials. J Trauma 2005; 59: 8–15, discussion 15–18

[59] Dutton RP, McCunn M, Hyder M et al. Factor VIIa for correction of traumatic coagulopathy. J Trauma 2004; 57: 709–718, discussion 718–719

[60] Harrison TD, Laskosky J, Jazaeri O, Pasquale MD, Cipolle M. "Low-dose" recombinant activated factor VII results in less blood and blood product use in traumatic hemorrhage. J Trauma 2005; 59: 150–154

[61] Stein DM, Dutton RP, Hess JR, Scalea TM. Low-dose recombinant factor VIIa for trauma patients with coagulopathy. Injury 2008; 39: 1054–1061

[62] Hauser CJ, Boffard K, Dutton R et al. CONTROL Study Group. Results of the CONTROL trial: efficacy and safety of recombinant activated Factor VII in the management of refractory traumatic hemorrhage. J Trauma 2010; 69: 489–500

[63] Little RA, Stoner HB. Body temperature after accidental injury. Br J Surg 1981; 68: 221–224

[64] Jurkovich GJ, Greiser WB, Luterman A, Curreri PW. Hypothermia in trauma victims: an ominous predictor of survival. J Trauma 1987; 27: 1019–1024

[65] Hayes JS, Tyler-Ball S, Cohen SS, Eckes-Roper J, Puente I. Evidence-based practice and heat loss prevention in trauma patients. J Nurs Care Qual 2002; 16: 13–16

[66] Bernardo LM, Henker R, Bove M, Sereika S. The effect of administered crystalloid fluid temperature on aural temperature of moderately and severely injured children. J Emerg Nurs 1997; 23: 105–111

[67] Prueckner S, Safar P, Kentner R, Stezoski J, Tisherman SA. Mild hypothermia increases survival from severe pressure-controlled hemorrhagic shock in rats. J Trauma 2001; 50: 253–262

[68] Wladis A, Hahn RG, Hjelmqvist H, Brismar B, Kjellström BT. Acute hemodynamic effects of induced hypothermia in hemorrhagic shock: an experimental study in the pig. Shock 2001; 15: 60–64

[69] Pepe PE, Dutton RP, Fowler RL. Preoperative resuscitation of the trauma patient. Curr Opin Anaesthesiol 2008; 21: 216–221

[70] Watts DD, Trask A, Soeken K, Perdue P, Dols S, Kaufmann C. Hypothermic coagulopathy in trauma: effect of varying levels of hypothermia on enzyme speed, platelet function, and fibrinolytic activity. J Trauma 1998; 44: 846–854

[71] Mikhail J. The trauma triad of death: hypothermia, acidosis, and coagulopathy. AACN Clin Issues 1999; 10: 85–94

[72] Boyd JH, Walley KR. Is there a role for sodium bicarbonate in treating lactic acidosis from shock? Curr Opin Crit Care 2008; 14: 379–383

[73] Jansen JO, Thomas R, Loudon MA, Brooks A. Damage control resuscitation for patients with major trauma. BMJ 2009; 338: b1778

4 Imaging of Thoracic Trauma

Mark S. Parker

4.1 Epidemiology

Trauma is the third leading cause of death in the United States and the most frequent cause of death in individuals less than 35 years of age.[1] The rate of thoracic trauma in the United States alone is ~ 12 per million per day resulting in more than 300,000 hospitalizations each year. Thoracic injuries account for 25 to 35% of trauma-related deaths or ~ 16,000 deaths per year.[1,2]

Thoracic trauma is broadly categorized as blunt and penetrating. Blunt trauma accounts for 90% of chest trauma and is most often the result of deceleration forces associated with motor vehicle collisions (i.e., 75–80%), automobile versus pedestrian collisions, falls, assaults, and blast and compression injuries. Injuries of the thorax are a major cause of morbidity (36%) and mortality (16%) in cases of blunt trauma.[3] The latter is usually due to aortic or great vessel injury.[1] Most penetrating injuries to the chest are by knives or handgun bullets.[4] Approximately 4 to 15% of admissions to major trauma centers are attributable to penetrating thoracic injuries. For every firearm-related death, it is estimated there are 3 to 5 other nonfatal firearm injuries.[4] Penetrating trauma can be further categorized as low- and high-energy injuries. All stabbings are considered low-energy injuries. Such hand-driven low-energy weapons damage tissue from their sharp cutting edge or point.[4]

The radiologist assessing the extent of underlying injuries must consider the length and width of the projectile or weapon, its depth of penetration and angle of entry, as well as the nature and mechanisms of the force applied (e.g., single thrust, repetitive thrust, and twisting and rotation with entry), etc. Gunshot wounds can be divided into low-energy (e.g., handguns, air-powered pellet guns) and high-energy injuries (e.g., rifles and military weapons). High-energy gunshot wounds have a muzzle velocity of 1,000 to 2,500 ft/s.[4] Most "civilian" penetrating trauma results from knife stabbings or handguns (i.e., low-energy injuries). The extent of tissue damage is more severe for high-energy projectiles, which are associated with the formation of "temporary" and "permanent" cavities resulting in substantial tissue damage along the wound tract and surrounding tissues and organ systems. This latter concept ("temporary cavity") is critical to the appropriate analysis of diagnostic imaging studies.[4] The temporary cavity may be 10 to 20 or more times larger than the permanent cavity.

4.2 Imaging Techniques

4.2.1 Conventional Chest Radiography

Supine chest radiography is the primary screening examination for most trauma patients.[1] The primary purpose of screening exams is the early detection of life-threatening thoracic injuries (e.g., esophageal intubation, mainstem bronchial intubation, large or tension pneumothoraces, hemothoraces). The chest radiograph is also an adjunct to the diagnosis of other important clinical conditions including, but not limited to, chest wall and diaphragmatic injuries, contusions, hemothorax,

mediastinal hematoma, etc. It may also detect delayed complications, not infrequent in stabbing victims. Delayed complications from chest stab wounds occur in 8 to 12% of asymptomatic patients with initially normal chest radiographs and usually occur 2 to 5 days after the injury.[4] The initial chest radiograph has a sensitivity of 93% and a negative predictive value of 87% in detecting stab wound-related injuries. The negative predictive value increases to nearly 100% at 6 hours allowing for potential outpatient management after this time. However, it is recommended that chest stab wound victims receive serial radiography at 4- to 6-hour intervals to detect the potential delayed presentation of some injuries (e.g., vascular injuries, hemothorax, pneumothorax, etc.).[4,5]

Chest radiography, on the other hand, is a relatively poor screening modality for acute aortic injury, given that subtle injuries may occur in the absence of significant mediastinal hematoma. Additionally, many factors adversely affect or alter the contour of the mediastinum in the absence of a true aortic injury (e.g., magnification from backboards, short target-to-film distances, aggressive volume resuscitation, pulmonary contusion, hemothorax, atelectasis) resulting in many false-positive chest radiographs.

4.2.2 Computed Tomography and Computed Tomography Angiography

The clinical role of invasive transcatheter aortography has substantially declined over the last decade, largely replaced by helical computed tomography (CT) and CT angiography (CTA). Computed tomography angiography is now the first-line imaging modality in the evaluation of trauma victims with suspected acute traumatic aortic injury (ATAI) with sensitivity and negative predictive values of nearly 100%.[6,7] State-of-the-art multidetector array CT (MDCT) scanners perform multiplanar evaluations of the thoracic aorta clearly depicting the extent of an injury, and its relationship to branch vessels, thus streamlining appropriate medical or surgical management and does so in a fraction of the time and expense of traditional transcatheter aortography. Computed tomography offers the additional benefit of detecting otherwise unsuspected concomitant injuries in 66% of patients with initially abnormal chest radiography, subsequently altering the clinical management in 20% of cases. Computed tomography detects chest injuries in 39% of trauma patients with a severe mechanism of injury, but a normal initial chest radiograph, prompting a change in clinical management in 5% of patients.[8–15]

In the setting of penetrating trauma, the presence of air, hemorrhage, bone or bullet fragments along a wound track on the CT allows the radiologist to identify the course of the projectile and thus the neighboring organ systems that may have been injured.[4] For example, penetrating injuries traversing the mediastinum (i.e., transmediastinal) or in proximity to vital mediastinal structures necessitate further investigation with esophagography, possibly esophagoscopy, and bronchoscopy, etc.

4.2.3 Thoracic Aortography

Helical CT and MDCT aortography in particular have replaced conventional transcatheter aortography in the evaluation of most trauma patients with suspected ATAI, either on the basis of chest radiography alone or the incurred mechanisms. Aortography is now reserved only for patients with either indeterminate or abnormal CT exams, thus eliminating up to 67% of invasive, time-consuming, costly, and labor-intensive angiography.[16,17] Furthermore, it is now accepted that patients with only an anterior or posterior mediastinal hematoma and an otherwise normal appearing aorta, do not need further evaluation with aortography.[18]

Prominent vessels adjacent to the aorta, atheromatous plaques that may mimic intimal flaps or ductus diverticula that may mimic a pseudoaneurysm and mediastinal hematoma, without direct evidence of aortic or great vessel injury, may occasionally create a diagnostic dilemma on older-generation CT scans. The former have become less of an issue with MDCT with its multiplanar and three-dimensional (3D) reconstruction capabilities. Supplementary aortography has been advocated in those latter indeterminate more problematic cases. However, recently it has been shown that in those cases in which MDCT is indeterminate. conventional aortography is unlikely to show an aortic or intrathoracic great vessel injury as well. Evidence now supports that these patients can be followed clinically, with subsequent cross-sectional imaging, or both without the need for catheter aortography.[19]

Branch vessel injuries at their origin from the aortic arch should be obvious on CT and MDCT. However, more distant or peripheral vascular injuries may be less apparent. The presence of a local hematoma should raise the suspicion of vascular injury warranting further investigation with selective angiography.[17]

In the 21st century, the emphasis of transcatheter aortography shifted primarily from a diagnostic to a therapeutic role.[20] Endovascular stent-graft repair to cover the injured aneurysmal segment of the aorta has emerged as an alternative for treating acute thoracic aortic injuries. In many practices, endovascular stent-grafts have become the procedure of choice for treating these otherwise lethal injuries.[20,21,22,23] This minimally invasive interventional radiology (IR) procedure employs self-expanding, fabric-covered metal stents, introduced in a retrograde fashion by a dedicated delivery system, ideally percutaneous via the common femoral artery. Advantages of this technique over that of a traditional open surgical repair include the ability to treat patients with contraindications to thoracotomy, an up to 75% reduction in postprocedural paraplegia, and more importantly up to a 50% reduction in mortality.[21,22,23] Significant advances in endovascular management of trauma with embolization and stent placement now allows for definitive repair of branch vessel and intercostal artery injuries as well.[24]

4.2.4 Ultrasound

Focused assessment with ultrasound for trauma (FAST) is a rapid, bedside study performed by radiologists, trauma surgeons, and emergency physicians to quickly assess for hemoperitoneum or hemopericardium after significant thoracic and or thoracoabdominal trauma. Four anatomic areas are rapidly scanned for free fluid. These are the perihepatic or hepatorenal space, perisplenic space, pericardium, and pelvis. Fluid in any one of these spaces suggests the presence of blood. Hypotensive patients with FAST scan findings are triaged directly to therapeutic laparotomy, without the need for CT.[25]

Increasingly, transesophageal echocardiography (TEE) is being used to assess the thoracic aorta after severe trauma. This modality is helpful when MDCT or even aortography have inconclusive findings. Transesophageal echocardiography may also demonstrate hemothorax, pneumothorax, a wide spectrum of acute cardiovascular abnormalities including myocardial contusion, valvular injuries, rupture of the chordae tendinae and papillary muscles, and hemopericardium or pericardial effusion with or without tamponade. Unfortunately, TEE is operator-dependent (as other ultrasound- (US-) based studies) and has "blind spots" created by the tracheal-bronchial bifurcation precluding adequate visualization of portions of the thoracic aorta. Additional blind spots include the distal ascending aorta and the aortic arch vessels.[26,27] Intravascular ultrasonography (IVUS) is also helpful in the evaluation of the thoracic aorta in patients with equivocal MDCT or aortography. On the other hand, in patients with suspected aortic injury along the lesser curvature of the archisthmus junction, TEE allows better vascular delineation than IVUS because of its multiplanar imaging capabilities.[27,28]

4.2.5 Magnetic Resonance Imaging

Although magnetic resonance imaging (MRI) can demonstrate the presence of mediastinal hematoma and acute aortic injuries, it currently has a limited role in the initial evaluation of critically ill, hemodynamically unstable trauma patients. Magnetic resonance imaging is, however, a very useful modality for the diagnosis of thoracic spine and spinal cord injuries, as well as suspected diaphragmatic injuries in hemodynamically stable patients. Delayed contrast-enhanced cardiac MRI may help differentiate myocardial contusion and acute peritraumatic myocardial infarction, thus appropriately directing patient management. Magnetic resonance imaging is also useful in the evaluation of chronic posttraumatic aortic pseudoaneurysms.[29,30]

4.2.6 Contrast Esophagography

Esophagography is indicated for patients with possible esophageal injuries in whom esophagoscopy is negative. Ideally, this study should be performed with the patient in a right lateral decubitus position. Despite its modest sensitivity (i.e., 60–75%), esophagography is first performed with water-soluble contrast media (e.g., Gastrografin). If this study is negative, further evaluation is then immediately performed with barium. Barium esophagography has a higher sensitivity (i.e., 90%) for detecting small perforation, but may induce a severe inflammatory response, most notably mediastinitis. If both water soluble and barium contrast esophagography are negative, an esophageal injury is reliably excluded.[31,32]

4.3 Nonvascular Thoracic Trauma

4.3.1 Pleura Injuries

Pneumothorax

Pneumothorax is a frequent complication after blunt or penetrating chest trauma.[13] In blunt trauma, it is the second most

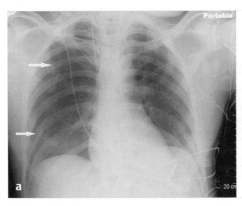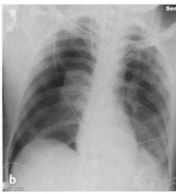

Fig. 4.1 A 38-year-old man with splenic trauma necessitating emergent laparotomy after a motor vehicle collision. Note the surgical packing in the left upper quadrant. (a) Baseline anteroposterior (AP) chest radiograph demonstrates appropriately positioned life-support tubes and lines, slight elevation of the left diaphragm, and a right lateral pneumothorax with 15 to 20 mm of pleural separation (arrows). (b) AP chest radiograph 12 hours later following an abrupt drop in oxygenation saturations shows progression of this pneumothorax to tension while on positive pressure ventilation.

common injury after rib fractures, occurring in 30 to 40% of patients.[33] Although often small in volume, the diagnosis is important because an unsuspected pneumothorax may rapidly enlarge and become symptomatic in patients receiving mechanical ventilation or undergoing general anesthesia (▶ Fig. 4.1).[14] The anatomical localization of pleural air depends on the position of the patient, the volume of intrapleural air, the presence or absence of pleural adhesions, and atelectasis.[13] Concomitant atelectasis and the presence of pleural adhesions may result in unusual and atypical pleural air collections.[13]

In the erect or semierect patient, pleural air rises to the most nondependent region of the hemothorax. That region is either the apex or the lateral hemithorax. The diagnosis of pneumothorax is easily made by identifying a thin curvilinear white visceral pleural reflection and the absence of vascular markings extending beyond its lateral border (▶ Fig. 4.2).[13] In the supine patient, the most nondependent region of the thorax changes and pleural air may accumulate in several recesses. The anteromedial recess becomes the most nondependent region, accumulates air earliest, and accounts for up to 30% of pneumothoraces, but may not be recognized on frontal supine chest radiographs in as many as 30 to 50% of trauma patients.[14,34] Left unrecognized and untreated, such pneumothoraces can progress to tension in one-third of affected patients.[13] Radiographic features of an anterior medial pneumothorax include the deep sulcus sign manifest by a deep lucent costophrenic sulcus (▶ Fig. 4.3a), a relative increase in lucency over the affected lung base (▶ Fig. 4.3b), and a double diaphragm sign in which air outlines the central dome and anterior insertion of the diaphragm.[13,14,33] The subpulmonic recess is the second most common region to accumulate pleural air and represents an extension of the anteromedial recess (▶ Fig. 4.3c). Both recesses may accumulate air simultaneously.[14] The apicolateral recess fills with pleural air in 22% of supine patients.[14] Air within the posteromedial recess may manifest radiographically as a lucent line sharply delineating the ipsilateral paraspinal line, descending thoracic aorta and or the posterior costophrenic sulcus.[13]

Air within the pulmonary ligament is infrequent and should not be misinterpreted as a posteromedial pneumothorax. The former is characterized by a linear lucent band with a convex lateral border and a superior border that curves toward the upper hilum. The latter has a triangular morphology.[13]

Tension pneumothorax is an emergent clinical and not a radiologic diagnosis that should be made and treated before acquiring any imaging studies. However, unexpected tension pneumothoraces are not infrequently encountered on imaging studies. Radiologic features include flattening or inversion of the ipsilateral diaphragm, contralateral mediastinal shift, widening of the ipsilateral intercostal spaces, collapse of the ipsilateral lung, and effacement of the ipsilateral heart border (▶ Fig. 4.4).[33]

Ultrasound is now being used to diagnose occult pneumothorax at the bedside and in unstable patients with problematic or nondiagnostic portable chest radiography. Three US signs of pneumothorax that may be observed along the anterolateral chest wall in supine patients include lung sliding, the A-line sign, and the lung point. The normal lung glides smoothly under the parietal pleura during respiration. For the diagnosis of occult pneumothorax, the abolition of the lung sliding alone has a sensitivity of 100% and a specificity of 78%. Absent lung

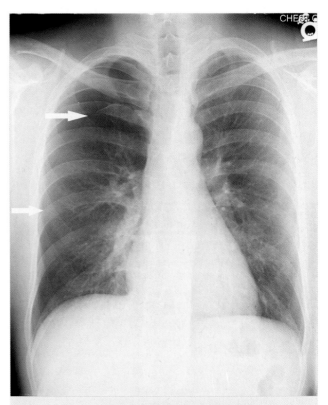

Fig. 4.2 A 46-year-old man stabbed in the right back. Erect posteroanterior chest radiograph reveals a modest-sized right apical and apical-lateral pneumothorax. Notice the white visceral line (arrows) and absence of vascular markings beyond its peripheral border.

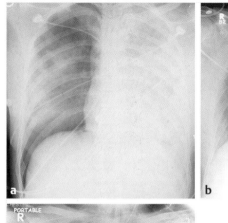
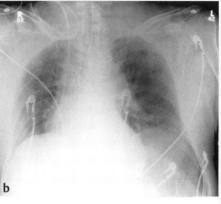

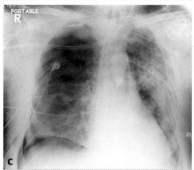

Fig. 4.3 Radiographic manifestations of pneumothoraces on supine chest radiography. (a) Supine radiograph in a young man with severe multifocal pulmonary contusions and increasing difficulty to mechanically ventilate demonstrates a spontaneous right tension pneumothorax manifest by a deep hyperlucent right costophrenic sulcus (deep sulcus sign). (b) Supine chest radiograph of another patient with a tension left pneumothorax characterized by a hyperlucent left lung base and upper quadrant (courtesy of Narinder Paul, MD; University of Toronto). (c) Supine chest radiograph of a middle-aged man with bilateral pulmonary contusions. There has been progression of the right pneumothorax while on mechanical ventilation, manifesting as a subpulmonic air collection extending from the anteromedial recess.

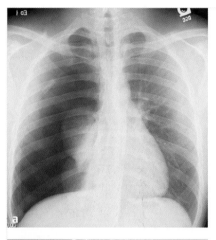
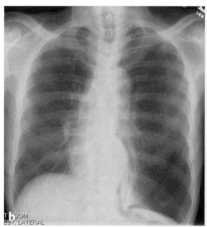

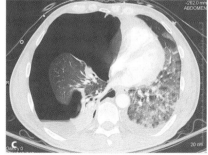
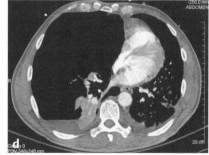

Fig. 4.4 Various radiologic imaging features of tension pneumothoraces. (a) Erect posteroanterior (PA) chest radiograph of a young man stabbed in the right back reveals a tension pneumothorax. There is total collapse of the entire right lung, widening of the ipsilateral intercostal spaces, effacement of the right heart border, and contralateral mediastinal shift. (b) Erect PA radiograph of a young man stabbed in the left back reveals a tension pneumothorax. Note the increased size of the left thorax relative to the right, the ipsilateral diaphragmatic inversion, and contralateral mediastinal shift. (c,d) Contrast-enhanced axial computed tomography (lung and mediastinal windows) demonstrate an unsuspected right tension hemopneumothorax. The right atrium and most of the right ventricle are effaced.

sliding plus the A-line sign has a sensitivity of 95% and a specificity of 94%. The lung point has a sensitivity of 79% and a specificity of 100%.[35] Either vertical (comet-tail artifacts) or horizontal reverberation artifacts arise from the lung-wall interface during respiration. Ultrasound is deemed positive for pneumothorax when only horizontal artifacts are visible and negative when artifacts arise from the pleural line and spread up to the edge of the screen (i.e., "comet-tail artifacts").[36]

Computed tomography is more sensitive than chest radiography for detecting pneumothoraces, especially in the supine

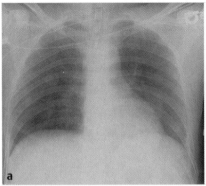
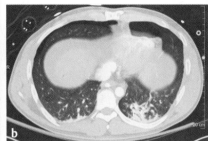

Fig. 4.5 Radiographically occult pneumothoraces detected on computed tomography (CT) in a young man who sustained both head and abdominal trauma following a motor vehicle collision. (a) Supine chest radiography reveals no conspicuous pneumothorax. (b) Contrast-enhanced abdominal CT (lung window) at the thoracoabdominal level demonstrates clinically and radiographically unsuspected bilateral pneumothoraces.

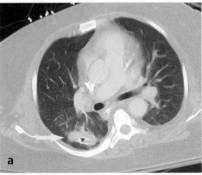
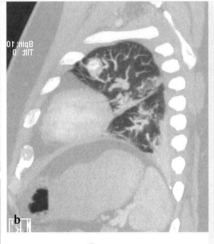

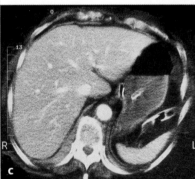
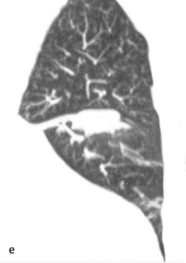

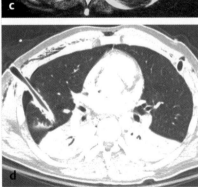

Fig. 4.6 Malpositioned thoracostomy tubes detected on chest computed tomography (CT). (a,b) Contrast-enhanced axial (a) and sagittal maximum intensity projection (MIP) (arrow) (b) CT (lung windows) show an intraparenchymal chest tube with parenchymal hemorrhage surrounding the tube. (c) Contrast-enhanced axial CT (mediastinal window) reveals inadvertent subdiaphragmatic insertion of a left pleural drain between the spleen and the stomach. (d,e) Contrast-enhanced axial (d) and sagittal MIP (e) CT (lung windows) show a right thoracostomy tube incorrectly positioned within the horizontal fissure.

patient. As many as 10 to 15% of blunt abdominal trauma patients may have unsuspected pneumothoraces detected on CT (► Fig. 4.5).[14,15,33] Therefore, imaging through the inferior one-third of the lung bases is routinely performed on abdominal CT scans in blunt-trauma patients.[37]

The failure of a pneumothorax to decompress following thoracostomy tube placement may be the result of tube malpositioning. Such malpositioning may be difficult to appreciate on chest radiography. Computed tomography is excellent for delineating thoracostomy tubes inadvertently placed in aberrant locations (e.g., extrathoracic chest wall soft tissues, below the diaphragm, intraparenchymal, intrafissural) (► Fig. 4.6).[38,39] Intraparenchymal tube placement can be difficult to recognize clinically and radiographically. Landay et al reported 26% patients in their series experienced clinical and radiographic improvement after the inadvertent placement of an intraparenchymal chest tube and

42% of such patients had no ill sequelae.[40] The authors postulated malpositioned tubes may evacuate pleural air and or fluid collections as they penetrate the pleural space to or from the lung parenchyma.[40] However, such tube thoracostomy lung penetration may produce air leaks or vascular injuries, resulting in pseudoaneurysm or bleeding (i.e., hemothorax).[41,42] A radiographic clue to possible intraparenchymal thoracostomy tube placement is the sudden onset of extensive extra-alveolar air (e.g., marked increase in size of a pre-existing pneumothorax or development of extensive subcutaneous air) following the pleural tube placement. Hemorrhage or hematoma manifest as ground-glass opacity or consolidation surrounding the intraparenchymal thoracostomy tube may be another radiographic clue, but is often difficult to appreciate in the setting of concomitant noniatrogenic pulmonary contusion, laceration, and or hemothorax. An abrupt or gradual increase in either parenchymal or pleural opacity following pleural tube placement is another helpful radiographic sign.[40] Multidetector array CT scanners and multiplanar reconstructions in sagittal, sagittal oblique, and coronal planes is much more sensitive for delineating the aberrant course and associated lung penetration (▶ Fig. 4.6a,b). All malpositioned subcutaneous, intraparenchymal, and subdiaphragmatic thoracostomy tubes need to be removed as soon as possible.[14,33] Extrathoracic subcutaneous pleural drains will not evacuate either pleural air or fluid and may be complicated by chest wall hematoma and subsequent infection. Many patients with intraparenchymal chest tube placements will only require tube removal. Others will require additional pleural tube placements or surgical repair of the parenchymal laceration.[40] Subdiaphragmatic pleural drain placements are rare, but more problematic, and may necessitate surgical repair of the diaphragm and or injured hollow and or solid subdiaphragmatic viscera (▶ Fig. 4.6c). An intrafissural thoracostomy tube may adequately decompress a pneumothorax, but is often less effective in evacuating hemothorax and other pleural fluid collections (▶ Fig. 4.6d,e).[15]

4.3.2 Pleural Effusions

Traumatic pleural fluid collections may result from bleeding of the chest wall, mediastinal, or diaphragmatic vessels; traumatic central venous catheter insertions; or thoracic duct injuries. Such fluid collections following chest trauma usually represent hemothorax. In fact, hemothorax occurs in ~ 50% of major trauma victims, especially those caused by penetrating trauma.[13,15,33] A small hemothorax also typically occurs in association with a posttraumatic ipsilateral pneumothorax.[13]

Venous injuries or direct injuries to the lung parenchyma result in low-pressure bleeding with little mass effect and are usually self-limited. On the other hand, arterial injuries (e.g., intercostals, subclavian, internal mammary) are under higher pressure, may continue to bleed and rapidly fill the affected hemithorax, and may be associated with lung compression and mediastinal displacement.[13,15,33] Continued bleeding may require tube drainage.[33] Closed drainage may be used for hemothorax with volumes of 500 to 1500 mL that stop bleeding after thoracostomy tube placement. Open thoracotomy may be necessary in up to 10 to 15% of patients. The latter usually reserved for hemothorax with volumes of more than 1500 to 2000 mL or for patients with continued bleeding and pleural tube output of more than 200 - 300 mL per hour.

Early evacuation of retained hemothorax by either video thoracoscopy or thoracotomy improves pulmonary function, prevents empyema and delayed fibrothorax and should ideally be performed within 3 days of the injury.[43] Massive bleeding from an intercostal artery or pulmonary artery laceration can also be managed by selective arteriography and transcatheter embolization. Embolization is an alternative to control hemorrhage from noniatrogenic and iatrogenic vascular injuries.[44,45]

Pleural effusions, under 200 to 300 mL, usually go undetected on supine chest radiography. As the effusion increases, it first collects posteriorly in the dependent hemithorax. The only radiographic clue may be a relative increased opacity with preserved vascular markings compared with the contralateral hemithorax (▶ Fig. 4.7a).[13] As the effusion increases, it collects laterally along the chest wall producing a band-like radiopacity and eventually spills into the ipsilateral apex forming an apical cap (▶ Fig. 4.7b).[13] Further increases are characterized by contralateral displacement of the cardiomediastinal silhouette and physiologically may behave similar to a tension pneumothorax (▶ Fig. 4.7c).[33] On upright chest radiography, pleural effusion first presents as an opaque meniscus obscuring the ipsilateral costophrenic and/or cardiophrenic recesses (▶ Fig. 4.7d).[13] Larger effusions increase the relative opacity of the hemithorax and extend along the lateral chest wall and eventually into the apex in a manner similar to that observed in supine chest radiography (▶ Fig. 4.7b).[13]

Pleural fluid may accumulate in the subpulmonic recess between the lung base and diaphragm forming a subpulmonic effusion. Bilateral subpulmonic effusions are infrequently diagnosed on chest radiography, often misinterpreted as hypoventilation or low lung volumes. Unilateral subpulmonic effusions may mimic an elevated diaphragm. However, on closer radiographic inspection, the resulting pseudodiaphragm shows a flattened contour adjacent to the cardiac border and the peak of this apparent diaphragm shifts lateral to its normal position. Additionally, the ipsilateral costophrenic angle often becomes less well defined and a small juxtaphrenic spur may be seen created by fluid extending into the caudal aspect of the oblique fissure (▶ Fig. 4.7e).[46]

Ultrasonography is increasingly used to exclude pleural effusion, evaluate its volume when present, assess its potential compositions, and as a guide for thoracentesis, as well as drain placement.[47,48,49] During respiration, an effusion demonstrates the fluid color sign, in which color Doppler signal is returned from within the effusion. This sign is useful in distinguishing pleural effusion from pleural thickening.[35] Sonographic appearances and patterns of pleural effusion can be subclassified as anechoic, complex nonseptated, complex septated, and homogeneously echogenic. Transudates are usually anechoic; however, in daily practice heterogeneous echogenic material is frequently present in transudative pleural effusions.[49] Complicated effusions (e.g., exudative and hemorrhagic) more often demonstrate complex nonseptated, complex septated, and homogeneously echogenic patterns (▶ Fig. 4.8).[50]

Computed tomography is superior to chest radiography in identifying traumatic pleural fluid collections. Whereas serous effusions often demonstrate attenuation coefficients similar to that of water, acute hemothorax is higher, ranging from 35 to 75 Hounsfield unit (HU) (▶ Fig. 4.9a). Focal areas of high attenuation within the pleural fluid collection usually represent clot

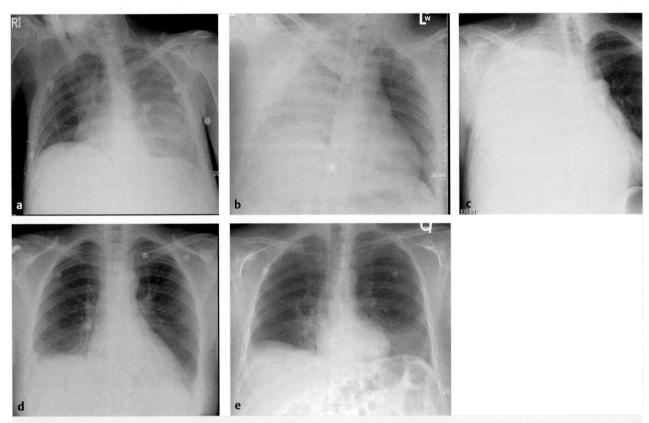

Fig. 4.7 Radiologic features of pleural effusion. (a) Anteroposterior (AP) portable supine radiograph demonstrates increased opacity of the left hemithorax due to a posteriorly layering effusion. Preserved conspicuity of vascular markings differentiates this effusion from air–space disease. (b) AP supine radiograph demonstrates an even larger right pleural effusion extending laterally along the chest wall to the apex. Again there is increased radiopacity, but vascular markings are preserved. (c) Chest radiograph reveals complete "white-out" from a massive right hemothorax, with contralateral displacement of the cardiomediastinal silhouette. (d) Erect AP chest radiograph shows a unilateral right pleural effusion characterized by a radiopaque meniscus that silhouettes the ipsilateral costophrenic recesses. (e) Erect chest radiograph illustrating typical features of a right-sided subpulmonic effusion. At first inspection, the right diaphragm appears elevated. However, lateral displacement of the peak of the apparent diaphragm and obscuration of the costophrenic sulcus indicate the presence of subpulmonic fluid.

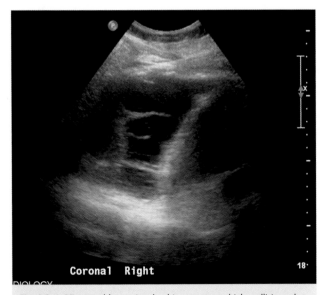

Fig. 4.8 A 27-year-old man involved in a motor vehicle collision who sustained significant chest wall trauma complicated by hemothorax incompletely evacuated by closed pleural drainage. Coronal ultrasound reveals a complex, multiseptated right pleural fluid collection. Video-associated thoracoscopic evacuation of the retained multiloculated hemothorax was subsequently performed.

or fibrin (▶ Fig. 4.9b). Hemothorax may also be associated with relaxation atelectasis, pulmonary contusion, pulmonary or vascular lacerations with active extravasation, and pneumothorax (▶ Fig. 4.9c,d).[13,33] Similar to US, small-bore caliber catheter placement under fluoroscopic or CT guidance may be used to drain loculated hemothoraces as well as pyohemothoraces (▶ Fig. 4.10).

An important clinical and radiologic caveat is that hemothorax often appears several hours after the traumatic insult.[13] That is, the initial chest radiograph following blunt chest trauma may demonstrate no pleural effusion or only a small one that markedly enlarges over the next several hours, in some cases even progressing into tension physiology.[14]

Central venous catheterization is routine in the management of trauma and hemodynamically unstable patients. Traumatic line placements may be complicated by vascular injury with hemothorax (▶ Fig. 4.11) or infusothorax (▶ Fig. 4.12). Iatrogenic hemothorax during unsuccessful catheter placement attempts are a serious complication due to laceration of the venous or arterial wall (e.g., subclavian artery or vein, internal jugular vein, common carotid artery, brachiocephalic artery, internal mammary system, aorta, pulmonary artery) (▶ Fig. 4.11).[50,51]

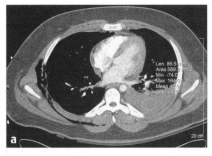
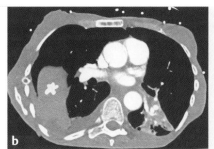
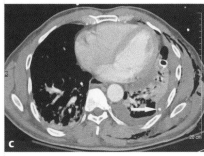
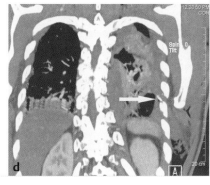

Fig. 4.9 Various presentations of hemothorax on chest computed tomography (CT). (a) Contrast-enhanced chest CT (mediastinal window) of a 19-year-old man involved in a motor vehicle collision demonstrates a high attenuation left effusion consistent with acute hemothorax. Attenuation estimated at 45 Hounsfield unit (HU). (b) Contrast-enhanced chest CT (mediastinal window) of a trauma victim with a complex, mixed attenuation loculated right hemothorax. There had been no chest tube output for the past 36 hours. Note the difference in attenuation between this complex loculated collection (annotation) and the more simple appearing fluid along the costovertebral pleura. (c,d) Contrast-enhanced axial and coronal maximum intensity projection CT (mediastinal windows) of a young man repeatedly stabbed in the chest demonstrates a left hemothorax and active extravasation of contrast media from a torn 8th intercostal artery (arrow). This artery was successfully embolized.

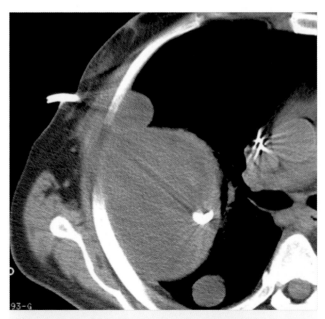

Fig. 4.10 Computed tomography- (CT-) guided drainage of complicated right effusion. Unenhanced axial CT (mediastinal window) show a well-positioned small-bore catheter in the loculated pyohemothorax. The combination of catheter drainage and intrapleural instillation of lytic agents successfully evacuated the collection over 5 days without the need for thoracotomy.

The incidence of iatrogenic vascular injuries can be reduced when access is performed under US or fluoroscopic guidance.[51,52,53] Rarely, the catheter tip may become adherent to the vessel wall and tear the vessel upon its removal resulting in vascular injury and an iatrogenic hemothorax.[54] The degree of bleeding from these iatrogenic injuries varies. Minor bleeding usually has no significant sequelae. However, major bleeding requires immediate treatment. When conservative treatment is ineffective (i.e., pleural drainage, volume resuscitation), surgical repair or stenting of the lacerated vessel and subsequent evacuation of the pleural space, must be performed (▶ Fig. 4.11b–d).[51] Infusothorax is the iatrogenic infusion of intravenous fluids, medications, and or blood products into an extravascular space (e.g., pleura, mediastinum, pericardium) resulting from perforation of a vessel wall and pleura overlying the mediastinum by the catheter tip (▶ Fig. 4.12). The two major risk factors for possible infusothorax include (1) left-sided catheter insertions, and (2) large-caliber central catheters. The distribution of insertion sites complicated by central venous perforation or erosion is as follows: left subclavian vein (46%), right subclavian vein (18%), left internal jugular vein (20%), and right internal jugular vein (5%). The average time interval from catheter perforation to the onset of symptoms is 2.0 days (range, 1–60 days), but symptoms also depend on the rate of the infusion. The average delay from the onset of symptoms to diagnosis is 3.0 days (range, 0–11 days). Clinical signs and symptoms may include dyspnea (82%), chest pain (46%), respiratory failure (18%), hypotension (13%), and cardiac arrest (5%).

Important radiographic clues supporting the diagnosis of infusothorax include (1) a rapidly evolving pleural or pericardial effusion or mediastinal widening in the presence of a central venous catheter, especially a left-sided approach and if the catheter tip abuts the lateral wall of the superior vena cava at a 45-degree angle, (2) loss of the pharmacologic action of the infusate, (3) inability to aspirate blood back through the catheter, and (4) chemical analysis of the pleural fluid resembling that of the infusate.[55] Although rare, this complication may be potentially fatal if unrecognized. Prompt discontinuance of the infusate and evacuation of the pleural fluid is necessary.

Chest radiography may reveal unilateral (i.e., ipsilateral or contralateral to the catheter insertion site) or bilateral pleural effusions with or without mediastinal widening (▶ Fig. 4.12a).[55] Unenhanced CT is helpful in depicting the site of vascular perforation and the extravascular course of the malpositioned catheter (▶ Fig. 4.12b). However, a catheter venography, or even

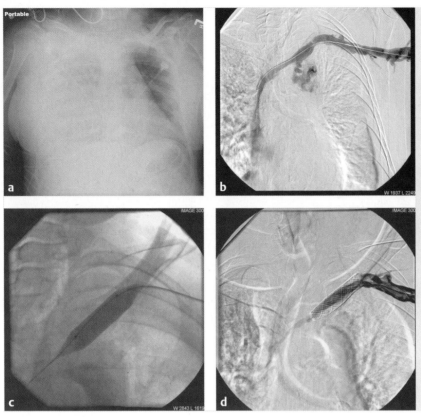

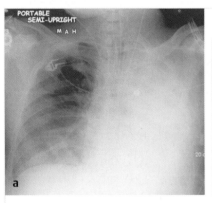

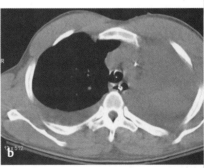

Fig. 4.11 Pleural fluid collections related to traumatic central line placements. (a) Antero-posterior chest radiograph obtained 1 hour following a difficult right internal jugular line placement demonstrates the acute onset of a large ipsilateral pleural effusion from iatrogenic laceration of the internal jugular vein. Note the medial deviation of the IJ catheter course at the level of the 1st posteromedial rib from the superior mediastinal hematoma. (b–d) Series of digital subtraction angiography (DSA) images of a man who sustained a left subclavian vein laceration following an unsuccessful central line placement attempt. (b) Reveals active extravasation of injected contrast media at the laceration. (c) Subsequent advancement of the balloon and endoluminal stent into the lacerated vein. (d) Deployment of the endoluminal stent and cessation of active bleeding from the laceration.

Fig. 4.12 Infusothorax following unsuccessful central line placement. (a) Anteroposterior semiupright chest radiograph several hours following an "uneventful" left internal jugular catheter placement. The patient developed shortness of breath and decreased left-sided breath sounds. The left hemithorax is completely opacified. The central venous catheter does not follow an expected vascular course. (b) Unen-hanced computed tomography (mediastinal window) reveals the extravascular catheter course relative to the mediastinal vasculature. Note the massive ipsilateral and smaller contra-lateral pleural effusion. Thoracentesis revealed fluid identical in composition to the infusate.

bedside Doppler venography may be more advantageous in the appropriate clinical setting. Repair of the perforated vessel may require the deployment of endovascular stents, embolization, or both by the interventional radiologist.

Chylothorax is the accumulation of chyle in the pleural space. Trauma is the second leading cause of chylothorax (25%). Although rare, iatrogenic injury to the thoracic duct has been reported with most invasive thoracic surgical procedures (e.g., central line and thoracostomy tube placements, coronary artery revascularization, thyroidectomy, lobectomy and pneumonectomy, esophagectomy, radical neck dissection, spinal surgery). Nonsurgical traumatic thoracic duct injury is very rare and secondary to penetrating trauma, but rarely is associated with fracture-dislocations of the thoracic spine.[56]

Thoracic duct disruption is complicated by the accumulation of lymph in the extrapleural mediastinum forming a mass-like collection called a chyloma, which eventually ruptures into the pleural space and causes the chylothorax. The anatomical course of the thoracic duct and the site of injury determine the situs of the chylous effusion. The thoracic duct originates off the cisterna chyli at the L2 level, courses to the right of the spine ventral and medial to the azygos vein. Therefore, injuries to the caudal half of the duct results in a right-sided effusion. Between T5–T8, the thoracic duct crosses the midline and ascends to the left of the spine and drains into the left subclavian vein near the entrance of the left internal jugular vein. Therefore, injuries to the cranial half of the duct result in a left-sided effusion.[57] The thoracic duct transports up to 4 L of chyle per day, thus a large volume of chyle may accumulate

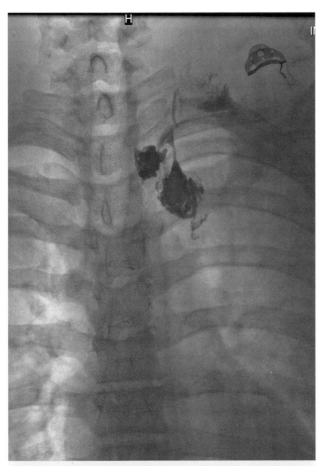

Fig. 4.13 A chylous leak as shown by lymphangiography. Pedal-ascending lymphangiography was performed following the infusion of 10 mL of Ethiodol (Savage Laboratory, Melville, NY). Coned-down inverted anteroposterior chest radiograph centered over the left hemithorax of a 17-year-old man with a chylous effusion refractory to conservative management shows diffuse extravasation of contrast in the left supraclavicular region. (Case courtesy of Sonya Bhole, BS, Department of Radiology, Division of Interventional Radiology, Medical College of Virginia Hospitals, Richmond, VA).

quite rapidly in the pleural cavity in cases of ductal injury. Although usually unilateral, chylous effusions can be bilateral.

Initial patient signs and symptoms are usually related to the presence of a large hydrothorax compressing the lung and most often manifest as dyspnea. However, cyanosis and hypotension may also occur. Lymphangiography is a highly specific and reliable imaging technique that best demonstrates the site of injury and may even assist with the percutaneous catheterization and occlusion of the damaged thoracic duct, thereby avoiding surgery (► Fig. 4.13).[58] Unfortunately, lymphoangiography is rarely done by most interventional radiologists today and the technique has become obsolete. Lymphoscintigraphy may also localize thoracic duct injuries and can be performed by the oral administration of I-123 β-methyl-iodophenyl pentadecanoic acid (BMIPP), as well as the intravenous administration of technetium-99 m human serum albumin or filtered sulfur colloid.[59,60,61] Computed tomography rarely provides much additional diagnostic information. The CT appearance of chylous effusions is similar to that of other pleural effusions. Prior to rupture, the

chyloma may be identified as a low or fluid attenuation mediastinal mass-like lesion. Magnetic resonance signal intensities are equivalent to that of proteinaceous fluid demonstrating increased signal on T1-weighted images and homogeneous signal intensity on T2-weighted images.[62]

Conservative management of chylothorax consists of pleural fluid drainage, supportive ventilation, fluid replenishment, elemental diet supplementation, and or total parenteral nutrition. If conservative management fails, CT-guided percutaneous needle ablation, video-assisted thoracoscopic duct ligation, laparoscopic duct ligation, or thoracotomy and or laparotomy may then be necessary.[63,64,65] Sometimes the ablation of these injuries is rather complicated and extremely frustrating for the trauma care team and the IR experts in lymphangiography.

4.3.3 Parenchymal Lung Injuries

Pulmonary Contusions

Pulmonary contusions are the most common pulmonary injury after severe blunt thoracic trauma present in 17 to 70% of patients with severe chest trauma.[10,13] Contusions result from either a direct blow immediately adjacent to normal lung parenchyma or from a contrecoup injury.[1] Such force disrupts small blood vessels and capillary alveolar membranes with subsequent extravasation of blood and edema into the interstitium and alveoli.[13] Contusions often occur in the parenchyma adjacent to rigid or solid structures (e.g., thoracic spine, ribs, heart, and liver) or at the lung bases (i.e., increased basilar mobility), and are one of the principal factors affecting patient morbidity and mortality, the latter of which varies from 14 to 40% depending upon the severity of the contusion and the presence of concomitant thoracic and nonthoracic injuries.[1,10,13] On chest radiography, contusions manifest as peripheral focal or multifocal nonsegmental ground glass opacities or consolidations that do not respect fissural boundaries (► Fig. 4.14a,b). Severe contusions can affect an entire lobe, lung, or both lungs. Air bronchograms may be absent because of airway obstruction by retained secretions and/or blood.[1,10,13] Severe contusions manifest early on chest radiography, often within 3 to 4 hours, become most conspicuous within 24 to 72 hours, and then gradually clear over 3 to 10 days. Air space opacities that fail to clear in this time frame or alternatively progress radiographically raise the specter of secondary infection or acute respiratory distress syndrome (ARDS).[1,10,13] Computed tomography more accurately demonstrates the size and extent of the lung injury, as well as the presence of concomitant lung laceration(s). Injuries to the interstitium with partial alveolar compromise manifest as diffuse, nonsegmental, heterogeneous ground glass opacities (► Fig. 4.14c,d).

The nonsegmental distribution of pulmonary contusion is often helpful in differentiating contusion from aspiration, which is usually segmental. In the setting of severe alveolar injury or concomitant pulmonary laceration, the air spaces fill with blood forming parenchymal consolidations (► Fig. 4.14e). Clinically, severe pulmonary contusions may be complicated by intrapulmonary shunts, reduced compliance, ventilation-perfusion mismatch, hemoptysis, tachypnea, hypoxemia, bronchorrhea, and reduced cardiac output.[13] Management is supportive therapy, pain control, and pulmonary toilet and supplemental oxygen. Severe contusions associated with significant pulmonary shunting may require mechanical ventilation.

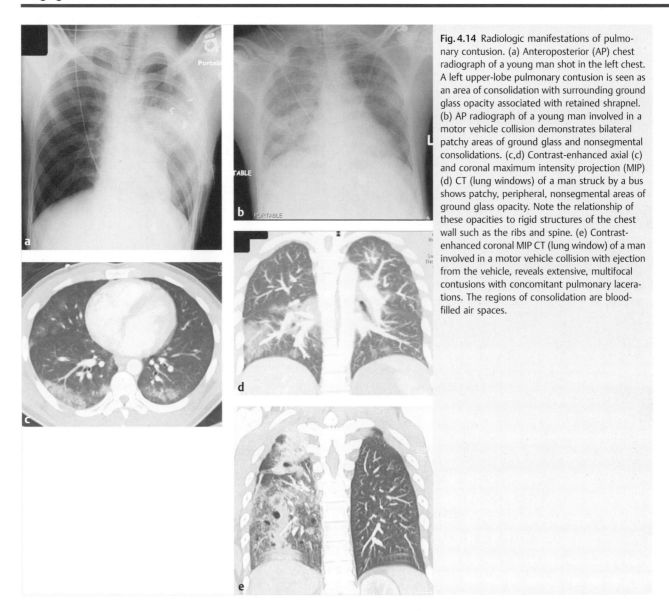

Fig. 4.14 Radiologic manifestations of pulmonary contusion. (a) Anteroposterior (AP) chest radiograph of a young man shot in the left chest. A left upper-lobe pulmonary contusion is seen as an area of consolidation with surrounding ground glass opacity associated with retained shrapnel. (b) AP radiograph of a young man involved in a motor vehicle collision demonstrates bilateral patchy areas of ground glass and nonsegmental consolidations. (c,d) Contrast-enhanced axial (c) and coronal maximum intensity projection (MIP) (d) CT (lung windows) of a man struck by a bus shows patchy, peripheral, nonsegmental areas of ground glass opacity. Note the relationship of these opacities to rigid structures of the chest wall such as the ribs and spine. (e) Contrast-enhanced coronal MIP CT (lung window) of a man involved in a motor vehicle collision with ejection from the vehicle, reveals extensive, multifocal contusions with concomitant pulmonary lacerations. The regions of consolidation are blood-filled air spaces.

Pulmonary Lacerations

Pulmonary lacerations represent serious sequelae of chest trauma and may be caused by perforation of the lung parenchyma or pleura (e.g., stab wounds, gunshot wounds, and rib fractures) or by inertial deceleration.[13] These may be inconspicuous or difficult to appreciate on initial chest radiography, often obscured by surrounding contusion, consolidation, and not infrequently, an ipsilateral hemothorax (▶ Fig. 4.15a).[13] Computed tomography more readily demonstrates lacerations as localized air collections of varying shapes and morphologies within areas of parenchymal consolidation. Pulmonary lacerations are classified into four categories based upon the nature of the applied force and the CT appearance. Type I lacerations (compression rupture) are the most common, result from chest wall compression causing an area of lung parenchyma to rupture, and are located centrally (▶ Fig. 4.15b). Type II lacerations (compression shear) are the result of a lateral compression force between the lung and the thoracic spine and are most often seen as paravertebral ovoid or elliptical lesions in the lung bases

(▶ Fig. 4.15c). Type III lacerations (rib penetration, tear) are usually small, rounded, peripherally located and often associated with rib fractures and a pneumothorax (▶ Fig. 4.15d). Type IV lacerations (adhesion tear) result from the shearing of peripheral lung from previously formed pleuropulmonary adhesions and are only diagnosed at surgery or on pathologic specimens. Multiple types may coexist in the same patient, lung, or even lobe.[1,10,13] A pneumatocele forms if the space created by the laceration fills with air from the tracheobronchial tree. A pulmonary hematoma forms if this space instead fills with blood originating from a disrupted lung vessel.[13] Pneumatocele and hematoma may coexist (i.e., hematopneumocele) and is characterized by an air-fluid level (▶ Fig. 4.15e).[13] Pulmonary lacerations usually resolve over 3 to 5 weeks. Complicated lacerations may persist for as long as one year. Lacerations may be complicated by bronchopleural fistulas, which can be further complicated by pneumothorax or tension pneumothorax. Post-traumatic pneumatoceles may progressively enlarge in patients on mechanical ventilation.[1,10,13]

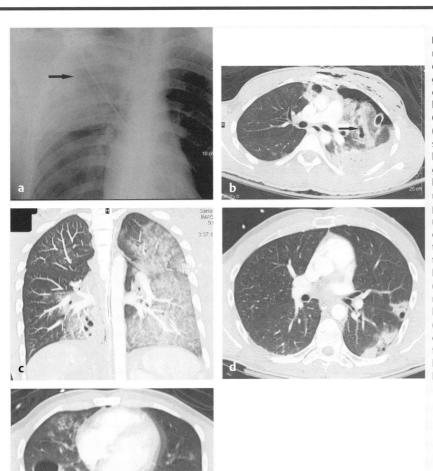

Fig. 4.15 Radiologic manifestations of pulmonary lacerations. (a) Coned-down, narrowly windowed supine chest radiograph reveals ground glass opacity throughout the right upper lobe delimited by the horizontal fissure. The eccentric lucency is a concomitant laceration (arrow). (b) Contrast-enhanced chest computed tomography (CT) (lung window) of a bicyclist struck by a car shows a type I left upper-lobe pulmonary laceration (arrow). Note the surrounding ground glass consistent with hemorrhage and the lower lobe consolidation and volume loss. Pneumomediastinum and a left pneumothorax are present. (c) Contrast-enhanced coronal maximum intensity projection CT (lung window) demonstrates extensive ground glass opacity throughout the left lung and right lower lobe due to hemorrhage and right-sided paravertebral lucent lesions of type II pulmonary lacerations. (d) Contrast-enhanced chest CT (lung window) reveals peripheral contusions in the lingula and left lower lobe with associated type III lacerations. (e) Contrast-enhanced chest CT (lung window) demonstrates extensive bibasilar consolidations, foci of ground glass in the middle lobe, and a hematopneumocele characterized by an air-fluid level in the superior segment of the lower lobe.

4.3.4 Traumatic Lung Hernia

Focal lung herniation is a rare complication that may result from acquired defects in the chest wall (e.g., rib fractures, sternoclavicular, or costochondral dislocations) following blunt chest trauma. Traumatic lung herniation most often occurs in the anterolateral chest wall, where there is minimal soft tissue support (e.g., intercostal muscles) and may be complicated by pneumothorax, hemothorax, lung incarceration, and strangulation (▶ Fig. 4.16). The latter requires prompt recognition and surgical reduction.[10]

4.4 Airway Injuries

4.4.1 Tracheobronchial Injury

Injuries of the tracheobronchial tree are relatively rare, but may occur after blunt or penetrating trauma. Iatrogenic injuries may result from traumatic intubation or overinflation of an endotracheal tube balloon cuff or tracheostomy placement. Blunt trauma usually produces shear forces that are associated with vertical tears in the membranous trachea, axially oriented tears in the cartilaginous rings or transections of the mainstem

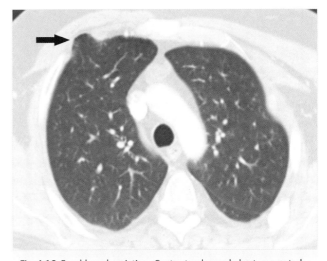

Fig. 4.16 Focal lung herniation. Contrast-enhanced chest computed tomography (lung window) of a 39-year-old man involved in a high-speed motor vehicle collision demonstrates a focal intercostal herniation of the anterolateral right upper lobe (arrow). The hernia was reduced at surgery.

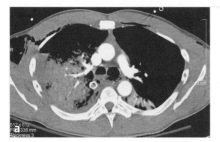

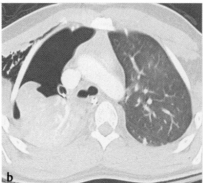

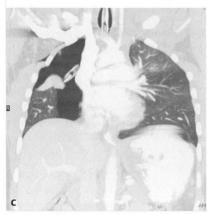

Fig. 4.17 Traumatic injury of the left main bronchus. (a) Contrast-enhanced chest computed tomography (CT) (mediastinal window) of a 30-year-old man involved in a motor vehicle collision demonstrates complete disruption of the posterior wall of the left main bronchus. Note the gross discrepancy in caliber of the right and left main bronchi. Foci of pneumomediastinum, extensive right upper lobe air-space disease, right hemothorax, and left lower lobe collapse are also present. (b,c), Contrast-enhanced axial and coronal maximum intensity projection chest CT (lung windows) of a 26-year-old man involved in a motor vehicle collision with ejection shows a "fallen-lung sign." Note the caliber change in the right main bronchus relative to the left, persistence of a large right pneumothorax despite the chest tube placement, and lateral inferior collapse of the detached right lung away from its hilum.

bronchi. Penetrating trauma usually involves the cervicothoracic trachea.[13,66] Bronchial injuries are more common than tracheal injuries, and more than 80% occur within 2 cm of the carina. Right-sided bronchial injuries are also more common than left-sided injuries.[13] Those bronchial injuries within the pleural envelope (i.e., distal to the insertion of the pulmonary ligament) more likely result in an ipsilateral pneumothorax, whereas those that occur outside the pleural envelope (i.e., medial to the pulmonary ligament) are associated with pneumomediastinum.[13] Additionally, because the left main bronchus has a longer mediastinal course than the right main bronchus, injuries to the left main bronchus injuries are more often associated with a pneumomediastinum and right main bronchus injuries are often associated with a pneumothorax.

A clinical characteristic of bronchial injury is a persistent pneumothorax or a persistent air leak, despite appropriate chest tube placement and functioning.[33] Chest radiography often demonstrates atelectasis and evidence of extra-alveolar air manifested as a persistent pneumothorax, pneumomediastinum, and/or subcutaneous air.[13] The "bayonet sign" is rare, but presents as a thin tapering air-filled structure at the proximal end of the ruptured bronchus.[13] The "double wall sign" manifests as intramural air in the proximal airways.[1] The "fallen lung sign" is caused by the detachment of the lung from the mainstem bronchus. The affected lung "falls" or collapses away from the hilum and toward the lateral chest wall into the most dependent portion of the thoracic cavity.[1,13,33] Computed tomography features of acute bronchial injury include an acute angulation or change in caliber of the tracheobronchial tree, tract(s) of air extending from the injured bronchus or trachea, or frank discontinuity of the affected airway (▶ Fig. 4.17). These findings are more readily appreciated on multiplanar reconstructions.[1,13,33] Virtual bronchoscopy complements CT and is a helpful adjunct to guide conservative medical or surgical management. Short lacerations of the upper one third of the

trachea may be treated with antibiotics and intubation beyond the level of the injury. Some small or peripheral bronchial tears can also be treated conservatively, but may be complicated by an eventual stenosis. Surgical repair is indicated for transmural tears > 1 cm and those associated with a persistent pneumothorax unrelieved by tube thoracostomy.

4.4.2 Pneumomediastinum

Pneumomediastinum is the presence of air in the mediastinal compartment. It occurs in ~ 10% of blunt chest trauma victims, but may also occur with penetrating chest injuries. In more than 95% of cases, pneumomediastinum results from alveolar rupture following an abrupt increase in intra-alveolar pressure. The extra-alveolar air then dissects along the pulmonary interstitium and peribronchovascular sheaths centrally to enter the mediastinum (i.e., Macklin effect).[3,13] Such abrupt increases in intra-alveolar pressure may occur with simple straining against a closed glottis (e.g., weightlifting, childbirth), mechanical ventilation with barotrauma or with the deep inhalation of illicit recreational drugs (e.g., crack cocaine, marijuana). Air may also enter the mediastinum from injuries to the aerodigestive tract (e.g., tracheobronchial tree, larynx, retropharynx) or via the retroperitoneum.[3,13,33] On imaging, air can be seen outlining various mediastinal structures such as the superior vena cava and the descending thoracic aorta (▶ Fig. 4.18a).

The abnormal presence of mediastinal gas collections about various mediastinal structures have created numerous radiologic signs. The "double bronchial wall sign" is present when air accumulates adjacent to the bronchial wall allowing visualization of both sides of the bronchial wall. The "continuous diaphragm sign" occurs when air becomes trapped posterior to the pericardium and the entire diaphragm becomes conspicuous (▶ Fig. 4.18b). The "tubular artery sign" manifests as air outlining the ascending aorta, the aortic arch, and or the major branches of the aorta. Lateral

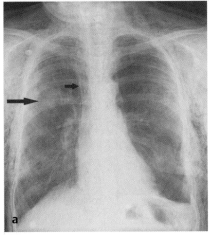
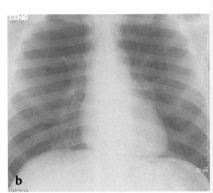
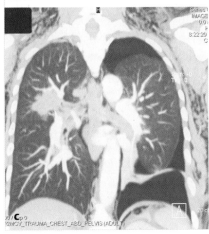

Fig. 4.18 Radiologic features of pneumomediastinum. (a) Anteroposterior (AP) chest radiograph of a 50-year-old woman who was assaulted demonstrates extensive pneumomediastinum. Air is seen outlining the branch vessel origins (short arrow) and the descending thoracic aorta. Note the extensive subcutaneous air. A right upper-lobe lung cancer was incidentally detected at the time of her injury (long arrow). (b) AP chest radiograph of a 27-year-old woman struck by a car shows complete visualization of the diaphragm from one side to the other, crisply delineated by the mediastinal air ("continuous diaphragm sign"). Normally, the central portion of the diaphragm is obscured by the heart and mediastinal soft tissue structures contacting the diaphragm. Mediastinal air is seen around the aorta and left heart border. (c) Contrast-enhanced coronal maximum intensity projection chest CT (lung window) demonstrates pneumomediastinum complicated by an ipsilateral pneumothorax as well as pneumoperitoneum and pneumoretroperitoneum.

chest radiography may reveal air outlining the pulmonary artery forming the "ring around the artery sign."[1,3,13,33] "Naclerio's V sign" is produced by air outlining the descending thoracic aorta and extending laterally between the parietal pleura and the medial left hemidiaphragm.

It may be difficult to differentiate pneumomediastinum from pneumopericardium or a medial pneumothorax. Pneumopericardium allows direct visualization of the pericardium. Intrapericardial air respects the normal pericardial borders. As the volume of air increases, it assumes a more ovoid as opposed to linear morphology.[1] Medial pneumothoraces are often characterized by additional signs of pleural air elsewhere in the affected hemithorax.[1] Lateral decubitus exams may aid in the differentiation in problematic cases. In the setting of both pneumothorax and pneumopericardium, air moves to the nondependent surface with manipulation of the patient. However, air within the mediastinum does not move with such manipulations.[13] When extensive, air from the mediastinum can rupture into the pleural space creating a pneumothorax, extend inferiorly into the retroperitoneum and rupture into the peritoneal space resulting in pneumoperitoneum or may impede venous return to the heart (i.e., tension pneumomediastinum with cardiac tamponade).[13,33]

4.4.3 Esophageal Injuries

Esophageal tears are uncommon in blunt thoracic trauma (1 per 1,000 cases), occurring more frequently with penetrating

injuries.[3,13] Blunt injuries result from increased intraluminal pressure induced by decompressive forces. Perforations may occur as sequelae of bone fragments from adjacent spine fractures, shrapnel, or the projectile itself.[1,33] About 52% of esophageal injuries involve the cervical or proximal thoracic esophagus.[3] Most patients have other significant concomitant thoracic injuries.[13] Chest radiography findings are nonspecific and include persistent or unexplained pneumomediastinum, left-sided pneumothorax, left-sided pleural effusion, and left lower-lobe atelectasis.[3,33]

Indirect CT findings include focal or asymmetric esophageal wall thickening at the site of perforation, periesophageal gas collections, deep cervical soft tissue emphysema, and left pleural effusion.[1,13,33] As discussed earlier, diagnosis should be confirmed with esophagography. Unrecognized and left untreated, esophageal injuries have a high morbidity and mortality, increasing from 10 to 25% within the first 24 hours to 40 to 60% when treatment is delayed > 48 hours.[1]

4.4.4 Cardiac and Pericardial Injuries

Cardiac and pericardial injuries are uncommon after blunt thoracic trauma, but may occur following severe blows to the anterior chest. Potential injuries include cardiac contusion, cardiac rupture, valvular injuries, coronary artery injuries, conducting system injuries, and pericardial tears. These injuries may be complicated by hemopericardium and resultant cardiac tamponade.[13,33] Acute tamponade may be caused by as little as

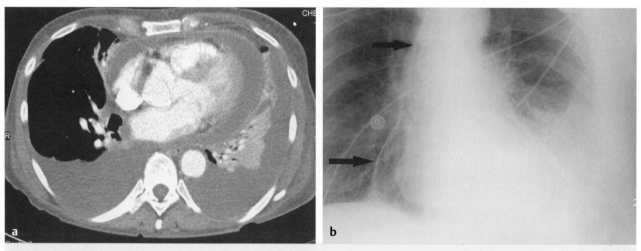

Fig. 4.19 (a) Contrast-enhanced axial chest computed tomography (CT) (mediastinal window) of a young man who sustained a crushing injury to his chest following collapse of a car jack shows high attenuation pericardial fluid enveloping the myocardium consistent with hemopericardium. Bilateral hemothoraces are also seen. (b) Anteroposterior chest radiograph of a young man stabbed in the chest demonstrates pneumopericardium. The trapped pericardial air forms a double contour along the cardiac borders (arrows) that surrounds the myocardium, but is limited superiorly by the attachment of the pericardial reflections differentiating it from pneumomediastinum. Left hemothorax is present.

250 to 300 mL of blood.[13] Contusion is the most common injury to the heart, occurring in up to 76% of blunt chest trauma victims. The anteriorly located right heart chambers are more commonly injured than the left heart chambers.[33] Cardiac laceration and rupture, although rare (0.21–2.0% incidence), often involve the right atrium, right ventricle, or both. Mortality rates range up to 54% for right atrial rupture and 29% for right ventricular rupture.[13] Chest radiography is of limited value for the detection of such injuries. Nonspecific radiographic findings may include cardiomegaly, heart failure, pneumopericardium, and abnormal cardiac contours. The universal finding of cardiac injury at CT is hemopericardium (▶ Fig. 4.19a). Additional CT findings may include compression of right-sided cardiac chambers, pneumopericardium, and active arterial extravasation.

Transthoracic (TTE) or transesophageal echocardiography (TEE) should be readily performed in any suspect cases without hesitation. Although MRI can demonstrate traumatic cardiac injuries, as well as valvular and possible coronary vessel injuries, echocardiography and DSA remain the modalities of choice for the evaluation of such injuries in the acute trauma patient.[13] Pneumopericardium secondary to blunt chest trauma is generally due to one of three mechanisms: (1) penetration along pulmonary venous perivascular sheaths from ruptured alveoli to the pericardium, (2) pneumothorax associated with a pleuropericardial tear, or (3) a direct tracheobronchial–pericardial communication. On imaging, pneumopericardium outlines the myocardium and is limited superiorly by the normal pericardial reflections (▶ Fig. 4.19b).[33]

4.4.5 Diaphragmatic Injuries

Most diaphragmatic injuries are caused by penetrating trauma.[13] The incidence of diaphragmatic injury among blunt trauma victims varies from 0.8 to 8.0%; it is more frequently from abdominal as opposed to thoracic trauma.[13,33] The postulated mechanism is a sudden increase in either intra-abdominal or intrathoracic pressure against a fixed diaphragm. Left-sided injuries are 3 times more common than right-sided injuries because of theoretical protection by the liver. However, ~ 4.5% of blunt trauma victims sustain bilateral injuries.[33] Most diaphragmatic tears are more than 10 cm in length and involve the muscular posterior or posterolateral aspects of the diaphragm. The majority of patients (< 94%) have concomitant injuries, such as multiple lower rib fractures, pulmonary contusions and lacerations, aortic injuries, and intra-abdominal organ injuries such as hepatic and splenic lacerations.[1,13] Initial chest radiography is diagnostic in 27 to 60% of left-sided diaphragmatic injuries, but in only 17% of right-sided injuries. Nonspecific chest radiographic findings may include poor delineation of the affected diaphragm, hemo-, pneumo-, and hemopneumothorax, lower-lobe opacification in the presence of an elevated diaphragm, contralateral mediastinal shift, and lower rib fractures. More specific signs include an abnormal course of the nasogastric tube and herniation of abdominal contents into the thorax (▶ Fig. 4.20a).[1,3,13,33] Multidetector array CT has a sensitivity of 50 to 100% and a specificity of 86 to 100% for diaphragmatic injury. Computed tomography findings include an abrupt discontinuity of the diaphragm with or without herniation of the stomach or other viscera into the thorax (▶ Fig. 4.20b); nonvisualization of the diaphragm in an area where it is not in contact with another organ, and should otherwise be seen (i.e., "absent diaphragm sign"); visualization of peritoneal fat, bowel, or viscera lateral to the lung or diaphragm or posterior to the diaphragmatic crus; loss of the superior support of the liver, stomach, and bowel allowing them to fall dependently against the posterior ribs (i.e., "dependent viscera sign"); and a focal constriction of herniated viscera, stomach, or bowel (i.e., "CT collar sign") (▶ Fig. 4.20c).

Additional CT findings may be an irregularly thickened diaphragm, reflective of either a partial- or full-thickness tear with associated hematoma and proximity trauma to the neighboring subdiaphragmatic hollow and solid viscera and or osseous structures.[67] Sagittal and coronal MRI planes nicely delineate the left diaphragm on T1-weighted imaging as a low signal intensity curvilinear band of soft tissue outlined by higher signal intensity abdominal and mediastinal fat. Evaluation of the

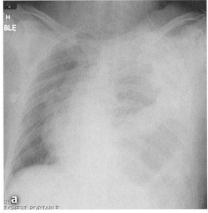

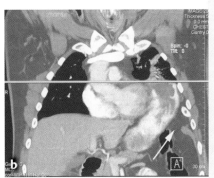

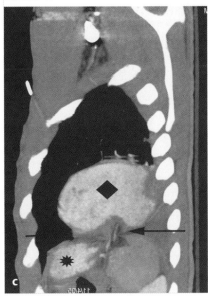

Fig. 4.20 Radiologic findings of acute diaphragmatic rupture. (a) Anteroposterior chest radiograph of a young man involved in a motor vehicle collision shows marked rightward displacement of the cardiomediastinal silhouette by herniated hollow viscera into the left thorax. A left-sided hemothorax extends into the apex. (b,c) Contrast-enhanced coronal (b) and sagittal maximum intensity projection (c) chest CT (mediastinal windows) of another young blunt trauma victim demonstrate herniation of the stomach into the left thorax. Focal disruption of the diaphragm is readily appreciated on the coronal image (arrow). The diaphragmatic defect creates a focal constriction (arrows) in the herniated stomach delineating portions of the herniated stomach above (•) and below (*) the diaphragmatic injury (CT collar sign). This gives the stomach a mushroom or hour-glass morphology (c).

right diaphragm by MRI is more problematic. Cardiac and respiratory gating should be employed to minimize motion artifacts.[13] An important caveat is that positive-pressure ventilation can prevent the herniation of bowel into the thorax, delaying the diagnosis of diaphragmatic tears in some patients until after extubation.[13,33] The mortality of diaphragmatic ruptures approaches 30% and may be adversely affected by delays in diagnosis and surgical repair.[1,13]

4.4.6 Thoracic Skeletal Injuries

Ribs

Rib fractures are the most common injury in blunt chest trauma, occurring in at least 50% of patients.[3] The location and number of fractured ribs serve as clues to possible concomitant injuries, and to the severity of the trauma. For example, ribs 1–3 are very stable, protected by the shoulder girdle and adjacent musculature. Therefore, fractures of the first three ribs require a substantial force. As a result, there is a high correlation of such fractures or fractures of the first two ribs and clavicle with maxillofacial, cranial, brachial plexus, branch vessel, and tracheobronchial injuries.[1,13,33] Fractures of ribs 4–9 are common and most significant when associated with flail chest.[1] Fractures of ribs 10–12 are less common, but may be associated

with traumatic injuries of the liver, spleen, kidneys, and diaphragm.[13,33] Initial chest radiography is of limited value, demonstrating only 40–50% of acute rib fractures, and even less sensitive in detecting costochondral fractures.[3] Multidetector array CT with 3D reconstruction is much more sensitive.

Flail chest is the most severe traumatic injury of the chest wall in blunt trauma. Clinically, it is characterized by chest wall instability and focal paradoxical chest wall motion during respiration that inhibits normal respiratory excursion and impairs ventilation. On imaging, there are anterior and posterior segmental fractures of more than three contiguous ribs or single fractures of more than four contiguous ribs (▶ Fig. 4.21).[1,3,13,33] Intercostal muscular injury may be more important to patient morbidity and long-term disability than the actual osseous trauma. Stabilization of the flail chest through surgical plating of the affected ribs, up to 6 days postinjury, may allow intercostal muscle healing, thus reducing or alleviating the discoordinated paradoxical chest wall motion and improving ventilation.[1]

Sternum

The incidence of sternal fracture as a result of motor vehicle collisions range between 3 and 10%, although the incidence may decrease in the setting of airbags.[3,13] The most common location is within 2 cm of the sternomanubrial joint. Most

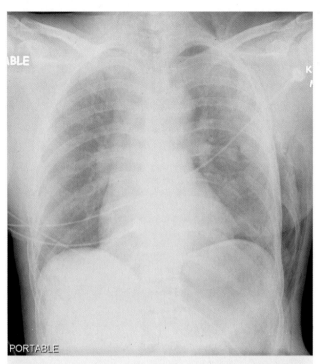

Fig. 4.21 Anteroposterior chest radiograph of a young man involved in a motorcycle collision demonstrates a bilateral flail chest. There are acutely displaced fractures of the left 3rd to 10th ribs and of the right 4th to 8th ribs. A left subpulmonic pneumothorax is also present characterized by a hyperlucent diaphragm. Extensive subcutaneous air is seen in the left chest wall.

Scapula

A significant, direct force is required to fracture the scapula. Therefore, an acute scapular fracture should alert the radiologist and clinicians to the possibility of additional important thoracic injuries. Up to 40% of patients with scapular fractures have associated pulmonary contusion, pneumothorax, or hemothorax. There is also a direct relationship between scapular fractures, thoracic spine fractures, and head injuries.[33] Multidetector array CT depicts scapular fractures not readily appreciated on chest radiography; also 3D reformatted images delineate intra-articular extension of fractures, helpful in planning surgical reconstruction and stabilization (▶ Fig. 4.23).

Scapulothoracic dissociation is a rare, but serious and devastating closed forequarter amputation of the upper extremity resulting from a direct blow to, or severe traction on, the shoulder girdle. Clinically, there is near complete disruption of the forequarter from the torso. Invariably, there is injury to the ipsilateral brachial plexus, subclavian artery, and/or subclavian vein. On imaging, this injury is characterized by lateral displacement of the scapula (i.e., thoracic spinous process to the medial scapular border distance is greater than 1.4 on a nonrotated chest radiograph), fracture of the clavicle with lateral displacement of the distal fragment, acrominoclavicular separation, and sternoclavicular fracture. There is a high prevalence of concomitant injuries. Upper-extremity CT angiography and/or arteriography are needed to assess for potential limb- and/or life-threatening vascular injuries.[13,33]

Clavicle

Clavicular fractures are common and comprise 4% of all fractures in adults. These fractures are classified according to their location. Type I involves the midclavicular shaft (80%), type II involves the distal one-third of the lateral clavicle (15%), and type III involves the medial one-third of the clavicle (5%). Most clavicular fractures have cephalad displacement of the distal fragment.

Closed fractures are typically managed conservatively. Distal fractures have a higher incidence of non-union requiring surgical reduction in symptomatic patients.[1]

fractures are associated with a retrosternal hematoma.[3] Simple sternal fractures are benign. Depressed, segmental fractures have an increased association with myocardial contusions, traumatic hemopericardium, coronary vessel lacerations, thoracic aortic lacerations, tracheobronchial tears, thoracic spine fractures, and head trauma.[3,13,33] Multidetector array CT with sagittal and coronal MIP reformations optimally display both the sternal fracture and the potentially associated injuries (▶ Fig. 4.22a). The presence of a preserved fat plane between the retrosternal hematoma and the aorta implies that the hematoma is not related to an acute aortic injury (▶ Fig. 4.22b).[3,33]

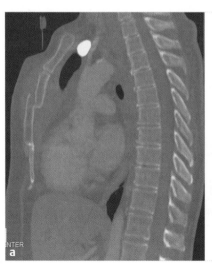
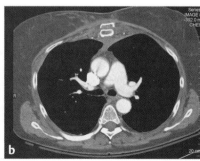

Fig. 4.22 Contrast-enhanced sagittal maximum intensity projection (bone window) (a) and axial (b) (mediastinal window) chest computed tomography of an unrestrained driver involved in a high-speed motor vehicle collision shows a markedly depressed midsternal body fracture. There is associated peristernal, parasternal, and retrosternal hematoma, as well as soft tissue stranding overlying the sternum. Note the preserved fat plane between the retrosternal hematoma and the aorta. The vehicle's steering wheel was severely deformed in the collision.

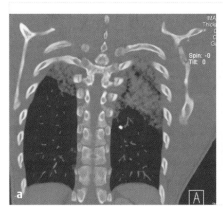

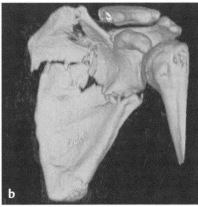

Fig. 4.23 Contrast-enhanced chest computed tomography coronal maximum intensity projection (bone window) (a) and three-dimensional reformatted image of the left scapula (b) (bone window) of a young patient struck by a car shows comminuted fracture of the scapula and bilateral upper-lobe pulmonary contusions. Three-dimensional reformations reveal the articular surface of the glenoid intact.

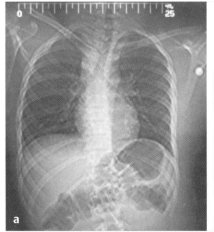

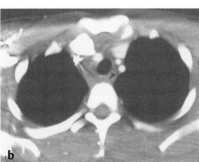

Fig. 4.24 A 15-year-old fell off his dirt bike while attempting to jump over an embankment and sustained a posterior dislocation of the right sternoclavicular joint. (a) A frontal chest computed tomography (CT) scout shows asymmetric alignment of the clavicles; the right clavicle lies lower than the left. (b) Contrast-enhanced chest CT (mediastinal window) reveals posterior displacement of the right clavicular head at the sternoclavicular joint with the medial edge abutting the brachiocephalic artery. Note the right paratracheal hematoma. (Used with permission from Parker MS, Rosado-de-Christenson, ML, Abbott GF. Chest Imaging Case Atlas. 2nd ed. New York, NY: Thieme;2012: 473.

Posterior sternoclavicular dislocation is relatively rare, accounting for < 1% of all dislocations. The proximity of the dislocated medial clavicular head to critical structures in the thoracic inlet (e.g., aerodigestive tract, great vessels, brachial plexus, and apical pleural reflections) can result in serious injuries the exclusion of which should be part of the radiologist's search pattern. Conventional chest radiography findings can be subtle and easily unappreciated and include an apparent asymmetry in clavicular head height and or alignment and lateral displacement of the proximal clavicle. However, posterior sternoclavicular dislocation is clearly depicted on CT and MDCT with sagittal and coronal MIP images readily demonstrates the presence of concomitant injuries (▶ Fig. 4.24).[1,3,13]

Spine

Fracture dislocations of the thoracic spine account for 30% of all spine injuries.[3,33] Most result from hyperflexion and axial loading. These injuries are clinically devastating. Neurologic deficits in patients with thoracic spine fractures are as high as 62%, far greater than those occurring with cervical spine (32%) or lumbar spine injuries (2%). The most vulnerable region of the spine is referred to as the functional thoracolumbar spine (i.e., T9–T11).[3,68] However, over 20% of patients have multilevel injuries, which are noncontiguous in up to 27% of cases, factors that radiologists must keep in mind during interpretation of trauma chest CT scans.[68] Only 12% of patients with thoracic spine fracture dislocations are neurologically intact at presentation. About 70% of acute thoracic spine fractures may be identified on conventional radiography. The conspicuity of these fractures is dependent upon many factors including radiographic technique, patient body habitus, concomitant pulmonary contusions, and hemothorax, etc. As a result, many fractures are not appreciated. Conventional radiography may reveal mediastinal widening and/or widening of paraspinal lines (▶ Fig. 4.25a), loss of vertebral body height, and or poor definition of the pedicle(s).[68] Multidetector array CT with coronal and sagittal thoracic spine reformations acquired from the chest CT data, with its superior spatial resolution, clearly demonstrates the extent of radiographically demonstrable fractures, but more importantly reveals unsuspected fractures and associated complications such as retropulsion to better advantage (▶ Fig. 4.25b,c). Additional CT imaging findings of thoracic spine trauma are paraspinal hematoma, mediastinal hematoma confined to the paravertebral compartment, and pneumorachis. Moreover, 3D volumetric reconstructions display complex fractures and fracture dislocations. Magnetic resonance imaging is indicated when neurologic deficits accompany fracture dislocation.[68] Early surgical stabilization and fixation (i.e., within 3 days of injury) of patients allows earlier mobilization and reduces the incidence of respiratory complications.[68]

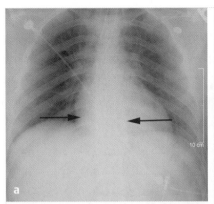

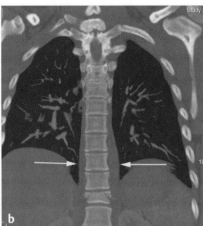

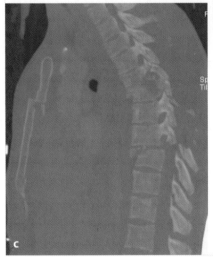

Fig. 4.25 Radiologic findings of acute thoracic spine trauma. (a) Anteroposterior supine chest radiograph of a young trauma patient shows widening of both paraspinal lines suggestive of paraspinal hematoma and/or occult thoracic spine trauma (arrows). Osseous detail is poor and a definitive fracture cannot be seen. (b) Contrast-enhanced coronal maximum intensity projection (MIP) chest computed tomography (CT) (bone window) reveals an acute T11 compression fracture, with associated paraspinal hematoma (arrows) that created the wide paraspinal lines on the chest radiograph. (c) Contrast-enhanced sagittal MIP chest CT (bone window) demonstrates multilevel, noncontiguous fractures of the thoracic spine. A subtle fracture is present in the superior end plate of T2. An acute hyperflexion fracture dislocation involves all three columns of T4 and T5 with retropulsion of osseous fragments into the spinal canal. There is another fracture in the superior end plate of T6 and a hyperflexion fracture dislocation at T8. The posterior columns are also disrupted at T6 and T7. Note the depressed proximal sternal and minimally displaced distal sternal fractures. Fractures of the sternum and thoracic spine are often seen in association.

4.5 Vascular Injuries

4.5.1 Acute Thoracic Aortic and Great Vessel Injury

Multidetector array CT has emerged as the definitive screening imaging for both diagnosis and exclusion of acute injuries to the thoracic aorta (ATAIs) and its great vessels branches without the need for transcatheter aortography or transesophageal echosonography. The latter studies are now typically only used in the infrequent setting of equivocal MDCT findings. In fact, the increased use of MDCT in trauma patients has led to the recognition of numerous vascular variants that may mimic acute vascular injuries, as well as to the diagnosis of more subtle vascular injuries (i.e., nonruptured, but injured), which heretofore likely went undiagnosed, often with little or no surrounding peribranch vessel or periaortic hematoma.[69]

The increasing use of nonsurgical therapies (e.g., blood pressure augmentation, endovascular stents) both for temporary and definitive management necessitates the accurate localization and characterization of these otherwise lethal injuries.[70,71] Thus, the radiologist must specifically describe (1) the nature of the lesion (e.g., pseudoaneurysm, intimal flap, dissection, luminal thrombosis, pseudocoarctation), (2) the diameter of the aorta or affected branch vessel immediately proximal and distal to the injury, (3) the length of the injury along the vascular axis, (4) the relationship between the injury and the nearest arterial

branch vessel, and (5) the presence of congenital vascular anomalies (e.g., aberrant right subclavian artery, direct origin of the left vertebral artery from the aortic arch, right-sided aortic arch with or without aberrant left subclavian artery, vascular slings, etc.) and their relationship to the site of injury.

Computed tomography features of aortic and great vessel injury are categorized as direct and indirect. Direct signs include pseudoaneurysm, intraluminal flap, focal contour abnormality, abrupt aortic caliber change, pseudocoarctation, intraluminal thrombus or debris, and frank contrast extravasation. The most specific direct signs are intimal flap and intraluminal thrombus or debris (100%), whereas an irregular aortic contour or a pseudoaneurysm is the most sensitive (100%). These signs do not require "confirmation" with angiography.[72] Additionally, a combination of ≥ 3 direct signs and periaortic contrast media extravasation significantly correlates with early aortic rupture and high mortality.[73]

Indirect signs include subtle contour anomalies, hemomediastinum, peribranch vessel, and periaortic blood.[74] Steenburg and Ravenel reported in their series that no trauma patient with equivocal or indirect CT findings needed surgical repair and that transcatheter angiography was of limited value for clarifying equivocal or indirect MDCT findings.[72]

Although most aortic injuries are associated with mediastinal hemorrhage, subtle injuries may occur with little or no hemomediastinum. When present, hemomediastinum is most often due to bleeding from small veins and arteries, or cervicothoracic

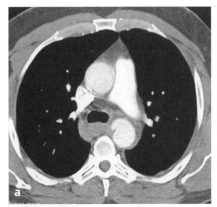
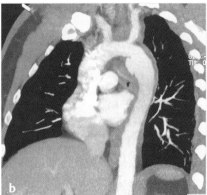
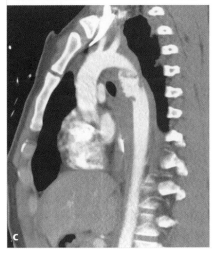

Fig. 4.26 A 40-year-old man involved in an all-terrain vehicle incident (ATV) with a typical acute posttraumatic aortic pseudoaneurysm. (a,b) Contrast-enhanced axial and sagittal oblique MIP CT (mediastinal windows) demonstrate the typical location and appearance of an acute aortic injury. The pseudoaneurysm projects from the anteromedial aorta at the level of the left main stem bronchus and distal to the left subclavian artery. Note the associated hemomediastinum. (c) Contrast-enhanced sagittal oblique MIP CT (mediastinal window) of a 30-year-old man involved in a high-speed motor vehicle collision shows a severe acute injury involving the entire circumference of the aorta extending for several centimeters in length. Note the extensive mediastinal hemorrhage.

spinal or sternal fractures, and does not originate directly from an injury to the aorta.[74] However, the presence of hemomediastinum requires close scrutiny of the adjacent vasculature for occult vascular injury.

4.6 Pseudoaneurysm

Most acute aortic injuries will manifest as a well-defined rounded bulge with irregular margins arising from the anterior or anteromedial aspect of the proximal descending thoracic aorta, distal to the ligamentum arteriosum, that is at the level of the left mainstem bronchus and proximal left pulmonary artery (▶ Fig. 4.26a,b). Such injuries may involve the entire circumference of the aorta and may extend several centimeters in length (▶ Fig. 4.26c). This finding is often better appreciated on sagittal and sagittal oblique MIP images than on the axial scans. Invariably, linear intimal flaps project across the base of the pseudoaneurysm.

4.6.1 Contour Anomalies

An obvious pseudoaneurysm may not be evident in all cases of aortic injury. Acute injuries may also be characterized by an abrupt alteration in luminal diameter or as an irregular change in shape or contour of the aorta (▶ Fig. 4.27). Such variations are more readily appreciated on sagittal, coronal, and sagittal

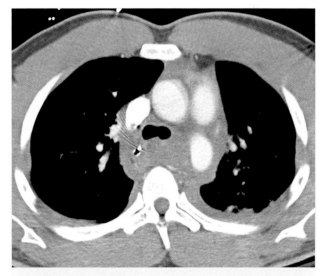

Fig. 4.27 A 41-year-old man involved motor vehicle collision with an acute aortic injury manifesting as a contour abnormality in the absence of a pseudoaneurysm or intimal flap. Contrast-enhanced axial computed tomography (mediastinal window) shows effacement of the medial wall of the descending aorta at the level of the left main stem bronchus. Note the rightward displacement of the nasogastric tube by the hemomediastinum and the left hemothorax.

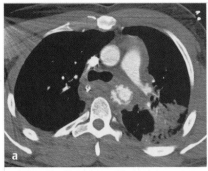
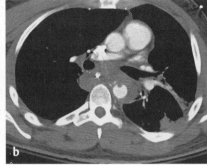

Fig. 4.28 (a) Contrast-enhanced axial computed tomography (CT) (mediastinal window) of a 40-year-old man involved in an all-terrain vehicle incident with an acute aortic injury characterized by gross irregularity in the descending aorta and an intimal flap from 5:00 to 11:00. Note the concomitant mediastinal hemorrhage and left upper-lobe contusion. (b) Contrast-enhanced axial CT (mediastinal window) of a 30-year-old man involved in a motorcycle collision with a tree demonstrates an aortic injury with intraluminal thrombus at the site of injury. Significant mediastinal hemorrhage is present.

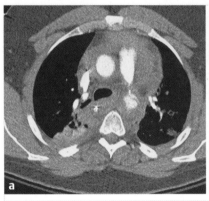
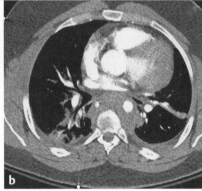

Fig. 4.29 A 27-year-old man involved in a motorcycle collision with an acute injury of the aorta characterized by pseudocoarctation distal to the injury. (a) Contrast-enhanced axial computed tomography (CT) (mediastinal window) demonstrates a severe injury to the aorta characterized by an anterior pseudoaneurysm and an intimal flap. The residual aortic lumen at this site of injury is small, compressed by the pseudoaneurysm. (b) Axial CT several centimeters distal shows the small caliber of the descending aorta lumen relative to the ascending aorta at the same level. Periaortic hematoma is present.

oblique MIP images. Remember, that aside from the mild narrowing at the isthmus of the aorta, the luminal diameter of the normal aorta changes very little from the origin of the left subclavian artery through the upper abdomen. Acute blood dissecting in the aortic wall or circumferential tears of the entire lumen, along the weakened wall of the aorta may be responsible for this imaging finding.

4.6.2 Intimal Flaps, Luminal Debris, and Thrombus

Torn flaps of intima may project into the lumen of the acutely injured aorta and thrombus may form along these flaps, which can subsequently embolize to solid and hollow visceral organs and the distal extremity arteries resulting in ischemia and even infarction (▶ Fig. 4.28a,b).

4.6.3 Pseudocoarctation

Acute aortic injuries such as those thus far described can adversely alter blood flow to the aorta distal to the site of injury, physiologically resulting in an aortic pseudocoarctation. Clinically, affected patients may have diminished lower extremity blood pressures and pulses.[75] Computed tomography findings include compression of the aortic lumen by an adjacent pseudoaneurysm or narrowing of the lumen by a focal dissection or thrombus, or encroachment upon the lumen by the circumferential tear in the intima and media. The thoracic aorta distal to the site of injury is usually small in caliber (▶ Fig. 4.29a,b).

4.6.4 Contrast Media Extravasation

Active extravasation of contrast media from an injured aorta during the acquisition of the CT images fortunately is rarely seen. Affected patients usually have a severely injured aorta, significant hemomediastinum and are at risk for imminent exsanguination (▶ Fig. 4.30). Only rarely do such patients survive.

4.7 Periaortic and Peribranch Vessel Hematoma

Mediastinal hemorrhage in the form of periaortic and/or peribranch vessel hematoma is present in most cases of acute aortic and great vessel injuries, respectively. Not infrequently, the mediastinal blood dissects along the descending aorta to the level of the diaphragm and may present as a retrocrural hematoma on abdominal CT scans. Therefore, a retrocrural hematoma, on an abdominal CT in a trauma patient, in the absence of neighboring spine trauma, indicates an acute thoracic aortic injury until proven otherwise and mandates emergent imaging of the thoracic aorta.[76]

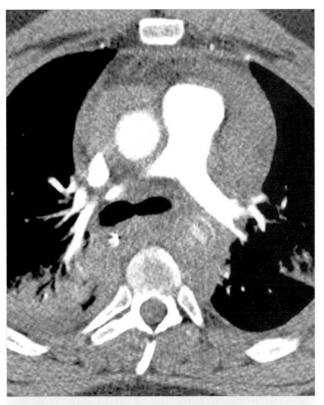

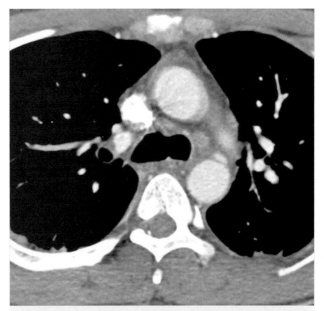

Fig. 4.31 A 27-year-old man involved in a motor vehicle collision with a subtle aortic injury. Contrast-enhanced axial computed tomography (mediastinal window) reveals a subtle intimal flap and posttraumatic pseudoaneurysm originating from the anterior wall of the descending aorta at the aortic pulmonary window level. No mediastinal hematoma.

Fig. 4.30 A young man involved in a sky-diving accident with a completely transected aorta. Contrast-enhanced axial computed tomography (mediastinal window) demonstrates near complete absence of opacification of the descending aorta at the site of injury. There is an amorphous blush of contrast media extravasating from the transected aorta. Note the hemomediastinum. Blood is also intimately related to the ascending aorta. Bilateral pulmonary contusions are present. The patient did not survive.

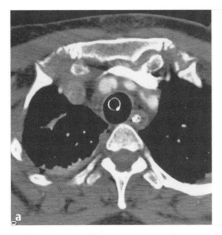

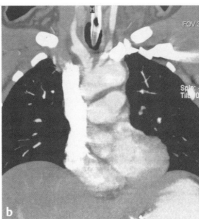

Fig. 4.32 A 49-year-old man involved in a motor vehicle collision with a subtle injury of the brachiocephalic artery. (a,b) Contrast-enhanced axial and coronal maximum intensity projection (MIP) computed tomography (mediastinal windows) demonstrate a subtle intimal flap and posttraumatic pseudoaneurysm involving the medial wall of the brachiocephalic artery extending from 12 to 6 o'clock. No superior mediastinal or peribranch vessel hematoma is present.

However, it is also imperative that radiologists and trauma team members be cognizant of the fact that subtle vascular injuries may indeed occur in the absence of mediastinal hemorrhage. The lack of mediastinal hemorrhage should never be an exclusionary criterion of injury when an abnormal appearing aorta or branch vessel is present (▶ Fig. 4.31, ▶ Fig. 4.32a,b).

Mediastinal hematoma isolated to either the anterior mediastinum and or the paravertebral space that is not in direct contact with the aorta is rarely associated with an acute vascular injury.[18] However, a superior mediastinal, peribranch vessel, and/or periaortic hematoma in the absence of obvious direct signs of vascular injury requires a thorough interrogation of these vessels in multiple planes to exclude an occult vascular injury that may otherwise go unrecognized (▶ Fig. 4.33). Selective arteriography may be necessary in such cases both for diagnosis and endovascular management (▶ Fig. 4.34).

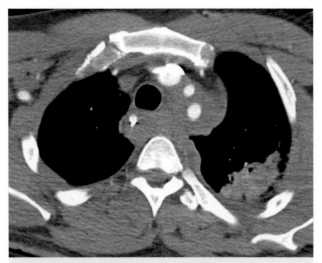

Fig. 4.33 A 32-year-old man involved in a motor vehicle collision with significant mediastinal hemorrhage. Contrast-enhanced axial computed tomography (mediastinal window) demonstrates a significant amount of peribranch vessel blood intimately related to the aortic great vessels. Additional multiplanar images of the branch vessels and aorta (not illustrated) revealed no vascular injury.

4.8 Atypical Aortic Injury Locations

Although most acute aortic injuries occur at the level of the left main stem bronchus and proximal left pulmonary artery, the radiologist should evaluate the aorta and its branch vessels in their entirety. About 10% of acute aortic injuries occur in less commonly recognized locations in the thoracic and proximal abdominal aorta. Also, multiple noncontiguous, injuries to the aorta are rare, but well described.[77]

4.9 Unsuspected Chronic Traumatic Aortic Pseudoaneurysm

About 2 to 5% of patients with unrecognized and untreated posttraumatic pseudoaneurysms of the thoracic aorta survive and develop a chronic pseudoaneurysm.[78] Affected patients may be asymptomatic, although 42% of them eventually will develop signs or symptoms within 5 years and 85% do so within 20 years.[78] Symptoms may include chest pain, hoarseness, dyspnea, dysphagia, and asystolic cardiac murmurs. Chronic pseudoaneurysms can rupture. However, open repair has a mortality rate of 5 to 18% and a morbidity rate of 11 to 50%.[79] Endovascular stenting has recently become recognized as an equally effective treatment option for chronic posttraumatic pseudoaneurysms with a markedly reduced morbidity and mortality.[80] On imaging, chronic pseudoaneurysms present as well-defined, often partially calcified lesions, located in the descending aorta at the level of the left main stem bronchus and proximal left pulmonary artery. Acute mediastinal hemorrhage is not present (▶ Fig. 4.35). The diagnosis is rather easy and straightforward. Such patients usually have a history of a severe car accident. Some patients, however, must be carefully and repeatedly questioned for such an occurrence.

4.10 Anatomical Variants Simulating Acute Injury

4.10.1 Ductus Diverticulum

The ductus diverticulum is either a remnant of the ductus arteriosum or the right dorsal aortic root.[81] The most common diagnostic challenge for the radiologist is differentiating a posttraumatic aortic isthmus pseudoaneurysm from a normal type III ductus diverticulum.[82] Both occur in roughly the same

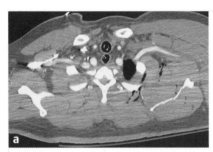

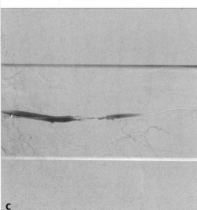

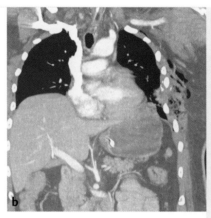

Fig. 4.34 A 27-year-old man with a left axillary artery injury after a motorcycle collision. (a,b) Contrast-enhanced axial and coronal maximum intensity projection computed tomography (mediastinal windows) demonstrate peribranch hematoma paralleling the left axillary artery, which is attenuated in caliber, suggesting an occult vascular injury. Note the ipsilateral axillary hematoma, rib fractures, and subcutaneous air. (c) Selective arteriography of the left axillary artery reveals a long segmental injury characterized by multifocal luminal irregularities with distal reconstitution. By the time the patient reached the angiography suite, left upper extremity distal pulses were fading. The injury was subsequently stented with return of distal circulation.

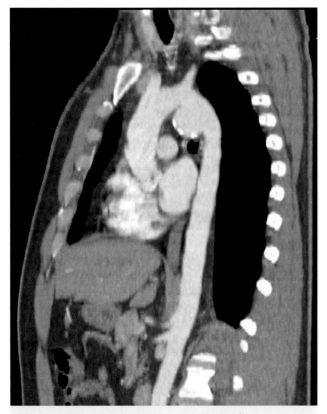

Fig. 4.35 A 48-year-old man who presented to his primary care physician with complaints of nonspecific chest pain has a chronic posttraumatic pseudoaneurysm of the thoracic aorta. Contrast-enhanced axial computed tomography (mediastinal window) demonstrates a well-defined partially calcified pseudoaneurysm located just distal to the left subclavian artery origin. No mediastinal hematoma is present. The patient had been involved in a severe boating accident with a prolonged hospitalization 20 years earlier.

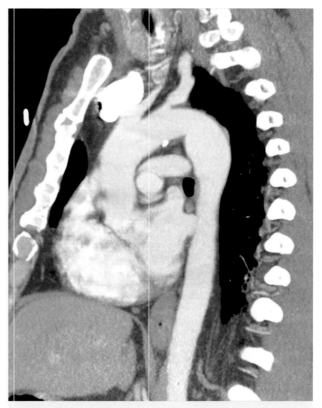

Fig. 4.36 A 46-year-old man with a type III ductus diverticulum who was involved in a motor vehicle collision. Contrast-enhanced sagittal oblique maximum intensity projection computed tomography (mediastinal window) demonstrates a focal convex bulge in the aortic isthmus (type III ductus). Note the smooth contour and the obtuse margin formed with the aortic lumen and the absence of an intimal flap and hemomediastinum.

location often leading to diagnostic confusion. Goodman describes the contour of the aortic isthmus as follows: type I—a concave contour, type II—mild straightening or convexity without a discrete bulge, and type III—a discrete focal bulge referred to as the *ductus diverticulum*.[83]

The ductus diverticulum is best appreciated on sagittal and sagittal oblique MIP CT. It is characterized as a focal convex bulge with a smooth contour forming an obtuse angle with the aortic lumen (▶ Fig. 4.36). Intimal flaps and hemomediastinum are not present. In contrast, a true traumatic pseudoaneurysm manifests as an irregular outpouching from the aortic lumen, displaying more acute margins. In addition, intimal flaps and/or mediastinal hemorrhage are usually present (▶ Fig. 4.26, ▶ Fig. 4.27, ▶ Fig. 4.28, ▶ Fig. 4.29). On axial CT, the ductus diverticulum demonstrates a smooth transition between contiguous slices, whereas a posttraumatic pseudoaneurysm is variable in shape with sharp and more irregular margins.[81] Further, an atypical ductus diverticulum may cause even more diagnostic dilemma. It is characterized superiorly by a shorter, steeper slope and inferiorly by a more typical, gentler slope, and is smooth. The smooth uninterrupted margins aid in differentiation from a true posttraumatic aortic pseudoaneurysm (▶ Fig. 4.37).

4.10.2 Aortic Spindle

The aortic spindle manifests as a fusiform dilatation of the aorta immediately distal to the isthmus (i.e., region between the left subclavian artery origin and the point of attachment of the ligamentum arteriosum). On imaging, the spindle is characterized by mild, fusiform enlargement of the distal aortic arch (▶ Fig. 4.38). Multiplanar reformation (MPR) and MIP reformations acquired along the vascular axis are helpful adjuncts, given that they show a normal caliber arch and proximal descending thoracic aorta.

4.10.3 Branch Infundibula

Infundibula of the aortic branches, including the brachiocephalic, bronchial, intercostal (most commonly the right third), left common carotid and left subclavian arteries, may simulate acute traumatic injuries or pseudoaneurysms. Infundibula are recognized by their triangular anatomic morphology, smooth margins, and by the presence of a vessel originating from their apex. Maximum intensity projection and 3D reformations are useful confirmatory images that can nicely delineate the origin and course of the vessel related to the infundibulum.

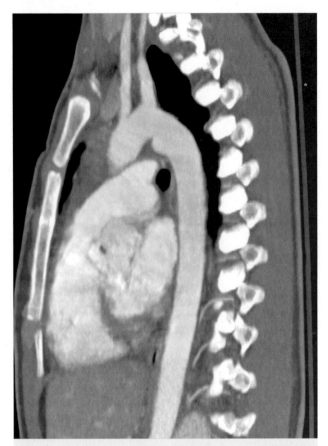

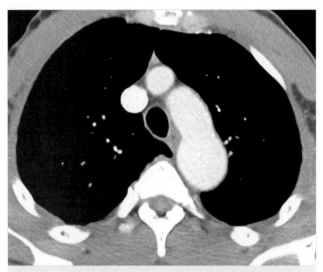

Fig. 4.38 A 26-year-old man with an aortic spindle who was involved in a motor vehicle collision. Contrast-enhanced axial computed tomography (mediastinal window) demonstrates mild, fusiform enlargement of the distal aortic arch characteristic of an aortic spindle.

Fig. 4.37 A 27-year-old man with an atypical ductus diverticulum who was involved in a motor vehicle collision. Contrast-enhanced sagittal oblique maximum intensity projection computed tomography (mediastinal window) demonstrates a focal convex bulge in the aortic isthmus. Note the shorter, steeper slope superiorly and the gentler appearing slope inferiorly. The margins appear smooth and uninterrupted. No mediastinal hemorrhage is present.

4.10.4 Placement of Endoluminal Stent Grafts

Endoluminal stent-graft placement has emerged as an alternative to traditional surgery for repair of posttraumatic aortic pseudoaneurysms. Conventional open surgical therapy carries a mortality rate between 3% and 26%, but can be as high as 75% in emergency repairs.[84] The high mortality is partially due to the frequency of coexisting serious nonaortic injuries and the morbidity that accompanies open thoracotomy. Endoluminal stent-graft deployment is associated with an overall 30-day mortality rate of 6%. The mortality decreases to 3% with elective treatment and increases to 13% with more-emergent treatment.[84] Moreover, the rates of spinal cord paralysis in surgical repair range from 1.5% to 19%.[84] Because aortic cross clamping and reperfusion is avoided, this alternative has a much lower incidence of spinal cord ischemia. In fact, Piffaretti et al reported no cases of paraplegia or paralysis in their patients treated with stent grafts.[84]

The stents successfully bridge and occlude the pseudoaneurysm and isolate it from the circulation forming a tight seal with the aortic wall proximally and distally.[85] Because most aortic injuries occur at the isthmus just beyond the left subclavian artery take-off, the origin of this great vessel must often be covered by the stent graft to obtain a tight proximal seal. This often necessitates a preprocedural left-carotid-to-subclavian arterial bypass graft or surgical transposition of the left subclavian artery to the left carotid artery.[85] The uncovered orifice of the left subclavian artery is then often occluded with either embolization coils or an Amplatzer vascular occluder to reduce the risk of thromboembolism with resultant upper limb claudication or tissue loss (▶ Fig. 4.39).

4.10.5 Endoleaks

The longitudinal flexibility of the stent-graft design and its ability to adequately conform to the curvature of the distal arch and/or proximal descending aorta and form a tight seal may predispose the stent graft to leakage. Such endoleaks after thoracic endoluminal therapy are a serious complication.

Endoleaks are a complication of endoluminal stent-graft therapy and represent one of the limitations of this surgical alternative. These leaks are characterized by blood flow outside the stent-graft lumen, but within the aneurysm or pseudoaneurysm. Lifelong surveillance (e.g., CTA, MRA, DSA, and US) is necessary to detect endoleaks and to assess the long-term durability of these devices. Computed tomography angiography is the imaging of choice for this purpose.

A classification system has been developed that organizes endoleaks into one of five categories based on the source of blood flow.[86] The radiologist must be cognizant that it is the source of blood flow into the endoleak that defines the specific type of endoleak which subsequently affects patient management.[86]

Type I endoleaks represent attachment-site leaks. These are further separated based upon whether the endoleak site is proximal (type Ia) or distal (type Ib). In either case, separation occurs between the stent graft and the native aortic wall,

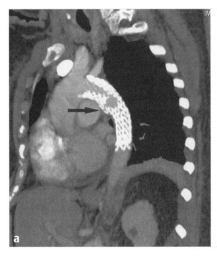
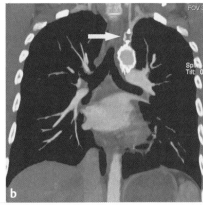

Fig. 4.39 (a) A 62-year-old man with acute aortic injury treated with placement of a stent graft. Contrast-enhanced sagittal oblique computed tomography (mediastinal window) demonstrates coverage of the posttraumatic pseudoaneurysm (arrow) and occlusion of the left subclavian artery origin. (b) A 46-year-old man with an aortic injury treated with an endoluminal stent graft. The endoluminal stent graft is seen en face, covering the left subclavian artery origin. An Amplatzer is seen in the left subclavian artery (arrow). A left carotid-to-subclavian arterial bypass graft was performed the day before (not illustrated).

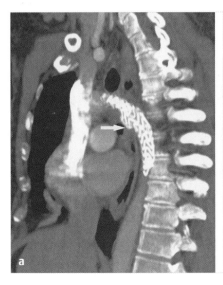
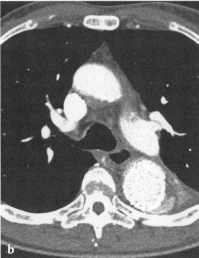

Fig. 4.40 A 52-year-old man with acute aortic injury treated with an endoluminal stent graft 12 months earlier and now complicated by a type III endoleak. (a) Contrast-enhanced sagittal oblique computed tomography (CT) (mediastinal window) demonstrates coverage of the post-traumatic pseudoaneurysm; however, contrast media can be identified both medially (arrow) and laterally between adjacent contiguous stent grafts. No endoleak was identified at this level 6 months earlier (not illustrated). (b) A 47-year-old man with acute aortic injury treated with contiguous endoluminal stent-graft deployments 14 months earlier and now demonstrating a type III endoleak.Contrast-enhanced axial CT (mediastinal window) demonstrates a lentiform collection of contrast media posterolaterally at 4 to 6 o'clock between adjacent contiguous stent grafts and the partially collapsed left lower lobe.

allowing direct communication between the aneurysm or pseudoaneurysm and the systemic arterial circulation. Type I endoleaks most commonly occur after endoluminal repair of thoracic aortic aneurysms.[86] These leaks should be repaired immediately after diagnosis and may be corrected by securing the attachment sites with balloons, stents, stent-graft extensions, and/or embolization coils.[86]

Type II endoleaks represent a collateral vessel leak. That is, there is retrograde blood flow through aortic branch vessels into the aneurysm or pseudoaneurysm. As with type I endoleaks, a direct communication from the systemic arterial circulation to the aneurysm or pseudoaneurysm is established. Type II endoleaks are most commonly encountered following endoluminal repair of abdominal aortic aneurysms.[86] The treatment of these leaks remains debatable. Up to 40% of these endoleaks will spontaneously thrombose. The remainder may require repair.[86]

Type III endoleaks represent structural failures in stent-graft integrity. This includes stent-graft fractures, holes that form in the fabric of the device, and junctional separations between multiple devices. Repetitive stresses placed on the grafts from arterial pulsations may be responsible for this type of leak (▶ Fig. 4.40). Type III endoleaks are the most dangerous endoleak and should

be repaired immediately at the time of diagnosis with a stent-graft extension.[86]

Type IV endoleaks are caused by stent-graft porosity. These leaks are uncommon, but are most often seen at the time of implantation and manifest as a "blush" on the immediate postimplantation angiogram, when patients are fully anticoagulated. These endoleaks are self-limited and resolve spontaneously.[86]

Type V endoleaks are commonly referred to as *endotension*, and are characterized by expansion of the aneurysm or pseudoaneurysm without the presence of an obvious leak. The exact cause is unknown, but may be related to a radiologically occult type I, II, or III endoleak. Treatment typically requires conversion to an open vascular repair.[86]

4.11 Nonaortic Vascular Injuries

4.11.1 Azygos Injury

The azygos vein ascends along the thoracic spine and drains into the superior vena cava at T4. In addition to penetrating injuries, violent axial or rotary forces applied to the mobile azygos arch by sudden deceleration, sudden increases in venous

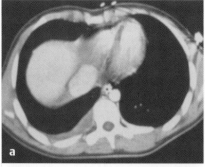
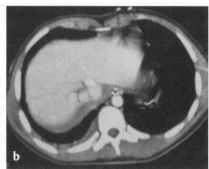
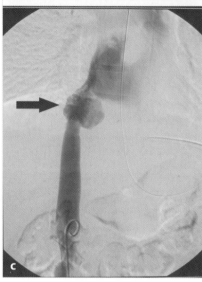

Fig. 4.41 (a–c) Young woman involved in a serious motor vehicle collision with a posttraumatic pseudoaneurysm of the retrohepatic and intrapericardial segments of the inferior vena cava (IVC). (a,b) Contrast-enhanced axial computed tomography (mediastinal windows) at the thoracoabdominal level shows marked enlargement of the IVC immediately inferior to the right atrium. The concomitant hemopericardium is not illustrated, but note the small right hemothorax and the free fluid surrounding the proximal IVC. (c) A venacavogram shows aneurysmal dilatation of the IVC (arrow) without contrast extravasation. (Used with permission from Parker MS, Rosado-de-Christenson, ML, Abbott GF. Chest Imaging Case Atlas. 2nd ed. New York, NY: Thieme; 2012: 473.)

pressure resulting from myocardial compression between the sternum and thoracic spine, and fracture dislocations of the midthoracic spine can lacerate the azygos vein.[87,88] Although isolated traumatic laceration of the azygos vein is rare, it has a morbidity and mortality similar to that of other great vessel injuries.[87,88] Chest radiographic findings include mediastinal widening, right hemothorax, and the delayed presentation of right hemothorax. Contrast-enhanced CT may demonstrate an eccentric right-sided hemomediastinum, right hemothorax, and extravasation of iodinated contrast media at the origin of the azygos arch vein.[88] Surgical exploration and venous ligation needs to be performed emergently.[87]

4.11.2 Superior Vena Cava Injury

Injuries of the superior vena cava (SVC) are due to penetrating or iatrogenic trauma. Blunt traumatic injury is rare. Contrast-enhanced chest CT may reveal mediastinal hemorrhage and active extravasation of contrast media at the site of injury. Stenting is the procedure of choice, if feasible. Otherwise, emergency thoracotomy is needed for repair.

4.11.3 Inferior Vena Cava Injury

The inferior vena cava (IVC) is protected by its anatomical location, but remains vulnerable to trauma. Inferior vena cava injuries are most frequently due to penetrating gunshot wounds, or rarely due to blunt trauma.[89] About one third of patients die before reaching the hospital. Moreover, the mortality of those reaching the hospital is 50%.[89] Concomitant injuries of the thoracic and/or abdominal aorta, liver, and bowel are frequent.[89] Anatomically, the IVC is divided into five segments: infrarenal, perirenal, suprarenal, retrohepatic, and intrapericardial. The intrapericardial and retrohepatic segments are the most vulnerable to blunt trauma.

A relationship between the segment injured and mortality rate exist. The closer the injury is to the heart, the worse the outcome. Infrarenal IVC injuries have 33% mortality while injuries of the intrapericardial IVC have 50 to 100% mortality.[90] Death is commonly caused by intraoperative exsanguination during attempted surgical repair of the injured cava. Venous complications in survivors are common and include venous hypertension, IVC thrombosis, IVC syndrome, and pulmonary embolism.[89] Contrast-enhanced CT findings include hemopericardium (with intrapericardial IVC disruption); aneurysmal-, irregular-, or amorphous-appearing IVC (i.e., pseudoaneurysm); contrast extravasation at the laceration; right-sided hemothorax; hemoperitoneum; and retrohepatic or retroperitoneal hematomas (▶ Fig. 4.41).

Venography or magnetic resonance venogram (MRV) is used to evaluate the pseudoaneurysm, contrast extravasation, and on occasion, intraluminal filling defect.[89] Management depends on the IVC segment injured. The retrohepatic and intrapericardial are the most difficult to repair: Primary venorrhaphy, IVC ligation, prosthetic grafting, atriocaval bypass, etc., and recently endoluminal stent graft.[90]

4.12 Conclusion

Imaging is of paramount importance in the diagnosis and management of patients with thoracic trauma. Noninvasive imaging modalities include duplex US, MDCT, CTA, MRI, MRA, and MRV. More invasive, but often necessary imaging studies include transesophageal ultrasound, intravascular ultrasound, and transcatheter angiography/venography. The interventional radiologist plays a crucial role in the nonsurgical diagnosis and many times treatment and management of these often critically ill and hemodynamically unstable patients. Rapidly evolving techniques in vessel ligation, embolization, vessel repair, and endovascular stent deployment performed by interventional radiologists continue to have a dramatic impact on the outcome of these patients.

References

[1] Costantino M, Gosselin MV, Primack SL. The ABC's of thoracic trauma imaging. Semin Roentgenol 2006; 41: 209–225

[2] Tocino I, Miller MH. Computed tomography in blunt chest trauma. J Thorac Imaging 1987; 2: 45–59

[3] Primack SL, Collins J. Blunt nonaortic chest trauma: radiographic and CT findings. Emerg Radiol 2002; 9: 5–12

[4] Shanmuganathan K, Matsumoto J. Imaging of penetrating chest trauma. Radiol Clin North Am 2006; 44: 225–238, viii

[5] Ordog GJ, Wasserberger J, Balasubramanium S, Shoemaker W. Asymptomatic stab wounds of the chest. J Trauma 1994; 36: 680–684

[6] Dyer DS, Moore EE, Mestek MF et al. Can chest CT be used to exclude aortic injury? Radiology 1999; 213: 195–202

[7] Parker MS, Matheson TL, Rao AV et al. Making the transition: the role of helical CT in the evaluation of potentially ATAR. AJR Am J Roentgenol 2001; 176: 1267–1272

[8] Kuhlman JE, Pozniak MA, Collins J, Knisely BL. Radiographic and CT findings of blunt chest trauma: aortic injuries and looking beyond them. Radiographics 1998; 18: 1071–1084

[9] Parker MS, Matheson TL, Rao AV et al. Spiral CT in blunt thoracic trauma: detection of "unsuspected" concomitant injuries. Radiologist 2000; 7: 137–146

[10] Sangster GP, González-Beicos A, Carbo AI et al. Blunt traumatic injuries of the lung parenchyma, pleura, thoracic wall, and intrathoracic airways: multidetector computer tomography imaging findings. Emerg Radiol 2007; 14: 297–310

[11] Omert L, Yeaney WW, Protetch J. Efficacy of thoracic computerized tomography in blunt chest trauma. Am Surg 2001; 67: 660–664

[12] Exadaktylos AK, Sclabas G, Schmid SW, Schaller B, Zimmermann H. Do we really need routine computed tomographic scanning in the primary evaluation of blunt chest trauma in patients with "normal" chest radiograph? J Trauma 2001; 51: 1173–1176

[13] Gavelli G, Canini R, Bertaccini P, Battista G, Bnà C, Fattori R. Traumatic injuries: imaging of thoracic injuries. Eur Radiol 2002; 12: 1273–1294

[14] Primack SL, Collins J. Blunt nonaortic chest trauma: radiographic and CT findings. Emerg Radiol 2002; 9: 5–12

[15] Rivas LA, Fishman JE, Múnera F, Bajayo DE. Multislice CT in thoracic trauma. Radiol Clin North Am 2003; 41: 599–616

[16] Gavant ML, Flick P, Menke P, Gold RE. CT aortography of thoracic aortic rupture. AJR Am J Roentgenol 1996; 166: 955–961

[17] Gavant ML, Menke PG, Fabian T, Flick PA, Graney MJ, Gold RE. Blunt traumatic aortic rupture: detection with helical CT of the chest. Radiology 1995; 197: 125–133

[18] Mirvis SE, Shanmuganathan K, Miller BH, White CS, Turney SZ. Traumatic aortic injury: diagnosis with contrast-enhanced thoracic CT—five-year experience at a major trauma center. Radiology 1996; 200: 413–422

[19] Sammer M, Wang E, Blackmore CC, Burdick TR, Hollingworth W. Indeterminate CT angiography in blunt thoracic trauma: is CT angiography enough? AJR Am J Roentgenol 2007; 189: 603–608

[20] Demetriades D, Velmahos GC, Scalea TM et al. Diagnosis and treatment of blunt thoracic aortic injuries: changing perspectives. J Trauma 2008; 64: 1415–1418, discussion 1418–1419

[21] Mohan IV, Hitos K, White GH et al. Improved outcomes with endovascular stent grafts for thoracic aorta transections. Eur J Vasc Endovasc Surg 2008; 36: 152–157

[22] Ott MC, Stewart TC, Lawlor DK, Gray DK, Forbes TL. Management of blunt thoracic aortic injuries: endovascular stents versus open repair. J Trauma 2004; 56: 565–570

[23] Hoffer EK, Forauer AR, Silas AM, Gemery JM. Endovascular stent-graft or open surgical repair for blunt thoracic aortic trauma: systematic review. J Vasc Interv Radiol 2008; 19: 1153–1164

[24] Malloy PC, Richard HM. Thoracic angiography and intervention in trauma. Radiol Clin North Am 2006; 44: 239–249, viii

[25] Lee BC, Ormsby EL, McGahan JP, Melendres GM, Richards JR. The utility of sonography for the triage of blunt abdominal trauma patients to exploratory laparotomy. AJR Am J Roentgenol 2007; 188: 415–421

[26] Mandavia DP, Joseph A. Bedside echocardiography in chest trauma. Emerg Med Clin North Am 2004; 22: 601–619

[27] Patel NH, Hahn D, Comess KA. Blunt chest trauma victims: role of intravascular ultrasound and transesophageal echocardiography in cases of abnormal thoracic aortogram. J Trauma 2003; 55: 330–337

[28] Uflacker R, Horn J, Phillips G, Selby JB. Intravascular sonography in the assessment of traumatic injury of the thoracic aorta. AJR Am J Roentgenol 1999; 173: 665–670

[29] Descat E, Montaudon M, Latrabe V, Surcin B, Morales P, Laurent F. MR imaging of myocardial haematoma after blunt chest injury. Eur Radiol 2002; 12 Suppl 3: S174–S176

[30] Southam S, Jutila C, Ketai L. Contrast-enhanced cardiac MRI in blunt chest trauma: differentiating cardiac contusion from acute peri-traumatic myocardial infarction. J Thorac Imaging 2006; 21: 176–178

[31] Buecker A, Wein BB, Neuerburg JM, Guenther RW. Esophageal perforation: comparison of use of aqueous and barium-containing contrast media. Radiology 1997; 202: 683–686

[32] Back MR, Baumgartner FJ, Klein SR. Detection and evaluation of aerodigestive tract injuries caused by cervical and transmediastinal gunshot wounds. J Trauma 1997; 42: 680–686

[33] Lomoschitz FM, Eisenhuber E, Linnau KF, Peloschek P, Schoder M, Bankier AA. Imaging of chest trauma: radiological patterns of injury and diagnostic algorithms. Eur J Radiol 2003; 48: 61–70

[34] Tocino IM, Miller MH, Fairfax WR. Distribution of pneumothorax in the supine and semirecumbent critically ill adult. AJR Am J Roentgenol 1985; 144: 901–905

[35] Koh DM, Burke S, Davies N, Padley SPG. Transthoracic US of the chest: clinical uses and applications. Radiographics 2002; 22: e1

[36] Lichtenstein D, Mezière G, Biderman P, Gepner A. The comet-tail artifact: an ultrasound sign ruling out pneumothorax. Intensive Care Med 1999; 25: 383–388

[37] Wolfman NT, Gilpin JW, Bechtold RE, Meredith JW, Ditesheim JA. Occult pneumothorax in patients with abdominal trauma: CT studies. J Comput Assist Tomogr 1993; 17: 56–59

[38] Lim KE, Tai SC, Chan CY et al. Diagnosis of malpositioned chest tubes after emergency tube thoracostomy: is computed tomography more accurate than chest radiograph? Clin Imaging 2005; 29: 401–405

[39] Baldt MM, Bankier AA, Germann PS, Pöschl GP, Skrbensky GT, Herold CJ. Complications after emergency tube thoracostomy: assessment with CT. Radiology 1995; 195: 539–543

[40] Landay M, Oliver Q, Estrera A, Friese R, Boonswang N, DiMaio JM. Lung penetration by thoracostomy tubes: imaging findings on CT. J Thorac Imaging 2006; 21: 197–204

[41] Etoch SW, Bar-Natan MF, Miller FB, Richardson JD. Tube thoracostomy. Factors related to complications. Arch Surg 1995; 130: 521–525, discussion 525–526

[42] Jaillard SM, Tremblay A, Conti M, Wurtz AJ. Uncommon complications during chest tube placement. Intensive Care Med 2002; 28: 812–813

[43] Ambrogi MC, Lucchi M, Dini P, Mussi A, Angeletti CA. Videothoracoscopy for evaluation and treatment of hemothorax. J Cardiovasc Surg (Torino) 2002; 43: 109–112

[44] Kessel B, Alfici R, Ashkenazi I et al. Massive hemothorax caused by intercostal artery bleeding: selective embolization may be an alternative to thoracotomy in selected patients. Thorac Cardiovasc Surg 2004; 52: 234–236

[45] Carrillo EH, Heniford BT, Senler SO, Dykes JR, Maniscalco SP, Richardson JD. Embolization therapy as an alternative to thoracotomy in vascular injuries of the chest wall. Am Surg 1998; 64: 1142–1148

[46] Fraser RS, Müller NL, Coleman N, Paré PD. Radiologic signs of chest disease: pleural abnormalities. In: Fraser RS, Müller NL, Coleman N, Paré PD, eds.

Fraser and Paré's Diagnosis of Diseases of the Chest. 4th ed. Philadelphia, PA: Saunders, 1999: 566–572

[47] Bouhemad B, Zhang M, Lu Q, Rouby JJ. Clinical review: bedside lung ultrasound in critical care practice. Crit Care 2007; 11: 205

[48] Akhan O, Ozkan O, Akinci D, Hassan A, Ozmen M. Image-guided catheter drainage of infected pleural effusions. Diagn Interv Radiol 2007; 13: 204–209

[49] Chen HJ, Tu CY, Ling SJ et al. Sonographic appearances in transudative pleural effusions: not always an anechoic pattern. Ultrasound Med Biol 2008; 34: 362–369

[50] Harrer J, Brtko M, Zácek P, Knap J. Hemothorax–a complication of subclavian vein cannulation. Acta Medica (Hradec Kralove) 1997; 40: 21–23

[51] Pieters PC, Tisnado J, Mauro MA. Complications of central venous access. In: Pieters PC, Tisnado J, Mauro MA. Venous Catheters: A Practical Manual. New York: Thieme, 2003: 253–254

[52] Turba UC, Uflacker R, Hannegan C, Selby JB. Anatomic relationship of the internal jugular vein and the common carotid artery applied to percutaneous transjugular procedures. Cardiovasc Intervent Radiol 2005; 28: 303–306

[53] Tercan F, Oguzkurt L, Ozkan U, Eker HE. Comparison of ultrasonography-guided central venous catheterization between adult and pediatric populations. Cardiovasc Intervent Radiol 2008; 31: 575–580

[54] Collini A, Nepi S, Ruggieri G, Carmellini M. Massive hemothorax after removal of subclavian vein catheter: a very unusual complication. Crit Care Med 2002; 30: 697–698

[55] Thurnheer R, Speich R. Impending asphyxia in a 27-year-old woman 14 days after a gynecologic operation. Chest 1995; 107: 1169–1171

[56] Silen ML, Weber TR. Management of thoracic duct injury associated with fracture-dislocation of the spine following blunt trauma. J Trauma 1995; 39: 1185–1187

[57] Gray H. The lymphatic System: the thoracic duct. In: Goss CM, ed. Gray's Anatomy: Anatomy of the Human Body. 29th ed. Philadelphia, PA: Lea & Febiger; 1973: 738–739

[58] Kos S, Haueisen H, Lachmund U, Roeren T. Lymphangiography: forgotten tool or rising star in the diagnosis and therapy of postoperative lymphatic vessel leakage. Cardiovasc Intervent Radiol 2007; 30: 968–973

[59] Sugiura K, Tanabe Y, Ogawa T, Tokushima T. Localization of chyle leakage site in postoperative chylothorax by oral administration of I-123 BMIPP. Ann Nucl Med 2005; 19: 597–601

[60] Stavngaard T, Mortensen J, Brenoe J, Svendsen LB. Lymphoscintigraphy using technetium-99 m human serum albumin in chylothorax. Thorac Cardiovasc Surg 2002; 50: 250–252

[61] Bybel B, Neumann DR, Kim BY, Amin K, Rice T. Lymphoscintigraphy using (99m)Tc filtered sulfur colloid in chylothorax: a case report. J Nucl Med Technol 2001; 29: 30–31

[62] Fraser RS, Müller NL, Coleman N, Paré PD. Traumatic chest disease: penetrating and nonpenetrating trauma. In: Fraser RS, Müller NL, Coleman N, Paré PD, eds. Fraser and Paré's Diagnosis of Diseases of the Chest. 4th ed. Philadelphia, PA: Saunders, 1999: 2634–2636

[63] Litherland B, Given M, Lyon S. Percutaneous radiological management of high-output chylothorax with CT-guided needle disruption. J Med Imaging Radiat Oncol 2008; 52: 164–167

[64] Buchan KG, Hosseinpour AR, Ritchie AJ. Thoracoscopic thoracic duct ligation for traumatic chylothorax. Ann Thorac Surg 2001; 72: 1366–1367

[65] Pandey R, Lee DF. Laparoscopic ligation of the thoracic duct for the treatment of traumatic chylothorax. J Laparoendosc Adv Surg Tech A 2008; 18: 614–615

[66] Ketai L, Brandt MM, Schermer C. Nonaortic mediastinal injuries from blunt chest trauma. J Thorac Imaging 2000; 15: 120–127

[67] Parker MS, Rosado de Christenson ML, Abbott GF. Traumatic rupture of the left hemidiaphragm. In: Parker MS, Rosado de Christenson ML, Abbott GF, Teaching Atlas of Chest Imaging. New York, NY: Thieme, 2006: 383–387

[68] Parker MS, Rosado de Christenson ML, Abbott GF. Vertebral compression fracture. In: Parker MS, Rosado de Christenson ML, Abbott GF. Teaching Atlas of Chest Imaging. New York: Thieme, 2006: 397–399

[69] Downing SW, Sperling JS, Mirvis SE et al. Experience with spiral computed tomography as the sole diagnostic method for traumatic aortic rupture. Ann Thorac Surg 2001; 72: 495–501, discussion 501–502

[70] Symbas PN, Sherman AJ, Silver JM, Symbas JD, Lackey JJ. Traumatic rupture of the aorta: immediate or delayed repair? Ann Surg 2002; 235: 796–802

[71] Xenos ES, Abedi NN, Davenport DL et al. Meta-analysis of endovascular vs open repair for traumatic descending thoracic aortic rupture. J Vasc Surg 2008; 48: 1343–1351

[72] Steenburg SD, Ravenel JG. Acute traumatic thoracic aortic injuries: experience with 64-MDCT. AJR Am J Roentgenol 2008; 191: 1564–1569

[73] Ng CJ, Chen JC, Wang LJ et al. NG CJ. Diagnostic value of the helical CT scan for traumatic aortic injury: correlation with mortality and early rupture. J Emerg Med 2006; 30: 277–282

[74] Fishman JE, Nuñez D, Kane A, Rivas LA, Jacobs WE. Direct versus indirect signs of traumatic aortic injury revealed by helical CT: performance characteristics and interobserver agreement. AJR Am J Roentgenol 1999; 172: 1027–1031

[75] Mirvis SE. Thoracic vascular injury. Radiol Clin North Am 2006; 44: 181–197, vii

[76] Wong H, Gotway MB, Sasson AD, Jeffrey RB. Periaortic hematoma at diaphragmatic crura at helical CT: sign of blunt aortic injury in patients with mediastinal hematoma. Radiology 2004; 231: 185–189

[77] Gavant ML. Helical CT grading of traumatic aortic injuries. Impact on clinical guidelines for medical and surgical management. Radiol Clin North Am 1999; 37: 553–574, vi

[78] Creasy JD, Chiles C, Routh WD, Dyer RB. Overview of traumatic injury of the thoracic aorta. Radiographics 1997; 17: 27–45

[79] Gawenda M, Landwehr P, Brunkwall J. Stent-graft replacement of chronic traumatic aneurysm of the thoracic aorta after blunt chest trauma. J Cardiovasc Surg (Torino) 2002; 43: 705–709

[80] Andrassy J, Weidenhagen R, Meimarakis G, Lauterjung L, Jauch KW, Kopp R. Stent versus open surgery for acute and chronic traumatic injury of the thoracic aorta: a single-center experience. J Trauma 2006; 60: 765–771, discussion 771–772

[81] Grollman JH. The aortic diverticulum: a remnant of the partially involuted dorsal aortic root. Cardiovasc Intervent Radiol 1989; 12: 14–17

[82] Macura KJ, Corl FM, Fishman EK, Bluemke DA. Pathogenesis in acute aortic syndromes: aortic aneurysm leak and rupture and traumatic aortic transection. AJR Am J Roentgenol 2003; 181: 303–307

[83] Goodman PC, Jeffrey RB, Minagi H, Federle MP, Thomas AN. Angiographic evaluation of the ductus diverticulum. Cardiovasc Intervent Radiol 1982; 5: 1–4

[84] Piffaretti G, Tozzi M, Lomazzi C, Rivolta N, Caronno R, Castelli P. Complications after endovascular stent-grafting of thoracic aortic diseases. J Cardiothorac Surg 2006; 1: 26

[85] Kato N, Dake MD, Miller DC et al. Traumatic thoracic aortic aneurysm: treatment with endovascular stent-grafts. Radiology 1997; 205: 657–662

[86] Stavropoulos SW, Charagundla SR. Imaging techniques for detection and management of endoleaks after endovascular aortic aneurysm repair. Radiology 2007; 243: 641–655

[87] Drac P, Manak P, Klein J, Kral V. Azygos vein injury in blunt chest trauma. Biomed Pap Med Fac Univ Palacky Olomouc Czech Repub 2007; 151: 347–348

[88] Bowles BJ, Teruya T, Belzberg H, Rivkind AI. Blunt traumatic azygous vein injury diagnosed by computed tomography: case report and review of the literature. J Trauma 2000; 49: 776–779

[89] Parker MS, Rosado de Christenson ML, Abbott GF. Vena cava injury. In: Parker MS, Rosado de Christenson ML, Abbott GF. Teaching Atlas of Chest Imaging. New York, NY: Thieme, 2006: 364–366

[90] Buckman RF, Pathak AS, Badellino MM, Bradley KM. Injuries of the inferior vena cava. Surg Clin North Am 2001; 81: 1431–1447

5 Imaging of Abdominal Trauma

Robert A. Halvorsen and Jinxing Yu

The evaluation of patients who have sustained blunt abdominal trauma remains difficult. Physical examination alone has a reported sensitivity for the detection of significant intraperitoneal injury of 50 to 60%.[1] The accuracy of physical examination is hampered by the presence of intoxicants or head injuries, both of which are not uncommonly encountered in blunt abdominal trauma patients. Consequently, diagnostic modalities other than physical examination are frequently necessary.

The options for detection of intraperitoneal injuries are numerous. An early report of a novel technique to diagnose bowel injury was reported in the American Medical Association's *The Medical News* in 1888 in an article entitled, "Rectal Insufflation of Hydrogen Gas as an Infallible Test in the Diagnosis of Visceral Injury of the Gastro-intestinal Canal in Penetrating Wounds of the Abdomen without Laparotomy," by a surgeon from the Milwaukee Hospital, Dr. Senn.[2] In this article, he describes his technique which includes inserting a rectal tube and insufflating hydrogen into the body. Then he recommends holding a lit taper (now called a candle) in front of the abdomen. If a small explosion occurred, then the test was positive and there was perforation of the bowel and the abdominal wall. Although this test never achieved widespread clinical usage, many other tests have been developed to help detect bowel injury.

5.1 Diagnostic Peritoneal Lavage

Diagnostic peritoneal lavage (DPL) was introduced by Root in 1965[3] and was the primary means for evaluating the abdomen after blunt trauma for years. Diagnostic peritoneal lavage is very sensitive in detecting intraperitoneal hemorrhage, but has a poor specificity for the site and the severity of organ injury.[4] Computed tomography (CT) has replaced DPL as the primary tool for assessing the abdomen in blunt trauma patients (▶ Fig. 5.1). But CT also has its limitations. Patients must be clinically stable enough to be taken from the trauma bay to the CT scanner. The sensitivity of CT for the detection of hollow viscus injury is less than optimal, from 50 to 88%.[5] Radiation dose is another consideration.

5.2 Ultrasound

Ultrasound is among the newer technologies available to evaluate the abdomen in trauma patients. A sonogram can be performed rapidly at the bedside and is often readily available. Ultrasound has a reported sensitivity for the detection of intraperitoneal fluid of 86 to 98%.[1] Although ultrasound may detect solid organ injury, the sensitivity is suboptimal (40–87%).[1,6,7] Further, the ability of ultrasound to detect hollow viscus injury is very limited.

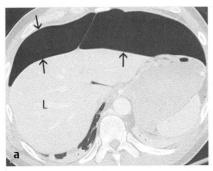
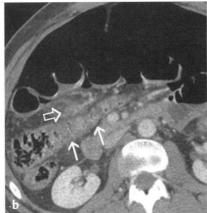
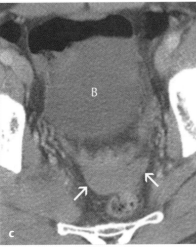

Fig. 5.1 Bowel perforation in a blunt abdominal trauma patient. (a) Axial computed tomography (CT) with lung window demonstrates a large amount of free air (arrows) anterior to the liver (L). (b) Axial CT shows thickened transverse colon (arrows) with fat stranding (open arrow) in the mesentery. (c) Axial CT shows complex fluid (higher than water density) in the pelvis (arrows) posterior to the bladder (B). Surgery confirmed perforation of the transverse colon.

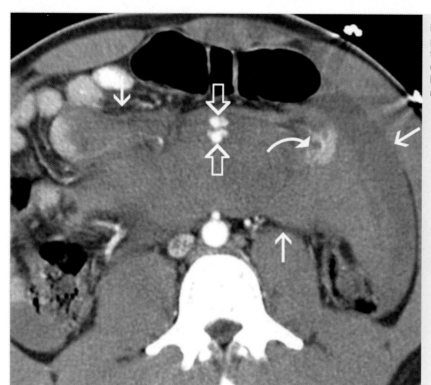

Fig. 5.2 Active bleeding in the mesentery with perforation of jejunum. Axial computed tomography demonstrates high density foci (open arrows) in the mesentery surrounded by a large hematoma (arrows). A loop of jejunum was ruptured (curved arrow).

5.2.1 Focused Assessment with Sonography for Trauma

The role of FAST (focused assessment with sonography for trauma) in the evaluation of trauma victims is controversial. A FAST scan is a rapid, noninvasive, portable, and inexpensive screening test for blunt abdominal trauma. Ultrasound can detect as little as 100 cc of peritoneal fluid.[8] A FAST scan sequentially surveys for the presence of blood in the pericardial sac, and dependent regions of the abdomen and pelvis including the right upper quadrant and left upper quadrant of the abdomen. A prospective comparison of adult trauma victims managed with and without FAST was reported by Boulanger et al.[9] In those patients managed without FAST, hemodynamically stable patients underwent CT and unstable patients had a DPL. They found that the diagnostic accuracy of the FAST and non-FAST groups and the rates of laparotomy were similar. The diagnostic cost and the mean time for diagnostic workup were much less for the FAST group. Another study found that FAST had a high rate of false-negative examinations in patients with pelvic ring-type fractures and recommended CT of the abdomen and pelvis in patients with pelvic ring fractures.[10]

The use of FAST varies from institution to institution and between the United States and Europe. The demographics of trauma patients in Europe is different from U.S. patients: Europeans report relatively higher rates of blunt trauma.[11] European countries, such as the United Kingdom, provide centralized emergency services predominately managed by multidisciplinary teams consisting of anesthetists and emergency physicians. Ultrasound is more frequently utilized in trauma patients in Europe in part due to the availability of trained sonographers in emergency departments, as well as a lower number of CT scanners compared with the United States.

5.3 Computed Tomography

5.3.1 Multidetector Computed Tomography

Multidetector computed tomography (MDCT) has several advantages over DPL and FAST in the evaluation of trauma patients. It is the most comprehensive modality, allowing evaluation of solid and hollow organs, bones, and soft tissues. Multidetector computed tomography can detect active bleeding when intravenous contrast is given (▶ Fig. 5.2).[12]

5.3.2 Penetrating Trauma

Some trauma patients with penetrating trauma to the abdomen or pelvis will require immediate operative intervention. Computed tomography can be useful in patients when it is unclear if the peritoneum has been violated. Computed tomography criteria have been developed to determine if penetration has reached the peritoneum and include
1. Visible wound tract into the peritoneum
2. Intraperitoneal fluid, free air, or bullet fragment
3. Intraperitoneal organ injury

With penetrating trauma, the CT technique is modified to include triple contrast, including oral, intravenous, and rectal contrast (▶ Fig. 5.3). Computed tomography utilizing the above

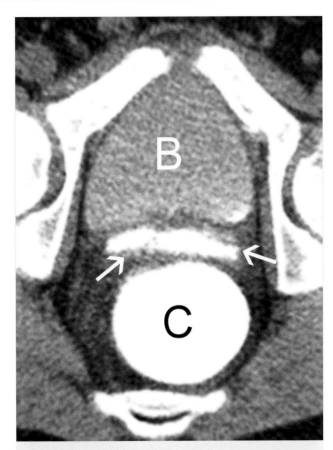

Fig. 5.3 Perforation of rectum with rectal contrast extravasation in a patient with foreign body injury to the rectum. Axial computed tomography with rectal contrast demonstrates extravasated contrast (arrows) anterior to the rectum (C) and posterior to the bladder (B), consistent with rectal perforation.

three criteria with triple-contrast CT has a reported sensitivity of 97%, specificity of 98%, and an accuracy of 98% in diagnosing penetrating injuries.[13]

5.3.3 Blunt Trauma

Hemodynamically unstable blunt trauma patients are usually considered candidates for emergent operative intervention. Computed tomography of the abdomen and pelvis is usually restricted to relatively stable patients. In the majority of trauma centers, the CT is located separately from the trauma bay where the initial assessment and treatment occurs. To perform a CT study, the patient must be stable enough for transportation to the CT suite, the time required for the performance of the CT, and the time of transport from CT. A few institutions have incorporated CT scanners into the trauma resuscitation room, but this has not been practical in the majority of institutions.

5.3.4 Technique for MDCT

The optimal technique for MDCT in trauma patients for evaluation of the abdomen and pelvis has yet to be established. Currently, different institutions use different techniques. Some

centers, such as Massachusetts General Hospital, advocate the use of "whole-body" CT in the trauma patient.[14] The whole-body technique utilizes a continuous scanning of the head, the cervical spine, the chest, the abdomen, and the pelvis. The whole body scanning technique still requires two separate CT studies. First, the patient has a head and spine CT performed with the patient's arms at his or her sides to decrease artifacts. Then a second CT is performed with the arms elevated alongside the head for the chest, abdomen, and pelvic CT.

The group from Maryland Shock Trauma Hospital have evaluated single-pass continuous whole-body MDCT and concluded that this technique can decrease examination times for patients of polytrauma, and has improved image quality compared with conventional serial MDCT scan protocols.[15] They found that the median acquisition times for the single-pass protocols were significantly shorter (-42.5%) than the acquisition time for the conventional protocol. The time reductions were achieved by avoiding image reconstruction delays between segmental scans, and by reducing the need to reposition the patient, the number of scout images, and the time needed for scan programming.

Other centers, such as ours, continue to perform separate MDCT studies for each area of the body. For instance, a polytrauma patient in our emergency department will have the cervical spine, chest, and abdominal CTs performed separately as three independent studies. This allows for optimal timing of contrast enhancement of each of the organ systems. For instance, scanning of the chest is optimized for aortic enhancement to detect aortic injuries. Timing for the abdominal CT is optimized to detect solid organ injury. Anecdotally, we have seen several cases where hepatic and splenic injuries could not be detected on the chest CT and were detected on the abdominal CT obtained ~ 15 seconds later. We have seen cases in which arterial bleeding of a splenic injury was better detected on the chest CT, which is obtained during the arterial phase of enhancement (▶ Fig. 5.4).

The routine use of oral contrast during MDCT is controversial. Some authors describe unnecessary delays, and increased risk of vomiting and aspiration; they claim that there is no significant improvement in diagnostic capability.[16,17] Other authors have demonstrated that administration of oral contrast in trauma patients is safe and improves visualization of bowel injuries.[18,19]

Step-by-Step Approach to MDCT Interpretation

Interpretation of the MDCT obtained in trauma patients requires attention to detail. The use of a rigorous routine in the interpretation of these studies can significantly diminish missing traumatic lesions.[20] To avoid misses, review all trauma CTs with five settings:
1. Lung window
2. Soft tissue windows
3. Liver window
4. Bone window
5. Sagittal and coronal multiplanar reconstruction (MPR)

The following is one possible detailed routine for interpretation of abdominal and pelvic MDCT in trauma patients.

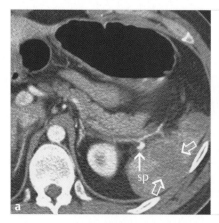
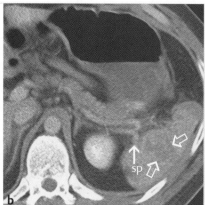

Fig. 5.4 Splenic arterial pseudoaneurysm only seen on chest computed tomography (CT). (a) Axial contrast-enhanced CT demonstrates a small pseudoaneurysm from the splenic artery (arrow) with a large laceration (open arrows) in the spleen (sp). The abdominal CT (not shown) failed to demonstrate the pseudoaneurysm. (b) Axial contrast-enhanced CT on a slightly delayed image demonstrates the small pseudoaneurysm from the splenic artery (arrow) is poorly visualized. The large laceration (open arrows) in the spleen (sp) is again seen.

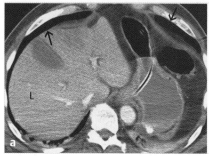
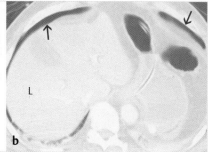

Fig. 5.5 Pneumothorax overlooked by abdominal soft tissue window in a trauma patient. (a) Axial computed tomography (CT) with soft tissue window demonstrates air density (arrows) in the anterior aspect of abdomen simulating lung. (L, liver) (b) Axial CT with lung window at the same level as (a) shows air density in the anterior aspect of abdomen is consistent with pneumothorax. (L, liver)

Lung Window

In our experience, the most frequently overlooked finding in trauma CT of the abdomen is the pneumothorax (▶ Fig. 5.5). We use lung windows to search not only for pneumothorax, but also for pneumoperitoneum. The entire abdomen and pelvis is scanned from top to bottom using lung windows for the detection of free intraperitoneal air, intraperitoneal air adjacent to bowel loops, or retroperitoneal air.

Soft Tissue Windows

After scrolling through the abdomen and pelvis using lung windows, we switch to soft tissue windows and scroll from the bottom back to the top. This primary initial soft tissue survey is performed to search for free intraperitoneal fluid. More than a small amount of intraperitoneal fluid in a trauma patient is most likely due to either solid organ or bowel injury and is a good indicator of injury severity. Careful attention should be made to the presence or absence of pelvic free fluid where small amounts of fluid are easily overlooked. When fluid is encountered on an MDCT of a trauma patient, an analysis of fluid density is very helpful. Clotted blood next to or adjacent to the bleeding site is called a *sentinel clot* (▶ Fig. 5.6).[21] This clotted blood is of higher density than more serous blood further away from the site of bleeding. Identification of the higher-density sentinel clot is helpful in identifying the site of bleeding.

After evaluation of the abdomen and pelvis for blood, individual organs are scrutinized. We scroll through the spleen twice. First, we look within the splenic parenchyma for areas of low or high density, with low-density areas representing splenic lacerations or fractures, and high-density foci material representing

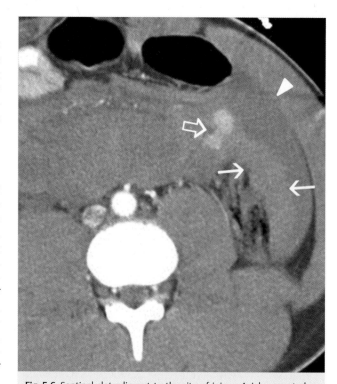

Fig. 5.6 Sentinel clot adjacent to the site of injury. Axial computed tomography shows high-density fluid collection (arrows) consistent with hematoma (sentinel clot) adjacent to the site of bowel injury (open arrow). The more lateral fluid collection is low in attenuation (arrowhead).

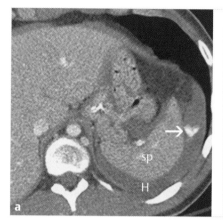
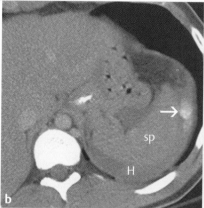

Fig. 5.7 Active bleeding of splenic injury. (a) Axial contrast-enhanced computed tomography (CT) demonstrates high attenuation focus (arrow) in the perisplenic hematoma (H) lateral to the spleen (sp). (b) Axial contrast-enhanced CT in a delayed phase demonstrates increase in size of the active bleeding (arrow) in the perisplenic hematoma (H) lateral to the spleen (sp).

active bleeding. A fracture of a solid organ is defined as a laceration that extends from one capsular surface to the other. Splenic lacerations are usually identified because of the hematoma within the splenic parenchyma. Whenever a hematoma is identified in or near the spleen, we then search for the presence of active extravasation of the contrast material (▶ Fig. 5.7), which usually signifies arterial bleeding. Recognition of active bleeding has dramatically increased with the introduction of MDCT with rapid administration of high-concentration contrast media. Sivit et al[22] first reported the demonstration of active intra-abdominal arterial bleeding in 1989 in a patient with splenic rupture from blunt trauma. Since then, multiple authors have emphasized the usefulness of detecting active bleeding in predicting the need for surgical intervention or embolization.[23,24,25,26] Detection of active extravasation on CT is usually considered an indication for splenic arteriography with possible embolization or surgery.

Splenic Injury Scoring System

The American Association for the Surgery of Trauma (AAST) Scoring System has been modified using MDCT information to classify the severity of splenic and hepatic injuries (▶ Fig. 5.8). With splenic injuries, Mirvis et al in 1989[27] proposed the following system:

- Grade I: Subcapsular hematoma or laceration < 1 cm
- Grade II: Larger subcapsular hematoma or laceration 1–3 cm
- Grade III: Capsular disruption or laceration > 3 cm
- Grade IVA: Shattered spleen or active extravasation into the spleen, subcapsular
- hematoma, pseudoaneurysm, or arteriovenous fistula
- Grade IVB: Active intraperitoneal bleeding

This scoring system has been criticized; several authors have found it unhelpful.[28,29,30] Others have found the scoring system useful in patients with massive splenic injury; most patients with grades IVA or IVB splenic injuries will require either surgery or embolization.[31]

Liver Window

The liver is the most frequently injured organ in trauma patients in general when both blunt and penetrating trauma is considered. In blunt trauma alone, the spleen is the most

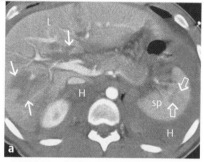
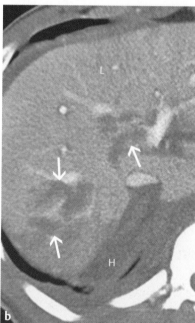

Fig. 5.8 Severe hepatic and splenic injury. (a) Axial contrast-enhanced computed tomography (CT) demonstrates a large perisplenic hematoma (H) with ill-defined low densities in the spleen (sp) consistent with a grade II injury. Again, noted are the lacerations (arrows) in the liver (L) with a hematoma (H) posterior to the inferior vena cava. (b) Axial contrast-enhanced CT demonstrates multiple low densities (arrows) in the liver (L) with subsapsular hematoma (H), consistent with a grade III injury.

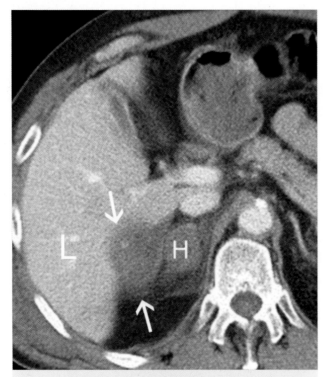

Fig. 5.9 Deep hepatic laceration. Axial contrast-enhanced computed tomography (CT) demonstrates a hematoma (arrows) in the posterior aspect of the right lobe of liver (L) consistent with laceration. Hematoma (H) is also noted in the right adrenal gland.

of great concern in hepatic trauma. Although injuries to the hepatic veins are rarely seen with blunt trauma, retrohepatic caval injuries have a high mortality rate. Venous injury is suggested on MDCT when lacerations extend to the inferior vena cava (IVC) or into the porta hepatis. With many venous injuries, the liver parenchyma itself compresses the laceration of the vein and no large hematoma may be detected. However, if a surgeon elevates the patient's liver, the tamponading effect of the liver parenchyma against the bleeding site is removed and the patient may exsanguinate on the operating room table. Therefore, if the MDCT suggests possible hepatic vein or IVC injury (▶ Fig. 5.10), the surgeon should be alerted to the finding prior to any operative intervention. The surgeon can then control the IVC prior to elevating the liver to prevent excessive bleeding.[32]

Hepatic Injury Scoring System

A hepatic classification system has been proposed.
- Grade I: Hematoma: subcapsular: < 1 cm
  - Laceration: Capsular tear: < 1 cm
- Grade II: Hematoma: 1–3 cm diameter subcapsular or
  - Intraperitoneal: < 3 cm diameter
  - Laceration: 1–3 cm
- Grade III: Hematoma: subcapsular: > 3 cm
  - Laceration: > 3 cm deep
- Grade IV: Hematoma: > 10 cm
  - Lobar tissue destruction (maceration) or devascularization
- Grade V: Bilobar tissue destruction (maceration) or devascularization

commonly injured organ. A survey of the liver is similar to that of the spleen, but requires more attention due to the complexity of the shape and the size of the organ. The initial review is of the deep hepatic parenchyma in the search for laceration or hematoma (▶ Fig. 5.9). A second scrolling through the liver is performed to evaluate the margin of the liver in the search for subtle lacerations or perihepatic blood. Finally, the right paracolic gutter in a trauma patient should be surveyed for a small amount of fluid. Occasionally in MDCT, subtle hepatic injuries may not be detectable, but perihepatic blood can be seen.

If a hepatic injury is identified, it is important to look for active extravasation. But besides arterial injury, venous injury is

Mirvis et al proposed a CT-based liver injury severity scale adapting the American Association for the Surgery of Trauma (AAST).[33] The ability of this CT system to predict the need for intervention either by surgery or by angioembolization has been questioned. One study that compared CT results with operative findings concluded that CT could underestimate the degree of liver injury.[34] They found that a large hemoperitoneum and the need for more than two units of blood predicted the need for operative intervention. Another study compared CT findings with outcome and concluded that the CT-based scoring system did not predict which patients required surgery or had complications.[30]

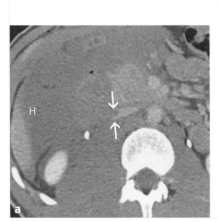
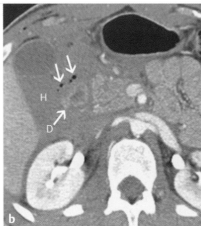

Fig. 5.10 Injury to the inferior vena cava (IVC) with perforation of the duodenum. (a) Axial contrast-enhanced computed tomography shows an irregular contour of IVC (arrows) with a large hematoma (H) nearby. (b) Axial contrast-enhanced CT shows air collection (arrows) adjacent to the thickened duodenum (D) in the center of a large hematoma (H). Surgery confirmed the diagnosis of IVC injury and perforation of the duodenum.

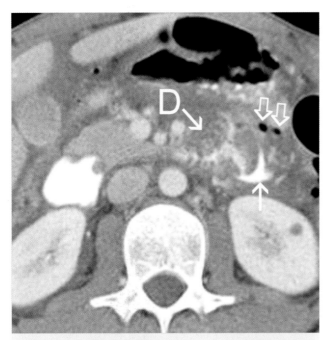

Fig. 5.11 Perforation of the duodenum. Axial contrast-enhanced computed tomography shows air collection (open arrows) and oral contrast extravasation (lower arrow) adjacent to the mildly thickened duodenum (D) (upper arrow). Surgery confirmed perforation of the duodenum.

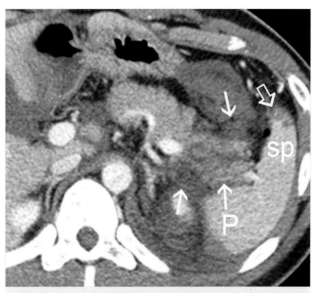

Fig. 5.12 Pancreatic and splenic injuries. Axial contrast-enhanced CT shows low densities in the pancreatic tail (P) surrounded by a hematoma (arrows). Low densities (open arrow) are noted in the anterior aspect of spleen (sp). Surgery confirmed injuries to the pancreatic tail and spleen.

5.3.5 Hepatic Bleeding

The diagnosis of active arterial bleeding in the liver with CT is more difficult than in the spleen. In a study comparing CT to angiographic or surgical findings in 77 patients, detection of increased intrahepatic attenuation for depicting active bleeding had a sensitivity of only 56%, a specificity of 83%, and an accuracy of 74%.[35] When an additional criterion of hematoma/laceration extending to the portal vein or hepatic vein was added to the presence of contrast extravasation, they found that 85% of patients with both findings had arterial bleeding. Patients that had neither finding of active extravasation or laceration extending to a major vein had the most reliable evidence to exclude hepatic arterial bleeding with 100% sensitivity, 92% specificity, and 95% accuracy.

5.3.6 Pancreatic and Duodenal Injury

Due to anatomical proximity, any injury to the pancreas or duodenum warrants careful scrutiny of the adjacent structures. Duodenal hematomas may be difficult to identify with only mild thickening present in the duodenal wall (▶ Fig. 5.11). Serosal tears of the duodenum producing a paraduodenal hematoma often have a triangular, pointed shape.

Pancreatic lacerations are often associated with duodenal or splenic injuries (▶ Fig. 5.12), but can occur without a detectable duodenal hematoma or splenic injury. Pancreatic lacerations may not manifest on the initial trauma MDCT. Traumatic pancreatitis requires time to produce edema within the pancreas; therefore, the initial CT may fail to show pancreatic injury

unless a laceration within the pancreas is large enough to be visualized or there is peripancreatic bleeding. One trick is to always look for fluid density between the pancreas and the splenic vein; normally, only fat is found between the pancreas and the splenic vein. If fluid is present between these structures, then there is either traumatic pancreatitis or actual bleeding into the pancreatic space. Larger pancreatic injuries will be detected as a linear laceration extending through the tissue of the pancreas. Pancreatic injuries often occur with a sheering injury slightly to the right or to the left of midline where the pancreas is sheered against the side of the vertebral body (▶ Fig. 5.13). Therefore, lacerations frequently occur either at the junction of the head and body of the pancreas to the right of the spine or within the body just to the left of the vertebral body.

The severity of a pancreatic injury is dependent upon the status of the main pancreatic duct. Although contusions to the pancreas may be treated conservatively, a laceration or transection of the main pancreatic duct usually requires either stenting or a surgical resection.

Any indication of injury to the pancreas warrants careful monitoring. Serum amylase may be used to detect changes in the amylase level, although the initial amylase obtained in the emergency department may be misleading. For instance, patients who have been subjected to head and neck injury may have an elevated amylase because of injury to the salivary glands, while the initial amylase in a pancreatic injury may be normal to only rise later.

In patients with possible pancreatic injuries, especially if the amylase becomes elevated on serial laboratory examinations, magnetic resonance cholangiopancreatography (MRCP) (▶ Fig. 5.14), or occasionally an endoscopic retrograde cholangiopancreatography (ERCP) may be useful to better assess the main pancreatic duct.

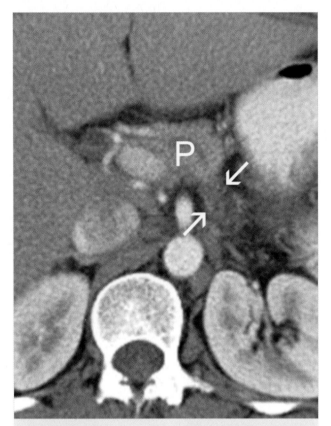

Fig. 5.13 Pancreatic injury occurring to the left of midline. Axial contrast-enhanced CT demonstrates marked atrophy of the proximal portion of the pancreatic tail and body (arrows) with an abrupt transition (left of midline) to the normal pancreas (P), consistent with prior pancreatic injury.

5.3.7 Kidneys

Evaluation of patients with possible renal injuries requires a different technique than with injuries to the liver or spleen. Injury to the kidney can produce bleeding or urinary leak. Although perihepatic or perisplenic fluid is usually due to blood,

perinephric fluid may represent either urine or blood. When renal trauma is suspected, it is essential to obtain delayed CT images (▶ Fig. 5.15). On delayed images, the perirenal fluid will remain unchanged if it is due to blood, but will become densely enhanced if it represents urinoma. If the CT is obtained after a sufficient length of time for contrast to have been excreted into the renal collecting system, the detection of urinomas is facilitated. A 2- to 3-minute delay is typically adequate. Multidetector computed tomography of abdominal trauma patients should include initial evaluation of the abdominal CT prior to removing the patient from the CT table. If there is any abnormality of the kidney, then delayed imaging is obtained. Likewise, if the patient is known to have hematuria prior to the CT, then delayed images are programmed prior to the initiation of the CT examination.

5.3.8 Retroperitoneal Structures and Evidence of Shock

Adrenal injuries can occur as isolated phenomena, but frequently are associated with renal or other organ injury. Adrenal hematoma usually manifests as a simple adrenal mass.

Analysis of the IVC is important in the detection of shock. When the IVC is flat or "slit-like" on at least three slices of the infrahepatic IVC, shock is suggested (▶ Fig. 5.16). We typically look at the IVC at the level of the left renal vein. A flat or "slit-like" IVC can be seen in normals when a rapid inspiration occurs, sucking blood out of the abdomen into the thorax. For instance, if the patient gasps during the CT examination, a flat-like cava may occur. Therefore, analysis requires seeing a narrowed IVC on at least three slices to increase the specificity of this finding.

A small spleen is also suggestive of shock. In a recent review of our experience of hypotensive patients in our emergency department studied with CT, we identified that the small spleen is an additional finding of hypotension. In patients who were hypotensive either in the ambulance during transportation to or on arrival in the emergency department, we found that mean spleen volume in hypotensive patients was 142 cc. Following fluid resuscitation, the spleen in the same patients was noted to increase to a mean volume of 227 cc.

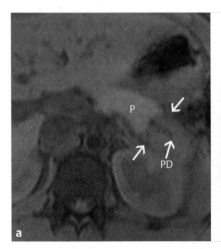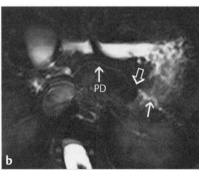

Fig. 5.14 Pancreatic injury demonstrated on magnetic resoance imaging (MRI) and magnetic resonance cholangiopancreatography (MRCP). (a) Axial T1-weighted MRI demonstrates marked decreased T1 signal of the pancreatic tail (arrows) with a dilated proximal pancreatic duct (PD) and an abrupt transition to the normal pancreas (P), consistent with pancreatic injury. (b) Axial MRCP demonstrates termination of the pancreatic duct at the junction of the pancreatic body and tail (open arrow), with a dilated upstream pancreatic duct (arrow) and a normal downstream pancreatic duct (PD), consistent with pancreatic ductal injury.

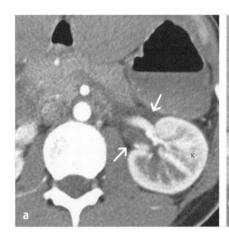
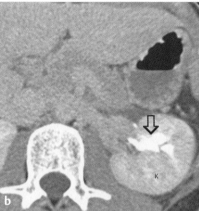

Fig. 5.15 Renal collecting system injury detected on delayed images. (a) Axial contrast-enhanced computed tomography (CT) demonstrates a small amount of fluid surrounding the renal hilum (arrows) of the left kidney (K). (b) Axial contrast-enhanced CT at the same level of (a) on a delayed image demonstrates contrast extravasation (open arrow) surrounding the renal pelvis of the left kidney (K), consistent with injury to the collecting system.

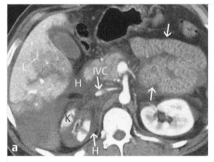
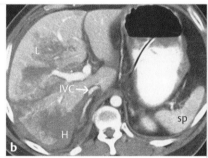

Fig. 5.16 Evidence of shock on multidetector computed tomography (MDCT). (a) Axial contrast-enhanced computed tomography (CT) demonstrates a small inferior vena cava (IVC), vivid enhancement of small bowel mucosa (arrows), perinephric and perihepatic hematoma (H) with extensive lacerations of liver (L) and right kidney (K). (b) Axial contrast-enhanced CT demonstrates a small spleen (sp). Again noted are the small IVC (IVC), perihepatic hematoma (H) with extensive lacerations of liver (L), consistent with shock.

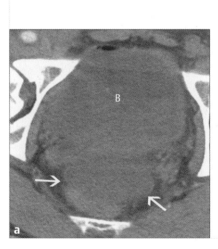
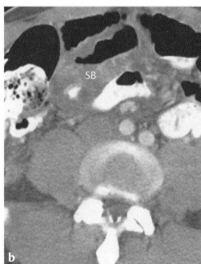

Fig. 5.17 Small bowel injury following blunt abdominal trauma. (a) Axial contrast-enhanced computed tomography (CT) demonstrates a moderate amount of complex fluid in the deep pelvis (arrows) posterior to the bladder. (b) Axial contrast-enhanced CT demonstrates a loop of ileum with marked wall thickening (SB). Surgery confirmed injury of the ileum.

5.3.9 Bowel and Mesenteric Injury

Detection of bowel injury with MDCT has improved significantly in recent years. Delay in the diagnosis of bowel injury is serious. In a study of patients who suffered small bowel injury from blunt trauma, the mortality rate was 2% if the diagnosis was made in less than 8 hours, increasing to 31% if the delay was over 24 hours.[36] In a multicenter study of 198 patients who suffered small bowel injury, it was reported that delaying diagnosis of small bowel injury was directly responsible for almost one half of deaths and even brief delays of 8 hours resulted in significant morbidity and mortality. In another study of blunt trauma

patients, 10% of patients who had solid organ injury also had hollow viscus injury. They also found that patients that had more than one solid viscus injury had a much higher rate of bowel injury representing 34.4%.[37] The solid organ with the highest frequency of associated bowel injury was the pancreas. If the pancreas was injured alone, 18% of patients also had bowel injury. If there is a pancreatic injury and any other solid organ, the rate of bowel injury was greater than 33%. Findings that are suggestive of bowel injury include free intraperitoneal air (▶ Fig. 5.1), free intraperitoneal fluid and wall thickening of the bowel (▶ Fig. 5.17).

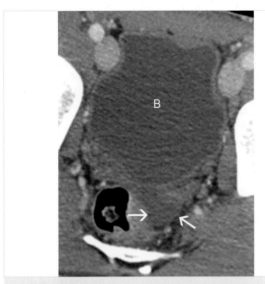

Fig. 5.18 Small amount of isolated pelvic free fluid in a male patient following blunt abdominal trauma. Axial contrast-enhanced computed tomography demonstrates a small amount of simple fluid in the deep pelvis (arrows) posterior to the bladder. Follow-up revealed no injury to the abdomen or pelvis.

Unfortunately, extraluminal gas is frequently not detectable even with a complete transection of the bowel. When a loop of bowel is fluid filled without air and is ruptured, there will be no initial release of gas into the peritoneum. Therefore, an MDCT obtained soon after a bowel injury will often fail to detect extraluminal gas. Free air has been reported as detectable on MDCT in 20 to 55% of blunt trauma patients with bowel injury.[33, 38,39,40] Extraluminal oral contrast is even less frequent than free intraperitoneal air. In one study, extraluminal contrast was detected in only 19% of cases.[41] In some institutions, oral contrast is not routinely administered to trauma patients and therefore in those patients extravasated contrast will not be seen.

Detection of intraperitoneal fluid is critical in identification of bowel injury,[42] but peritoneal fluid seen in a trauma patient can be either normal or abnormal. There are many nontraumatic causes of intraperitoneal fluid—the most problematic being "physiologic fluid" in women of childbearing age. In an unpublished ongoing study from our institution, we reviewed 175 CT scans of women of childbearing age who had been subjected to blunt abdominal trauma. Of those patients who had no evidence of injury on CT and required no operative management of abdominal injury, ~ 50% were identified to have at least a small amount of intraperitoneal fluid.

In the past, the detection of free intraperitoneal fluid in the male blunt trauma victim without identifiable source necessitated exploratory laparotomy to exclude occult mesenteric or bowel injury.[40,43] Recently, Drasin et al reviewed a one-year experience at a level 1 trauma center and found that 3% of male blunt trauma victims had free intraperitoneal fluid detected by MDCT.[44] All 19 patients with other CT detectable injuries to the abdomen or pelvis, but with free fluid were admitted for observation and none required surgery. In a study from our institution, we found that 4.9% (49 of 1,000) male blunt trauma patients had free fluid (▶ Fig. 5.18).[45] None had bowel or mesenteric injury. The four findings we described as required to ensure that the fluid is not result of bowel and/or mesenteric injury are (1) presence of fluid must be an isolated finding, (2) small in amount (seen on fewer than five contiguous 5 mm sections), (3) simple fluid in attenuation (less than 20 HU), and (4) located in the deep pelvis.

Besides nontraumatic causes of intraperitoneal fluid, there are a variety of fluid collections that could be related to trauma. Obviously, blood from bowel or solid organ injuries is a possibility. Traumatic causes of intraperitoneal fluid include not only blood, but also bowel contents, bile from a ruptured gallbladder or biliary tree, or urine from a ruptured urinary bladder. If a cystogram is performed, contrast extravasation from the injured bladder may be evident (▶ Fig. 5.19). Peritoneal fluids seen in a trauma patient can also arise from a combination of more than one injury.

The location of intraperitoneal fluid is very helpful in identifying the site of bleeding. Sentinel clots can be useful in identifying the site of bleeding. With solid-organ injuries, the initial bleeding occurs at the injury site and then extends further away from the site as bleeding continues. Therefore, hepatic or splenic injury blood will often extend into the pericolic gutters and then later into the pelvis. Only after the dependent locations in the peritoneum are filled, will fluid extend between the leaves of the mesentery. With a large amount of intraperitoneal blood from a solid organ injury, "interloop" fluid may be detectable (▶ Fig. 5.20). However, if bleeding occurs due to a bowel injury, the initial bleeding occurs into the interloop space and the dominant hematoma may occur adjacent to the

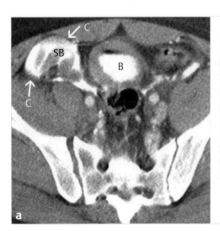

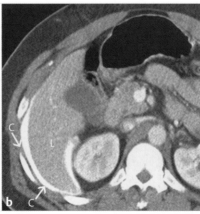

Fig. 5.19 Intraperitoneal bladder rupture following blunt abdominal trauma. (a) Axial contrast-enhanced computed tomography (CT) with CT cystogram demonstrates extravasated contrast (C) surrounding small bowel loop (SB) in the right lower quadrant. Bladder (B) is filled with contrast. (b) Axial contrast-enhanced CT with CT cystogram demonstrates extravasated contrast (C) surrounding the liver (L).

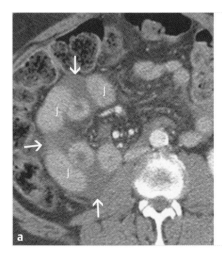

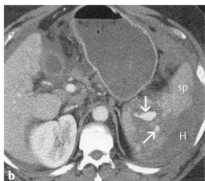

Fig. 5.20 Hematoma between the loops of jejunum due to a splenic injury. (a) Axial contrast-enhanced computed tomography (CT) demonstrates hematoma (arrows) between the loops of jejunum (J). (b) Axial contrast-enhanced CT demonstrates active bleeding (arrows) in the spleen (SP) with lacerations and perisplenic hematoma (H).

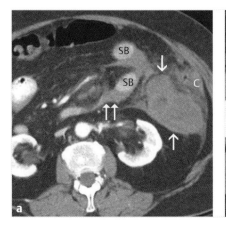

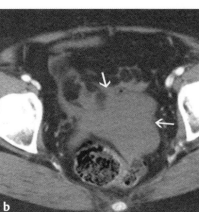

Fig. 5.21 Dominant hematoma adjacent to the descending colonic injury. (a) Axial contrast-enhanced computed tomography (CT) demonstrates a large hematoma (arrows) adjacent to the thickened descending colon (C). Hematoma (double arrows) in the interloop space of the mesentery. The small bowel (SB) is noted. (b) Axial contrast-enhanced CT demonstrates a large amount of complex fluid in the pelvis. Surgery confirmed perforation of the descending colon.

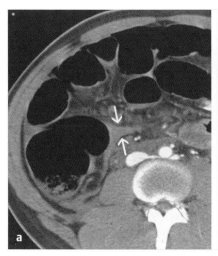

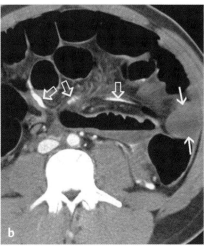

Fig. 5.22 Triangular-shaped fluid collection versus more-rounded shape of fluid within bowel loop. (a) Axial contrast-enhanced computed tomography (CT) demonstrates a triangular-shaped fluid collection (arrows) between the leaves of mesentery. (B) Axial contrast-enhanced CT demonstrates a more-rounded shape of fluid in the left abdomen (arrows), consistent with fluid within a small bowel loop. High-density foci (open arrows) in the mesentery indicate active bleeding.

site of bowel injury (▶ Fig. 5.21). Therefore, if blood is seen only between the leaves of the mesentery with no blood in the pericolic gutters or pelvis, then bleeding is likely from a bowel injury and not a solid organ injury.

The shape of abdominal fluid collections can be useful in differentiating fluid collection from unopacified bowel. Mesenteric or interloop fluid often manifests as V- or triangular-shaped fluid collection between the leaves of mesentery that are easily discerned from the more rounded shape of fluid within bowel loops (▶ Fig. 5.22).[46] The V or triangular shape is caused by the convergence of the mesenteric leaves at the root of the mesentery with fluid caught between the leaves tending to have a point or apex of a triangle that points toward the mesenteric root.

Bowel wall thickening is an important finding in the identification of bowel injury. However, because most small and large

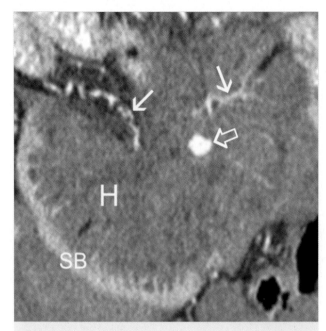

Fig. 5.23 "Beaded appearance" of mesenteric vessels in mesenteric vascular injury. Coronal reformatted computed tomography of the abdomen with intravenous contrast material demonstrates beading (arrows) of jejunal branches of the superior mesenteric artery. A large hematoma in the mesentery (H) with active bleeding (open arrow) was noted and was surrounded by a loop of small bowel (SB). At surgery, a large mesenteric hematoma with active bleeding and perforation of jejunum were found.

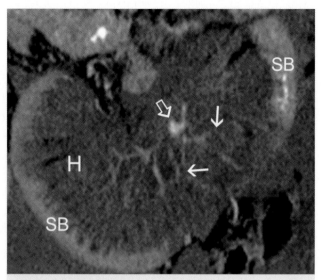

Fig. 5.24 "Abrupt termination" of mesenteric vessels in mesenteric vascular injury. Coronal reformatted computed tomography image of the abdomen with intravenous contrast material demonstrates abrupt termination (arrows) of jejunal branches of the superior mesenteric artery. A large hematoma in the mesentery (H), active bleeding (open arrow), and wall thickening of a loop of small bowel (SB) are noted. A large mesenteric hematoma with active bleeding and perforation of jejunum were found at surgery.

bowel loops are not opacified with oral contrast on a trauma patient's CT, identification of bowel wall thickening with confidence can be difficult. One useful trick is to consider that bowel wall thickening is almost always circumferential in a trauma patient. Therefore, if the anterior portion of the bowel loop is thin and the posterior appears thickened, this is likely due to underdistension or bowel contents, and not injury. Another trick is to use the concept that bowel injury is usually not a short segment, but often extends over 2 to 3 cm. Therefore, bowel wall thickening should only be called when it is seen in the same bowel loop on at least two contiguous slices.

Other MDCT signs of bowel or mesenteric injury besides free air, free fluid, and bowel wall thickening include mesenteric air, mesenteric hematoma, mesenteric fluid and/or stranding, active extravasation in the mesentery and two newly described findings, mesenteric vessel beading and abrupt vessel termination. Atri et al reported a case control study of 96 blunt trauma patients who underwent laparotomy and had MDCT.[47] They described the sign of "beaded appearance" of mesenteric vessels defined as an irregular contour of the vessels (▶ Fig. 5.23). The second sign was called "abrupt termination" of mesenteric vessels evidenced by lack of continuity or tapering of a mesenteric artery or vein (▶ Fig. 5.24). Of all the various signs on MDCT, the combination of the vessel beading or irregularity and abrupt termination of mesenteric vessels showed the best combination of sensitivity and specificity in identifying surgically important bowel and/or mesenteric injuries. Mesenteric vessel beading had a sensitivity of 50% and a specificity of 95%, whereas abrupt vessel termination was 45% and 93%, respectively.

The correct identification of bowel injury is important. In a report from San Francisco General Hospital, there were 46 patients that were reported with bowel injury who had a delay in diagnosis resulting in more than 6 hours from the time of injury to operative intervention.[38] The mortality rate was 4.3%.

5.4 Conclusion

Imaging of the abdomen with CT has become a part of the standard of care in the evaluation of most stable blunt trauma victims. Imaging is useful in selected unstable blunt trauma patients and occasionally with patients subjected to penetrating trauma. Familiarity with the CT findings of trauma is essential for radiologists and trauma surgeons.

References

[1] Branney SW, Moore EE, Cantrill SV, Burch JM, Terry SJ. Ultrasound based key clinical pathway reduces the use of hospital resources for the evaluation of blunt abdominal trauma. J Trauma 1997; 42: 1086–1090

[2] Senn N. Rectal insufflation of hydrogen gas as an infallible test in the diagnosis of visceral injury of the gastro-intestinal canal in penetrating wounds of the abdomen without laparotomy. The Medical News 1888; 52: 767–777

[3] Root HD, Hauser CW, McKinley CR, Lafave JW, Mendiola RP. Diagnostic peritoneal lavage. Surgery 1965; 57: 633–637

[4] Henneman PL, Marx JA, Moore EE, Cantrill SV, Ammons LA. Diagnostic peritoneal lavage: accuracy in predicting necessary laparotomy following blunt and penetrating trauma. J Trauma 1990; 30: 1345–1355

[5] Mirvis SE, Gens DR, Shanmuganathan K. Rupture of the bowel after blunt abdominal trauma: diagnosis with CT. AJR Am J Roentgenol 1992; 159: 1217–1221

[6] Brown MA, Casola G, Sirlin CB, Patel NY, Hoyt DB. Blunt abdominal trauma: screening US in 2,693 patients. Radiology 2001; 218: 352–358

[7] Dolich MO, McKenney MG, Varela JE, Compton RP, McKenney KL, Cohn SM. 2,576 ultrasounds for blunt abdominal trauma. J Trauma 2001; 50: 108–112

[8] Goldberg BB, Goodman GA, Clearfield HR. Evaluation of ascites by ultrasound. Radiology 1970; 96: 15–22

[9] Boulanger BR, McLellan BA, Brenneman FD, Ochoa J, Kirkpatrick AW. Prospective evidence of the superiority of a sonography-based algorithm in the assessment of blunt abdominal injury. J Trauma 1999; 47: 632–637

[10] Ballard RB, Rozycki GS, Newman PG et al. An algorithm to reduce the incidence of false-negative FAST examinations in patients at high risk for occult injury. Focused Assessment for the Sonographic Examination of the Trauma patient. J Am Coll Surg 1999; 189: 145–150, discussion 150–151

[11] Kinross J, Warren O, Darzi A. ATLS versus ETC: Time for a decision? Letter to the Editor. Ann Emerg Med 2006; 48: 761–762

[12] Yao DC, Jeffrey RB, Mirvis SE et al. Using contrast-enhanced helical CT to visualize arterial extravasation after blunt abdominal trauma: incidence and organ distribution. AJR Am J Roentgenol 2002; 178: 17–20

[13] Shanmuganathan K, Mirvis SE, Chiu WC, Killeen KL, Hogan GJF, Scalea TM. Penetrating torso trauma: triple-contrast helical CT in peritoneal violation and organ injury—a prospective study in 200 patients. Radiology 2004; 231: 775–784

[14] Novelline RA, Rhea JT, Rao PM, Stuk JL. Helical CT in emergency radiology. Radiology 1999; 213: 321–339

[15] Nguyen D, Platon A, Shanmuganathan K, Mirvis SE, Becker CD, Poletti P-A. Evaluation of a single-pass continuous whole-body 16-MDCT protocol for patients with polytrauma. AJR Am J Roentgenol 2009; 192: 3–10

[16] Tsang BD, Panacek EA, Brant WE, Wisner DH. Effect of oral contrast administration for abdominal computed tomography in the evaluation of acute blunt trauma. Ann Emerg Med 1997; 30: 7–13

[17] Stuhlfaut JW, Soto JA, Lucey BC et al. Blunt abdominal trauma: performance of CT without oral contrast material. Radiology 2004; 233: 689–694

[18] Mirvis SE, Whitley NO, Vainwright JR, Gens DR. Blunt hepatic trauma in adults: CT-based classification and correlation with prognosis and treatment. Radiology 1989; 171: 27–32

[19] Federle MP, Courcoulas AP, Powell M, Ferris JV, Peitzman AB. Blunt splenic injury in adults: clinical and CT criteria for management, with emphasis on active extravasation. Radiology 1998; 206: 137–142

[20] Halvorsen RA Jr McCormick VD, Evans SJ. Computed tomography of abdominal trauma: a step by step approach. Emerg Radiol 1994; 1: 283–291

[21] Orwig D, Federle MP. Localized clotted blood as evidence of visceral trauma on CT: the sentinel clot sign. AJR Am J Roentgenol 1989; 153: 747–749

[22] Sivit CJ, Peclet MH, Taylor GA. Life-threatening intraperitoneal bleeding: demonstration with CT. Radiology 1989; 171: 430

[23] Gavant ML, Schurr M, Flick PA, Croce MA, Fabian TC, Gold RE. Predicting clinical outcome of nonsurgical management of blunt splenic injury: using CT to reveal abnormalities of splenic vasculature. AJR Am J Roentgenol 1997; 168: 207–212

[24] Jeffrey RB Jr Cardoza JD, Olcott EW. Detection of active intraabdominal arterial hemorrhage: value of dynamic contrast-enhanced CT. AJR Am J Roentgenol 1991; 156: 725–729

[25] Federle MP. Splenic trauma. In: Federle MP, Jeffrey RB, Woodward PJ, Borhani A, eds. Diagnostic Imaging: Abdomen. Salt Lake City, UT: Amirsys; 2004: chap 6:20–21

[26] Stephen DJ, Kreder HJ, Day AC et al. Early detection of arterial bleeding in acute pelvic trauma. J Trauma 1999; 47: 638–642

[27] Mirvis SE, Whitley NO, Gens DR. Blunt splenic trauma in adults: CT-based classification and correlation with prognosis and treatment. Radiology 1989; 171: 33–39

[28] Umlas SL, Cronan JJ. Splenic trauma: can CT grading systems enable prediction of successful nonsurgical treatment? Radiology 1991; 178: 481–487

[29] Kohn JS, Clark DE, Isler RJ, Pope CF. Is computed tomographic grading of splenic injury useful in the nonsurgical management of blunt trauma? J Trauma 1994; 36: 385–389, discussion 390

[30] Becker CD, Spring P, Glättli A, Schweizer W. Blunt splenic trauma in adults: can CT findings be used to determine the need for surgery? AJR Am J Roentgenol 1994; 162: 343–347

[31] Federle MP. Diagnosis of intestinal injuries by computed tomography and the use of oral contrast medium. Ann Emerg Med 1998; 31: 769–771

[32] Halvorsen RA. MDCT of abdominal trauma. In: Saini S, Rubin GD, Kalra MK, eds. MDCT A Practical Approach. New York, NY: Springer; 2006:185–195

[33] Mirvis SE, Gens DR, Shanmuganathan K. Rupture of the bowel after blunt abdominal trauma: diagnosis with CT. AJR Am J Roentgenol 1992; 159: 1217–1221

[34] Durham RM, Buckley J, Keegan M, Fravell S, Shapiro MJ, Mazuski J. Management of blunt hepatic injuries. Am J Surg 1992; 164: 477–481

[35] Poletti PA, Mirvis SE, Shanmuganathan K, Killeen KL, Coldwell D. CT criteria for management of blunt liver trauma: correlation with angiographic and surgical findings. Radiology 2000; 216: 418–427

[36] Fakhry SM, Brownstein M, Watts DD, Baker CC, Oller D. Relatively short diagnostic delays (<8 hours) produce morbidity and mortality in blunt small bowel injury: an analysis of time to operative intervention in 198 patients from a multicenter experience. J Trauma 2000; 48: 408–414, discussion 414–415

[37] Nance ML, Peden GW, Shapiro MB, Kauder DR, Rotondo MF, Schwab CW. Solid viscus injury predicts major hollow viscus injury in blunt abdominal trauma. J Trauma 1997; 43: 618–622, discussion 622–623

[38] Harris HW, Morabito DJ, Mackersie RC, Halvorsen RA, Schecter WP. Leukocytosis and free fluid are important indicators of isolated intestinal injury after blunt trauma. J Trauma 1999; 46: 656–659

[39] Sherck J, Shatney C. Significance of intraabdominal extraluminal air detected by CT scan in blunt abdominal trauma. J Trauma 1996; 40: 674–675

[40] Breen DJ, Janzen DL, Zwirewich CV, Nagy AG. Blunt bowel and mesenteric injury: diagnostic performance of CT signs. J Comput Assist Tomogr 1997; 21: 706–712

[41] West OC. Intraperitoneal abdominal injuries. In: West OC, Novelline RA, Wilson AJ, eds. Emergency and Trauma Radiology. Washington, DC: American Roentgen Ray Society; 2000:87–98

[42] Dowe MF, Shanmuganathan K, Mirvis SE, Steiner RC, Cooper C. CT findings of mesenteric injury after blunt trauma: implications for surgical intervention. AJR Am J Roentgenol 1997; 168: 425–428

[43] Cunningham MA, Tyroch AH, Kaups KL, Davis JW. Does free fluid on abdominal computed tomographic scan after blunt trauma require laparotomy? J Trauma 1998; 44: 599–602, discussion 603

[44] Drasin TE, Anderson SW, Asandra A, Rhea JT, Soto JA. MDCT evaluation of blunt abdominal trauma: clinical significance of free intraperitoneal fluid in males with absence of identifiable injury. AJR Am J Roentgenol 2008; 191: 1821–1826

[45] Yu J, Fulcher AS, Turner MA, Cockrell C, Halvorsen RA. Blunt bowel and mesenteric injury: MDCT diagnosis. Abdom Imaging 2011; 36: 50–61

[46] Halvorsen RA, McKenney K. Blunt trauma to the gastrointestinal tract: CT findings with small bowel and colon injuries. Emerg Radiol 2002; 9: 141–145

[47] Atri M, Hanson JM, Grinblat L, Brofman N, Chughtai T, Tomlinson G. Surgically important bowel and/or mesenteric injury in blunt trauma: accuracy of multidetector CT for evaluation. Radiology 2008; 249: 524–533

6 Imaging of Peripheral Vascular Trauma

Mark Foley, Felipe Munera, Kim M. Caban, and Michelle Ferrari

Vascular injuries to the extremities are serious complications following both penetrating and blunt trauma. An early diagnosis of injuries is mandatory because delays in treatment can result in ischemia or subsequent compartment syndrome.[1] In the past, the radiologic evaluation of the vascular supply to the extremities was with conventional angiography beginning in the 1970s, and subsequently advanced with the advent of digital subtraction angiography (DSA), which to this day remains the gold standard for the detection of vascular injury. The significant benefits of DSA are twofold: to reduce the number of negative exploratory surgeries, which have a higher morbidity and mortality when compared with DSA, and in many cases to manage vascular injuries with less risks than surgical explorations. Angiography is invasive and has complications. The literature reports a morbidity of 1 to 2% of complications from the procedures, including vessel thrombosis, intimal dissection or plaque embolization, and arteriovenous fistulas (AVFs), as well as other complications.[2] Additionally, there are other indirect risks of DSA related to time needed to do the procedure, sedation and/or anesthesia risks, and the need of excessive moving and manipulation of a traumatized patient.

The introduction of angiography resulted in reducing the high percentage of negative explorations for suspected vascular injury; however, a high number of angiograms subsequently turned out to be negative for vascular injuries.[3] In attempts to decrease the number of negative angiograms, treatment algorithms using clinical assessment in combination with duplex ultrasound (US) and/or with ankle brachial index evaluation have been developed in most trauma centers (particularly trauma level I) with reported success in excluding clinically significant major vascular injuries.[4,5,6]

Computed tomography angiography (CTA) of the extremities, an imaging modality developed over the past decade offers a method to accurately evaluate noninvasively the extremities for vascular injuries. Computed tomography (CT) scanning has developed from a single-slice scan to helical CT and now multidetector CT (MDCT) scans. Currently, our ability to image noninvasive arteries and veins of the extremities has markedly improved. An MDCT (64 detection) scan is now widely available in most, if not all, trauma centers, allows faster scanning than ever before, and we can now acquire submillimeter isotropic datasets along the whole body including the extremities. This equipment allows true three-dimenaional (3D) volumetric reconstructions as well as diagnostic quality multiplanar reformatted images, with improved visualization of small vessels (such as the leg arteries and veins) below the knee to the level of the ankle. The fast speed of scanning allows us to image the entire body and extremities while the contrast arterial bolus remains in the arterial system.[7] We now can accurately diagnose vascular injuries to the neck, mediastinum, chest, abdomen, pelvis, as well as extremities.

Many studies have validated CTA as a highly accurate, noninvasive modality to assess injuries from penetrating, blunt, and iatrogenic trauma. Sensitivities of 95 to 100% and specificities of 87 to 10% have been reported in the literature.[8–13]

In our institute, we prefer CTA as an initial study in the workup of patients with suspected vascular injuries, both for patients with discrete penetrating traumatic injuries such as knife or gunshot wounds, as well as the blunt polytrauma patient involved in a motor vehicle crash or crush injuries who do not immediately require surgery. The advantages and disadvantages of CTA when compared with DSA are listed in the Box Advantages and Disadvantages of Computed Tomography Angiography (p. 54).

Advantages and Disadvantages of Computed Tomography Angiography

Advantages of Computed Tomography Angiography

- Less invasive than conventional digital subtraction angiography
- Fast and readily available in most emergency departments (24/7)
- Assessment of multiple areas and organs with a single study, which is of critical importance in the polytrauma patient
- Simultaneous evaluation of the perivascular and adjacent soft tissues and organs
- Less radiation—this is enhanced by development of automated dose-modulation methods
- Cheaper

Disadvantages of Computed Tomography Scan

- Limited evaluation of the smaller caliber vessels of the foot and hand secondary to the inherent spatial resolution capabilities of computed tomography angiography
- Intervention not possible if injury identified
- Not always possible to obtain diagnostic quality images
- Artifacts

6.1 Ultrasound

Vascular ultrasound (US) evaluation of the injured extremity is a modality with varying degrees of acceptance at trauma centers. It has some advantages over CT and DSA in that no iodinated contrast material is necessary and ionizing radiation is not utilized. It is portable and real-time information about arterial and venous flow is provided. Furthermore, intimal injuries, pseudoaneurysms, dissections, thromboses, AVFs, and vessel spasm have been demonstrated on duplex US. However, as an imaging modality it is very operator-dependent and can be limited in the evaluation of patients with extensive soft tissue injuries, open fractures, splints, or other foreign objects in the vicinity of the vessel to be examined. Although studies have shown a high sensitivity and specificity of US for the detection of arterial injuries (95–100% sensitive and 99% specific), most of these studies were performed with well-trained sonographers and in the constant presence of a physicians,[14] circumstances that are not always readily available in many trauma centers, particularly in the emergency situation and after "regular" working

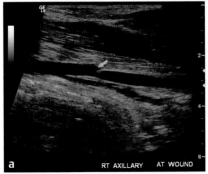
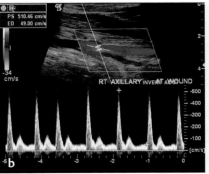
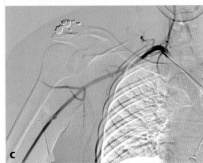

Fig. 6.1 A 26-year-old man with a right brachial artery injury resulting from a gunshot wound to the right axillary region. (a) Gray-scale ultrasound image demonstrating an intimal flap (arrow) along the proximal third of the brachial artery. (b) Color Doppler and spectral waveforms showing focal high-peak systolic velocities indicating high-grade stenosis along the lesion. (c) Digital subtraction angiography confirms findings. Bullet fragments are noted overlying the acromioclavicular joint.

hours. Another study involving 258 patients with penetrating trauma demonstrated a high specificity (100%) for vascular injury, although a lower sensitivity (72.5%).[15]

We use US in evaluating suspected vessel injuries in patients with an equivocal CTA and when DSA is not indicated, or if the clinical suspicion for vessel injury remains low. A focused US examination, in conjunction with the CT findings and the clinical examination may be sufficient for these patients. However, depending on the CT findings, a low threshold for proceeding to DSA should be maintained and discussed by the trauma team (▶ Fig. 6.1).

6.2 Clinical Evaluation of Arterial Injury

6.2.1 Role of CTA in Suspected Arterial Injuries

During triage of the trauma patient with a suspected vascular injury, the conventional treatment for unstable patients with obvious active hemorrhage and absent distal pulses is immediate surgical intervention. However, in more stable patients, a combination of clinical assessment and imaging studies are used to determine the further course of management.

The clinical assessment of extremities for arterial injuries, classically, has been and may still be classified into hard and soft signs. Hard signs include pulsatile bleeding, expanding hematoma, absent distal pulses, palpable thrill, audible bruit, and a cold, pale limb. In almost all cases, the presence of hard signs requires immediate surgical exploration and repair. Soft signs include hematoma, unexplained hypotension, peripheral nerve deficit, injury site in close proximity to a vessel, or a reported history of hemorrhage at the scene of trauma.

Some special injury patterns also have frequent association with vessel injuries such as posterior dislocations of the knee, tibial plateau fractures (Schatzker IV, Schatzker VI), "floating" knee injuries, supracondylar femur fractures, and elbow fractures or dislocations. These usually necessitate further vascular imaging.[16]

In patients with apparently normal distal pulses, the ankle/brachial index (A/BI) is another very useful adjunct in the workup for suspected lower extremity vascular injuries. This is done by obtaining the systolic blood pressure (BP) in the dorsalis pedis or posterior tibial artery and dividing by the systolic BP in the brachial artery. In a healthy patient, without peripheral vascular disease, the systolic BP in the lower extremities should be higher than in the upper extremities. In cases where the A/BI is > 0.9, most authors advocate conservative management, observing the patient and intervening only if the clinical course changes. Patients with A/BIs < 0.9 are suspected of having a clinical significant vascular injury and further evaluation is usually recommended.[17] Our suggested algorithm for evaluation of the injured extremity is provided in ▶ Fig. 6.2.

6.3 Technique of Extremity CTA

At our institute, most of the vascular injury patients have multiple other injuries such as in motor vehicle accidents, multiple gunshot wounds, stab wounds, or crush injuries. Therefore, in most cases CTA of the extremities is performed at the same time as whole-body CTA (WBCTA). Whole-body CTA is the routine method for scanning severe blunt polytrauma patients who had indications for cervical spine imaging, as well as contrast-enhanced body CT. Our protocol with a 64-slice scanner images the body from the Circle of Willis to the symphysis pubis. Scanning begins 20 to 25 seconds (depending on the patient's age) after administration of 100 mL of intravenous contrast material at a rate of 4 mL/s followed by a 40-mL saline "chaser" at

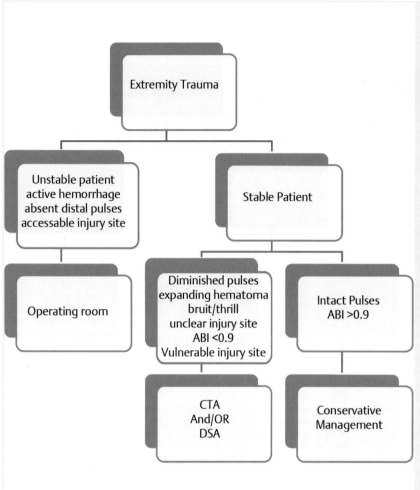

Fig. 6.2 Algorithm for the management of extremity vascular trauma. (CTA, computed tomography angiography; DSA, digital subtraction angiography)

Extremity Trauma

Unstable patient active hemorrhage absent distal pulses accessable injury site

Stable Patient

Operating room

Diminished pulses expanding hematoma bruit/thrill unclear injury site ABI <0.9 Vulnerable injury site

Intact Pulses ABI >0.9

CTA And/OR DSA

Conservative Management

a rate of 4 mL/s. A "portal vein" phase of the upper abdomen is usually obtained at 70 seconds. The scan can be extended in the early phase as required if the suspected extremity injury is proximal. If the injury is below the knee, our protocol requires imaging the extremity in question prior to WBCTA.

All images are reviewed on a PACS workstation. All source images, as well as multiplanar reconstructions are reviewed; routinely coronal and sagittal reformats are performed. Post-processed volume-rendered (VR) and maximum intensity projections (MIP) images are also reviewed on a color-display monitor. Additional postprocessing with 3D reconstructions as well as two-dimensional (2D) orthogonal, oblique, and curved linear plane images can be reconstructed from the source data by the on-call radiologist using thin client software. These images are available minutes after image acquisition. It is our experience that in the setting of extremity CTA, a dedicated orphan workstation is impractical for the purposes of the study. In cases where the patient has an isolated limb injury without clinical suspicion of thoracoabdominal injuries, a dedicated CTA of the extremities can also be performed (▶ Fig. 6.3).

6.3.1 Upper Extremities

Computed tomography angiography of the upper extremities is technically more challenging than CTA of the lower extremities.

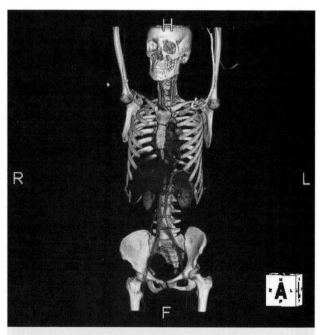

Fig. 6.3 Demonstration of a typical three-dimenional reconstruction of a whole-body computed tomography angiography performed routinely at our institution.

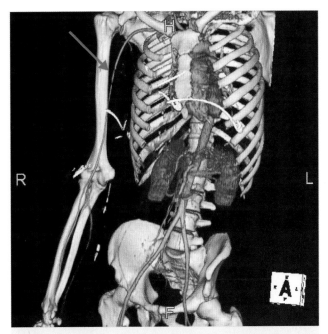

Fig. 6.4 A three-dimensional volume-rendered reformatted image of the upper-extremity computed tomography angiography runoff. Intimal injuries are seen in the right proximal to midbrachial artery (arrow).

Consideration must be made to position the patients' arms for optimal imaging of the vessels. If the patients have their arms above their head, CT imaging is less noisy, less degraded by adjacent attenuation, and subjects less radiation to the patient than if their arms are down by their sides. Positioning the patient with the arms up increases motion artifacts and in many cases it may not be possible due to the patient's clinical condition and cooperation for scanning. Contrast material bolus timing for the upper extremities consists of a 20-mL test bolus injected at 5-mL per second and images acquired every 2 seconds. Subsequent imaging must commence at 5 to 8 seconds after bolus arrival to completely opacify the upper extremity arterial system (▶ Fig. 6.4).

6.3.2 Lower Extremities

For the lower extremities, our institution prefers a 64-slice MDCT, with the following parameters: 0.6-mm-slice thickness, a pitch of 0.8, and interpolated slices of 1.3 mm with 50% of overlap (isotropic images). We image both lower extremities, even if only one is injured and our coverage includes the joint above and below the injuries. Contrast material bolus consists of 60 to 100 mL (Optiray, Mallinckrodt Inc., Hazelwood, MO; 350 mg of iodine per mL) injected through an 18- or 20-gauge cannula via an antecubital vein at a rate of 5 cc/s with 40-cc saline chaser to follow at 5 mL/s. The majority of our CTA studies of the lower extremities are performed as WBCTA studies, we prefer automatic triggering centered on the ascending aorta. If WBCTA is not being performed, then an "empiric" pause of 25 seconds prior to commencement of scanning of the lower extremities is adequate for good imaging (▶ Fig. 6.5).

6.4 CT Findings of Vascular Injury

A spectrum of vascular injuries occurs because the arteries and veins have several layers that can be injured independently or

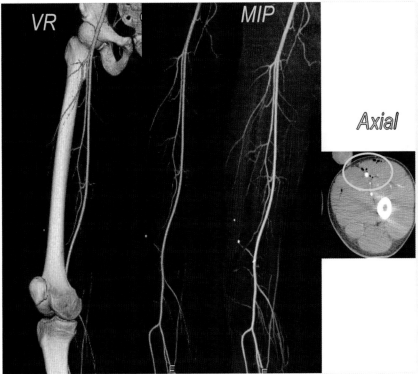

Fig. 6.5 Lower-extremity reconstruction using volume rendering, volume rendering after bone removal, and maximum intensity projection. The corresponding axial image shows a region of soft tissue injury with subcutaneous gas. However, the artery is intact.

Table 6.1 Types and site of vessel injury

Types of injury	Layers affected
Intimal	Intima
Intramural hematoma	Media
Dissection	Intima ± media
Pseudoaneurysm	Intima, intima and media, intima, media and adventitia
Transection	Intima, media and adventitia
Arteriovenous fistula	Intima, media and adventitia, and associated venous injury

together. The intima is a thin layer of endothelial cells in direct contact with the blood within the lumen. The media is the middle layer composed of smooth muscle cells and elastin, of varying thickness. The outermost layer is the adventitia, composed of connective tissue. The types of vessel injury are listed in ► Table 6.1 and described in detail below. Computed tomography angiography can identify all of these different lesions with high sensitivity and specificity.

6.4.1 Intimal Injury

Sometimes the only layer that is injured is the intima. In these cases, no extravasation of contrast is seen. Imaging abnormalities are, therefore, manifested as contour abnormalities, or focal, linear, or rounded filling defects within the lumen of the vessel on CTA. However, injuries to the intima may have intramural hematomas on occasion, resulting in enlargement of the vessel caliber, either isodense or hyperdense on CT imaging. However, usually in intimal injuries the caliber of the vessel remains normal. Intramural hematomas can also occur in the absence of intimal injuries due to traumatic injuries and rupture of the vasa vasorum. Due to its antithrombotic properties, the intimal injuries are prone to thrombosis and subsequent vessel occlusion (► Fig. 6.6). Treatment of intimal injuries and associated spasm, if present, is close clinical observation with a low threshold to proceed to DSA.[18] Anticoagulation may be given, if necessary. On occasion, surgical intervention may be necessary. Either primary repair or grafting is done. The choice is by the surgical team.

Arterial Dissection

Occasionally, results from an intimal injury can progress to involve a portion of the media and then propagate distally and/or proximally to separate (dissect) the layers of the artery. Computed tomography angiography demonstrates a longitudinal split of the wall layers with a linear or serpiginous filling defect within the lumen representing the flap. These findings taper much less smoothly and are more focalized than spasm (► Fig. 6.7).

Pseudoaneurysm

A pseudoaneurysm occurs when one, two, or three layers of the artery are injured. Usually the intima and media are damaged and the adventitia, the most resistant and tough layer is intact. However, on occasion, the adventitia is also lacerated and then

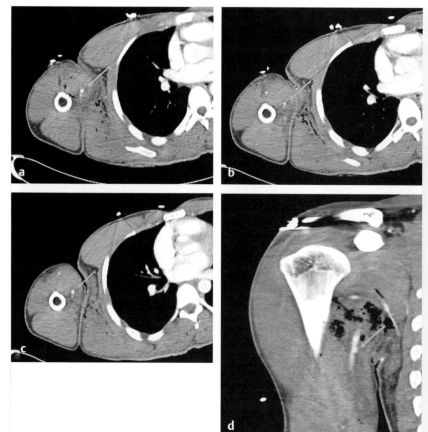

Fig. 6.6 Demonstrates the computed tomography angiography images of the patient injured. Axial images show an abrupt short segment caliber narrowing of the brachial artery (arrows) and the surrounding soft tissue swelling, edema, and air tracks, suspicious for spasm. (a-c) The coronal reformatted images demonstrate to better advantage the presence of irregularities of contour an intimal injury in addition to spasm. (d) This illustrates the contribution of isometric datasets.

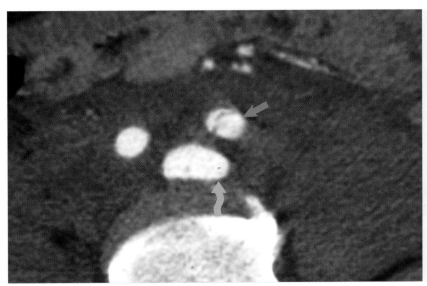

Fig. 6.7 Arterial phase of a contrast-enhanced computed tomography scan showing a traumatic intimal flap of the left common iliac artery (arrow). The oval hyperdensity anterior to the vertebral body is a traumatic pseudoaneurysm of the distal aorta (curved arrow).

frank extravasation occurs. Eventually the bleeding is contained by the adjacent tissues and a fibrous capsule may form in the chronic state. A pseudoaneurysm is formed when active bleeding is contained by surrounding fascia and the blood is eventually encased by a capsule of fibrous tissue, analogous in consistency to the adventitia of normal vessels. Some pseudoaneurysms present acutely, others chronically months to years later. Presenting symptoms include compression neuropathy, peripheral embolism, or soft tissue mass that represents the growing pseudoaneurysm. The risk of rupture of pseudoaneurysms is high because of the thin walls. Management includes US compression, US-guided thrombin injection para pseudoaneurysm injection or saline, or surgical repair. At this time, IR management is an alternative. The procedure is to embolize the lesion or to insert covered stents. Computed tomography angiography usually demonstrates a focal "ballooning" of the vessel wall filled with contrast material or a localized collection of contrast material adjacent to a vessel, artery, or vein (▶ Fig. 6.8).

Vessel Transection

Most trauma patients in whom a major artery is transected are hemodynamically unstable, requiring immediate surgical intervention. Penetrating injuries to the femoral, popliteal, or brachial arteries usually present with active hemorrhage, shock, or pulseless extremity. Some patients can present with vascular injury both proximally and distally to a complex fracture site. When evaluation of the entire extremity is necessary, and the patient's clinical condition permits, then CTA is useful for identifying any additional injuries. A complete transection disrupts all three layers of the vessel. Additionally, as large arteries function under constant longitudinal traction, transected vessels can go in spasm and retract as the hemostatic functional response. Therefore, no bleeding may be present upon admission (▶ Fig. 6.9).

Computed tomography angiography, in these situations, may demonstrate rapid extravasation of contrast into surrounding structures. On the other hand, absence of extravasation is not unusual for the reasons mentioned. Even in the presence of complete transection, the distal lumen may opacify due to collateral flow through uninjured branches. Other findings such as

an expanding hematoma or bone fractures could well be demonstrated.

6.5 Arteriovenous Fistulas

Arteriovenous fistulas are formed when both the artery and an adjacent vein are injured, and usually result from penetrating and iatrogenic trauma. The high-pressure arterial flow is directed into the low-pressure vein, diverting the blood supply to the distal tissues and causing engorging or distal veins. The flow through the relatively narrow fistulous connection is turbulent. Physical examination demonstrates palpable thrills and audible bruits. The clinical presentation may be delayed if the AVF is small and may manifest months to years later, as a pulsatile mass frequently associated with high output cardiac failure. Arteriovenous fistulas are suspected on CTA when the draining vein adjacent to an artery (such as the superficial femoral vein or subclavian vein) opacifies rapidly in the arterial phase. Computed tomography angiography may also demonstrate other signs of vessel injury, although in some cases, no other associated signs of injury may be present. Therefore, DSA may be necessary for a correct diagnosis (▶ Fig. 6.10).

6.6 Traumatic Occlusion

Traumatic occlusion is a relatively common injury after penetrating trauma to the lower extremities. Computed tomography angiography demonstrates lack of enhancement to the affected arterial segment, if completely occluded. On the other hand, a partial occlusion, often secondary to a dissection, will show marked narrowing of the vessel lumen with associated local signs of penetrating and blunt injury including venous injuries, hematomas, and others (▶ Fig. 6.11). Treatment options include interposition of graft, primary vessel repair, embolization, and different types of revascularization.

6.6.1 Vasospasm

In vasospasm, there is bone and soft tissue injury, the surrounding hematoma and soft tissue edema/swelling can occasionally

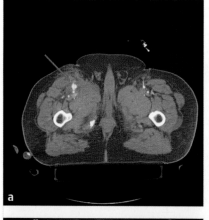
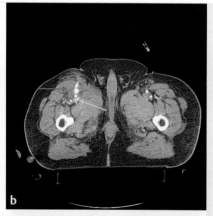
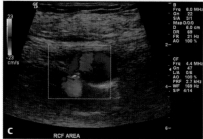
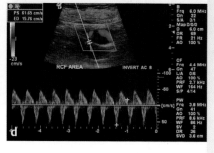
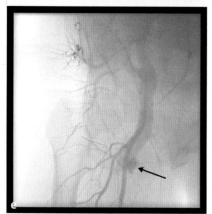

Fig. 6.8 A 68-year-old man fell 15 feet and sustained multiple pelvic fractures. (a) Computed tomography angiography demonstrates a localized collection of contrast material from the right superficial femoral artery (red arrow). (c) Duplex ultrasound demonstrates the typical ying/yang appearance of the pseudoaneurysm caused by to and fro flow of blood within the sac, seen both on color Doppler and spectral waveforms. (d) Digital subtraction angiography demonstrates the pseudoaneurysm and early filling of the common femoral vein indicating an arteriovenous fistula (AVF). (e) The AVF is noted on the computed tomography images given the density of the right superficial femoral vein is much higher than the contralateral side (black arrow). The superficial femoral artery is the rounded enhanced vessel between the two arrows.

cause external compression of an adjacent artery or spasm of the artery (▶ Fig. 6.12a). Computed tomography angiography may only demonstrate a diffuse narrowing of the caliber of the artery without focal filling defects (▶ Fig. 6.12b,c). Computed tomography angiography cannot rule out vessel injuries. If necessary, a DSA may still be required.

6.6.2 Indirect Signs of Vessel Injury

Some findings are demonstrable by CTA, which can suggest a vessel injury, even if no injury is visualized. These include signs such as a perivascular hematoma and injury trajectory leading to a blood vessel or bone/metallic fragments within 5 mm of a vessel. In these cases, evaluation with conventional angiography should be considered. ▶ Fig. 6.13 demonstrates an axial image of the pelvis in a patient who sustained a gunshot wound to the pelvis. The presence of a perivascular hematoma suggests a vascular injury.

Imaging Pitfalls

Unfortunately, many factors may limit the successful interpretation of CTA. These can be divided into technical factors and patient or injury factors. These pitfalls in diagnosis can be avoided with knowledge of the factors, proper technique, and multiplanar reconstruction and volume rendering, which can significantly reduce the number of nondiagnostic CTAs to ~ 1% (▶ Table 6.2).

Table 6.2 Pitfalls in computed tomography angiography

Technical factors	Patient or injury factors
Incorrect region of interest	Streak from bullet/metal or hardware
Poor bolus timing	Surrounding tissue injury/hematoma
Venous contamination	Patient motion
Spatial resolution of computed tomography limiting evaluation of small caliber vessels	

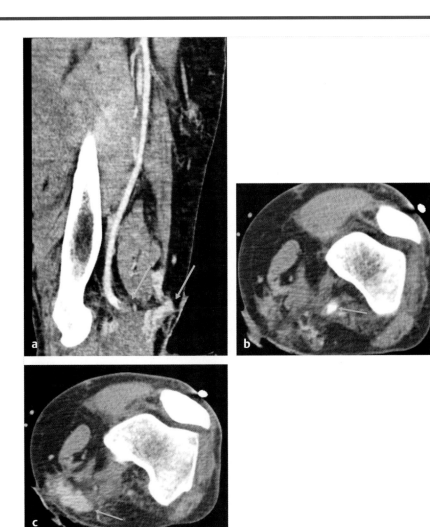

Fig. 6.9 (a) A 24-year-old man who fell from a ladder presented with absent pulses on Doppler ultrasound. There was also increasing left lower-extremity swelling, numbness, and pain. Computed tomography angiography demonstrates acute occlusion of the midsuperficial femoral artery and a small area of contrast extravasation (arrows). (b) Arterial and (c) delayed phases demonstrates extensive active extravasation medially in the midthigh (arrow). There is also absence of left popliteal artery enhancement, even during the delayed venous phase. At surgery, transections of the superficial femoral artery and veins were found.

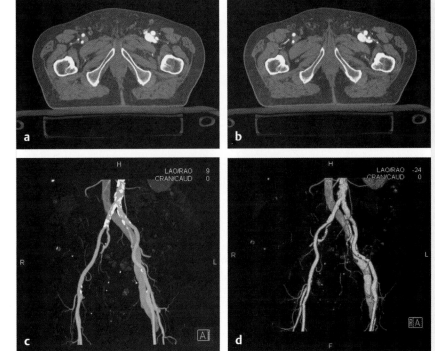

Fig. 6.10 A 93-year-old woman status post motor vehicle crash. Axial computed tomography angiography demonstrates early enhancement and enlargement of the left superficial femoral and common femoral veins. The density remains the same in the vein as the adjacent artery. There is direct communication between the profunda femoral artery and vein. An arteriovenous fistula is well redemonstrated on maximum intensity projection and volume-rendered reformats.

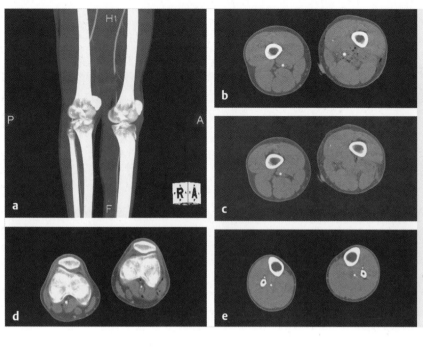

Fig. 6.11 (a) Volume-rendered reformatted images show traumatic occlusion of the left popliteal artery with distal reconstitution secondary to collateral flow through the profunda femoral branches. (b–e) Axial source images show the caliber change from above the injury to the level of the occlusion and gradual reconstitution of a normal vessel caliber at the level of the tibioperoneal trunk. Computed tomography angiography is useful in evaluating the adjacent soft tissues, identifying bullet tracts, and excluding osseous fractures.

6.7 Technical Factors

Regarding technical factors, operator-dependent factors can be improved with continued education and training of the technologists. We must select the appropriate region of interest and correct timing of the bolus administration and time of scan acquisition. Venous contamination can result from poor bolus timing, but can have physiological effects resulting from hyperdynamic circulation. It can limit or affect interpretation of the studies. Conversely, the scanning may "outrun" the bolus resulting in nonopacification of the mid- to distal vessels. This can be operator dependent or result from a poor cardiac output. The CTA findings are delayed opacification of the blood vessels. Last but not least, the evaluation of small caliber vessels in the hand and distal to the ankle is below the resolution of CTA.

6.7.1 Factors Inherent to the Patients

Streak artifacts from bullet fragments, metallic shards, shrapnel, or orthopedic or other hardware (pacemakers, ports, indwelling tubes) can result in limitation of the CTA study. Some of these limitations can be partially overcome with volume rendered and multiplanar reconstructions. But in some other cases, vessel injuries cannot be excluded; therefore, DSA is the study of choice, as has been in the past, before the advent of CTA (▶ Fig. 6.14). One tends to forget that DSA still remains the gold standard for vascular imaging regardless of the patient's condition and the size and caliber of the vessels to be evaluated.

Also, patient motion during image acquisition, a common occurrence in the setting of trauma, can render the CTA nondiagnostic, or limit the diagnostic accuracy for detection of arterial injuries. Unfortunately, due to venous contamination, as well as concerns about repeat contrast material administration, CTA is not usually repeated with a second bolus. However, in patients with normal renal function, a repeat CTA may be preferred to an "invasive" DSA. Although delayed imaging can

evaluate venous injuries in the pelvis,[19] there are no available reports of extremely venous injuries. Early venous filling can simulate a vascular injury such as an AVF, but the contrast material in the veins has the same density as in the arteries, whereas in venous contamination the density of the veins is lower than the density of the adjacent arteries.

Finally, difficulties in peripheral vascular evaluation are encountered in the elderly and diabetic patients with significant atheromatous disease and calcifications of the arteries (▶ Fig. 6.15a). Fortunately, vascular traumas affect younger patients with little or no arteriosclerosis or diffuse diabetic calcifications.[20]

In an elderly diabetic patient, lower-extremity CTA can show runoff. An MIP can demonstrate artificial occlusion of the mid-superficial arteries (▶ Fig. 6.15b). In a repeat scan, immediately afterwards, there may be increased visualization of the more distal arteries. The midcalf arteries can appear to be occluded. An aneurysmal dilatation of both superficial femoral arteries (arteriomegaly) can appear (▶ Fig. 6.15c).

6.8 Conclusion

Vascular injuries to the extremities are common occurrences in trauma victims, both penetrating and nonpenetrating, and also iatrogenic. If the patients are unstable or have "hard" signs of vessel injury, immediate surgical intervention remains the mainstay of treatment. The type of operation is dependent on the individual situation and the preference of the operators. This is beyond the scope of the textbook.

In more stable patients with a clinical suspicion of vascular extremity injury, CTA offers a safe, noninvasive, easy, and practical method for evaluating the arteries, as well as veins, the perivascular soft tissues, and bony structures with a high degree of sensitivity and specificity. At the present time, DSA is reserved for nondiagnostic or equivocal cases or when endovascular intervention is warranted.

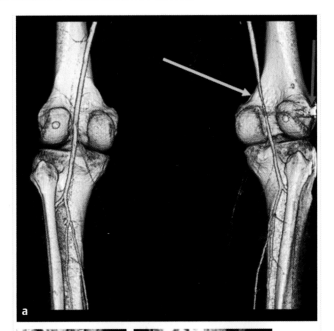

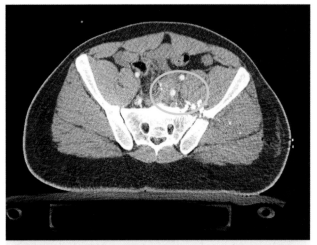

Fig. 6.13 An axial image of the pelvis in a patient who sustained a gunshot wound to the pelvis. The bullet tract is seen in the left gluteal region extending into the left iliac bone, which is fractured. Although no obvious vessel injury is identified, the presence of a perivascular hematoma (yellow circle) suggests a vascular injury.

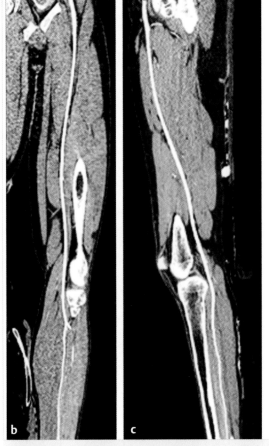

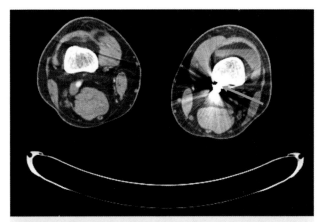

Fig. 6.14 Streak artifacts from bullet fragment (arrow) behind the tibia. The contralateral popliteal is well visualized. The left popliteal artery cannot be clearly distinguished from the adjacent bullet fragments. Digital subtraction angiography must be obtained. The associated finding is effusion with fluid level in the left knee joint.

Fig. 6.12 (a) A three-dimensional volume-rendered reconstruction of the popliteal arteries demonstrates spasm (yellow arrow) of the right popliteal artery with distal opacification secondary to gunshot wound. The bullet is lateral to the lateral femoral condyle (red arrow). (b,c) Multiplanar reformatted image demonstrates no focal injury to the artery despite the presence of an adjacent fracture in the distal femur and bullet tract. Therefore, multiplanar reformats can sometimes allow us to evaluate arteries even in the presence of streak artifact.

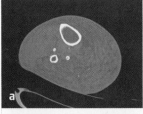
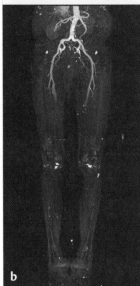
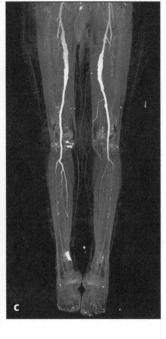

Fig. 6.15 (a) Computed tomography angiography (CTA) at the midcalf in 59-year-old man with diabetes demonstrating dense calcifications of the vessel walls, limiting intimal evaluation. These calcifications are usually not seen or identified during DSA. Therefore, in isolated cases of severe vascular disease, DSA will be required to exclude vascular injuries if there is clinical suspicion and CTA is nondiagnostic or equivocal. (b) Maximum intensity projection (MIP) images of a 74-year-old diabetic patient during lower-extremity CTA runoff. The first MIP demonstrates artificial occlusion of the midsuperficial arteries generated by the scanner outrunning the contrast material bolus. (c) A repeat scan, immediately afterward demonstrates increased visualization of the more distal arteries. The midcalf arteries appear to be occluded. In the setting of such baseline vascular disease, it was uncertain if the distal occlusion on the second study was also due to slow flow from poor cardiac output (although favored) or related to true vessel occlusion. There is aneurysmal dilatation of both superficial femoral arteries (arteriomegaly).

References

[1] Gonzalez RP, Scott W, Wright A, Phelan HA, Rodning CB. Anatomic location of penetrating lower-extremity trauma predicts compartment syndrome development. Am J Surg 2009; 197 Issue 3: 371–375

[2] Agaba AE, Hardiment K, Burch N, Imray CH. An audit of vascular surgical intervention for complications of cardiovascular angiography in 2324 patients from a single center. Ann Vasc Surg 2004; 18 Issue 4: 470–473

[3] Geuder JW, Hobson RW, Padberg FT, Lynch TG, Lee BC, Jamil Z. The role of contrast arteriography in suspected arterial injuries of the extremities. Am Surg 1985; 51: 89–93

[4] Johansen K, Lynch K, Paun M, Copass M. Non-invasive vascular tests reliably exclude occult arterial trauma in injured extremities. J Trauma 1991; 31: 515–519, discussion 519–522

[5] Kuzniec S, Kauffman P, Molnár LJ, Aun R, Puech-Leão P. Diagnosis of limbs and neck arterial trauma using duplex ultrasonography. Cardiovasc Surg 1998; 6: 358–366

[6] Mills WJ, Barei DP, McNair P. The value of the ankle-brachial index for diagnosing arterial injury after knee dislocation: a prospective study. J Trauma 2004; 56: 1261–1265

[7] Pieroni S, Foster BR, Anderson SW, Kertesz JL, Rhea JT, Soto JA. Use of 64-row multidetector CT angiography in blunt and penetrating trauma of the upper and lower extremities. Radiographics 2009; 29: 863–876

[8] Fishman EK, Horton KM, Johnson PT. Multidetector CT and three-dimensional CT angiography for suspected vascular trauma of the extremities. Radiographics 2008; 28: 653–665, discussion 665–666

[9] Soto JA, Múnera F, Cardoso N, Guarín O, Medina S. Diagnostic performance of helical CT angiography in trauma to large arteries of the extremities. J Comput Assist Tomogr 1999; 23: 188–196

[10] Soto JA, Múnera F, Morales C et al. Focal arterial injuries of the proximal extremities: helical CT arteriography as the initial method of diagnosis. Radiology 2001; 218: 188–194

[11] Busquets A, Acosta J, Colon E, Alejandro K, Rodriguez P. Helical computed tomographic angiography for the diagnosis of traumatic arterial injuries of the extremities. J Trauma 2004; 56: 625–628

[12] Núñez DB, Torres-León M, Múnera F. Vascular injuries of the neck and thoracic inlet: helical CT-angiographic correlation. Radiographics 2004; 24: 1087–1098, discussion 1099–1100

[13] Inaba K, Potzman J, Munera F et al. Multi-slice CT angiography for arterial evaluation in the injured lower extremity. J Trauma 2006; 60 Issue 3: 502–506, discussion 506–507

[14] Fry WR, Smith RS, Sayers DV et al. The success of duplex ultrasonographic scanning in diagnosis of extremity vascular proximity trauma. Arch Surg 1993; 128: 1368–1372

[15] Nassoura ZE, Ivatury RR, Simon RJ, Jabbour N, Vinzons A, Stahl W. A reassessment of Doppler pressure indices in the detection of arterial lesions in proximity penetrating injuries of extremities: a prospective study. Am J Emerg Med 1996; 14: 151–156

[16] Redmond JM, Levy BA, Dajani KA, Cass JR, Cole PA. Detecting vascular injury in lower-extremity orthopedic trauma: the role of CT angiography. Orthopedics 2008; 31: 761–767

[17] Levy BA, Zlowodzki MP, Graves M, Cole PA. Screening for extremity arterial injury with the arterial pressure index. Am J Emerg Med 2005; 23: 689–695

[18] Foster BR, Anderson SW, Soto JA. CT angiography of extremity trauma. Tech Vasc Interv Radiol 2006; 9: 156–166

[19] Anderson SW, Soto JA, Lucey BC, Burke PA, Hirsch EF, Rhea JT. Blunt trauma: feasibility and clinical utility of pelvic CT angiography performed with 64-detector row CT. Radiology 2008; 246: 410–419

[20] Miller-Thomas MM, West OC, Cohen AM. Diagnosing traumatic arterial injury in the extremities with CT angiography: pearls and pitfalls. Radiographics 2005; 25 Suppl 1: S133–S142

7 The Role of Nuclear Medicine Imaging in Trauma

Paul R. Jolles

Although other imaging modalities such as plain film radiographs, computed tomography (CT), and angiography/interventional radiology play a major role in the evaluation of the acute trauma patient, scintigraphy can provide useful information in some clinical situations. Here some of these contributions are described.

7.1 Musculoskeletal Trauma

7.1.1 Radiopharmaceuticals

The bone-seeking radiopharmaceuticals, mainly Tc-99 m methylene diphosphonate (MDP) and Tc-99 m hydroxymethylene diphosphonate (HMDP), are injected intravenously in an average adult dose of 20 millicurie (mCi; 740 megabecquerel [MBq]) and bind to the hydroxyapatite (HA) crystal within bone.[1] Tracer uptake is generally dependent upon perfusion and the degree of osseous reaction or remodeling.[2] These agents are cleared rapidly from the blood. Approximately 45 to 55% of the tracer localizes in the skeleton at 3 hours, with most of the residual tracer being excreted by the kidneys.[3] The skeleton receives the highest radiation dose, followed by the urinary bladder. The effective dose equivalent (based on a 20 mCi dose of Tc-99 m MDP) is 0.44 rem (roentgen equivalent in man).[4] The radiation dose may be reduced with frequent voiding and increased fluid intake.

7.1.2 Fractures

Bone scintigraphy is useful in evaluating trauma patients with suspected multiple fractures, those with a solitary skeletal injury (stress injury and insufficiency fractures) (▶ Fig. 7.1), and children with possible nonaccidental injuries (battered child syndrome). Bone scintigraphy can be a valuable tool for detecting fractures not radiographically apparent. One advantage of this modality is that after the patient receives the radiopharmaceutical dose, there is no extra radiation exposure regardless of the number of images necessary to help detect the abnormality.

Planar imaging is usually performed 2 to 3 hours after injection of the tracer. Three-phase imaging (arterial blood flow, blood pool, and delayed phases) can be utilized to evaluate the acuity or age of a fracture, with tracer uptake on the first two phases subsiding with progressive healing. Cross-sectional imaging with single photon emission computed tomography (SPECT) is a more sensitive technique that also provides better anatomic localization. This can be made even more powerful with the addition of concurrent CT (SPECT/CT).[5]

The sensitivity of bone scintigraphy for detection of fractures is ~ 95%, with scans appearing abnormal as early as a few hours after injury.[5,6] There is some evidence that fractures in patients over age 65 (who are prone to osteoporosis) might require as long as 3 days to show increased tracer uptake on scintigraphy[5]; this should be taken into consideration when planning patient imaging studies. Utility for demonstrating scaphoid fractures has been documented.[7] Single photon emission computed tomography is a more sensitive, cross-sectional technique that is particularly useful in the evaluation of the spine, such as in pars interarticularis stress injuries,[8] as well as in the distal extremities. Enhanced capability for anatomical localization is achieved with the addition of SPECT/CT.[9]

Bone scintigraphy provides valuable information in pediatric trauma. Children with battered child syndrome have been studied prospectively with radiographic skeletal surveys and bone scintigraphy. In a group of 50 children who had both imaging tests performed, one study[10] reported that the skeletal survey detected 54% of the fractures, while bone scintigraphy detected 88%. It was recommended that children receive both tests if either one is initially negative.

7.1.3 Heterotopic Ossification

Heterotopic ossification (HO) refers to the development of mature bone in locations outside of the skeleton. It has a tendency to occur in patients with a history of trauma that includes head injury and spinal cord injury,[11] and more often in head injury and femoral shaft fractures.[12] Ostensibly, the appearance of HO is related to some change in the tissue biochemical milieu following a traumatic injury, although the exact underlying mechanisms have yet to be identified. Differentiation of mesenchymal cells into osteogenic cells, whose products result in

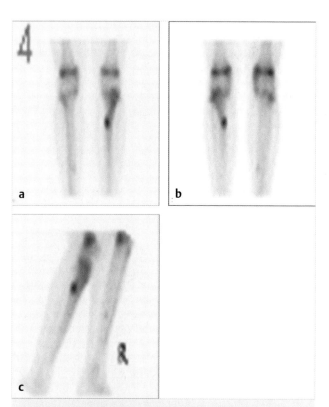

Fig. 7.1 Tc-99 m methylene diphosphonate bone scan. Delayed imaging showing a left tibial stress fracture and early stress injury of the right tibia. Plain film radiographs were negative.

collagen and subsequent bone formation, has been proposed as an initiating factor.[13] The "triple phase" bone scan can detect HO formation at the earliest stage, about 2 weeks following trauma, with the typical findings of increased blood flow, blood pool activity and delayed tracer uptake seen up to 4 weeks prior to radiographic abnormality. With maturity, the flow and blood pool phases recede in tracer intensity.[14] Early detection for initiation of therapy is important, given that progression can lead to joint immobilization. Also, surgical resection prior to maturity typically results in recurrence. A retrospective study of patients with traumatic brain injury (TBI) indicated a poorer functional outcome in those with HO; however, it was not clear as to whether HO caused the decreased function, or served as an indicator of those patients who would not progress as far or as rapidly during rehabilitation.[15]

7.1.4 Complex Regional Pain Syndrome Type 1

Complex regional pain syndrome type 1 (CRPS-1), also known as reflex sympathetic dystrophy, is a syndrome consisting of an instigating event (such as trauma); continuing pain that is disproportionate to any inciting event; evidence at some point of edema, changes in blood flow or abnormal sudomotor activity in the region of pain; the absence of conditions that would otherwise account for degree of pain and dysfunction.[16,17] Nontraumatic initiating events have also been noted, including stroke, spinal spondylosis, and disk herniation.[18] Three-phase bone scintigraphy can be useful in helping establish the diagnosis of CRPS-1, typically showing increased periarticular uptake of the radiopharmaceutical.[19] Scintigraphy changes generally predate radiographic abnormality, which usually consists of osteoporosis.[20] In the early stages, increased flow, blood pool activity and delayed uptake have been described in the bones of the upper extremity, particularly the hands.[21] Later, decreased or normal perfusion may be seen, with a decrease in delayed uptake.[22]

There are varying opinions regarding the sensitivity and specificity of bone scintigraphy for CRPS-1, both favorable[23] and unfavorable.[24]

7.1.5 Rhabdomyolysis

Rhabdomyolysis is the breakdown of muscle fibers resulting in the release of muscle fiber contents (myoglobin) into the bloodstream. It is a potentially life-threatening condition arising from the development of acute renal failure, compartment syndrome, cardiac arrhythmias, and coagulopathy.[25] Although the cause is not always related to direct trauma, it is known to occur as a result of crush injury and other traumatic mechanisms.[26,27] Early diagnosis and treatment are important for a satisfactory patient outcome.[28] Although usually diagnosed by laboratory abnormalities such as an elevated serum creatine phosphokinase (CPK),[28] it has been noted that bone radiotracers localize in regions of muscle injury.[29] In a study of patients with early mild rhabdomyolysis,[30] it was suggested that bone scintigraphy might help distinguish between traumatic and nontraumatic etiologies. Asymmetric localized soft tissue uptake was found to be associated with traumatic lesions, and negative findings were found in those with mild nontraumatic lesions.

Myocardial Contusion

Blunt thoracic trauma may result in injury to the myocardium. Of the commonly available clinical and diagnostic tests, troponin levels and electrocardiographic findings appear to be the most useful indicators.[31] Echocardiography is a useful tool in identifying areas of regional dysfunction.[32] However, the populations of patients sustaining chest trauma are quite diverse, and neither the sensitivity nor specificity of these tests may be optimal.[33,34] Radio-labeled myocardial perfusion agents, most recently thallium-201 chloride with SPECT technique, have been employed to assess for evidence of myocardial contusion. These studies have not yielded results to justify routine utilization, although there are reports that perfusion defects may be predictive of the development of arrhythmias.[35,36,37] A case report has described the use of fluorine-18 fluorodeoxyglucose (FDG) (in combination with thallium-201 chloride SPECT) to detect nonviable myocardium.[38]

Renal Injury

Renal injury in trauma patients is often detected by multidetector CT in the emergency department. The CT findings are used to determine the grade of renal injury, such as has been described in the American Association for the Surgery of Trauma (AAST) scale.[39] The grade of renal injury is directly correlated with the need for nephrectomy in cases of penetrating trauma, and predictive of nephrectomy, dialysis, and even death in patients with blunt injury.[40] More recently, it has been found that the decrease in renal function as depicted with the cortical renal imaging agent Tc-99 m dimercaptosuccinic acid (DMSA) is directly correlated with the AAST injury grade.[41] Therefore, renal cortical scintigraphy may be a valuable adjunct in evaluating trauma patients with kidney injury. Functional renal evaluation with Tc-99 m DMSA is useful in children after kidney trauma, providing information about the extent of the injury and helping guide follow-up.[42] In addition, scintigraphy permits the noninvasive quantitatation of global and regional renal function, a unique feature which is highly informative when comparing baseline and follow-up studies. Another tracer that exhibits renal cortical binding (although not to the degree of Tc-99 m DMSA) is Tc-99 m glucoheptonate (GH), which may be utilized if desired.

Scrotal Trauma

While only associated with trauma in ~ 4 to 12% of cases,[43,44,45] untreated testicular torsion can result in loss of the testis and therefore early diagnosis is essential. Scrotal scintigraphy was introduced nearly forty years ago,[46] and subsequently was found to have an ~ 93 to 98% sensitivity and 100% specificity[47,48] for the detection of testicular torsion. Typically, the study consists of flow and blood pool imaging of the scrotum after the intravenous injection of Tc-99 m pertechnetate, with testicular torsion manifesting as a photon deficit. Conversely, inflammatory conditions cause hyperemia on the involved side. However, in most cases, initial imaging evaluation of the painful scrotum following trauma is with ultrasound (US). Routinely available in the emergency department and not utilizing ionizing radiation, US with Doppler capability generally provides an excellent and rapid assessment of testicular perfusion and

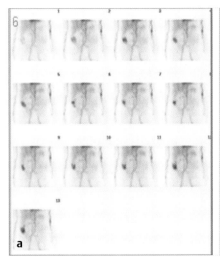 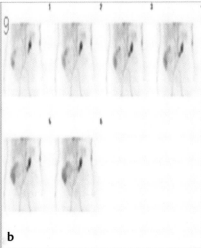

Fig. 7.2 Gastrointestinal bleeding scan. Tc-99 m labeled red blood cells. (a,b) Sequential imaging shows an active ascending colonic bleed, with movement into the splenic flexure.

depiction of anatomic abnormality.[49,50,51] Practice guidelines have recently been published by the American Institute of Ultrasound in Medicine.[52] Scrotal scintigraphy is easily performed and can be a useful imaging when US results are indeterminate.

Gastrointestinal Bleeding

Trauma patients may present with, or subsequently develop, gastrointestinal (GI) bleeding. Although immediate surgery or angiography may be indicated for patients with catastrophic bleeding, there is a more stable population in which noninvasive diagnostic testing is appropriate to help localize the sites of bleeding. In general, DSA can detect GI bleeding at a rate of ~ 0.5 to 1 mL/min. However, a less invasive study to confirm active bleeding would be preferable prior to DSA. Early scintigraphy GI bleeding studies in an animal model[53] employed the intravenous injection of Tc-99 m sulfur colloid, an agent rapidly taken up by the reticuloendothial system. With active bleeding, there is extravasation into the bowel, which is detected by serial sequential imaging. This technique was able to depict GI bleeding at a rate of ~ 0.1 ml/min. Tc-99 m sulfur colloid imaging has some limitations because it is rapidly cleared from the blood pool with a half-time of ~ 2 to 3 minutes[54] and is therefore best suited to localize active bleeding at the time of tracer injection. A technique employing a much longer circulating tracer, Tc-99 m labeled autologous red blood cells, was developed, and later shown to have a similar sensitivity in detecting active GI bleeding.[55,56,57] Sequential imaging is typically performed for 1 to 2 hours, increasing the capability to detect intermittent bleeding (▶ Fig. 7.2). Because of the relatively long half-life of circulating labeled red blood cells, imaging up to 24 hours is possible; however, the diagnostic accuracy at that time is usually suboptimal and of questionable clinical utility. More recently, improved accuracy in localizing the site of bleeding was reported using Tc-99 m labeled red blood cells and SPECT/CT.[58]

7.1.6 Bile Leaks

The spectrum of traumatic liver injuries ranges from mild to severe, associated with an increasing incidence of morbidity and mortality.[59] Patients sustaining trauma to the liver may

develop a bile leak, typically manifested as a fluid collection on CT or US. Some bile leaks do not require surgical repair. A minimally invasive approach can be taken after blunt trauma in children, utilizing operative endoscopy, interventional radiology, and laparoscopic surgery.[60] During hospitalization, there may be a clinical interest in determining whether the leak is active. This is easily done noninvasively with radiotracers that are in the chemical class of iminodiacetic acid compounds, mainly Tc-99 m disofenin and Tc-99 m mebrofenin, and are actively taken up into the hepatocytes similar to bilirubin, but do not subsequently undergo conjugation. After excretion into the biliary cannaliculi, the tracers accompany the flow of bile into the gall bladder (if the cystic duct is patent) and then into the duodenum via the common duct.[61] However, if there is a bile leak, extravasation is noted, with the radioactivity taking a course that appears extraluminal. Often, the tracer will progress into the dependent portions of the abdomen, such as the paracolic gutters. A diffuse peritoneal pattern can also be seen. However, if the bile leak is contained or loculated, a focal progressive accumulation will be noted.[62] Typically, planar sequential imaging over the anterior abdomen is performed for at least one hour, although a longer period of surveillance can be chosen. As in other scintigraphic applications, adding SPECT/CT may allow more precise anatomic localization.[63] Biliary scintigraphy have a major positive impact on the diagnosis and management of bile leaks associated with abdominal trauma, resulting in less invasive drainage procedures and a shorter hospital stay.[64,65]

7.2 Cerebral Perfusion: Brain Death

Some patients with catastrophic injuries may subsequently require evaluation for brain death. The determination of brain death in adults is made using clinical criteria, with the most recently updated evidence-based guidelines published in the report of the Quality Standards Subcommittee of the American Academy of Neurology in 2010.[66] Although procedures may vary in different states, the practical guidance is as follows: (1) establish irreversible and proximate cause of coma; (2) achieve core temperature; (3) achieve normal systolic blood pressure; and (4) perform one neurologic examination (sufficient to

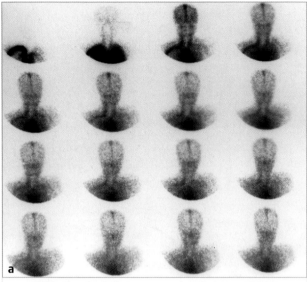

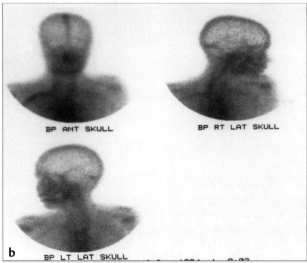

BP ANT SKULL   BP RT LAT SKULL

BP LT LAT SKULL

Fig. 7.3 Planar Tc-99 m diethylene triamine penta-acetic acid (DTPA) cerebral perfusion studies. (a,b) Normal arterial perfusion and venous sinus blood pool activity in a patient with intact brain perfusion.

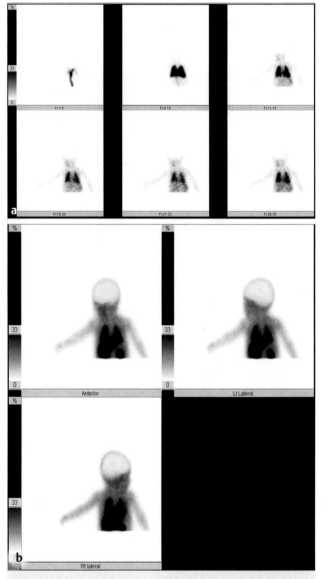

Fig. 7.4 Planar Tc-99 m diethylene triamine penta-acetic acid (DTPA) cerebral perfusion studies. (a,b) Absent arterial and venous sinus activity in a 2-month-old patient with a history of head injury and diagnosis of brain death.

pronounce brain death in most U.S. states; some states may require two examinations). The neurologic assessment includes confirming coma, the absence of brainstem reflexes and apnea.

Although these measures usually suffice to determine brain death, ancillary tests may be used in cases of uncertainty. Preferred tests as noted in the above report include electroencephalography (EEG), cerebral angiography, and nuclear scanning.

For over 40 years, radiopharmaceuticals have been used to assess cerebral perfusion in the setting of clinically suspected brain death. Early techniques focused on the arterial and venous phases of cerebral perfusion, with radiopharmaceuticals such as Tc-99 m pertechnetate,[67] Tc-99 m diethylene triamine pentaacetic acid (DTPA), and Tc-99 m GH, which are not ordinarily taken up into the brain parenchyma. Following the injection of radiotracers, serial dynamic images are first obtained over the upper chest, neck, and head in the anterior projection.

In patients with intact cerebral perfusion, tracer activity can be identified progressing up the carotid arteries in the neck and into the anterior and middle cerebral artery distributions in the brain. Subsequently, blood pool imaging exhibits tracer activity in the venous sinuses (▶ Fig. 7.3). Patients with absent cerebral perfusion will typically show tracer distribution in the cerebral arteries distributions on the arteriography phase, as well as absent venous sinus activity (▶ Fig. 7.4).[68] It has been observed that tracer activity may be seen in the venous sinuses in the absence of cerebral arterial perfusion, likely due to collateral circulation.[69]

In recent years, lipophilic (diffusible) radiotracers that cross the blood–brain barrier and localize in the brain parenchyma have been employed for the assessment of cerebral perfusion in cases of suspected brain death. These agents include Tc-99 m hexamethylpropyleneamine oxime (HMPAO) and Tc-99 m bicisate (ECD), which have similar brain uptake.[70] Patients with

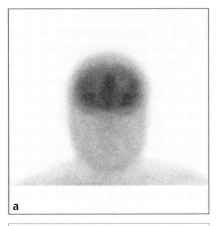
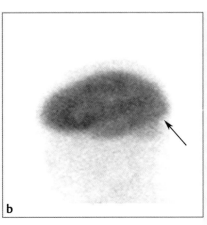

Fig. 7.5 Planar Tc-99 m bicisate brain perfusion study showing bilateral cerebellar hypoperfusion in a patient with computed tomogtaphy evidence of cerebellar ischemia (arrows). Intact cerebral hemispheric perfusion.

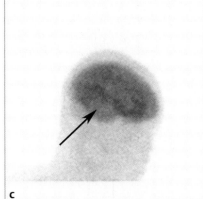

intact cerebral perfusion will exhibit immediate tracer activity in the anterior and middle cerebral circulations, and delayed uptake within the cerebral and cerebellar hemispheres, as well as the brain stem. Single photon emission computed tomography imaging can also be performed, if more anatomical detail is desired.[68] No tracer uptake is seen in the cerebral or cerebellar hemispheres, or the brainstem, in patients with brain death.

Occasionally, it may be found that only certain portions of the brain exhibit tracer uptake, indicating blood flow (▶ Fig. 7.5). Given that the diffusible tracers permit a more detailed picture of perfusion to the brain and brainstem, the use of these agents is preferred over the nondiffusible agents such as Tc-99 m DTPA. However, one study directly comparing Tc-99 m DTPA and Tc-99 m HMPAO for the evaluation of brain death showed identical results.[71] Regarding the diffusible tracers, a review of the literature from 1980 to 2008 reported that the sensitivity of absent blood flow on planar imaging for clinically confirmed brain death was 77.8%, and the specificity was 100%. With SPECT imaging, the sensitivity was 88.4%, and the specificity was 100%.[72]

7.3 Traumatic Brain Injury

Initial imaging evaluation of patients presenting with TBI typically involves CT and, perhaps also, magnetic resonance imaging (MRI). As a general rule, brain scintigraphy plays no major role in the clinical management of acute traumatic brain injury. However, perfusion (SPECT) and metabolic (8-fluoro-deoxyglucose positron emission tomography [FDG PET]) brain studies may have some utility in patients with a history of mild head injury and persistent symptoms. However, FDG PET abnormalities may be larger than the corresponding anatomic lesions, and metabolic abnormalities may exist in the absence of anatomic lesions.[73,74] However, the relationship of metabolic abnormalities to structural damage may be unclear.[75] Although negative SPECT brain perfusion findings generally predict a good prognosis for the TBI patient, positive (abnormal) findings lack specificity, and may not be clinically helpful.[76] In summary, perfusion SPECT and FDG PET brain imaging might be more sensitive techniques than CT or MRI, but the specificity of functional changes directly attributable to mild TBI is limited.[77] Therefore, these studies should be interpreted cautiously, with full clinical data and correlative CT or MRI findings available.

7.4 Cerebrospinal Fluid Leaks

Cerebrospinal fluid (CSF) leaks often manifest as rhinnorrhea or otorrhea. Both traumatic (related to accidental or iatrogenic causes) and nontraumatic etiologies have been recognized, with traumatic etiologies predominating. Patients with blunt or penetrating head trauma may develop a CSF leak, particularly those with fractures of the basilar skull, temporal bone, or sinuses (frontal, ethmoid).[78,79,80,81] Although a large proportion of post-traumatic CSF leaks resolve spontaneously, those who develop fistulas may develop meningitis, the incidence of which increases with the length of time the fistula remains open.[81] Therefore, surgical repair may be required, and finding the source of the leak becomes important for ensuring a good patient outcome.

Most patients undergo high-resolution CT and/or MRI, sometimes including contrast myelography, to help localize the site of CSF leaks, particularly in the identification of basal skull defects.[82,83] When no obvious anatomical site is evident, scintigraphy can be utilized as a very sensitive technique to confirm leakage. Detection of CSF leaks is performed with Indium-111 DTPA, injected aseptically into the lumbar subarachnoid space. Imaging over the posterior spine and head/neck is performed up to 6 hours, including initial imaging to confirm tracer activity in the subarachnoid space. Given that the actual site of leakage may be difficult to resolve by gamma camera imaging (or, if the rate of leakage is quite slow or intermittent), cotton pledgets can be placed in the nasal passages about 2 hours after tracer injection, and, after removal at ~ 6 hours, counted to determine whether either side contains a significant amount of tracer activity. This technique involves measuring the counts in the pledgets, and then comparing them to the counts in plasma. Maximal pledgets-to-plasma ratios in normal patients have ranged from 1.3:1[84] to 2:1.[85]

References

[1] Subramanian G, McAfee JG. A new complex of 99mTc for skeletal imaging. Radiology 1971; 99: 192–196

[2] Hoving J, Roosjen HN, Brouwers JRBJ. Adverse reactions to technetium-99 m methylene diphosphonate. J Nucl Med 1988; 29: 1302–1303

[3] Davis MA, Jones AL. Comparison of 99mTc-labeled phosphate and phosphonate agents for skeletal imaging. Semin Nucl Med 1976; 6: 19–31

[4] Stabin MG, Stubbs JB, Toohey RE. Radiation Dose Estimates for Radiopharmaceuticals. Oak Ridge, TN: Radiation Internal Dose Information Center, Oak Ridge Institute for Science and Education (ORISE); 1996

[5] Matin P. The appearance of bone scans following fractures, including immediate and long-term studies. J Nucl Med 1979; 20: 1227–1231

[6] Holder LE, Schwarz C, Wernicke PG, Michael RH. Radionuclide bone imaging in the early detection of fractures of the proximal femur (hip): multifactorial analysis. Radiology 1990; 174: 509–515

[7] Beeres FJP, Hogervorst M, Rhemrev SJ, den Hollander P, Jukema GN. A prospective comparison for suspected scaphoid fractures: bone scintigraphy versus clinical outcome. Injury 2007; 38: 769–774

[8] Bellah RD, Summerville DA, Treves ST, Micheli LJ. Low-back pain in adolescent athletes: detection of stress injury to the pars interarticularis with SPECT. Radiology 1991; 180: 509–512

[9] Scharf S. SPECT/CT imaging in general orthopedic practice. Semin Nucl Med 2009; 39: 293–307

[10] Jaudes PK. Comparison of radiography and radionuclide bone scanning in the detection of child abuse. Pediatrics 1984; 73: 166–168

[11] Garland DE. Clinical observations on fractures and heterotopic ossification in the spinal cord and traumatic brain injured populations. Clin Orthop Relat Res 1988; 233: 86–101

[12] Garland DE, O'Hollaren RM. Fractures and dislocations about the elbow in the head-injured adult. Clin Orthop Relat Res 1982; 168: 38–41

[13] Buring K. On the origin of cells in heterotopic bone formation. Clin Orthop Relat Res 1975; 100: 293–301

[14] Freed JH, Hahn H, Menter R, Dillon T. The use of the three-phase bone scan in the early diagnosis of heterotopic ossification (HO) and in the evaluation of Didronel therapy. Paraplegia 1982; 20: 208–216

[15] Johns JS, Cifu DX, Keyser-Marcus L, Jolles PR, Fratkin MJ. Impact of clinically significant heterotopic ossification on functional outcome after traumatic brain injury. J Head Trauma Rehabil 1999; 14: 269–276

[16] Reinders MF, Geertzen JHB, Dijkstra PU. Complex regional pain syndrome type I: use of the International Association for the Study of Pain diagnostic criteria defined in 1994. Clin J Pain 2002; 18: 207–215

[17] Merskey H, Bogduk N. Classification of Chronic Pain: Descriptions of Chronic Pain Syndromes and Definitions of Terms. Seattle, WA: IASP Press; 1994

[18] Schwartzman RJ, McLellan TL. CRPS-1: a review. Arch Neurol 1987; 44: 555–561

[19] Kozin F, Ryan LM, Carerra GF, Soin JS, Wortmann RL. The reflex sympathetic dystrophy syndrome (RSDS). III. Scintigraphic studies, further evidence for the therapeutic efficacy of systemic corticosteroids, and proposed diagnostic criteria. Am J Med 1981; 70: 23–30

[20] Kozin F, Soin JS, Ryan LM, Carrera GF, Wortmann RL. Bone scintigraphy in the reflex sympathetic dystrophy syndrome. Radiology 1981; 138: 437–443

[21] Holder LE, Mackinnon SE. CRPS-1 in the hands: clinical and scintigraphy criteria. Radiology 1984; 152: 517–522

[22] Ruffins D. Natural history of CRPS-1. J Nucl Med 1984; 25: 423–429

[23] Wüppenhorst N, Maier C, Frettlöh J, Pennekamp W, Nicolas V. Sensitivity and specificity of 3-phase bone scintigraphy in the diagnosis of complex regional pain syndrome of the upper extremity. Clin J Pain 2010; 26: 182–189

[24] Lee GW, Weeks PM. The role of bone scintigraphy in diagnosing reflex sympathetic dystrophy. J Hand Surg Am 1995; 20: 458–463

[25] Knochel JP. Mechanisms of rhabdomyolysis. Curr Opin Rheumatol 1993; 5: 725–731

[26] Malinoski DJ, Slater MS, Mullins RJ. Crush injury and rhabdomyolysis. Crit Care Clin 2004; 20: 171–192

[27] Knottenbelt JD. Traumatic rhabdomyolysis from severe beating—experience of volume diuresis in 200 patients. J Trauma 1994; 37: 214–219

[28] Bagley WH, Yang H, Shah KH. Rhabdomyolysis. Intern Emerg Med 2007; 2: 210–218

[29] Chang HR, Kao CH, Lian JD et al. Evaluation of the severity of traumatic rhabdomyolysis using technetium-99 m pyrophosphate scintigraphy. Am J Nephrol 2001; 21: 208–214

[30] Esnault VLM, Nakhla M, Delcroix C, Moutel M-G, Couturier O. What is the value of Tc-99 m hydroxymethylene diphosphonate scintigraphy for the etiological diagnosis of mild rhabdomyolysis? Clin Nucl Med 2007; 32: 519–523

[31] Velmahos GC, Karaiskakis M, Salim A et al. Normal electrocardiography and serum troponin I levels preclude the presence of clinically significant blunt cardiac injury. J Trauma 2003; 54: 45–50, discussion 50–51

[32] Maenza RL, Seaberg D, D'Amico F. A meta-analysis of blunt cardiac trauma: ending myocardial confusion. Am J Emerg Med 1996; 14: 237–241

[33] Mori F, Zuppiroli A, Ognibene A et al. Cardiac contusion in blunt chest trauma: a combined study of transesophageal echocardiography and cardiac troponin I determination. Ital Heart J 2001; 2: 222–227

[34] Collins JN, Cole FJ, Weireter LJ, Riblet JL, Britt LD. The usefulness of serum troponin levels in evaluating cardiac injury. Am Surg 2001; 67: 821–825, discussion 825–826

[35] McCarthy MC, Pavlina PM, Evans DK, Broadie TA, Park HM, Schauwecker DS. The value of SPECT-thallium scanning in screening for myocardial contusion. Cardiovasc Intervent Radiol 1991; 14: 238–240

[36] Holness R, Waxman K. Diagnosis of traumatic cardiac contusion utilizing single photon-emission computed tomography. Crit Care Med 1990; 18: 1–3

[37] Godbe D, Waxman K, Wang FW, McDonald R, Braunstein P. Diagnosis of myocardial contusion. Quantitative analysis of single photon emission computed tomographic scans. Arch Surg 1992; 127: 888–892

[38] Pai M. Diagnosis of myocardial contusion after blunt chest trauma using 18F-FDG positron emission tomography. Br J Radiol 2006; 79: 264–265

[39] Santucci RA, McAninch JW, Safir M, Mario LA, Service S, Segal MR. Validation of the American Association for the Surgery of Trauma Organ Injury Severity Scale for the kidney. J Trauma 2001; 50: 195–200

[40] Kuan JK, Wright JL, Nathens AB, Rivara FP, Wessells H American Association for the Surgery of Trauma. American Association for the Surgery of Trauma Organ Injury Scale for kidney injuries predicts nephrectomy, dialysis, and death in patients with blunt injury and nephrectomy for penetrating injuries. J Trauma 2006; 60: 351–356

[41] Tasian GE, Aaronson DS, McAninch JW. Evaluation of renal function after major renal injury: correlation with the American Association for the Surgery of Trauma Injury Scale. J Urol 2010; 183: 196–200

[42] Moog R, Becmeur F, Dutson E, Chevalier-Kauffmann I, Sauvage P, Brunot B. Functional evaluation by quantitative dimercaptosuccinic Acid scintigraphy after kidney trauma in children. J Urol 2003; 169: 641–644

[43] Anderson JB, Williamson RCN. Testicular torsion in Bristol: a 25-year review. Br J Surg 1988; 75: 988–992

[44] Leape LL. Torsion of the testis. Invitation to error. JAMA 1967; 200: 669–672

[45] Elsaharty S, Pranikoff K, Magoss IV, Sufrin G. Traumatic torsion of the testis. J Urol 1984; 132: 1155–1156

[46] Nadel NS, Gitter MH, Hahn LC, Vernon AR. Preoperative diagnosis of testicular torsion. Urology 1973; 1: 478–479

[47] Lutzker LG, Zuckier LS. Testicular scanning and other applications of radionuclide imaging of the genital tract. Semin Nucl Med 1990; 20: 159–188

[48] Melloul M, Paz A, Lask D, Manes A, Mukamel E. The value of radionuclide scrotal imaging in the diagnosis of acute testicular torsion. Br J Urol 1995; 76: 628–631

[49] Blaivas M, Brannam L. Testicular ultrasound. Emerg Med Clin North Am 2004; 22: 723–748, ix

[50] Gunther P, Schenk JP, Wunsch R et al. Acute testicular torsion in children: the role of sonography in the diagnostic workup. Eur Radiol 2006; 16: 2527–2532

[51] Yagil Y, Naroditsky I, Milhem J et al. Role of Doppler ultrasonography in the triage of acute scrotum in the emergency department. J Ultrasound Med 2010; 29: 11–21

[52] American Institute of Ultrasound in Medicine. American College of Radiology. Society of Radiologists in Ultrasound. AIUM practice guideline for the performance of scrotal ultrasound examinations. J Ultrasound Med 2011; 30: 151–155

[53] Alavi A, Dann RW, Baum S, Biery DN. Scintigraphic detection of acute gastrointestinal bleeding. Radiology 1977; 124: 753–756

[54] Harper PV, Lathrop KA, Richards P. Tc-99 m as a radiocolloid(abstract) J Nucl Med 1964; 5: 382–386

[55] Pavel DG, Zimmer M, Patterson VN. In vivo labeling of red blood cells with 99mTc: a new approach to blood pool visualization. J Nucl Med 1977; 18: 305–308

[56] Winzelberg GG, McKusick KA, Strauss HW, Waltman AC, Greenfield AJ. Evaluation of gastrointestinal bleeding by red blood cells labeled in vivo with technetium-99 m. J Nucl Med 1979; 20: 1080–1086

[57] Smith R, Copely DJ, Bolen FH. 99mTc RBC scintigraphy: correlation of gastrointestinal bleeding rates with scintigraphic findings. AJR Am J Roentgenol 1987; 148: 869–874

[58] Schillaci O, Spanu A, Tagliabue L et al. SPECT/CT with a hybrid imaging system in the study of lower gastrointestinal bleeding with technetium-99 m red blood cells. Q J Nucl Med Mol Imaging 2009; 53: 281–289

[59] Cogbill TH, Moore EE, Jurkovich GJ, Feliciano DV, Morris JA, Mucha P. Severe hepatic trauma: a multi-center experience with 1,335 liver injuries. J Trauma 1988; 28: 1433–1438

[60] Castagnetti M, Houben C, Patel S et al. Minimally invasive management of bile leaks after blunt liver trauma in children. J Pediatr Surg 2006; 41: 1539–1544

[61] Wistow BW, Subramanian G, Heertum RL et al. An evaluation of 99mTc-labeled hepatobiliary agents. J Nucl Med 1977; 18: 455–461

[62] Siddiqui AR, Ellis JH, Madura JA. Different patterns for bile leakage following cholecystectomy demonstrated by hepatobiliary imaging. Clin Nucl Med 1986; 11: 751–753

[63] Tan KG, Bartholomeusz FD, Chatterton BE. Detection and follow up of biliary leak on Tc-99 m DIDA SPECT-CT scans. Clin Nucl Med 2004; 29: 642–643

[64] Fleming KW, Lucey BC, Soto JA, Oates ME. Posttraumatic bile leaks: role of diagnostic imaging and impact on patient outcome. Emerg Radiol 2006; 12: 103–107

[65] Mittal BR, Sunil HV, Bhattacharya A, Singh B. Hepatobiliary scintigraphy in management of bile leaks in patients with blunt abdominal trauma. ANZ J Surg 2008; 78: 597–600

[66] Wijdicks EFM, Varelas PN, Gronseth GS, Greer DM American Academy of Neurology. Evidence-based guideline update: determining brain death in adults: report of the Quality Standards Subcommittee of the American Academy of Neurology. Neurology 2010; 74: 1911–1918

[67] Goodman JM, Mishkin FS, Dyken M. Determination of brain death by isotope angiography. JAMA 1969; 209: 1869–1872

[68] Zuckier LS, Kolano J. Radionuclide studies in the determination of brain death: criteria, concepts, and controversies. Semin Nucl Med 2008; 38: 262–273

[69] Lee VW, Hauck RM, Morrison MC, Peng TT, Fischer E, Carter A. Scintigraphic evaluation of brain death: significance of sagittal sinus visualization. J Nucl Med 1987; 28: 1279–1283

[70] Léveillé J, Demonceau G, Walovitch RC. Intrasubject comparison between technetium-99m-ECD and technetium-99m-HMPAO in healthy human subjects. J Nucl Med 1992; 33: 480–484

[71] Spieth ME, Ansari AN, Kawada TK, Kimura RL, Siegel ME. Direct comparison of Tc-99 m DTPA and Tc-99 m HMPAO for evaluating brain death. Clin Nucl Med 1994; 19: 867–872

[72] Joffe AR, Lequier L, Cave D. Specificity of radionuclide brain blood flow testing in brain death: case report and review. J Intensive Care Med 2010; 25: 53–64

[73] Alavi A, Mirot A, Newberg A et al. Fluorine-18-FDG evaluation of crossed cerebellar diaschisis in head injury. J Nucl Med 1997; 38: 1717–1720

[74] Alavi A, Newberg AB. Metabolic consequences of acute brain trauma: is there a role for PET? J Nucl Med 1996; 37: 1170–1172

[75] Langfitt TW, Obrist WD, Alavi A et al. Computerized tomography, magnetic resonance imaging, and positron emission tomography in the study of brain trauma. Preliminary observations. J Neurosurg 1986; 64: 760–767

[76] Davalos DB, Bennett TL. A review of the use of single-photon emission computerized tomography as a diagnostic tool in mild traumatic brain injury. Appl Neuropsychol 2002; 9: 92–105

[77] Wortzel HS, Filley CM, Anderson CA, Oster T, Arciniegas DB. Forensic applications of cerebral single photon emission computed tomography in mild traumatic brain injury. J Am Acad Psychiatry Law 2008; 36: 310–322

[78] Ommaya AK, Di Chiro G, Baldwin M, Pennybacker JB. Non-traumatic cerebrospinal fluid rhinorrhoea. J Neurol Neurosurg Psychiatry 1968; 31: 214–225

[79] Yilmazlar S, Arslan E, Kocaeli H et al. Cerebrospinal fluid leakage complicating skull base fractures: analysis of 81 cases. Neurosurg Rev 2006; 29: 64–71

[80] Friedman JA, Ebersold MJ, Quast LM. Post-traumatic cerebrospinal fluid leakage. World J Surg 2001; 25: 1062–1066

[81] Brodie HA, Thompson TC. Management of complications from 820 temporal bone fractures. Am J Otol 1997; 18: 188–197

[82] Stone JA, Castillo M, Neelon B, Mukherji SK. Evaluation of CSF leaks: high-resolution CT compared with contrast-enhanced CT and radionuclide cisternography. AJNR Am J Neuroradiol 1999; 20: 706–712

[83] Aydin K, Terzibasioglu E, Sencer S et al. Localization of cerebrospinal fluid leaks by gadolinium-enhanced magnetic resonance cisternography: a 5-year single-center experience. Neurosurgery 2008; 62: 584–589, discussion 584–589

[84] McKusick KA, Malmud LS, Kordela PA, Wagner HN. Radionuclide cisternography: normal values for nasal secretion of intrathecally injected 111 In-DTPA. J Nucl Med 1973; 14: 933–934

[85] Schicha H, Voth E, Emrich D. Detection of occult and intermittent rhinorrhea using 111 In-DTPA. Eur J Nucl Med 1985; 11: 76–79

8 The Role of the Interventional Radiology Technologist

Carol Provost, Jaime Tisnado, and Christine Craft

8.1 The Interventional Radiology Suite

The interventional radiology (IR) suite is one of the most important places in a hospital, especially in a trauma level 1 center (▸ Fig. 8.1, ▸ Fig. 8.2, ▸ Fig. 8.3). An IR suite has many special requirements to promote the effficiency of the IR team; therefore, it is imperative to ensure that the unique needs of an IR suite are met.

First, a spacious well-designed IR procedure room should have ergonomically designed cabinetry to house the vast array of supplies and equipment (▸ Fig. 8.4, ▸ Fig. 8.5, ▸ Fig. 8.6). There must be one or more carts for supplies, also a large well-organized supply room to accommodate the extensive inventory of procedural supplies purchased from specialized vendors, as well as the basic supplies that are available in the hospital's central supply area.

The IR suite requires a scrub sink with cabinetry above, housing surgical caps and masks, shoe covers, and other items needed for scrubbing. There must be a lead apron rack and a vast supply

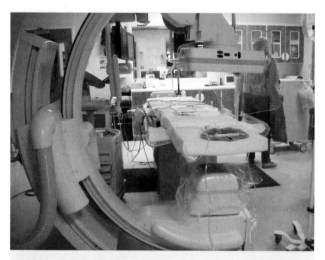

Fig. 8.1 General view of the interventional radiology suite showing the angiographic equipment and monitors, monitors, cabinets, tables, and supplies.

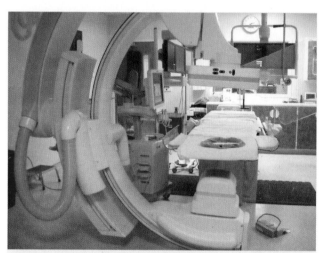

Fig. 8.2 Another view of the interventional radiology room.

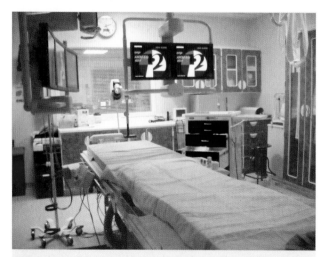

Fig. 8.3 Another view of the fully equipped Interventional Radiology (IR) room.

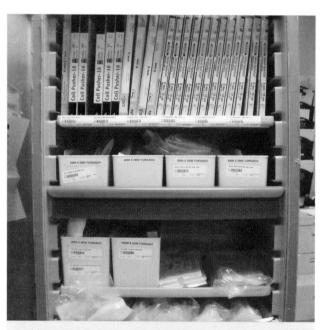

Fig. 8.4 Different arrangements of cabinets and supplies. Some newer cabinets are computerized to keep track of the inventory.

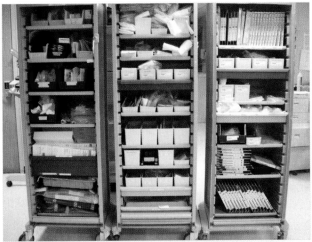

Fig. 8.5 Different arrangements of cabinets and supplies.

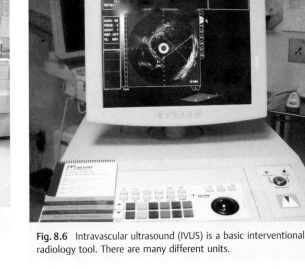

Fig. 8.6 Intravascular ultrasound (IVUS) is a basic interventional radiology tool. There are many different units.

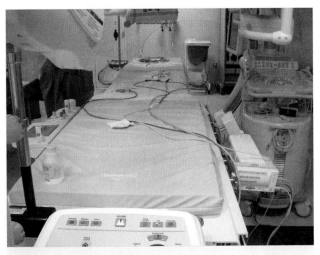

Fig. 8.7 The intravascular (IVUS) is ultrasound at the foot of the table in this particular angiographic and Interventional Radiology (IR) laboratory.

of scrub clothes readily available. The IR suite should be equipped with a "pyxis-type" pharmaceutical system beneficial for a busy department providing easy access to pharmacoangiography drugs. Also, a code cart with emergency drugs for adults and children, an automatic defibrillator (AED) with the appropriate pads for adults and children, the new "auto pulse" oxygen tanks, a portable heart monitor with pulse oximeter is needed, as well as electrocardiogram (ECG) and blood pressure (BP) monitoring for transporting patients in and out of the IR suite. A portable CO_2 tank is required for CO_2 angiography in patients with deteriorating renal function, to eliminate or decrease the amount of iodinated contrast media to be administered.

The IR suite should also have an isolation/personal protective equipment (PPE) cart, a "dirty" room or area to place used, resterilizable metal or glass items, and a hopper to dispose of liquid or other waste. Other necessary equipment includes a portable

12-lead ECG system, at least one or more color Doppler ultrasound (US) units, IVUS (intravascular ultrasound) (▶ Fig. 8.6, ▶ Fig. 8.7), and different thrombectomy thrombolysis apparatus. A vacuum or compressed-air tube system is helpful to send and receive laboratory work, blood products, and small central supply items.

A busy IR suite must have an attached recovery room (RR) to hold pre- and postprocedure patients, manned with dedicated intensive care unit (ICU) nurses, patient care technologists, and transport personnel to facilitate the turnaround of patients in the IR procedure room.

8.1.1 Mobile Carts

Other important considerations include the use of several mobile carts that are quickly accessible to the team with items needed for emergent situations.

A mobile embolization cart should be stocked with all types of embolizing agents, both temporary and permanent, such as Gelfoam® (Pfizer, Inc., New York, NY), Oxicell® (Apex Energetics, Irvine, CA), and Avitene™ (Bard Davol, Warwick, RI), as well as a variety of different coils and microcoils ranging from 0.010" to 0.035" to include straight, Hilal, interlocked fibered, tornado, nester, and vortex shapes. Amplatzer plugs; polyvinyl alcohol (PVA) sponges; embolization spheres and microspheres; "coil pushers"; catheters for deployment of the coils ranging from 0.010" to 0.018"; microcatheters; a vast array of diagnostic, guide, and balloon occlusion catheters, and introducer sheaths should be included. As primary devices for trauma management, stents of all types, such as covered and uncovered, self-expanding or balloon expandable, should be in generous supply.

A mobile trauma cart should also be available, providing emergency supplies for patients who begin to crash, which is not unusual in severely traumatized patients. The hospital trauma team, if it is called, is usually unfamiliar with the IR room layout; therefore, it is very important to keep these emergent supplies in one specific place, without making too many changes in the IR suite.

8.1.2 Resource Information

An important consideration and a valuable tool is a "resource" or "go-to" book containing pertinent, all-inclusive information because in emergent situations it may be difficult to locate necessary information in a timely manner. It should document the following procedures: code, emergency, and fire procedures; personnel recourse after exposure to blood or body fluids; and documentation of patient injuries while in the IR suite or in the OR. This book should contain phone listings (and locations where appropriate) for a code blue, fire alert, the police, the emergency room, the operating room (OR), the postanesthesia care unit (PACU), the ICU, the blood gas laboratory, the blood bank, the main and ICU pharmacy, the respiratory unit, and the anesthesia department, as well as all IR staff including IR attendings and on-call imaging residents. In addition, information about relevant hospital employees such as technologists, nurses, physician extenders, tech support, security, risk management, and the pastoral care team, as well as administrative and maintenance services such as the elevator, transport, EVS, and the hospital paging system should be provided.

The book should also contain an inventory of all the IR supplies, pharmacoangiography medications and doses and how to mix them, and an iodinated contrast media premedication guide. Injection rate and filming guidelines, and trouble-shooting guides for the various types of equipment must also be available. Information about companies whose equipment is routinely used in the IR unit may also be necessary. Locate all the book's information on a shared drive in the hospital's computer system, making it accessible to all IR staff members on any hospital computer that has login capabilities. Include any and all information that may be needed in special situations; the resource book is special and unique for each institution. It is called the "Bible" of our IR suite

8.2 Room and Equipment Requirements

The IR procedures in the setting of trauma are constantly changing—becoming more and more sophisticated; therefore, additional equipment requirements necessitate a large well-organized suite. Ideally, space for growth in IR should be planned in advance. For the team to function well, the ideal IR rooms need to be large and OR compatible for various procedures including endograft procedures.

Room dimensions and layout and cabinetry location are important considerations. It is reasonable to locate the cabinets and some countertop space at the foot end of the table and/or on the patient's right side. These must be easily accessible and strategically placed to allow access without disrupting the administration of care to the patient during the procedure.

There needs to be plenty of room on both sides of the angiographic table to allow ample workspace for the IR team to work and manage the tray, as well as the ability to open cabinet doors to access products without contaminating or disrupting the IR team. This is particularly important when the patient is unstable because there is additional equipment needed such as a ventilator or anesthesia equipment and carts, intravenous (IV) warming systems, multiple IV poles, the code cart, etc.

It is imperative to have sufficient space to monitor vital signs and airways, and possibly to perform cardiopulmonary resuscitation (CPR) while the diagnostic or IR procedure continues in an effort to stabilize the patient. Caution: Remember to always position the patient over the base of the IR table before beginning chest compressions. There are usually several trauma team members caring for the patient while the IR staff is trying to expedite the procedure in a relatively chaotic and crowded environment.

In general, it is better if the anesthesia equipment, ventilators, IV poles, ventilator connections, and lines are at the head or at the left side of the IR table. It is helpful to have ceiling and/or wall mounted setups to include at least two suction setups and two O_2 setups. Air lines and an evacuation line should be located near the patient's left shoulder when possible because a right femoral puncture is usually the best approach.

It is also necessary to instruct the medical team upon arrival to the IR suite, that the C-arm may also be in that area, and it will move around the table. The surgical trauma staff must avoid patient or personnel injury or crushing of the equipment when the C-arm is moving or rotating.

Cabinetry design and proper labeling are important considerations for an IR suite to expedite retrieval of items used in the procedures. Cabinets with translucent doors from ceiling to floor with individual designs are ideal. Cabinets should have pullout racks with hooks to hang a variety of catheters and sheaths and balloon catheters up to 130 cm in length. Other cabinets should contain shelves and drawers with dividers to accommodate numerous supplies such as guidewires, micropuncture sets, sheaths, dilators, power injector syringes, injector tubings, IV pressure tubings, closure devices, embolization kits, and various sizes of plastic, polycarbonate, and even glass syringes. Also included are assorted sizes and types of sterile and nonsterile gloves, sterile drapes, sterile gowns, sterile towels, sutures, and basic central supply items including hats, masks, PPE, and linens.

The cabinet setup should flow so that the sterile items are in close proximity and easily accessible. The basic central supply department (CSD) items can be grouped together slightly away from the tray so any members of the IR team can locate and obtain them as needed.

The oxygen and suction tubing should be in close proximity to the wall or ceiling-mounted connections for quick access. We have found it convenient to have at least one or more cabinets designated with trauma supplies and equipment in case the patient becomes unstable, which is common. These cabinets should contain a variety of emergency items that are easily accessible for all personnel.

The trauma cart may include stethoscopes, manual blood pressure cuffs, ECG leads, blood collection and culture tubes, arterial blood gas (ABG) kits, IV access setups along with scissors, clamps, tape, stopcocks, additional IV tubing, and blood tubing.

The IR suite must have many triple-lumen catheter insertion trays, arterial line insertion trays, and catheters and transducers. Oral airways, nasal trumpets, nonrebreather devices, trachea insertion trays, trachea collars, and trachea ties are also needed as are oxygen connectors and tubing, nasogastric tubes, suction catheters, connectors, and all types of tubing for respiratory issues. Another cabinet should contain urinary catheter

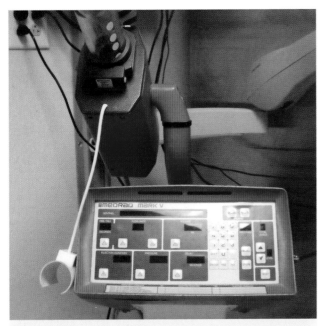

Fig. 8.8 The power injector is mounted on the table or ceiling. Indispensable equipment.

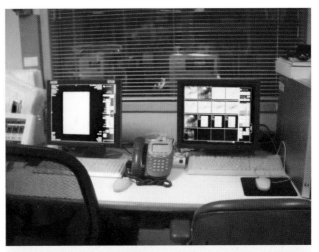

Fig. 8.9 In-room power control console with monitors, phones, etc. Ample room for working is mandatory.

insertion kits, specimen containers, irrigation trays, and syringes of different types and tips. Various sizes of trocar catheters; chest tube insertion trays; pleural vacuum-type setups; thoracentesis trays; hemothorax drainage catheters and valves, etc.; IV solution bags of normal saline and lactated Ringer, and all other fluids are necessary also.

The power injector (▶ Fig. 8.8) seems to function better if attached to the tableside; the use of additional injector tubing is necessary. This limits the possibility of catheter dislodgement from the vessel when the tabletop is moved because the injector moves with the table. On the other hand, when using a ceiling- or floor-mounted power injector, the injector must be moved manually and simultaneously with the angiographic table.

Ultrasound equipment is required for vascular and non-vascular access. Portable or table-mounted IVUS equipment is placed around the table. The surgical team is usually on one side of the patient while the IR team is on the opposite side. Skytron-type lighting and/or portable OR lights are necessary.

A heart monitor with pulse oxymetry, ECG, BP, two pressure-monitoring cables, several IV poles, a warming IV unit, a Bear Hugger patient warming device, and Ambu bags for both adults and children, are all mandatory equipment.

In-room computer access for charting, paging, and documentation increases the efficiency of the staff to complete the procedures. Additional Internet connections for the OR team and anesthesia documentation are important features. An intercom, phone, or personal digital communication devices should be considered, especially for larger departments. These are particularly useful when the patient suddenly becomes unstable and additional staff need to be called immediately.

The radiographic equipment should minimally include a single-plane C-arm with trifocal spot, and a large heat capacity tube including an image intensifier with at least a 9" screen (14" is preferred for vascular procedures) or better, a flat-screen detector. A biplane system has many advantages, especially for neuroangiographic procedures, given that we obtain two views with only one contrast injection.

The digital imaging system should be capable of imaging with a maximum rate of 4 frames per second (4 fps) in the biplane mode or 7.5 fps in the single-plane mode. Other options include "perivision" or step table imaging, "dynavision" or rotational angiography, three-dimensional (3D) rotation, and Dyna computed tomography (CT).

"RadCare" positioning allows for collimating the X-ray field without fluoroscopic exposure. It allows collimating the beam, as well as the placement of filters in a multidirectional fashion over areas of uneven densities, particularly where there is air in the field. It is important not to place the filter over vital organs because it may decrease the visualization of the opacified vessels and may also increase the exposure to the patient or operator.

An in-room tableside control console allows the operator to capture, review, and manipulate images on the fly. An additional work console in the control room enables the IR technologist to enter pertinent data and manipulate and send the images to the workstation. Both the in-room and work consoles should be equipped with various functions to simplify the procedures, allowing the selection of various capabilities such as road mapping, fluoro fade, last image hold, reference imaging, and the ability to store single fluoro images, store monitor, and fluoro scenes. It is also capable of storing C-arm and table positions.

A technologist workstation is necessary to perform vessel measurements, manipulate, and postprocess images and create 3D reconstructions and Dyna CT images, while the procedure is being performed. It also has the ability to send to and receive images from the work console, picture archiving and communication system (PACS), "Stentor," CT or magnetic resonance imaging (MRI) workstations, directly into the procedure room.

Two separate monitor cranes strategically placed in the IR room allows visualization from all over the room; this is important because patients are studied by accessing all parts of the body and the C-arm can be positioned in many different positions (▶ Fig. 8.9, ▶ Fig. 8.10, ▶ Fig. 8.11). It makes sense that the TV monitors have a wide range of maneuverability. One two-monitor crane on one side (generally parallel to the table on the patient's left with the ability to maneuver to the head of the

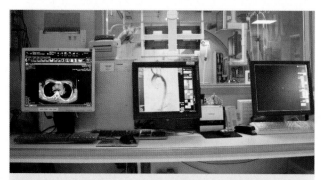

Fig. 8.10 Additional work consoles in the control room are necessary. The more the better as it makes the work of IR technologists, nurses, and physicians much easier and complete.

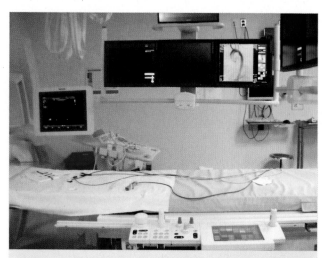

Fig. 8.11 3-crane fluoro monitors are ideal, especially for neuroradiology work and to facilitate trauma diagnostic and intervention.

table) should have one monitor with live fluoroscopy and "last image hold," and the other monitor as a reference image. The second three-monitor crane on the opposite side, perpendicular at the foot end of the table to visualize both sides of the patient, consists of a primary monitor for live fluoroscopy and last image hold, one monitor for reference images, and the third monitor for reviewing PACS images from the "Leonardo" or workstation, or to select US or IVUS, if available.

The IR procedure rooms are always stocked and ready for multiple studies at all times. A list of necessary supplies to be stored in each room is ideal. The appropriate cabinetry must be labeled, keeping all of the IR rooms similar enabling the staff to locate things efficiently. The cabinetry is designed to allow room for catheters, guidewires, micropuncture access sets, vascular sheaths, dilators, and necessary tray add-ons.

The rooms require additional items such as vinyl-coated angle positioning devices to include 45-degree-angle sponges, head sponges, knee bolsters, and the "face-down pillows." Also a Muniz prone-positioning headholder is recommended. Radiolucent arm boards that can be slid under the table pad for supporting a limb or used as an armrest when the patient is prone such as during a nephrostomy procedure, are also recommended. Trauma scissors to cut small fixation devices for groin exposure and safety and restraint devices to include Velcro straps and 3-inch silk tape are routinely stored there.

8.3 Room Setup

Rapid action by an experienced IR team is the key for the severely traumatized patient's survival. The IR team must arrive promptly and set up the room expeditiously. It is important to have as many tasks completed and anticipated as possible before the patient's arrival to the IR suite because patients may suddenly become unstable. In IR we have a dictum: "The sooner the patient is cared for, the better the chance of survival."

In over three decades of practice we have found that we never underestimate the stable, nonemergent, probably negative diagnostic angiogram.

It is common that the requested study by the referring physician may only be a small portion of what actually needs to be performed. The experience and skills of the IR and the surgical trauma teams, and their review of the clinical situation, laboratory, and radiology findings, along with the mechanisms of

injury, the type of accident or trauma, the weapon utilized, etc., will help determine the optimal patient's care and outcome. In general, the more we (the team) know the better.

An experienced IR technologist will turn on the angiographic equipment as soon as possible. He or she will also compile the paperwork and enter the available patient data into the work console. The IR technologist and nurse must quickly review the patient's laboratory work, allergies, pregnancy status, isolation, contact and/or precaution status, and will make sure the order for the procedures to be performed, and the signed consents are in order. Once these items are reviewed, the technologist or nurse calls for the patient and then immediately prepares the room for the intended procedure.

The technologist sets up and labels the power injector with two 150-mL injector syringes of nonionic iodinated contrast media. Some waste of contrast may occur, but this is acceptable to save precious time. Visipaque 320% is preferred by our team because of the possibility of high-contrast material volume used in CT before. Also, it is the best contras material to avoid movement by the patient because of its low osmolarity, thereby decreasing the pain sensation. Sometimes utilizing one-half- to two-third-strength nonionic contrast media is possible and acceptable according to the sensitivity of the digital angiographic imaging. Thereafter, we cover the power injector with a sterile bag so that it can be connected to the catheter in a sterile fashion and remain close to the sterile field.

The IR technologist also sets up the IR tray with basic items on the angiographic table. This table can be simple, metal, wheel-mounted, ~ 24-inch width by 48-inch length, or an elaborate rolling cart containing drawers and cabinet space for additional storage with an attached IV pole to hang saline bag solution and a bottle of contrast material.

Designing a custom, disposable, multipurpose IR tray to use for the majority of IR procedures greatly streamlines the setup time and breakdown, and addresses storage issues. The IR tray that we designed consists of three sterile disposable gowns—one to set the sterile tray just prior to the patient procedure and two for the actual procedure—a sterile femoral angiography drape with femoral fenestrations and clear plastic sides to cover as well as visualize the tableside controls, 8 to 10 towels, one or

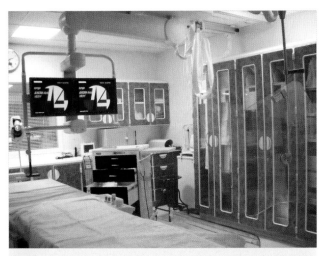

Fig. 8.12 A 2-monitor crane of fluoro monitors is evident. The supply cabinets are useful supplied with all needed for an efficient care of the severely traumatized patients.

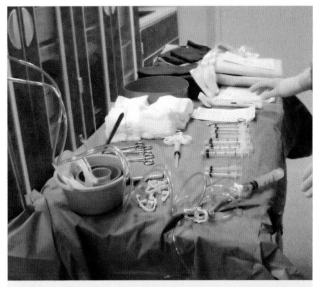

Fig. 8.13 A close view of the Multi-purpose I-R tray. All the basic equipment is ready for the diagnostic and Interventional Radiology (IR) procedure. The additional supplies are added as needed, so no waste of expensive equipment occurs.

more sharps containers, 18-gauge and 25-gauge 1 1/2" needles and an 18-gauge single-wall access needle, a medicine cup for local anesthetic, a small and large bowl with lids, a 26-mL Chloraprep applicator, a no. 11 scalpel with handle, scissors, mosquito and straight forceps, needle drivers, tissue forceps, five towel clamps, sterile gauze, a telfa pad, a Tegaderm dressing, and a plastic tray cover that is wrapped in a sterile back table cover. Our particular tray also contains assorted 5-mL and 20-mL plastic syringes we label and fill with heparinized saline (5,000 units of heparin per liter of normal saline). We use 10-mL syringes for diluted contrast material, and a 10-mL plastic control syringe for Lidocaine 1% that can be buffered with sodium bicarbonate (▶ Fig. 8.12, ▶ Fig. 8.13).

A customized manifold kit utilizing a closed system with a one-way valve and a stopcock to fill syringes with the saline solution and/or contrast material, designed to empty the "dirty" syringes into an attached disposable waste bag, is included. A one-way high-pressure stopcock, customized labels to make the syringes and bowls, injector tubing, sterile image intensifier or flat-screen detector band bag, and a sterile bag to cover the power injector head to allow the scrubbed technologist to connect the injector tubing to the catheter with the radiologist, are also included.

We routinely prefer 5-French (F) micropuncture sets, a 0.035" Bentson guidewire, a 0.035" angled glidewire, a torque vise, a 5F vascular sheath, and sterile vented IV tubing with a drip chamber to be connected to a pressure bag, which is attached to the side port of the vascular sheath and the catheter or catheters of choice.

We flush all catheters, dilators, and glidewire housing and sheaths with the heparinized saline. The arterial sheath is flushed through the side port and then the sheath is assembled with the stopcock turned off to the tubing to avoid blood from exiting the side port. We use a pressurized bag with heparinized saline (1,000 units of heparin per liter) that will be attached to the side port of the arterial sheath and remove the air from the pressurized saline bag as well as the tubing.

When preparing the pressurized heparinized bag, we insert the bag of heparinized saline into the pressure bag and turn it upside down. The scrubbed IR technologist will hand to a nurse or to another nonsterile helper, the drip chamber to be inserted into the heparinized saline bag while the bag is upside down. The helper inflates the pressure bag until one-third of the drip chamber is filled with saline. The scrubbed IR technologist closes the clamp and the helper turns and hangs the pressure bag upright onto an IV pole located on the same side of the table. The helper inflates the pressure bag to 300 mm Hg ensuring that the drip chamber is adequately filled to avoid air passing through the tubing, and the ability to adjust the flow rate. (Other devices to keep high pressure in the fluid bags are available, but we no not use them.) The scrubbed technologist slowly opens the clamp and clears the line of any air, moving the clamp while pinching the tubing because air bubbles get trapped in the location of the clamp. This process can be done prior to the patient's arrival after the pressurized bag is hung on the angiographic table pole. Once the patient is prepped, a helper can walk the tubing over to the table with the assistance of the scrubbed technologist.

Additional supplies in the room or in the near proximity are 0.035" routine flush and selective catheters for the organ of interest, 0.010" to 0.018" microcatheters and microguidewires. We already mentioned the need to have the mobile embolization cart with supplies to include different embolizing particles, prelabeled embolization kits (appropriate small prelabeled syringes and stopcocks), steristrips, sterile small bowls, sterile scissors and knives, and finally all the preferred types of vascular closure devices.

Plastic bags should be placed over the foot pedal and X-ray tube to protect against any type of fluids, and a back table cover placed on the angiographic table to help contain some of the fluids and debris that may be present, which, (1) i easily keeps the room clean upon completion of the procedure, and (2) it protects and maintains the operation of the table pad and the equipment.

It is obvious that all monitoring devices should be fully operational and completely set up and ready to be attached to the patient. This includes a minimum of two O_2 setups, two suction setups, a heart monitor with ECG, SAO_2, and pressure monitoring with recording and printing capabilities, etc., as mentioned above. There must be a defibrillator or (AED), a code cart, and a trauma cart along with the autopulse readily available for any type of emergency to include resuscitation, chest tube insertion, and/or thoracotomy. We suggest a dedicated individual mobile trauma cart with emergency supplies as an efficient and practical method to have supplies and equipment accessible, especially for the surgical trauma team, and other caregivers not familiar with the IR suite.

8.4 Patient Procedures

As soon as the patient arrives, we must quickly perform the verification and "time out protocol" and recheck the patient's fractures, injuries, precaution status, laboratory work, allergies, pregnancy status, and organs or systems to be studied. We use a backboard or flexible smooth mover to move the patient to the angiographic table. We assign one person to control the head to minimize or avoid cervical spine movement. This person usually directs the patient transfer to the IR table. Another person should monitor and assist with the IVs and chest tubes. Once the patient is on the table, we make sure that the table pad is in place and secure the patient to the IR table with safety devices and radiolucent removable curved arm boards, Velcro straps, and/or adhesive tape.

We then position the respiratory and/or anesthesia equipment, IV poles, and other equipment away from the C-arm to maintain tube angle flexibility, and free motion to optimally visualize the TV monitors around the room. Most times, the patient's right groin will be accessed, so the respiratory equipment and/or anesthesia equipment is located to the patient's left side.

We have developed a useful method: If the C-arm is parallel to the patient and the plan is to image from the diaphragm to cephalad, the respiratory and anesthesia equipment should be caudad to the patient's left shoulder. If the C-arm is perpendicular to the table to image from the diaphragm to caudad, the respiratory and anesthesia equipment should be cephalad on the left side of the patient. We try to relocate wires and tubings away from parts of the patient to be imaged and away from the imaging equipment. When possible, we place a Bear Hugger to keep the patient warm. A cool patient and a cool room are not conducive to a good outcome, particularly if the studies are prolonged, especially in children. Unfortunately, the use of a Bear Hugger can be bulky and time consuming, so it is not always utilized. A blanket warmer is a good alternative. Every institution must have one of these practical devices.

Another method we have used is to place an additional back table cover on the angiography table prior to the patient's arrival to minimize table clean up, and to cover the patient with blue pads (Chux) or a plastic tray cover to retain the patient's body temperature. We have found that the plastic from the "Chux" will hold and keep the patient's heat. A warming IV infusion pump is also recommended to maintain the fluid at

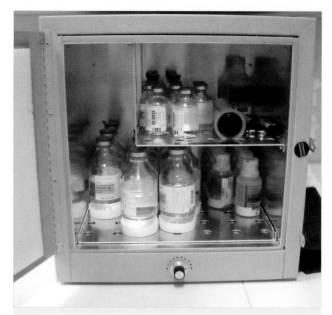

Fig. 8.14 A Warmer for fluids is standard equipment in modern Interventional Radiology (IR) suites. Also a warmer unit for drapes and linens is useful.

body temperature particularly when blood loss is great (▶ Fig. 8.14).

The team must shave, prep, and drape both groins for all trauma patients unless a brachial approach is deemed necessary. If that is the case, a high brachial approach is our preference. Placing a sheath of "Ioban" over the prepped area is a great option to maintain sterility. If the groin pulses are absent, it is wise to palpate all brachial/axillary pulses and seek advice from the IR if the brachial/axillary areas should be prepped as well. Ultrasound must be set up in advance to access the vessels in these patients because the pulses can be very weak and difficult to palpate in many trauma patients.

If a pelvic girdle has been applied prior to the patient's arrival, cutting an opening to work in the vicinity of the femoral pulses with "trauma" scissors is usually appropriate. We then prep the entire groin area including the girdle as well. Sometimes a sheet has been wrapped around the pelvis, knotted, and held with clamps or forceps for external fixation. We try to relocate the metallic instruments away from the area of interest, or sometimes we use silk tape to secure the knot and remove the forceps or clamps to make the approach easier and to avoid severe artifacts on the angiograms. It is important to have the assistance of members of the surgical trauma unit.

When confronted with an obese patient (not uncommon in our patient population), with a large fat abdominal pannus, we tape the belly up and away from the groin as best we can, avoiding excessive tension, which could cause skin damage. Remember to shave and prep well cephalad to the groin crease because it is well known that in obese patients the groin crease is well below or caudad to the site of puncture of the common femoral arteries.

Once the patient is prepped and draped, we take a scout image of the area of interest to assess any pre-existing abnormalities or radiologic findings. It is also helpful to document the location of central lines, endotracheal, orogastric, nasogastric, and/or chest tubes.

Here we perform the final time-out protocol with the IR who is doing the procedure and reaffirm the patient's injuries, precaution status, laboratory work, allergies, pregnancy status, and organs or systems to be studied once more, before starting the procedure.

Once vascular access is obtained utilizing a micropuncture set, the sheath is inserted and the side port of the sheath is connected with a pressurized heparinized saline solution free of air. The pressurized heparinized saline bag should be connected to the side port of the sheath prior to inserting the 5F catheter into the 5F sheath, to allow the side port to clear the sheath with heparinized saline. The diagnostic angiographic catheter is placed in the desired vessel and the test injection is made. Next we connect the catheter hub to the power injector and position the patient in a way that includes the largest area of injury site and vicinity, by increasing the focal-film distance (FFD).

Sometimes the table needs to be raised to its maximum height and the image intensifier or flat-screen detector is to be lowered. These maneuvers decrease the magnification and the radiation exposure to the patient. It may be necessary to do the opposite—increase the magnification factor to focus attention on the primary site of injury. This can be done by changing the magnification factor selection, or by deviating, raising, or lowering the table—the so-called air-gap technique.

Many times it may be necessary to increase the rate of image acquisition to visualize rapid blood flow or organs in motion. Some examples include the identification of an arteriovenous fistula, the site of a vessel actively bleeding, or to limit motion such as when the patient is breathing or moving, and especially when patients are uncooperative or have altered mental status. Suspending the respirations in a ventilated patient during the exposures is usually helpful as well.

Sometimes it is necessary to prolong the filming time and/or decrease the frame rate to demonstrate reconstitution or collateral flow distally to a transected vessel. Filming with the smallest focal spot possible to demonstrate fine detail is advised. Most of the new imaging systems usually provide a console to set up multiple selections with a variety of tailored acquisitions. This can be done during the installation of new IR equipment.

Once the procedure is completed, we consider the following options: (1) Remove the catheters/sheath and use a closure device, or (2) maintain the arterial sheath access connected to a transducer for monitoring. Maintaining an arterial sheath usually requires the patient to go to the ICU or PACU.

It is well known that traumatized patients are at risk of developing deep vein thrombosis (DVT) and/or pulmonary embolus (PE). Placing a retrievable inferior vena cava (IVC) filter may be necessary, particularly in patients with multiple fractures, head injuries, etc., or who are at risk for developing DVTs. With the availability of optional IVC filters, the use of filters is rather common. Furthermore, because the patients will probably be hospitalized for long periods requiring IV access, the insertion of a central catheter, peripherally inserted central catheter (PICC), or other catheter is usually recommended at this time while the patient is on the IR table.

During an IR procedure in trauma patients, it is also not uncommon to be asked to perform additional exams "as long as you are there," such as a kidney, ureter, and bladder (KUB) X-ray,

a modified chest X-ray to document a line placement or pneumothorax, a retrograde cystogram, or an esophagram to avoid moving the patient to another room and wasting valuable time.

Next, it is time to select the images for PACS, taking the time necessary to appropriately and carefully label the images as to right or left, preprocedure, postprocedure, embolization, nitroglycerin, stent, etc. We need to manipulate the images with peak opacification, unsubtracted, remasking pixel shifting or flexible pixel shifting. Flexible pixel shifting is a fairly new postprocessing feature, which is ideal for areas with multidirectional motion such as breathing. It may take an extra minute, but we are better able to realign the pixels to smooth out the background, thereby increasing our ability to visualize the contrast-enhanced vessels.

It is helpful to send to PACS subtracted images as well as a few native (unsubtracted) or anatomical background images with contrast-filled vessels and analyze its relationship to the bony structures. This capability usually helps the surgeons to get better information about the area of interest. We always send all of the images to PACS as soon as possible, before leaving the department because patients may require surgery or other clinical management as soon as we finish their diagnostic and/or IR procedures.

8.5 Multiple Simultaneous Traumatized Patients

On occasion, there are situations in which multiple traumatized patients may require IR procedures at the same time. We therefore set up a second room with the basic supplies as time allows. If more than one patient is in a critical condition, it is wise to organize a "second call team" as soon as possible, earlier rather than later, to facilitate the immediate treatment of the additional victims.

Some of our severe victims may require head-to-toe or full body angiography especially when multiple trauma patients arrive at the hospital simultaneously.

It is important to quickly review the imaging studies and even perform additional studies to ensure that the preliminary diagnosis is correct. This is particularly important given that on occasion, the area of suspected injury leads to a negative study. The requesting physician may have neglected to relay the pertinent patient information or may not have been able to clinically examine the patient for whatever reason, especially in the case of too many patients. No matter how busy and/or overwhelmed the IR staff may be, it is necessary to take the time to individualize patient care, to appropriately manage the patient quickly and even, perhaps, save his or her life.

If it is difficult to stay focused on the job (due to exhaustion or other factors) for only one IR to manage the case, the IR should not hesitate or be afraid to call for help: The patient's life is in our hands.

8.6 Professional Requirements and Experience of the IR Technologist

The IR technologist must have an extensive knowledge of the vascular anatomy (arteries, veins, lymphatics), normal and abnormal and variations. The technologist must know the inventory of supplies as well as how, when, and why to use them, along with their location in the carts, cabinets, trays, etc.

It is mandatory for the IR technologist to be familiar in all of the functions and capabilities of the digital imaging equipment, the power injector and other important apparatus like US, IVUS, thrombolytic devices, etc. The IR technologist working in a level 1 trauma unit must know all of the filming protocols and injection rates for different studies and when to vary their baseline protocols.

One of the most valuable assets in an IR technologist is the ability think on the "fly" and problem solve because every procedure in severely traumatized patients is unique and requires quick thinking, initiative, creativity, and rapid action.

In the past, before the availability of digital technology and multidirectional C-arms, it was rather a difficult task to obtain certain special views. Today there is no limit in our ability to demonstrate the injury. There are instances that necessitate the use of accessory items like positioning sponges, adhesive tape or Velcro straps, and even radiolucent extensions or arm boards to separate the lower extremities off the main IR table.

It is important to obtain as much information as necessary as to the mechanisms of injury: what happened, how it happened, what are the patient's suspected injuries and complaints; in the case of falls, how high and where they landed (concrete or wood), and how did they land (feet, head, back, or side); in cases of penetrating injuries such as stabbings or gunshots, the entrance site and/or exit, how long or large the knife was or what type of weapon (handgun or rifle) was used and whether the bullet ricocheted or passed through the body. In motor vehicle collisions, it is important to know whether the patients were a driver or passenger, wearing a seat belt or not, and where in the car they were seated. These questions help us to understand the nature and types of injuries and upon the patient's arrival to the IR suite; we begin to strategize accordingly.

We foster an open communication between all members of the trauma care team because different people process knowledge and information differently. An open dialogue encourages and challenges the health care team to perform a thorough investigation of the problem thereby enhancing the quality of patient care.

For example, a middle-aged patient presents with multiple pelvic and femur fractures and requires orthopedic surgery post an IR procedure. A discussion should include angiography of the pelvis with selective injections of both the internal and external iliac arteries, superficial femoral artery (SFA), and lower extremity arteries to the ankle or dorsalis pedis and posterior tibial to ensure that at least one vessel runoff is patent and enough to support the extremity's viability. A decision must be made as to one injection for a single leg step-table runoff perivision, or a series of multiple injections made with single-station imaging. The flow rates of contrast are decreased and the filming rate slowed to demonstrate vessel injury or vessel spasm.

Vasodilators and other drugs are often used for pharmacoangiography. It is the IR technologist's responsibility to adjust the filming to image at a lower frame rate for a longer period and to place a time delay on the injector to demonstrate the vessels eventually. On the contrary, nitroglycerin may be given to relieve spasm and hasten the flow to the extremity. Sometimes, if there is a partial transection or other injury to an artery, it may be necessary to cross the lumen of the injured vessel to insert a stent. This obviously will require measuring the diameter of the vessel and length of the injury before gathering the supplies for stent placement.

8.7 The Role of the Interventional Radiology Nurse

The nurses in the IR suite should make sure they have the needed equipment available in the room, including equipment to rescue an airway. There should be bag valve masks (BVM), nonrebreathers (NRB), nasal cannula, and suction equipment. The correct oxygen valves should be in place and in proper working order. Mandatory in all rooms are code carts, as well as a defibrillator. The defibrillator must always be checked prior to patient arrival. Telemetry should be in proper working condition. Cables for BP, a pulse oximeter, cardiac monitoring, central venous pressure monitoring (CVP), arterial pressure monitoring, and possible temperature monitoring should all be readily available to monitor the patient: all in working condition, sterile and ready for use.

Laboratory tubes are needed to draw appropriate laboratory work, as many times as needed throughout the procedure. There should be an adequate number of tubes to draw multiple laboratory studies during a long case. There should be tubes for hemoglobin (HB), hematocrit (Hct), a metabolic panel, lactate, coagulation, arterial blood gas, type and screen. In case of chest trauma, the nurse should anticipate drawing cardiac enzymes as soon as possible. Moreover, there should also be rapid infuser sets that are ready for use before the patient arrives to the suite. Spare tubing for the infuser is needed because the infuser has an increased likelihood of clotting in the tube.

Once the patient has entered the IR suite, the IR nurse must be given a recent patient report. This includes the mechanisms of injury, as well as the initial treatment provided in the trauma bay. Upon patient arrival, the nurse must communicate with the trauma team including the different physicians and the IR team. It is important to name a physician who will be communicating the orders, thus avoiding the possibility of conflicting orders.

We suggest that the nurse have an individual acting as a "runner." This person can assist getting needed items and transporting samples to the laboratory so that the patient will never be left alone. One of the initial tasks of the IR nurse is a baseline assessment of the patient's airway, breathing, circulation (ABCs). After the initial assessment is complete and satisfactory in the IR suite, the patient can be moved to the procedure table. Telemetry is applied with audible alarms set. Baseline vital signs are obtained. The IVs must be patent and infusing without signs of infiltration. The patient should be covered with blankets, or better, warming blankets because shock is possible. Furthermore, the IR rooms are always cold.

At this time, we get baseline laboratories. The nurse must communicate with the IR team to let everybody know if the procedure will be lengthy or there was a complication with significant bleeding, so the nurse is prepared to send laboratory work.

Patient comfort is very important. The nurse discusses the type of sedation to be used throughout the procedure so the reversal agents will be readily available, if needed. At the beginning of the procedure, the nurse checks to make sure that the patient is prepped using sterile technique, the IR team is sterile, and that sterile technique is maintained throughout. Otherwise, the nurse mentions that sterility has been compromised, and acknowledges to the team that the patient must be reprepped and a new tray opened.

The starting time is recorded and vital signs checked every 5 minutes or per facility protocol. If at any time there is a change in baseline, the nurse must communicate and discuss this with the IR team. If the patient is receiving sedation, there may be a small drop in blood pressure. A proper understanding of IR procedures is a must for the nurse. There may be "floating" wires in the heart. This could cause arrhythmias, such as ventricular tachycardia. Of concern is the fact that if the wires are removed, the rhythm does not resolve to baseline. Nurses and physicians must know how to treat arrhythmias that resolve spontaneously.

Adequate patient sedation and comfort is the nurse's goal throughout the procedure. There is a thin margin between sedation, oversedation, and complication.

The nurse must also monitor the airway at all times. At the first sign that the oxygen levels are decreasing, the nurse must attempt to improve the oxygen level. A nasal cannula is used in a slight oxygen deprivation. A NRB is used for moderate oxygen deprivation, and BVM can be used for severe oxygen deprivation. If the nurse determines that the patient is in severe distress, one member of the team bags the patient, as another person checks to see if there is a palpable pulse. The nurse must not relay on the monitor because the patient could be in pulseless electrical activity (PEA). Again, we cannot emphasize that communication with the physicians and the IR care team is a must. As soon as the airway is starting to be compromised, it must be resolved quickly. The nursing staff should be prepared and qualified to administer blood products per hospital policy. A thorough understanding of medications and contraindications is a must for the nurse. When in doubt, the nurse needs to look up the medication in a formulary. The nurse must understand the onset of the medication and the half-life, meaning the time that it takes for one half of the medication to be broken down and eliminated from the body. The duration is also important, to be prepared for adverse reactions. Most medications have antidotes to reverse its effects. Knowing the antidotes is life saving for the patient. Obviously, all drugs must be ready and handy in the IR room.

Throughout the entire procedure the nurse should be reassessing the patient. Reassessing the patient in the IR suite can be very challenging to say the least. The patient is on the table dressed with sterile drapes and the skin has been prepped with sterile solution as well. Here is where the nurse shines. The nurse makes sure the patient is stable and there are no complications. The entire IR team is the advocate for the patient to make sure that the patient is getting the best of care. After the procedure is finished, the IR team will most times use a closure device. The type and the time that the device is deployed should be noted.

The IR nurse should always communicate any nursing considerations or concerns to the nurses assuming care postprocedure. These include the type of dressing in place, appearance of dressing, how long the patient should lie flat, how often should the pulses be checked, and the character of pulses palpable or heard by Doppler. The nurse should document the IR team's assessment as well as perform and document their assessments. The patient or the bed is then moved.

The patient must be reassessed from head to toe, as if you are performing the preprocedure survey. Reporting can then be called to the floor as follows: patient name, age, allergies, history, what brought the patient to the hospital, mechanisms of injury, medications given, IV access, IV fluids given and the amount, any blood products given, condition of the airway, breath sounds, circulation, what is wrong with the patient, procedure performed, closure devise, nursing considerations, and laboratory values.

In summary, the role of the nurse in the trauma care team is a very important one and the nurse must be very experienced in the care of the traumatized patient. The nurse must communicate all the information about the patient at all times, and be aware of the patient's condition at all times as well. Communication between all members throughout the time of administering care is essential.

8.8 Inventory Considerations

The IR inventory is a very challenging responsibility of knowing where the products are located, how they are used and what other devices are compatible with each other in size, diameter, and other aspects. For example, a trauma patient is actively bleeding and is sent to the IR suite. The procedure begins with arterial access using a 21-gauge micropuncture needle. Once vascular access is obtained, a 0.018 guidewire is inserted through the 2-gauge needle and the needle is removed. The 5F coaxial micropuncture catheter is inserted over the 0.018-inch guidewire and the inner catheter of the 5F coaxial micropuncture catheter is removed, then the 0.035-inch Bentson guidewire is advanced into the vessel. The coaxial micropuncture catheter is removed and the 5F introducer sheath is inserted followed by a 5F diagnostic catheter advanced over the 0.035-inch guidewire through the 5F sheath. There is bleeding from this small vessel so embolization is planned (▶ Fig. 8.4 ▶ Fig. 8.6).

We now need to determine whether the 5F catheter system will navigate the small vessel to embolize the vessel with 0.035-inch embolization coils, spheres or Gelfoam, or which particular microcatheter will fit into this particular catheter, and then which coils are needed for embolization. If the wrong embolization coil is used, the wrong coil could become lodged in the catheter, requiring a removal and exchange of a catheter, which may have required 30 minutes or more to selectively place, and we would have to start again. An even worse scenario would be to deploy a coil into the wrong vessel requiring retrieval in a patient who continues to bleed. This scenario is not rare in dealing with severely traumatized patients.

8.8.1 Power Injector

The IR technologist must be knowledgeable of the varied functions of the power injectors, and must be able to quickly troubleshoot problems. We have found that the power injector functions best when attached to the IR table avoiding catheter dislodgement from the vessel upon the movement of the IR table. Failure to monitor the power injector during the table movement with a ceiling-mounted or floor-mounted power injector may result in dislodging the catheter.

The first and foremost consideration is to make sure to never leave air in a contrast-filled injector syringe. If the IR technologist does not know or did not load the injector syringe properly with iodinated contrast material, then the syringe should not be put into the plunger of the injector. Air, if any, must be completely expelled decreasing the possibility of an air embolus. Thereafter, we attach 48" to 72" injector tubing and remove the air again. Prior to connecting the injector to the catheter we must turn the injector head down so any air bubbles will rise to the plunger side of the contrast filled syringe. When connecting the injector tubing to the catheter hub, it is important to hold the catheter hub steady and rotate the injector tubing, not the catheter hub, to make the connection. Otherwise, the catheter tip may be dislodged from the vessel. We prefer injector tubing with a rotating connector to avoid this problem (▶ Fig. 8.8).

The next step is to aspirate blood into the tubing. We must be sure that no air bubbles are aspirated into the tubing. If there is difficulty when aspirating, the catheter tip may be against the sidewall of the vessel creating a vacuum and therefore aspiration of air bubbles. We must move or "shake" the catheter slightly under fluoroscopy. This may solve the problem. Otherwise, it is necessary to disconnect and reposition the catheter correctly in the desired vessel before reconnecting. If it still does not work, inject the contrast material by hand.

In general, the IR technologist must know injection rates for the different vessels. Injecting too much could damage the vessel, whereas injecting too little will waste contrast and result in a poor nondiagnostic study. The technologist must understand the settings of a "rate rise" and pressures of injection in (psi) pounds per square inch. The rate rise is used for selective injections because it controls the rate of delivery of contrast into the catheter. The higher the rate rise, the slower the contrast will be initially injected during the first second of injection to decrease catheter whipping and dislodgement from the selected vessel. The psi function relates to the pressure exerted upon the catheter. All catheter packaging is labeled with the maximum flow rate and the psi that the catheter can withstand under ideal conditions. High psi settings are used for aortic or IVC injections, while a selective injection requires a smaller bolus of contrast. A too high setting may dislodge the catheter from the selected vessel. A good rule of thumb for aortic flush procedures is to set the rate rise at 0.1 seconds and 900 psi. For visceral injections, we set the rate rise at 0.5 seconds and 600 psi.

The power injector is very easy to use, for a majority of the procedures, but it is commonly plagued with technical errors, usually created by the IR technologist. The injector is usually connected to the X-ray equipment and can be programmed in two different ways, such as injection delay or X-ray delay.

The injection delay is set at a predetermined time during the acquisition of images. The injection delay of 1.5 seconds is our normal setting. In this mode, the filming sequence begins producing several noncontrast enhanced images. After 1.5 seconds, the injection begins and the vessels are enhanced with contrast. This is the normal process, which is used as a postprocessing tool for the IR technologist to create high-quality images. It is particularly helpful when patient motion is a factor.

The X-ray delay is set to inject contrast prior to initiating the filming sequence. It is used when the contrast material has a long way to travel through the vessels to get to the area that needs to be imaged. To determine the X-ray delay, we review the previous run and determine the time for the contrast material to arrive at the area of interest and factor an X-ray delay that is at least two seconds prior to obtain the noncontrast images. This process decreases the radiation exposure to the patient and is also helpful to decrease the motion on the images.

The X-ray delay will vary if the catheter is moved or if a vasodilator is used. After the run is performed, we set the injector back to the standard injection delay of 1.5 seconds, otherwise problems may occur, and the next patient could receive an unnecessary amount of contrast material.

Both injection and X-ray delay features help the IR technologist in postprocessing functions. The concept is to create a mask image, which is the image without contrast material that is acquired immediately prior to visualizing contrast material on the image. By creating a mask image and superimposing it over the contrast images (a normal postprocessing function of the digital equipment), the end result is a subtracted image that has the least amount of motion.

Today's digital equipment has several different features to manipulate and smoothen the images. These include remasking, peak opacification, edge enhancement, pixel shifting, and flexible pixel shifting. An experienced IR technologist uses these postprocessing tools to create the highest quality images.

8.9 Troubleshooting Ideas

There is a list of problems that may arise during any procedure. The last resort is to move the patient to another room to complete the procedure. The more-experienced IR technologist will troubleshoot or circumvent a problem and will get the equipment operational quickly. Having a troubleshooting guide and access to technical support personnel is helpful. If an IR workstation is not functioning appropriately for any reason, it is a good idea to have a back-up system to accommodate transfer of the images directly from the work console.

The power injector may malfunction for various other reasons as well. Some errors that have prevented an injection include the turret which holds the injector syringe is not aligned properly or the lever located next to the manual dial on the bottom injector arm on a particular injector has been moved. When this occurs, the black plunger of the injector syringe disables the ability to check for air bubbles. Another problem that may occur is the toggle switch on the main injector control panel might have been switched to only allow manual injections with the handheld injector control.

8.10 Conclusion

The IR technologist and nurse are important members of the trauma team. The technologist and nurse need to have the experience to take great care of the trauma patient beginning well before the patient comes to the IR suite, then during the actual procedure and thereafter, when the patient has gone to the next location. A high degree of care, attention to detail and knowledge of the IR suite, X-ray equipment, supplies, procedures, and protocols are important. The trauma team is composed of technologists, nurses, physician assistants, physicians, and equipment. All people and machines work together for the purpose of providing first-quality care to the traumatized patient.

9 Interventional Radiology Techniques

Carol Provost and Jaime Tisnado

Advances in interventional radiology (IR) are constantly changing the field and the scope of practice. In this chapter we will deal with different regions of the body where IR has revolutionized our concepts and will introduce some basic interventional techniques used in daily practice.

9.1 Thoracic Aortography

Emergency imaging of the thoracic aorta is performed for various reasons in the setting of trauma. The interventional radiologist must have wide flexibility in positioning, the rate of injections, and film imaging sequences based on the nature and type of the injury.

When one is imaging a patient with a stab wound, gunshot wound, or rib fractures, it is important to include in the filming not only the aorta and great vessels, but also other possibly injured vessels such as the internal mammary and/or intercostal arteries, particularly on the side of the injury.

When evaluating a possible aortic dissection it is beneficial to use a marker pigtail catheter to determine the extent and character of the dissection and especially to determine the diameter, length, and type of the stent graft to be used. Intravascular ultrasound (IVUS) is useful at this time and must be ready to be used.

We position the patient supine on the angiographic table, positioning the electrocardiogram (ECG) leads, ventilator lines, intravenous (IV) lines, and other monitoring devices away from the thorax, if possible. The C-arm must be positioned to obtain anteroposterior (AP) and steep oblique views. Filming sequences and injection rates are set and reviewed with the IR physician just prior to obtaining the arteriogram. Once the pigtail or flush catheter is positioned into the ascending aorta, a test injection is made, and the injector is connected to the catheter. The C-arm is then positioned in the 35- to 45-degree left anterior oblique (LAO) view, centered at the nipples with the least degree of magnification to visualize the thorax from C5 to the diaphragm to include the ascending, aortic arch, aorta, great vessels, and the descending aorta. The second view should be an AP or slight right anterior oblique (RAO) centered slightly lower to include from C7 to the origin of the celiac axis. The images should be acquired on deep inspiration if possible. The filming and positioning can be altered to include the area of injury (▶ Fig. 9.11,▶ Fig. 9.1).

It is important to carefully review the images of the aorta and branches particularly in the vicinity of the injury. An average injection rate for thoracic aortography is 20 to 25 mL/s for a total volume of 40 to 50 mL. The filming is 4 frames per second (fps) for 4 seconds, 2 fps for 6 seconds, and 1 fps for 20 seconds, or 4/4, 2/6, 1/20 in our "lingo" for a total time of 30 seconds. Other pertinent factors include a rate rise no longer than 0.1 second, an injection delay of 1.5 seconds, and a psi of 900. The maximum psi and flow rate for each catheter is on the catheter package. If aortic injury is suspected or the heart rate increases, the filming rate may be increased to 7.5/4, 2/6, and 1/20, and the injection rate increased to 25 to 30 mL/s for a total of 50 mL (▶ Fig. 9.1, ▶ Fig. 9.2, ▶ Fig. 9.3).

9.2 Abdominal Aortography

When imaging the abdominal aorta, we place the side holes of the pigtail catheter at the level of the celiac axis. We set the injection rate at 20 mL/s for 40 mL, a rate rise of 0.1 second, and a psi of 900. A typical filming rate is 4/4, 2/6, 1/20, positioning the top of the image 1 to 2 fingerbreadths above the diaphragm. Ideally, we use the least degree of magnification by raising the table to the maximum height and then lowering the image intensifier or flat-screen detector as close to the patient as possible. We film on expiration if possible (▶ Fig. 9.4, ▶ Fig. 9.5).

With the patient on the table, we do fluoroscopy to locate the level of the diaphragm, and then place a filter horizontally over the lung bases. It is important to even out the densities across the image such as the lung so as not to get "burnout" artifacts. However, too much filtering may fade the contrast resolution over the denser bony structures or organs. This maneuver increases the radiation exposure to the patient because a filter is added to an already dense area. We always film long enough to visualize the portal, renal, and other veins when possible (▶ Fig. 9.4, ▶ Fig. 9.5, ▶ Fig. 9.6).

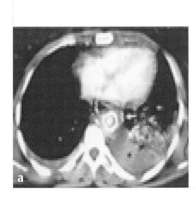
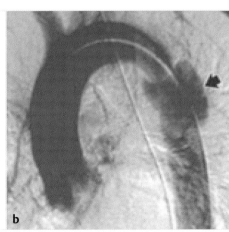

Fig. 9.1 (a) A chest computed tomography and a (b) thoracic aortogram in the left anterior oblique position show the characteristic disruption of the thoracic aorta distally to the origin of the left subclavian artery—the typical appearance of an acute traumatic rupture of the thoracic aorta.

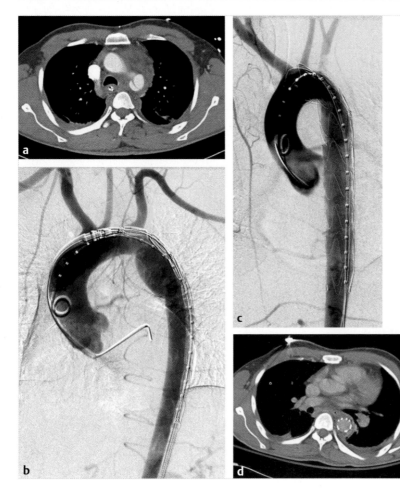

Fig. 9.2 (a) A 17-year-old boy involved in a high-speed motor vehicle collision with evidence of traumatic rupture of the thoracic aorta on chest computed tomography. The patient also had a subdural hematoma, bilateral pneumothorax, a liver laceration, as well as fractures of the T-spine, left scapula, multiple ribs, and facial bones. He was treated for his other injuries, stabilized in the surgical trauma intensive care unit with strict blood pressure control, and taken for thoracic endovascular aortic repair on hospital day 15. (b,c) The pseudoaneurysm was covered with a Talent 22 × 116 mm stent graft, with planned exclusion of the left subclavian artery origin. He recovered from his other injuries and was eventually discharged home. (d) Postoperative CT angiography confirmed exclusion of the pseudoaneurysm with no evidence of endoleak. He remains stable at 4-year follow-up.

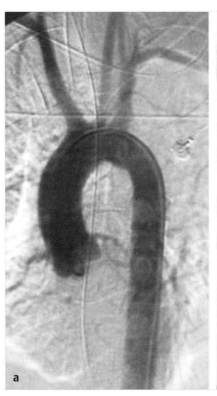
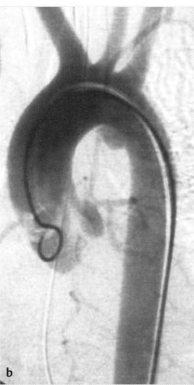

Fig. 9.3 (a,b) Thoracic aortogram in left anterior oblique shows a pseudoaneurysm of the aortic arch just distal to the origin of the left subclavian artery.

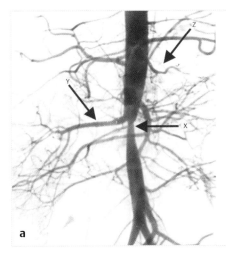

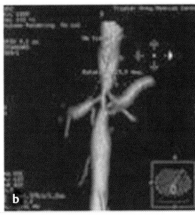

Fig. 9.4 (a) An abdominal aortogram and (b) corresponding computed tomography reformat in three-dimensional surface rendering in a young patient with acute abdominal pain and leg claudication. There is evidence of a lesion, so-called "mid-aortic stenosis". By pass surgery is therefore indicated.

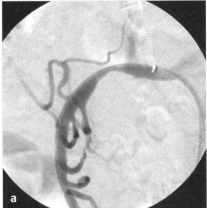

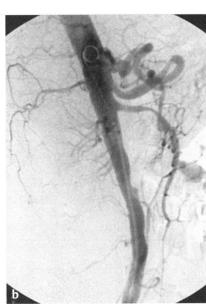

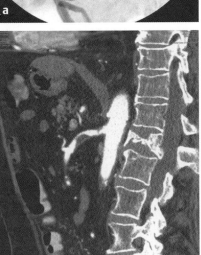

Fig. 9.5 (a–c) An elderly woman with symptoms and signs of chronic mesenteric ischemia. Marked stenosis of both the superior and inferior mesenteric arteries is noted anteriogram and CT scanning. Angioplasty and stenting was done.

After filming, we select the best images of the arterial, capillary, and venous phases. We manipulate the images by remasking, pixel shifting, and window and leveling as needed to see through the celiac axis, superior mesenteric artery (SMA), and renal arteries in both subtracted and native or "landmarked" images.

If selective arteriography is necessary a landmarked or "anatomical background" image on the in-room monitor may help the interventional radiologist. Preferred selective catheters are RC2, C2, Sos Omni Select, VS1, Chung C, Rim, Levin, or others. We always store a kidney, ureter, and bladder (KUB) image for gross evaluation of the gastrointestinal (GI) and genitourinary (GU) systems (▸ Fig. 9.7).

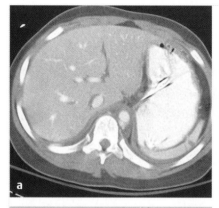

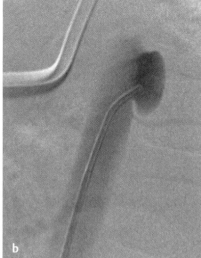

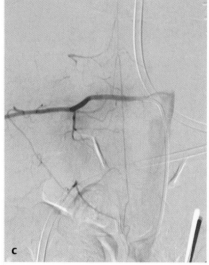

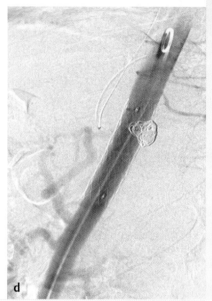

Fig. 9.6 An 11-year-old boy s/p all-terrain vehicle accident. He suffered extensive injuries including traumatic brain injury, pulmonary contusion, liver and splenic lacerations, as well as multiple fractures. (a) He was found to have acute traumatic aortic injury on computed tomography. (b) Emergent intraoperative angiogram confirmed a pseudoaneurysm of the aorta at the T10 level. (c) After the artery of Adamkiewicz was identified originating from the right T8 intercostal artery, the pseudoaneurysm was packed with multiple detachable microcoils to prevent a possible endoleak followed by placement of a 14-mm limb extension from an endovascular aneurysm repair graft across the region of injury. (d) Completion angiogram confirmed no further filling of the pseudoaneurysm. The patient was eventually discharged in stable condition with no focal neurologic deficits. He was followed closely for signs of pseudocoarctation for 5 years, but eventually moved out of state and was lost to follow-up.

9.3 Pelvic Arteriography

Patients with severe pelvic fractures usually have immobilization devices in place upon arrival in the IR suite. Prepping both groins is ideal, but not always possible. The interventional radiologist must choose the groin with the least apparent injuries or with the best arterial pulse, unless an axillary approach is to be chosen. The immobilization devices always create a challenge to the IR technologist as they are located across both groins.

External fixation devices include a sheet wrapped and knotted or with metal clamps, or nylon pelvic compression restraint, or a girdle with a shoestring tightening apparatus. We usually do not remove the immobilization devices but we work around the situation. Our preferred method is to remove the metal clamps from the sheet, twist the sheet tight, and tape it or wrap it with adhesive tape toward the shoulder, away from the groin accessed. This should be done after approval of the referring physicians and with the help of the IR and the trauma teams.

We must be sure to keep constant pressure on the pelvis at all times. The nylon restraint can be partially cut with trauma scissors to remove and create a notch in the groin area to be punctured. We must prep the groin area and the restraint device as this area is not a very sterile one. If possible we place Ioban over the site to maintain sterility.

A careful review of the CT and other diagnostic images prior to the arteriogram is very important to determine the area to be examined. We usually perform an AP pelvic arteriogram with a pigtail or Sos Omni flush catheter, which can be used next for selective arteriography. We film the entire pelvis from the aorta-iliac bifurcation to below the symphysis pubis and from the midline to the gluteal area with both obliques. Sometimes it may be necessary to obtain a "high" and "low" pelvis according to the extension of the pelvic injuries. We make sure to have a landmarked reference image on the in-room monitor.

A "midstream" pelvic arteriogram may not show signs of active bleeding or extravasation, but it will delineate the vasculature or provide an accurate roadmap of the pelvic vessels.

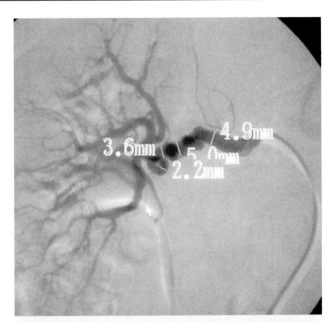

Fig. 9.7 A middle-aged woman with medial fibromuscular dysplasia (FMD). Stenosis severity determined by qualitative angiography has poor correlation with hemodynamic significance. Pressure gradients measured with special wire are ideal. 20 mmHg is significant. Transluminal gradient plus intravascular ultrasound is very good for the evaluation of Percutaneous Transluminal Angioplasty (PTA) in FMD.

Whether or not active bleeding is seen, we proceed to select bilateral internal iliac arteriography. We look for completely or partially transected vessels and/or active extravasation of contrast material. It is always a good idea to have the IR nurse to insert a Foley catheter, if one is not in place, before the procedure to drain the bladder and improve visualization of small bleeding sites.

9.4 Lower Extremity Arteriography

Lower extremity (LE) angiography can be performed in several ways dependent upon interventional radiologist's preferences, the presentation and size of the patient, the obvious deformities of the extremity, the extent of the injuries, and whether there are distal pulses or not. There are several methods to image the lower extremities: (1) the "stepping" or "runoff" approach, (2) perform single-station images with the catheter at the aortic bifurcation, and (3) two separate single LE runoffs by placing the catheter into the contralateral external iliac or common femoral artery and imaging the first LE followed by removing the catheter and connecting the injector directly into the arterial sheath for imaging the ipsilateral LE.

A single extremity leg runoff is done if the extremity is fairly straight, can be placed near the center of the table to visualize the entire LE from the hip to the foot, and the blood flow is continuous to monitor the table-stepping without missing the flow of contrast.

Sometimes it is quicker and easier to do single stations because of the extra equipment and devices in the room that may interfere with the movement of the table and/or C-arm.

It is necessary to position the leg and move the table with the center lock on, move the leg into position, and collimate and add filters side to side to each area as the stepping process is engaged. If the flow is disrupted, very slow due to vasospasm, or the leg is not straight, it will be necessary to make separate injections over each area with a 1- to 2-inch overlap so as not to miss any portion of the vessel due to parallax. We need to raise the table to maximum height, oblique the tube 20 to 25 degrees in the ipsilateral oblique, and start with the top of the field just above the hip, making sure to collimate and filter slightly side to side to include the soft tissues. If no injury exists in the proximal extremity, a rapid manual injection can be made and a last image hold or a roadmap image taken to document the intact vascular anatomy.

We must maintain the angle or alter accordingly the C-arm throughout the various steps of the table for speed and to make sure the common femoral artery bifurcation is open and to separate and align three leg arteries away from the cortex of the tibia and fibula. Once the knee is imaged, the next station can begin at the top of the tibial plateau and include the "trifurcation." The last station should include from the mid tibia to the entire foot. It is also recommended to set a lateral view from the midtibia to include the foot for complete coverage. If there are fractures, we prefer to position the fracture in the middle of the filming area if possible and set orthogonal views of that area (i.e., AP and lateral).

Bilateral LE angiography or runoffs are easily performed by placing a pigtail or flush catheter into the distal aorta, obtain two oblique pelvic runs and then set up for the step-table runoff. Position both LE in the center of the table and close together, especially the knees. We prefer using the Octostop® (Laval, Quebec, Canada) rubberized leg filter devices on the sides and in between the legs keeping the legs in an AP to slight internally rotated with overlapping of the toes on both feet.

Depending on the type of equipment, it is important to raise the table to the maximum height; if using a flat-screen detector, and either landscape or portrait image, position the patient to visualize the maximum of vessels at every single station. Ideally, the top of the first station is at the level of the iliac crest centered on the table and engage the stepping program or the center lock mechanism, whichever is appropriate. Next, pan, move, or step the table or C-arm during fluoroscopy to finetune each step with collimators and filters ensuring that the LE are centered. Then we secure the feet and knees with a Velcro strap or adhesive tape to decrease movement. We connect the catheter to the injector making sure there is plenty of slack so the injector tubing or catheter will not get pulled during the stepping of the table. We must ensure that the LE are clear of tubing and ECG leads and try not to dribble contrast material on the sterile drapes over the LE to avoid unwanted artifacts. The injection rate varies with the different equipment. Our average table step runoff is 8 mL/s for a total of 80 mL. A slower C-arm stepping system may require 9 mL/s for a total of 108 mL.

In our three decades of experience, we have found some problems such as the metal components of the table obscuring the image and sometimes causing artifacts overlying the vessel. Also when a portion of vessels are not visualized, it may be because the images were not overlapped. This has already been mentioned, parallax is the main offender.

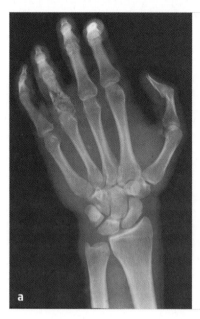

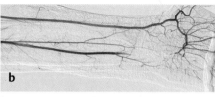

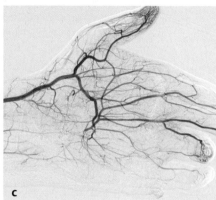

Fig. 9.8 (a–c) Forearm and hand arteriography in a patient with traumatic occlusion of the distal ulnar artery at the level of the wrist. There is also occlusion of the third common palmar digital artery and the proper palmar digital arteries to the index and little fingers.

The table sides have metal gear mechanisms to allow panning of the table in multiple directions. The metal usually shows when imaging steep oblique views of the distal LE. Therefore, it is important to keep the leg near or in the center of the table. When this occurs, we slightly rotate the leg internally or externally, if possible, and/or decrease the C-arm angulations.

If the opposite extremity is in the way, we place a straight flat radiolucent plexiglass board under the table pad and move the LE to the board and secure the leg with hook and loop fastener straps or adhesive tape.

If we note metal parts or artifacts on the fluoroscopic control, it is important to position the extremity away from the metal or opaque parts to visualize the vessels in at least two views to find injuries.

Most new IR rooms have either a round image intensifier (II) or a rectangular flat-screen detector. This influences vessel field of visualization and overlap. With a round II, we must have at least a 2" overlap because the diameter is the largest field of filming. If the vessel is not overlying the center of the II, a portion of the vessel is missed. On the other hand, with the flat-screen detector we can film in landscape or portrait modes. With a flat screen the overlap is consistent across the edges of the images.

9.5 Upper Extremity Arteriography

When we are dealing with upper extremity (UE) injuries (▶ Fig. 9.8-), we place the patient on the IR table, and insert a radiolucent straight arm board under the table pad, and adduct the affected extremity supine, flat, palm up, and secure with hook and loop fastener straps or wrap a small towel on the extremity and tape to the arm board for security. It is important to separate and extend the fingers on the board and tape them just enough to hold them still, but to not obstruct blood flow.

Once the arterial sheath is inserted in the femoral artery, a 5-French (F), 100-cm pigtail catheter is advanced into the ascending aorta and the patient positioned in a 30- to 45-degree left anterior oblique (LAO) view. If the injury is confined to one extremity, it is possible to off-center the filming on the aortic arch and the affected extremity.

We usually include the neck from C5 to midchest, from the midclavicle to include as much shoulder as possible, being careful to include the entire aortic arch.

Thereafter, we connect the injector to the catheter and set 15 mL/s for 30 mL with a 900 psi and a 0.1 rate rise. The filming rate is set at 4 fps/4 s, 2 fps/6 s, and 1 fps/20 s to visualize the vascular anatomy into the venous phase. Select the best aortic arch image for anatomical background and send it to the in-room monitor. The next step is to exchange the pigtail catheter for a 5-F, 100-cm DAV or other catheter and catheterize the subclavian artery. We film the vascular anatomy into the arm and identify the radial and ulnar arteries to rule out the possibility of a high radial or ulnar artery origin from the axillary or brachial artery. It will be necessary to skew or rotate the table to see the UE on the arm board. If a high origin is not found and the injuries are distal to the brachial artery, then the catheter can be positioned distally. Care must be taken to avoid spasm of the small arteries due to the catheter. Perhaps a microcatheter can be used in this situation. We always set two orthogonal views at the site of injury.

For the hand (▶ Fig. 9.8), we make sure the fingers are separated, extended and held in the AP position. Using an air-gap technique and the magnification setting we film the hand and wrist with magnification. We place filters over the fingers to even out the densities, if needed. A 250-mL or 500-mL saline plastic bag over the hand helps to secure the hand, and evens the densities, and improves image quality. It is wise to decrease the filming to 2 fps/4 s and 1 fps/5 s or 2 fps/4 s, 1 fps/10 s and 0.5 fps/40 s to capture the contrast filled arteries into the venous phase.

We usually use pharmacoangiography with nitroglycerin. We place a 3-way stopcock between the catheter and the injector tubing and inject 200 to 500 micrograms of nitroglycerin via the remaining port of the stopcock, just prior to the injection of contrast and filming with the same sequence. As the nitroglycerin is a vasodilator, the flow will be faster and comparison can be made with the other injections and the degree of spasm, if any, can be assessed.

Sometimes the patients cannot extend the UE so they are medicated to decrease the pain and then gently adduct the arm, rotate the tube, and skew or rotate the table to set two orthogonal views with cranial or caudal angulation as well as a LAO and a right anterior oblique (RAO). It may be possible to place an angled cushion between the patient's body and extremities to separate them enough to obtain a few views. If the arm can be built up on cushions, a lateral shoot-thru view can be obtained. It is important to obtain as much information as possible.

9.6 Arteriography for Knee Dislocation

Vascular injuries during trauma to the knee are common. Usually, posterior dislocation of the knee may result in intimal flap, dissection, transection, occlusion, stretching, and spasm of the popliteal artery. Venous injuries such as occlusion or thrombosis are rare, but potentially catastrophic. The contralateral femoral approach is preferred, but it is also possible to access the ipsilateral common femoral artery, either antegrade or retrograde, using a 5F dilator, sheath, or short catheter. We must be mindful of the timing for the arrival of contrast material to the area to be studied. The retrograde approach results in a short delay and dilution of the contrast compared with the antegrade access.

We use different methods to visualize the popliteal region. A single plane runoff is performed from the common femoral artery to the ankle. Then an orthogonal view is obtained over the knee. Another method can be single-step imaging from the groin to the knee with routine image acquisitions versus stored monitor images. Anteroposterior and lateral projections are the most beneficial to visualize the popliteal area. For the lateral view, the affected leg is placed in an external oblique position in the center of the table and the C-arm is rotated. If the patient is unable to move, we elevate the unaffected LE on a stool or cushions and set "shoot-thru" the lateral knee, centering at the joint space. A third method is to rotate the patient 30 to 40 degrees with positioning sponges, separate both legs, and then rotate the C-arm to be AP and lateral to the knee. The idea is to position the artery away from the bony structures and film from the midthigh to the midcalf, to include the three arteries of the leg.

If the blood flow distal to the "trifurcation" is slow, we decrease the frame rate to 2 fps/4 s, 1 fps/40 s or 2 fps/4 s, 1 fps/12 s, or 0.5 fps/24 s, unless we need to visualize the venous phase. Forty seconds is usually adequate, unless there is an injury or history of peripheral vascular disease.

It is important to send to the picture archiving and communication system (PACS) several images including the arterial, capillary, and venous phases and a native or unsubtracted image, in addition to images with peak opacification.

9.7 Head and Neck Trauma Arteriography

Head and neck injuries result from multiple types of mechanisms: motor vehicle, falls, gunshots, stabbings, etc. A biplane neuroradiology room is ideal. The biplane equipment saves time and contrast material. The patient is positioned on the table and attached to the monitors. Once the arterial access is obtained and a 5-F sheath is inserted, a 5-F 100-cm pigtail catheter is advanced into the ascending aorta above the aortic valve. In a single plane room the initial injection is in the LAO 30- to 45-degree projection centering at the base of the neck to include from aortic arch to the mandible. We inject 20 mL/s for 40 mL total for an average-sized adult or 25 mL/s for 50 mL total for a large adult. The usual filming is 4 fps/s for 4 seconds, 2 fps/s for 6 seconds, 1 fps/s for 20 seconds, terminating after the venous phase. In case of tachycardia, we increase the early rate to 7.5 fps for 4 seconds instead of 4 fps for 4 seconds to visualize the aorta without motion. The LAO projection usually shows the origin of the great vessels and the "opened" aortic arch. The images are on inspiration and collimated to the full size of the screen, to visualize the subclavian arteries and the internal mammary arteries, if injuries due to a clavicle or rib fractures are suspected. An AP projection and additional views (RAO, lateral) are necessary when rupture of the aorta or great vessels is suspected (▶ Fig. 9.9, ▶ Fig. 9.10).

The easiest way to perform two views in a biplane room is to position the lateral tube in the LAO projection, and the AP tube in an AP or mild RAO projection. It takes a few minutes to center both tubes adjusting the height of the table, as well as moving the table horizontally to center the filming in the aorta in the two planes.

After filming, we select an image with the aorta opacified and change it to a native or landmarked image and send it to the in-room reference monitor. Thereafter, we exchange the pigtail catheter to a selective catheter such as a DAV, vertebral, JB1, nontapered angled glide catheter or similar and proceed to selective injections of the appropriate head or neck vessels. The neck vessels in older patients are more tortuous and may require the use of a reversed curve catheter such as a Sims 2 or similar.

When the patients have a cervical collar, we must keep the head in a neutral position and secure the head by placing a hand towel over the forehead and 3" silk tape or a Velcro strap over the towel.

In general, during filming the patients are instructed to stop breathing in inspiration, hold still, and not talk or swallow.

When imaging for neck trauma we choose the appropriate common carotid and/or vertebral arteries and set two orthogonal views and an AP view to include the tip of the catheter from C7 to the sella turcica. When the mandible obscures the common carotid bifurcation, we angle the AP tube caudally 5 to 10 degrees to project the mandible above the bifurcation. Some interventional radiologists prefer an ipsilateral oblique 25- to 40-degree view. We review the arch injection and choose what may be the best angle to study the bifurcation. The lateral view is usually ideal for "opening" the bifurcation. We try to image from C7 to the sella turcica, including the catheter tip and center slightly anterior to the cervical spine using filters over the "bright areas" or "air" to obtain better images.

For the vertebral arteries in lateral projections, we center on C2 and image from C7 to the skull base.

For cranial views, the head is in a neutral position, the orbitomeatal line perpendicular to the table. For an AP carotid injection we position the superior orbital ridge at the top of the

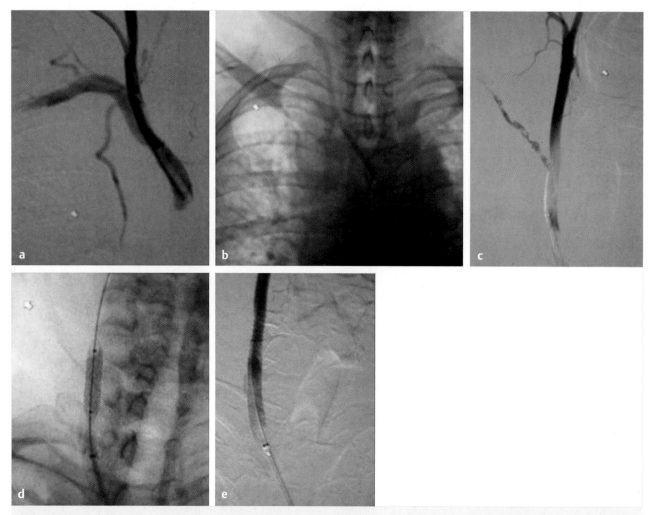

Fig. 9.9 A 50-year old man with end-stage kidney disease had depleted central venous accesses; therefore, a femoral venous catheter was inserted for hemogialysis (HD). The patient underwent HD with reported difficulty and pain for a couple of weeks until he was referred back to our institution for neck catheter exchange. (a) Upon fluoroscopy of the chest, it was obvious that the catheter was misplaced with its tip in the midline. (b) Contrast material was injected demonstrating that the catheter had been inserted into the right common carotid artery, with the tip located in the aortic arch. After consultation, the surgeons requested interventional radiology to remove the catheter and manually compress the puncture site to achieve hemostasis. Due to the potentially disastrous complications if manual compression failed, puncture was made of the right common femoral artery and wire access was obtained across the puncture site in the common carotid artery. However, upon catheter removal and manual compression, no hemostasis was achieved with evidence of an expanding neck hematoma. (c) A follow-up arteriogram demonstrated free extravasation of contrast from the common carotid artery through the catheter track in the neck, therefore the decision was made to place a covered stent across the lesion. (d, e) Using the right common femoral arterial approach, a 6 mm × 40 mm iCast, covered stent, was deployed at the site of the common carotid artery puncture. The stent was dilated with a 6-mm balloon. A small endoleak was noted at follow-up arteriogram; therefore, the stent was further dilated with a 7-mm balloon. The patient did well and is receiving chronic hemodialysis 5 years later.

petrous ridges to include the top of the skull to the nose. We select a micro focal spot and the highest magnification factor with the air-gap technique. We use filters, when necessary, to improve imaging.

For an intracranial vertebral arteriogram we increase the caudal tube angulation to 25 degrees and position the superior orbital ridges below the tops of the petrous ridges to include from the top of the skull to C2.

The lateral view is centered near the top of the ear, to include the base of the skull, superimposing the internal auditory canals and doing magnification as described above.

Sometimes we need transorbital oblique views so we angle the tube 25 degrees to the ipsilateral side and caudad ~ 15

degrees centering on the orbit. This view projects the optic canal in the center of the orbit and separates the anterior and middle cerebral arteries. If a lateral-oblique view is needed, we angle the tube LAO 25 degrees.

When facial views are needed a transorbital AP view to include from the mandible to just above the superior orbital ridge. The lateral projection includes from below the mandible to above the sella turcica (the Turkish saddle) and anteriorly to include the nose.

In cases of occlusion of the cervical or intracranial carotid and/or vertebral arteries, it is important to study the contralateral side to evaluate the circle of Willis supplying the occluded artery through the anterior or posterior communicat-

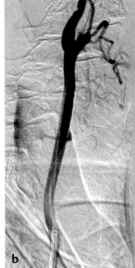
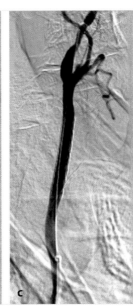
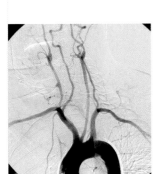

Fig. 9.10 An elderly individual had an attempted placement of a central catheter in the right internal jugular vein for hemodialysis. (a,b) Aortic arch arteriography and selective right carotid arteriography demonstrated a small pseudoaneurysm in the mid-common carotid artery. (c) Insertion of a covered stent was easily performed and the carotid blowout lesion managed by endovascular technique, the ideal choice method for these very serious iatrogenic traumatic injuries.

ing arteries. Sometimes external carotid arteriography is also needed to assess for collateralization. Certainly external carotid arteriography is done in all cases of injuries to the head, face, and when external carotid arteries and branches need to be embolized, and also in rare cases of arteriovenous fistula of traumatic origin.

9.8 Percutaneous Nephrostomy

Percutaneous nephrostomy (PCN) in trauma patients may present some challenges due to the different injuries elsewhere and the need to place the patient prone preferably, otherwise lateral or near prone. One of the main indications is an occluded or totally or partially transected ureter. Once the side to be studied is determined, we set up the tray with all of the needed supplies on the affected side.

The interventional radiologist marks the kidney for the PCN. We then place the ultrasound unit directly across the table on the contralateral side. Place the MizuhOSI ProneView Protective Helmet System or the face-down pillow on the table, if the patient is on a ventilator so the ventilator tubing may be connected through the openings of the device.

We place a radiolucent board under the table pad horizontally under the shoulders and rest the elbows on the arm board. It may be necessary to place folded towels or sheets under the patient's stomach to increase the accessibility of the kidney to be punctured. We image with single-shot imaging or last image hold or store monitor images (▶ Fig. 9.7).

Once the PCN is completed, we make sure to label the images correctly before sending the images to PACS.

9.9 Central Venous Access

Central venous access is necessary for fluid management, medication administration, blood draws, and can also facilitate power-injected CT scans. Although most trauma patients arrive at the IR suite with several IV sites and possibly a central line, some severely traumatized patients may require an extended hospital stay, so we make sure to consider inserting adequate access for the patient while in the IR suite.

It is fairly simple and quick to place a peripherally inserted central catheter (PICC) or a triple lumen catheter in IR with US guidance. The PICC is done by placing the arm on a radiolucent arm board and adducted, in the supine, palm-up position. We then raise the arm and prep the entire arm from just distal to the elbow to the axilla, and drape the patient in a sterile fashion.

Next is to place a sterile tourniquet under the arm, as close to the axilla as possible, and tighten. Utilizing US guidance, locate the basilic vein on the midarm to be accessed, inject a small amount of Lidocaine, and puncture the vein using a 4-cm echogenic micropuncture needle. Once accessed, gently insert a small 0.018" guidewire into the needle and advance it into the vein; with fluoroscopy position the tip of the wire into the superior vena cava (SVC)-right atrial junction. We then inject an additional amount of Lidocaine at the puncture site, make a small skin nick and remove the needle and insert a short Peel-Away. Determine the length of the PICC, cut it, and remove the inner dilator of the Peel-Away sheath and advance the PICC over the guidewire. Once in place, remove the wire, flush the catheter to ensure adequate blood return and either attach it to an IV for immediate use or block each port with heparin, if a dual-lumen PICC is inserted. We now document the PICC placement with a single shot or store monitor image. Secure the catheter in place with a suture or StatLock (Bard Davol, Warwick, RI) device. Fluoro and store an image of the chest to include to the shoulder to document the procedure. Finally, we label the images with the number of lumens, the length of the PICC, and if it can be power injected.

A triple lumen catheter is usually placed in the internal jugular vein in IR, but there are times when a common femoral vein approach is referenced. Ultrasound guidance is used for IJ venous access. If possible, turn the patient's head away and prep the anterior and lateral neck from below the ear to the level of the clavicle. Place a small sterile fenestrated drape over the area and locate the internal jugular vein with US. Inject a

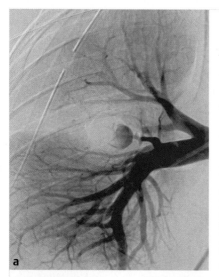

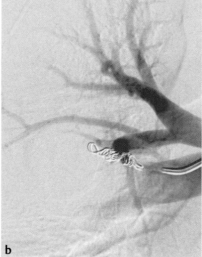

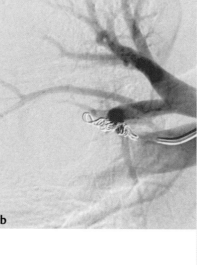

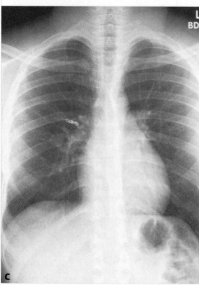

Fig. 9.11 Selective right pulmonary arteriogram in a child with a small pseudoaneurysm of the artery to the lingula secondary to a gunshot wound. The lesion was successfully embolized. (a) The patient received a bullet wound in the chest and was brought to the IR suite where a pseudoaneurysm arising from the right pulmonary artery was confirmed. (b) The apical superior segment of the right lower lobe pulmonary artery was catheterized and subsequently embolized with multiple 0.035 platinum coils. The patient was then taken to the operating room for evacuation of the hemothorax via video-assisted thoracoscopic surgery. (c) He was eventually discharged in stable condition with a normal follow-up chest radiograph. Catheter-directed embolization of pulmonary artery branches is a relatively straightforward and a much less-invasive technique to treat traumatic injury from penetrating or iatrogenic trauma, avoiding the significant morbidity and mortality associated with thoracotomy.

small amount of Lidocaine, and access the vein using a 4-cm echogenic micropuncture needle. Once accessed, gently slide a small 0.018" guidewire through the needle and advance it into the vein and with fluoroscopy position the tip of the wire into the SVC-right atrial junction. Inject additional Lidocaine at the puncture site, make a small skin nick and remove the needle and insert a short coaxial micropuncture catheter. Remove the 0.018 guidewire and inner catheter and advance a 0.035" guidewire to the SVC. Remove the outer micropuncture catheter and advance the triple lumen catheter over the 0.035" guidewire into position with fluoroscopic guidance. We then fluoro the chest and document the catheter placement with a single-shot image and secure in place with sutures and cover with a sterile dressing.

9.10 Inferior Vena Cava Filter Placement

Placement of inferior vena cava (IVC) filters may be beneficial for trauma victims that have multiple and extensive fractures of the pelvis and LE and/or are predisposed to deep vein thrombosis (DVT) or pulmonary embolism (PE) (▶ Fig. 9.11). It is important to determine whether a permanent or removable, temporary, optional IVC filter will be inserted. To insert an IVC filter while the patient is on the IR table, takes only a few minutes, particularly if the patient has just undergone an arteriogram from the femoral approach or requires an IJ triple-lumen catheter placement.

The groin is prepped and draped in a sterile fashion. Ultrasound guidance can be used for common femoral vein access, but it is not necessary. Once venous access is obtained, a 5F, 70-cm marker pigtail catheter is advanced into the common iliac vein and then inferior venacavogram filming is set from the top of the diaphragm to the iliac veins confluence slightly off centered toward the right with fluoroscopic monitoring.

The marker pigtail catheter is used to measure the diameter of the IVC because most IVC filters are recommended for a maximum diameter of 28 mm. Select a landmarked image and send it to the in-room monitor. From this point, we do not move the table until after the IVC filter is deployed. Next we advance a 0.035" guidewire through the pigtail catheter, remove the pigtail catheter, dilate the vein if necessary, and then advance the femoral IVC filter introducer catheter over the guidewire to the level of the renal veins. Depending upon which IVC filter is selected, the inner dilator is removed from the introducer and the IVC filter is advanced to the level just below the origin of the renal veins. While holding both hands steady, the introducer catheter is withdrawn releasing the IVC filter under careful fluoroscopic guidance. After deployment, the introducer is positioned in the distal IVC and an injection of contrast material is done by hand to confirm proper placement.

The jugular approach is performed by obtaining IJ venous access with a micropuncture set under US. A 0.035 guidewire is advanced distal to the common iliac vein bifurcation. The entire procedure is done under fluoroscopy. A 5-F, 100-cm marker pigtail catheter is advanced and inferior venacavogram obtained as stated above. The IVC jugular introducer sheath is positioned below the renal veins, the inner dilator removed, and the IVC filter is advanced through the introducer to the level below the origin of the renal veins. The filter delivery is similar, and once deployed, documentation with either a hand or a power injection is obtained.

Sometimes oblique views of 20 to 45 degrees are necessary pre- and postprocedure filter placement to visualize the IVC away from other structures such as bone or bowel gas to make sure the IVC is patent and free of clot. It may also be necessary to make several injections to determine IVC patency versus inflow or extrinsic compression. Finally, label and send contrast-enhanced and native images to PACS.

9.11 Conclusion

The most common diagnostic and IR procedures done in patients sustaining trauma have been mentioned and described briefly in this chapter. The interventional radiologist should be very familiar with all the necessary steps. The interventional radiology technologist works efficiently, quickly, and with a high degree of knowledge to obtain the best-quality studies considering the circumstances in each situation. The work is almost always done under extreme conditions with many people in the room; therefore, experience and special expertise and "touch" is needed by the IR technologists and ancillary personnel.

10 Interventional Radiology in Neck Trauma

Andre Biuckians and L.D. Britt

Traumatic injury to the neck has the potential for devastating morbidity and mortality due to its complex anatomical relationships of multiple vital structures. The major vascular structures at risk include the common carotid, internal carotid, external carotid, subclavian, and vertebral arteries. Blunt and penetrating trauma may result in vascular injuries. It is paramount that the trauma surgeons diagnose and properly manage such injuries.

Treatment for traumatic vascular injury dates back to Ambroise Pare's successful carotid ligation in 1510 for an injured soldier.[1,2] Ligation of blood vessels remained the mainstay of all vascular interventions until Mathieu Jaboulay, followed by Alexis Carrel who pioneered the vascular anastomosis.[3] Suture repair of a damaged blood vessel then became the foundation of open vascular surgery. Despite the continued improvement in surgical techniques, repair of traumatic injury to the blood vessels has remained a challenge to the surgeon.

Vascular surgery requires a meticulous operation in the best of circumstances and traumatic injury often includes several challenging variables. There can be local tissue destruction, other associated injuries, contaminated surgical fields, anatomically challenging locations of injured blood vessels and life-threatening physiologic disturbances. Any of these circumstances can hinder attempts at vessel repair or revascularization. For example, among the American casualties in World War II, there were 1,639 vessel ligations—compared with 59 vessel repairs in similarly grouped soldiers.[4]

The development of endovascular and catheter-directed interventions has changed the approach to the management of vascular disease, including vascular trauma. Routine use of angiography in trauma began in the early 1970s as an important diagnostic modality to localize vessel injury and has evolved to become an important treatment modality. In the United States from 1997 to 2003, there were 7,286 arterial repairs for traumatic injury and 281 catheter-based interventions.[5] Catheter-based interventions will continue to become more prevalent and are now common in the armamentarium of trauma care. In this chapter we will review the role of interventional radiology in cerebrovascular trauma.

10.1 Epidemiology

The overall incidence of a common carotid, internal carotid, or external carotid artery injury in all trauma patients is ~ 0.2%.[6] The true incidence of vertebral artery injury in all trauma patients is unknown. The mechanism of injury can be divided into two categories: penetrating and blunt.

In the civilian setting, penetrating injuries either involve low-velocity missile wounds or stab wounds, with stab wounds being the more common mechanism.[7,8,9] Vascular injuries due to low-velocity missile wounds more commonly have other significant injuries,[9,10] such as venous injury, cervical spine fractures, tracheobronchial injury, and alimentary tract injury. The overall mortality following penetrating trauma to the common carotid, internal carotid, or innominate artery ranges between 19 to 22%,[6,11] with 80% of these deaths due to stroke.[11] Stroke is seen in up to 15% of survivors.[11]

The incidence of blunt cerebrovascular injury among trauma patients ranges from 0.08 to 1.55%,[12,13,14,15] with the incidence of blunt common carotid or internal carotid artery injury reported as 1.11% and blunt vertebral artery injury as 0.77%.[15] The internal carotid artery is more commonly injured than the common carotid. Many authors believe that blunt cerebrovascular injury has been typically underdiagnosed because many patients remain asymptomatic or have a delayed onset of symptoms.[16] Some advocate aggressive screening for blunt cerebrovascular injury if cervical spine fractures are present.[17] Nearly all patients have other associated injuries, such as injuries to the brain, spine, chest, abdomen, and pelvis. Mortality can be as high as 26%, the majority of which is secondary to traumatic brain injury.[18] Up to 58% of survivors will have permanent neurologic deficits[19] and demonstrate more severe functional disability when compared with patients with penetrating carotid injury.[6]

10.2 Anatomical Considerations

The key to trauma surgery is damage control. There have been volumes written on the surgical experience when dealing with wartime and civilian trauma, and the first step is to stop hemorrhage. If the patient is stable, then there is an opportunity to proceed with a reparative operation. Anatomy and mechanisms of injury dictate the open approach to a vascular injury in the neck and understanding the anatomy provides the foundation on which endovascular interventions evolved.

The origins of the cerebrovascular vessels are confined to the mediastinum. The right common carotid is a branch of the innominate artery, whereas the left common carotid typically originates directly from the aortic arch. Injury to the proximal brachiocephalic vessels creates a challenge for the surgeon with regard to access and proximal control when attempting an open repair. Exposure of the innominate, right common carotid and left common carotid artery origins will often require a median sternotomy. Exposure of the left subclavian artery origin will require a high left thoracotomy.

Exposure and control of the distal internal carotid artery is of equal challenge. Maneuvers such as division of the posterior belly of the digastric muscle, mandibular subluxation, division of the stylohyoid ligament, and removal of styloid process may be used to gain exposure.[20] In some instances, exposure and control may not even be possible in distal cerebrovascular injury as the vessels disappear into the skull base. During aggressive distal exposure, there is a risk of injury to the hypoglossal, facial, and glossopharyngeal nerves. The distal branches of the external carotid artery are similarly surrounded by vital structures.

The vertebral artery is divided into four segments. The first (V1) vertebral artery segment starts at the origin, which typically is a branch of the subclavian artery and ends as the vertebral artery enters the transverse foramen of the cervical spine,

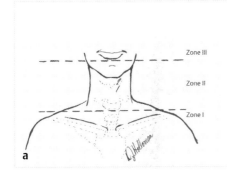

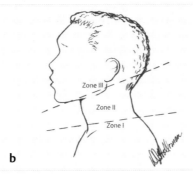

Fig. 10.1 The anatomical landmarks used to determine the three zones of neck injury. (Used with permission from Britt LD, Weireter LJ, Cole FJ. Management of acute neck injuries. In: Feliciano D, Mattox K, Moore E, eds. Trauma. 6th ed. New York, NY: McGraw-Hill; 2008)

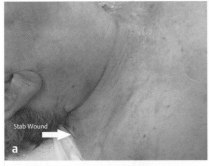

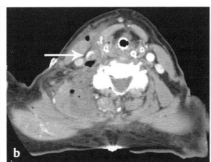

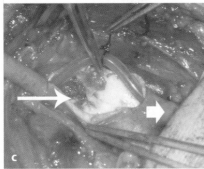

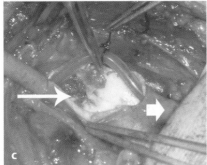

Fig. 10.2 (a) A stab wound to the right posterior neck (arrow). Note the lack of evidence of any vascular injury. (b) A computed tomography angiogram of the neck. The arrow marks the right common carotid artery which has been injured. (c) An intraoperative photograph of the same patient. The short arrow marks the right common carotid artery and the long arrow marks the intimal flap and thrombus due to the stab injury.

usually at C6. The second segment (V2) is the portion of the vessel that runs within the lateral cervical foramina. The third segment (V3) begins where the artery exits the lateral foramina of C1 and ends as it enters the skull base. The fourth segment (V4) is the intracranial portion. It is believed that 5 to 10% of individuals have hypoplasia of one of the vertebral arteries,[21,22] which becomes important in trauma if there is consideration of ligation versus repair. Ligation of a dominant vertebral artery may result in posterior cerebral ischemia.

It is well agreed that penetrating wounds superficial to the platysma do not require exploration.[8] Monson et al described an arbitrary division of the cervical region into three zones (► Fig. 10.1).[22] Zone I was described as the area from the sternal notch to the superior aspect of the sternoclavicular joint. Zone II was from the top of the sternoclavicular joint to the angle of the mandible. Zone III was the area from the angle of the mandible to the base of the skull. Modification of this scheme has evolved and describes zone I from the clavicles to the cricoid cartilage and zone II from the cricoid cartilage to the angle of the mandible.[23] Monson's original treatise proposed that penetrating injuries involving zone I and III require angiography, while all zone II penetrating injuries should undergo operative exploration.

10.3 Pathophysiologic Considerations

Trauma patients can be broadly fit into two categories: stable and unstable. The unstable trauma patient requires the concerted efforts of a highly trained trauma team and the use of the interventional radiology (IR) suite is limited.[24] Unstable patients may demonstrate hard signs of cerebrovascular injury such as active hemorrhage, a large pulsatile or expanding hematoma, or shock. Approximately 15 to 23% of patients present in this manner[7,8] and all must undergo operative exploration (► Fig. 10.2 a,c). Patients may present with "soft" signs of vascular injury that include a history of pulsatile bleeding, a small nonexpanding hematoma, or unexplained neurologic deficit. Other less common signs and symptoms that may be present with cerebrovascular injury include cervical bruit, radiographic evidence of cerebral infarction, unexplained focal neurologic deficits, and Horner syndrome. Further diagnostic testing is warranted and will be discussed below.

The mechanism of penetrating vascular injury is easily imagined and the artery is either lacerated or transected. Four mechanisms of blunt cerebrovascular injury have been described by Crissey et al[25]: Type 1 injury is a result of a direct blow to the neck; type 2 injuries result from hyperextension and rotation of the head and neck; type 3 results from intraoral trauma; type 4 is from a basilar skull fracture. Penetrating and blunt injuries may manifest as vessel thrombosis, pseudoaneurysm formation, arteriovenous fistula, dissection/intramural hematoma, or arterial disruption. When the injury stems from a penetrating trauma the tendency is toward repair whereas similar injuries in blunt trauma continue to be debated.

Biffl et al formalized an injury grading system in blunt carotid trauma.[26] Type I injuries either present with an irregular vessel lumen on angiogram or a dissection with < 25% stenosis. Type II injuries have either an intimal flap, intraluminal thrombus, or a dissection with > 25% stenosis. Type III injuries are pseudoaneurysms. Type IV includes thrombosed or occluded vessels. Type V injuries present with vessel disruption and hemorrhage. They reported that type I injuries typically heal, whereas type II and III injuries either progress or fail to heal. Type IV and V injuries are associated with a high rate of stroke and death.

10.4 Diagnosis

The diagnosis of vascular injury in neck trauma has been the focus of many debates and while a full discussion is beyond the scope of this chapter, there are a few salient points to be made. First, it is acceptable for the diagnosis of a cerebrovascular injury to be made in the operating room. An unstable trauma patient is typically not best served in the hallways of the radiology department, except in rare instances. In the majority of cases though there is an opportunity to perform diagnostic testing.

The gold standard diagnostic study in cerebrovascular trauma is the four-vessel carotid-vertebral angiogram. It is highly sensitive and specific. Its routine use though has been questioned because of the risks associated with an invasive diagnostic procedure (access site hematoma/pseudoaneurysm, contrast-agent nephrotoxicity, stroke) and a low clinical yield. North et al performed routine four-vessel angiography in 78 stable patients with penetrating neck trauma deep to the platysma with no other clinical findings, only to uncover two occult vascular injuries and neither one required operative treatment.[27] It can be argued that if a four-vessel angiogram reveals an injury, there is an opportunity for an endovascular treatment, but not every injury needs to be repaired.[1] In the setting of damage control, the goal should be to diagnose injury in the most efficient and effective manner with the least risk to the patient.

Duplex ultrasonography (DUS) has been shown to be an effective diagnostic tool in evaluating penetrating neck trauma. Fry et al found DUS detected clinically significant carotid injuries resulting from zone II penetrating trauma with 100% accuracy.[28] Demetriades et al reported a sensitivity of 91% and specificity of 98% when using DUS to evaluate patients with penetrating neck trauma.[29] Evaluation of blunt cerebrovascular injury using DUS has not been as effective with up to 14% of cerebrovascular injuries missed.[30] Also, DUS evaluation of the V2 and V3 segments of the vertebral artery is limited by its course through the lateral foramina and proximity to the skull base. Duplex ultrasonography use in penetrating or blunt vertebral artery trauma has not been fully evaluated.

The helical computed tomographic (CT) scan has become an important tool in the assessment of trauma patients (▶ Fig. 10.2b). It provides a quick radiographic assessment of a stable trauma patient and can diagnose bony, soft tissue, solid organ, and vascular injuries. Inaba et al performed helical CT angiography (CTA) on 91 stable patients with penetrating neck trauma and report a 100% sensitivity and 93% specificity in detecting vascular and aerodigestive injuries.[7] There were five false-positive scans, but only one was a falsely diagnosed vascular (vertebral artery) injury and the others were aerodigestive. Munera et al reported 98% specificity for CTA in penetrating neck trauma.[31] In these series, up to 1% of examinations were inadequate due to foreign body artifact and these patients underwent four-vessel angiogram. Malhorta et al performed helical CTA and digital subtraction angiogram on 92 patients with blunt neck trauma only to report 74% sensitivity and 86% specificity for detecting cerebrovascular injury due to blunt trauma.[32] Of note, this study was performed with a 16-detector CT scan and currently no studies have evaluated the newer 64-detector machines which may improve these results.

There have been reports of utilizing magnetic resonance imaging (MRI) or magnetic resonance angiography (MRA) in cerebrovascular trauma[13] but this must be approached with caution. There is absolutely no place for MRI/MRA evaluation of an acute trauma patient. Performing these diagnostic examinations takes time and isolates a potentially unstable patient in a room with limited monitoring capabilities. There are no acute injuries that cannot be diagnosed by the combination of examination, X-ray, duplex ultrasound, CT scan, or an open operation. If a trauma patient is stable after a full assessment, proceeding with an MRI/MRA may be reasonable.

In evaluating a stable patient with neck trauma, we perform either DUS, CTA, or both. In cases with suspected vertebral artery injury, if DUS and CTA are equivocal, then proceeding with a four-vessel angiogram is warranted. We typically do not utilize MRI/MRA except in special circumstances.

10.5 Treatment

The treatment of cerebrovascular injury in trauma continues to evolve especially with the advent of better diagnostic testing and less invasive treatments. This section will review the types of injuries, whether they should be treated, and whether they can be considered for an endovascular approach. When treating patients with neck trauma, airway management must always be a priority in all settings. A neck hematoma or oropharyngeal hemorrhage can immediately lead to airway loss and death. If there is any concern, airway control via intubation should be performed prior to any endovascular procedure. The presence of "hard" signs of vascular injury requires immediate operative exploration.

10.6 Vessel Disruption

Penetrating injury to the common carotid or internal carotid arteries with vessel disruption that present with exsanguinations or unstable hematoma must undergo operative repair or ligation. A percutaneous endovascular approach in this situation is ill-advised, but there are opportunities for endovascular adjuncts to open operative management. For example, Fogarty catheter balloon occlusion can be used for distal control if a distal vessel clamp cannot be applied,[33] which may occur in zone III injuries. Blunt carotid trauma resulting in a grade V lesion is typically fatal.[26]

External carotid injury is rare and open ligation of the external carotid artery is easily tolerated. Transcatheter embolization of external carotid artery injury has been successfully performed, but there are only a few reported cases.[34] Injury to the branches of the external carotid can present with severe refractory epistaxis. Luo et al successfully treated three patients with penetrating injuries to the internal maxillary artery with *N*-butyl-cyanoacrylate embolization with no postembolization complications.[35]

Penetrating injury to the vertebral artery rarely results in vessel disruption.[36] Operative management can be challenging due to vertebral anatomy as mentioned above. Proximal vessel ligation has been the typical approach given that unilateral vertebral artery ligation has a very low stroke risk.[37] But continued hemorrhage from the distal end can lead to further complications,[38] such as pseudoaneurysm or arteriovenous fistula formation. Lee et al report a successful transcatheter embolization of a transected vertebral artery due to penetrating trauma with proximal and distal coils.[36] To achieve this, they initially performed proximal coil embolization. Then a microcatheter was passed via the contralateral vertebral artery, across the vertebral artery confluence, and down the distal ipsilateral segment at which point detachable coils were utilized.

Repair of a vertebral artery injury is only reserved for patients with a hypoplastic, absent, or occluded contralateral vertebral artery because the risk for posterior ischemia is significant. There have been no reports of utilizing stent grafts in treating vertebral artery transection in lieu of open vessel repair or bypass, but it seems like a feasible option and warrants further investigation.

Vessel disruption often signifies a significant mechanism of injury and in most circumstances must be treated via open repair. Endovascular treatment seems feasible in two vessels. External carotid artery or vertebral artery disruptions may be amenable to transcatheter embolization. This avoids an extensive dissection required during an open ligation of these vessels and the four-vessel angiogram can diagnose other brachiocephalic injuries.

10.7 Pseudoaneurysm/Dissection/Arteriovenous Fistula

The bulk of endovascular treatments in cerebrovascular injury will treat pseudoaneurysm, dissection, or arteriovenous fistula. Treatment for traumatic pseudoaneurysm in neck trauma has continued to evolve and has included observation, anticoagulation, antiplatelet therapy, endovascular treatment, and open repair. Observation has been associated with worse neurologic outcomes and higher mortality,[16] and thus avoided. Despite better neurologic outcomes with anticoagulation, traumatic pseudoaneurysms do not spontaneously resolve.[16] Treatment decisions typically depend on the location of injury. For instance, zone II trauma with a pseudoaneurysm should undergo operative repair.[1,37] In many instances, an isolated

pseudoaneurysm in the neck will be treated with anticoagulation for a short time and then be considered for repair, or are discovered in follow-up diagnostic tests. This provides an opportunity to consider an endovascular approach.

Endovascular treatments for pseudoaneurysms include vessel preserving and vessel sacrificing coil embolization, stenting with either a noncovered or covered stent, or balloon occlusion. Location of the pseudoaneurysm plays a role in deciding which treatment to apply. A pseudoaneurysm of the common carotid or internal carotid artery should rarely be approached with coil embolization due to the risk of cerebral infarction, so stent repair seems logical.

Marin et al published one of the earliest series of stent graft repair of a pseudoaneurysm of a peripheral artery after penetrating trauma with no periprocedural complications and 100% patency at 14 months.[39] This series contained no cerebrovascular injuries. Edwards et al report the results of noncovered stent repair of 18 pseudoaneurysms from blunt carotid trauma.[18] Stents were placed in the internal carotid artery and all patients received either anticoagulation or antiplatelet therapy. Two patients died, two were lost to follow-up, and the remaining 14 patients had a patent stent confirmed by an angiogram with no neurologic sequelae. The follow-up ranged from 1 to 204 weeks; hence the long-term durability and patency cannot be determined.

10.8 Thrombosis

Cothren et al performed a randomized trial comparing anticoagulation versus antiplatelet therapy in patients with grade I–III blunt carotid injury.[40] At day 10, a repeat angiogram was performed and those with a new or persistent pseudoaneurysm were considered for noncovered stent placement. Twenty-three patients underwent stent repair with a 13% periprocedural stroke rate. Forty-five percent of the stents were occluded at follow-up. In a case report, Duane et al reported treatment of a pseudoaneurysm of the internal carotid artery with a covered stent graft, which was occluded at follow-up with no neurologic sequelae.[41] In another series, Cox et al reviewed endovascular treatments of traumatic pseudoaneurysms of the neck from war injuries.[42] One patient with an internal carotid artery pseudoaneurysm was treated with a self-expanding stent graft and antiplatelet therapy, but on follow-up was found to be occluded without neurologic sequelae.

The high rate of poststent occlusion is alarming and the reason is unclear. Hypercoagulable state secondary to the physiologic stress of trauma, accelerated intimal hyperplasia, reduced flow dynamics have all been suggested as mechanisms for the high occlusion rate.[40] There are a few case reports of combined coil embolization and stent deployment in these lesions.[43,44,45] This technique involves catheterizing the pseudoaneurysm, deploying a flexible stent, and then packing the aneurysm with coils. The stent acts as an intraluminal scaffold and cages the embolic agent in the pseudoaneurysm. This technique has not been fully investigated for use in the carotid artery pseudoaneurysm.

Lee et al performed coil embolization with stenting in vertebral pseudoaneurysms in five patients with a mean follow-up of 36 months.[36] There were no periprocedural complications. At follow-up, all the treated lesions remained occluded, the native vessel was patent, and there were no neurologic sequelae reported. The preservation of the native vessel is an additional advantage in this technique. Historically, vertebral artery ligation has been the typical approach to traumatic pseudoaneurysms.[46] Coil embolization and balloon occlusion is becoming an accepted modality in treating pseudoaneurysms of the vertebral artery.[1]

Blunt traumatic dissection of the carotid and vertebral artery should be treated with anticoagulation or antiplatelet therapy, which has been shown to prevent cerebral infarction with minimal complications.[16,18] Endovascular treatment for dissection should only be considered if a pseudoaneurysm forms as outlined above. There are some who advocate for stent repair of dissections that result in a critical common carotid or internal carotid artery stenosis. Assadian et al reported a 100% procedural success rate of stent graft repair of internal carotid dissections in six patients, four of which were due to trauma.[47] Four patients had a > 80% stenosis and the other two had aneurysmal degeneration of the dissection. One patient developed focal neurologic symptoms postoperatively but recovered. At follow-up, all patients were asymptomatic and the stents remained patent.

Endovascular treatment for traumatic cerebrovascular dissection remains controversial. There have been no randomized trials to determine best therapy. At this time anticoagulation or antiplatelet therapy remains as the first-line therapy and patients will require close follow-up with appropriate imaging. Endovascular treatment can be considered if the patient continues to be symptomatic or a pseudoaneurysm forms. If anticoagulation and antiplatelet therapies are contraindicated, then open repair may be the only solution. Stenting without antiplatelet therapy has a high risk of stent occlusion.

Arteriovenous fistulas (AVFs) have been successfully treated with coil embolization in a variety of anatomical locations.[48] Beaujeux et al treated 35 vertebral arteriovenous fistulas using detachable balloon embolization with no neurologic sequelae.[49] Complete obligation of the AVF was achieved in 94% of cases and those that resulted in partial occlusion had resolution of most symptoms. There were three vertebral artery occlusions postembolization and all three patients remained asymptomatic.

Endovascular treatment in the setting of thrombosis after common carotid or internal carotid artery trauma has a limited role. Thrombosis after penetrating carotid trauma should undergo open repair even in the asymptomatic patient.[37,50] Thrombosis after blunt carotid trauma requires anticoagulation.[16] Any attempt at endovascular recannulization or thrombolysis will surely be fraught with disaster.

Thrombosis of the vertebral artery after penetrating or blunt trauma remains controversial. Treatment with coil embolization has been advocated because arterial disruption is a common finding upon operative exploration.[38] On the other hand, several authors reported no significant sequelae after a limited follow-up period.[29,51]

10.9 Conclusion

In the acute setting, there seems to be a limited role for the endovascular approach to neck trauma. If the patient is unstable, the patient will be better served in the operating room or intensive care unit. Endovascular treatment has demonstrated effectiveness in treating traumatic pseudoaneurysms,

dissections, and arteriovenous fistulas. The role of endovascular therapy will likely continue to evolve and change. In the future, it will not be surprising to see increased utilization of endovascular therapies in the acute setting and in unstable patients. This will be aided by the carotid stent experience for the treatment of cerebrovascular atherosclerosis and will likely increase stent use in cerebrovascular trauma. A pertinent parallel might be made to the evolution of endovascular abdominal aortic aneurysm repair (EVAR). Initially, EVAR was performed in highly select individuals purely in an elective manner. As the EVAR experience has grown, now it is quite common for a patient with a ruptured abdominal aortic aneurysm to have an endovascular repair. Investigation in the use of endovascular treatments in neck trauma will continue.

References

[1] Ernst CB, Stanley JC. Current Therapy in Vascular Surgery. 4th ed. St. Louis, MO: Mosby; 2001

[2] Fogelman MJ, Stewart RD. Penetrating wounds of the neck. Am J Surg 1956; 91: 581–596

[3] Konner K. History of vascular access for haemodialysis. Nephrol Dial Transplant 2005; 20: 2629–2635

[4] Daniel C. Elkin MED. Vascular Surgery in World War II. Washington, DC: Office of the Surgeon General of the Army; 1955

[5] Reuben BC, Whitten MG, Sarfati M, Kraiss LW. Increasing use of endovascular therapy in acute arterial injuries: analysis of the National Trauma Data Bank. J Vasc Surg 2007; 46: 1222–1226

[6] Martin MJ, Mullenix PS, Steele SR et al. Functional outcome after blunt and penetrating carotid artery injuries: analysis of the National Trauma Data Bank. J Trauma 2005; 59: 860–864

[7] Inaba KMF, Munera F, McKenney M et al. Prospective evaluation of screening multislice helical computed tomographic angiography in the initial evaluation of penetrating neck injuries. J Trauma 2006; 61: 144–149

[8] Insull P, Adams D, Segar A, Ng A, Civil I. Is exploration mandatory in penetrating zone II neck injuries? ANZ J Surg 2007; 77: 261–264

[9] Biffl WL, Moore EE, Rehse DH, Offner PJ, Franciose RJ, Burch JM. Selective management of penetrating neck trauma based on cervical level of injury. Am J Surg 1997; 174: 678–682

[10] Medzon R, Rothenhaus T, Bono CM, Grindlinger G, Rathlev NK. Stability of cervical spine fractures after gunshot wounds to the head and neck. Spine 2005; 30: 2274–2279

[11] du Toit DF, van Schalkwyk GD, Wadee SA, Warren BL. Neurologic outcome after penetrating extracranial arterial trauma. J Vasc Surg 2003; 38: 257–262

[12] Berne JD, Norwood SH, McAuley CE, Vallina VL, Creath RG, McLarty J. The high morbidity of blunt cerebrovascular injury in an unscreened population: more evidence of the need for mandatory screening protocols. J Am Coll Surg 2001; 192: 314–321

[13] Biffl WL, Moore EE, Offner PJ, Burch JM. Blunt carotid and vertebral arterial injuries. World J Surg 2001; 25: 1036–1043

[14] McKinney A, Ott F, Short J, McKinney Z, Truwit C. Angiographic frequency of blunt cerebrovascular injury in patients with carotid canal or vertebral foramen fractures on multidetector CT. Eur J Radiol 2007; 62: 385–393

[15] Biffl WL, Ray CE, Moore EE et al. Treatment-related outcomes from blunt cerebrovascular injuries: importance of routine follow-up arteriography. Ann Surg 2002; 235: 699–706, discussion 706–707

[16] Fabian TC, Patton JH, Croce MA, Minard G, Kudsk KA, Pritchard FE. Blunt carotid injury. Importance of early diagnosis and anticoagulant therapy. Ann Surg 1996; 223: 513–522, discussion 522–525

[17] Cothren CC, Moore EE, Ray CE, Johnson JL, Moore JB, Burch JM. Cervical spine fracture patterns mandating screening to rule out blunt cerebrovascular injury. Surgery 2007; 141: 76–82

[18] Edwards NM, Fabian TC, Claridge JA, Timmons SD, Fischer PE, Croce MA. Antithrombotic therapy and endovascular stents are effective treatment for blunt carotid injuries: results from longterm followup. J Am Coll Surg 2007; 204: 1007–1013, discussion 1014–1015

[19] Biffl WL, Moore EE, Ryu RK et al. The unrecognized epidemic of blunt carotid arterial injuries: early diagnosis improves neurologic outcome. Ann Surg 1998; 228: 462–470

[20] Valentine RJ, Wind GG. Anatomic Exposures in Vascular Surgery. 2nd ed. Philadelphia, PA: Lippincott, Williams, & Wilkins; 2003

[21] Vilimas ABE, Vilionskis A, Rudzinskaite F, Morkunaite R. Vertebral artery hypoplasia: importance for stroke development, the role of the posterior communicating artery, possibility for surgical and conservative treatment. Acta Medica Lituanica 2003; 10: 1–10

[22] Monson DO, Saletta JD, Freeark RJ. Carotid vertebral trauma. J Trauma 1969; 9: 987–999

[23] Eddy VA. Is routine arteriography mandatory for penetrating injury to zone 1 of the neck? Zone 1 Penetrating Neck Injury Study Group. J Trauma 2000; 48: 208–213, discussion 213–214

[24] Agolini SF, Shah K, Jaffe J, Newcomb J, Rhodes M, Reed JF. Arterial embolization is a rapid and effective technique for controlling pelvic fracture hemorrhage. J Trauma 1997; 43: 395–399

[25] Crissey MM, Bernstein EF. Delayed presentation of carotid intimal tear following blunt craniocervical trauma. Surgery 1974; 75: 543–549

[26] Biffl WL, Moore EE, Offner PJ, Brega KE, Franciose RJ, Burch JM. Blunt carotid arterial injuries: implications of a new grading scale. J Trauma 1999; 47: 845–853

[27] North CM, Ahmadi J, Segall HD, Zee CS. Penetrating vascular injuries of the face and neck: clinical and angiographic correlation. AJR Am J Roentgenol 1986; 147: 995–999

[28] Fry WR, Dort JA, Smith RS, Sayers DV, Morabito DJ. Duplex scanning replaces arteriography and operative exploration in the diagnosis of potential cervical vascular injury. Am J Surg 1994; 168: 693–695, discussion 695–696

[29] Demetriades D, Theodorou D, Cornwell E et al. Penetrating injuries of the neck in patients in stable condition. Physical examination, angiography, or color flow Doppler imaging. Arch Surg 1995; 130: 971–975

[30] Cogbill TH, Moore EE, Meissner M et al. The spectrum of blunt injury to the carotid artery: a multicenter perspective. J Trauma 1994; 37: 473–479

[31] Múnera F, Cohn S, Rivas LA. Penetrating injuries of the neck: use of helical computed tomographic angiography. J Trauma 2005; 58: 413–418

[32] Malhotra AK, Camacho M, Ivatury RR et al. Computed tomographic angiography for the diagnosis of blunt carotid/vertebral artery injury: a note of caution. Ann Surg 2007; 246: 632–642, discussion 642–643

[33] Arthurs ZM, Sohn VY, Starnes BW. Vascular trauma: endovascular management and techniques. Surg Clin North Am 2007; 87: 1179–1192, x–xix-xi.

[34] Smith TP. Embolization in the external carotid artery. J Vasc Interv Radiol 2006; 17: 1897–1912, quiz 1913

[35] Luo CB, Teng MM, Chang FC, Chang CY. Transarterial embolization of acute external carotid blowout syndrome with profuse oronasal bleeding by N-butyl-cyanoacrylate. Am J Emerg Med 2006; 24: 702–708

[36] Lee YJ, Ahn JY, Han IB, Chung YS, Hong CK, Joo JY. Therapeutic endovascular treatments for traumatic vertebral artery injuries. J Trauma 2007; 62: 886–891

[37] Ballard JL, Teruya TH. Carotid and vertebral artery injuries. In: Rutherford RB, ed. Vascular Surgery. 6th ed. Philadelphia, PA: Elsevier Saunders; 2005:1006–1016

[38] Reid JD, Weigelt JA. Forty-three cases of vertebral artery trauma. J Trauma 1988; 28: 1007–1012

[39] Marin ML, Veith FJ, Panetta TF et al. Transluminally placed endovascular stented graft repair for arterial trauma. J Vasc Surg 1994; 20: 466–472, discussion 472–473

[40] Cothren CC, Moore EE, Ray CE et al. Carotid artery stents for blunt cerebrovascular injury: risks exceed benefits. Arch Surg 2005; 140: 480–485, discussion 485–486

[41] Duane TM, Parker F, Stokes GK, Parent FN, Britt LD. Endovascular carotid stenting after trauma. J Trauma 2002; 52: 149–153

[42] Cox MW, Whittaker DR, Martinez C, Fox CJ, Feuerstein IM, Gillespie DL. Traumatic pseudoaneurysms of the head and neck: early endovascular intervention. J Vasc Surg 2007; 46: 1227–1233

[43] Mericle RA, Lanzino G, Wakhloo AK, Guterman LR, Hopkins LN. Stenting and secondary coiling of intracranial internal carotid artery aneurysm: technical case report. Neurosurgery 1998; 43: 1229–1234

[44] Klein GE, Szolar DH, Raith J, Frühwirth H, Pascher O, Hausegger KA. Post-traumatic extracranial aneurysm of the internal carotid artery: combined endovascular treatment with coils and stents. AJNR Am J Neuroradiol 1997; 18: 1261–1264

[45] Assali AR, Sdringola S, Moustapha A et al. Endovascular repair of traumatic pseudoaneurysm by uncovered self-expandable stenting with or without transstent coiling of the aneurysm cavity. Catheter Cardiovasc Interv 2001; 53: 253–258

[46] Wiener I, Flye MW. Traumatic false aneurysm of the vertebral artery. J Trauma 1984; 24: 346–349

[47] Assadian A, Senekowitsch C, Rotter R, Zölss C, Strassegger J, Hagmüller GW. Long-term results of covered stent repair of internal carotid artery dissections. J Vasc Surg 2004; 40: 484–487

[48] Klein GE, Szolar DH, Karaic R, Stein JK, Hausegger KA, Schreyer HH. Extracranial aneurysm and arteriovenous fistula: embolization with the Guglielmi detachable coil. Radiology 1996; 201: 489–494

[49] Beaujeux RL, Reizine DC, Casasco A et al. Endovascular treatment of vertebral arteriovenous fistula. Radiology 1992; 183: 361–367

[50] Ramadan F, Rutledge R, Oller D, Howell P, Baker C, Keagy B. Carotid artery trauma: a review of contemporary trauma center experiences. J Vasc Surg 1995; 21: 46–55, discussion 55–56

[51] Yee LF, Olcott EW, Knudson MM, Lim RC. Extraluminal, transluminal, and observational treatment for vertebral artery injuries. J Trauma 1995; 39: 480–484, discussion 484–486

11 Interventional Radiology in Head Trauma

Emanuele Orrù, Sasikhan Geibprasert, Wen-Yuan Zhao, Marcus H.T. Reinges, and Timo Krings

11.1 Introduction

Trauma is the 10th cause of death worldwide[1] and was the leading cause of death in individuals under the age of 45 in the United States in 2010.[2] The predominant causes of death related to trauma are central nervous system (CNS) injuries and blood loss from hemorrhage. Head and neck trauma can lead to both these events, either in a direct or indirect way.

The American College of Surgeons National Trauma Databank of 2012 reported 773,299 traumas during 2011: falls and motor vehicle accidents accounted for the majority of these lesions. Other common causes of trauma include, but are not limited to gunshot wounds, stab wounds, and aggravated assault. The head and neck region was involved in 61.14% of these traumas.

In this chapter, we will focus on the diagnostic and therapeutic workup of traumatic damage to head and neck vasculature that can lead to additional secondary CNS injuries.

Traumatic injuries to the vessels of the head and neck are complications of head and neck trauma that can result in potentially devastating sequelae, both neurologic and systemic. To minimize the occurrence of these events an early diagnosis and a treatment tailored to each individual case are of utmost importance.

Depending on the cited source, the incidence of cerebral vascular trauma ranges from 0.18 to 1.55%[3,4,5,6,7] of all trauma patients with an approximate ratio of 2:1 for internal carotid artery (ICA) involvement compared with vertebral artery (VA) involvement. Traumatic injuries to head and neck arteries can lead to locoregional complications (i.e., intra- or extracranial hemorrhages with exsanguination and/or compression of nearby structures) and remote complications (i.e., ischemic lesions in the brain or spine).

The spectrum of cerebrovascular lesions resulting from head and neck traumas is broad and the lesions are dynamic in their evolution. Injuries can involve arteries, veins, or a combination of both. Arterial damage has been extensively studied and reviewed in the pertinent literature. Depending on how many layers of the vessel wall are involved in the injury and on the adjacent structures, intimal and/or medial tears with or without dissection, pseudoaneurysms, arteriovenous fistulas (AVFs), and vessel transection can occur. It is also important to understand that given the different types of cerebrovascular damage, patients may show a delayed clinical presentation, compared with the occurrence of the primary traumatic event. These different injuries can occur regardless of the pathomechanism of the trauma.

Neurovascular trauma can be divided according to their pathomechanisms in either penetrating or blunt with the latter being by far the most common one (see Box: Mechanisms of Arterial Cerebrovascular Trauma).

Mechanisms of Arterial Cerebrovascular Trauma

Penetrating trauma
- Direct injury to the arterial wall leading to disruption and false aneurysm (pseudoaneurysm) formation
- Disrupts only the tunica adventitia layer delayed aneurysm formation over years

Blunt trauma
- Pathomechanism
  - Direct force to the arterial wall
  - Indirect force, i.e., hyperextension-rotation injuries, shearing forces, enclosed head injuries
- Types of injury
  - Intimal tear, subintimal dissection (hematoma), stenosis, or occlusion
  - Subadventitia dissection only, Horner syndrome (wall thickening without narrowing of the lumen)
  - Hemorrhage into media + adventitia ± tear of the intima, fusiform dilatation
  - Tear of all layers
    - Into surrounding tissue false aneurysm
    - Adjacent vein arteriovenous fistula

11.2 Penetrating Trauma

Wounds that extend deep to the platysma are considered penetrating injuries of the neck. The most common causes of penetrating trauma are missile injuries from firearms and stab injuries, with the former usually causing a greater amount of damage than the latter. Other less usual events that lead to accidental penetrating traumas are falls and motor vehicle accidents. Up to 25% of penetrating neck injuries can result in arterial damage: Due to the more superficial location of the vessel, up to 80% involve the carotid arteries and up to 43% involve the VAs. Carotid artery injuries are particularly devastating, leading to stroke in as many as 15% of patients and death in 22%.[8] Landreneau et al found that patients with penetrating injuries involving both the carotid and vertebral arteries were subject to 50% mortality as compared with the mortality from penetrating trauma to either vessel alone.[9]

The neck has been divided for prognosis and treatment purposes into three zones.[10] Zone I extends from the clavicles to the cricoid cartilage, zone II from the cricoid cartilage to the angle of the mandible, and zone III from the angle of the mandible to the skull base. Although in the past zone II lesions have been considered an indication for surgical exploration and zone

I and III have been usually referred for therapeutic angiography, today the common initial approach to penetrating trauma, regardless of the affected anatomical zone, involves fast and widely available imaging studies such as computed tomography (CT) and CT angiography (CTA).

Penetrating trauma appears to be more related to vessel transection with pseudoaneurysm formation due to direct injury and disruption of the arterial wall, while dissections occur less frequently compared with blunt trauma.[8] In some cases, if the disruption involves only the tunica adventitita layer, a pseudoaneurysm can form over years.

11.3 Blunt Trauma

Blunt injury to the carotid or vertebral vessels (blunt cerebrovascular injury [BCVI]) has a prevalence that varies from 1.1 to 2.7% in patients hospitalized for blunt trauma in the United States, according to the severity of the injuries.[11] Damage to the vessels can occur by many means: direct force on the arterial wall due to compression with or without associated fractures and indirect forces secondary to stretching due to hyperextension-rotation injuries. Feiz-Erfan et al[12] noted that a neurovascular injury showed a statistically significant association with clival fractures and the tendency to be associated with fractures of the sella turcica-sphenoid sinus complex due to the close proximity of these regions to both the ICAs and the VAs. Skull base fractures should therefore be regarded as high-risk fractures for cerebrovascular injuries. Morbidity and mortality for carotid artery injuries range from 32 to 67% and from 17 to 38%, respectively. With VA lesions these values are lower, with a morbidity range of 14 to 24% and a mortality range of 8 to 18%.[13] Despite these high rates of morbidity and mortality BCVI can often present with few signs and symptoms, in contrast to the much more dramatic appearance of penetrating traumas. Given the aforementioned association with cervical/skull base fractures, imaging evaluation of the arterial system should be performed in the setting of high-impact mechanism injuries and in low-impact mechanism injuries if there are mandible fractures, basilar skull fractures, or cervical spine injuries.[13,14]

In 1999 Biffl et al[15] proposed a five-grade classification of blunt vascular injuries. In their experience, grade I injuries are mild intimal injuries with luminal narrowing < 25%; grade II injuries are intimal injuries, dissections, or intramural hematomas with luminal stenosis > 25%; grade III injuries have pseudoaneurysm formation; grade IV injuries are vessel occlusions; grade V injuries are complete transections. In their experience, the grade of the injury correlates with the clinical outcome. Two-thirds of mild intimal injuries (grade I) healed regardless of treatment, while grade II injuries progressed despite heparin in 70% of cases. Only 8% of pseudoaneurysms (grade III) injuries healed with heparin therapy, but 70% healed after stent placement. Grade IV injuries did not recanalize spontaneously in the early postoperative period, and grade V injuries were usually lethal and refractory to treatment. Overall, an increased stroke risk was consistent with injury grade.

The most common arterial injury after blunt trauma, at times minor or remote, is arterial dissection, whereas vessel wall irregularity, pseudoaneurysms, thrombi, and arterial occlusions are direct consequences of the dissection.[16]

11.4 Diagnostic Workup

Given the broad range of presentations of head and neck trauma, a detailed description of the emergency diagnostic approach to these patients is beyond the scope of this chapter. The clinical presentation of the patient may vary from the hemodynamically unstable polytraumatized patient to the individual that develops symptoms in a subtle way over a long time, sometimes months or even years after a minor traumatic event that can often go unnoticed.[16] Every patient should be thoroughly triaged and taken care of by a dedicated physician or team of physicians, which should then choose the most appropriate diagnostic modality.

In the acute trauma setting, after the trauma team has obtained a reasonable airway, breathing, and circulation (ABC) stability, CT should be the modality of choice since it is widely available throughout most hospitals and allows a fast assessment of large areas of the body including in the same exam an evaluation of bones, brain, soft tissues, and vasculature. In the event of a suspected or likely trauma-related vascular injury, the technique also allows for performing a CTA. In this case, a carefully timed contrast injection can give information on both the arterial and venous axis, on blood extravasations and on communications between the two systems (i.e., an AVF).

A noncontrast CT of the head is always the first imaging modality in the acute head trauma setting. The protocol should include the skull base through the vertex and can easily show the presence of intracerebral hemorrhages, parenchymal contusions, extra- or subdural hematomas, and subarachnoid hemorrhages (SAHs), thus guiding the indication for neurosurgical consultation and contraindicating antiplatelet/anticoagulating therapies. Also 1- to 1.25-mm-thick slices should be obtained to assess the presence of skull fractures, in which case a three-dimensional (3D) volume-rendered reconstruction is indicated. When the trauma involves the neck, an unenhanced CT can show vertebral fractures and soft tissue swellings. In some traumas, especially if penetrating, it can be helpful to localize foreign bodies like metallic fragments.

When needed, a CTA exam should be conducted from the aortic arch to above the circle of Willis, with an arterial trigger set at 80 Hounsfield unit (HU) on the aortic arch and with a 5- to 10-second delay. Submillimeter axial images allow for multiplanar reconstructions (MPR) and maximum intensity projections (MIP) in three planes, which provide an excellent representation of the head and neck vasculature and can guide the decision between conservative therapy and endovascular/surgical treatments.

In the past, digital subtraction angiography (DSA) has been the modality of choice for the evaluation of the head and neck vasculature, and is still considered the gold standard in the study of vessles. However, DSA has been essentially replaced by CTA because CTA is faster, much more available and does not have the 1% procedure risk related to DSA.[17] Digital subtraction angiography should therefore be reserved for unclear cases and for preoperative analysis of the vessels during endovascular therapeutic procedures.

Magnetic resonance imaging (MRI) is not routinely used in the acute setting because it is not always available, the examination takes longer than a CT, and because it is not compatible with certain life-support equipment. The possible presence of unknown metallic fragments or other paramagnetic foreign bodies constitutes another contraindication to this modality in the acute setting. Nevertheless, MRI is the modality of choice to detect recent ischemia (using diffusion weighted imaging [DWI]), for follow-up (i.e., in the case of dissections) and to study patients in nonemergent situations.

11.5 Therapy Options

Once a diagnosis has been established, the therapy options available to the treating physicians in the context of a cerebrovascular trauma are medical, surgical, and endovascular. In this chapter, we focus on the surgical and endovascular options. The aim of any therapeutic decision should be to stop ongoing active hemorrhages and to avoid/minimize cerebral ischemic damages.

11.5.1 Medical Therapy

Medical therapy in the form of observation and anticoagulation or antiplatelet drugs is the mainstay of conservative treatment in carotid dissections. Anticoagulants and antiplatelet drugs may prevent ischemic stroke, but bleeding from traumatized tissues may offset the benefits of antithrombotic treatment.[6]

When possible, in asymptomatic patients without pseudoaneurysms or other active bleeding spots, medical therapy should be favored.

11.5.2 Endovascular Therapy

When indicated, endovascular therapy guarantees a quick and minimally invasive approach to sites that would be difficult or impossible to reach with surgery. Neurointerventional techniques can be used alone or in combination with medical or surgical therapies. According to the case, it is possible to perform embolizations by means of particles, coils, Gelfoam (Pfizer, New York, NY), glue, or a combination of these agents or to restore/maintain patency of a vessel with conventional stents or covered stent grafts.

A diagnostic angiogram is always performed before starting any therapeutic procedure to visualize the precise anatomy of the vasculature, the exact location of the injury from an angiographic point of view, and to assess the presence and validity of a collateral circulation, especially when vessel sacrifice is contemplated. A standard cerebral DSA includes the study of the two ICAs and VAs, with the addition of the two external carotid arteries (ECAs) in selected cases. Multiple projections or 3D spins can be performed to better visualize the vascular anatomy and to choose the best working projection. After a thorough angiographic study of the head and neck vasculature, therapeutic procedures may require the use of microcatheters advanced over microguidewires in a coaxial fashion. The procedural approach and the choice of materials is highly dependent on the patient's vascular anatomy and on the therapeutic purpose, and must be approached on a case-by-case basis. In general, treatments can be categorized into deconstructive (occlusive) embolizations (temporary or permanent) and reconstructive treatments (vessel restorations).

11.5.3 Temporary Embolization: Polyvinyl Alcohol and Gelfoam

Polyvinyl alcohol (PVA) particles are the most commonly used nonabsorbable embolic agents, especially useful when dealing with ECA bleedings that require a fast embolization. Prepackaged PVA particles are provided in a range of sizes, typically 150 to 1,000 µm in particulate diameter. The most widely used sizes in the embolic therapy of head and neck traumas range between 150 µm and 500 µm. Smaller particles will embolize tiny vessels, with a slower recanalization, while the bigger ones will quickly stop the flow in bigger branches allowing subsequent faster recanalization through collaterals. The particles need to be suspended in contrast material to obtain a radiopaque solution that is easily visualized while injecting. Depending on the concentration of particles per ml of contrast, the solution will require different times to embolize the target. Denser solutions will achieve the desired occlusion in less time, but will require more control of the hand injection to avoid reflux in healthy branches, while the more diluted ones will embolize the lesion in a longer time but allow more control on reflux. In the PVA embolization technique, a microcatheter is advanced over a microguidewire to catheterize the injured vessels as selectively as possible, ideally at a safe distance from healthy branches to avoid unwanted reflux. Special attention should be paid to the danger zones of communication between ECA branches and ICA and especially VA small segmental branches.[18] The solution should be injected in the selected vessel under road map guidance; the operator should carefully assess flow reduction/slowing and stop the injection if there is presence or danger or reflux. A control angiogram will show the occlusion of the desired vessel branches. The microcatheter should be thoroughly flushed with saline to remove residual particles in the lumen before removal from the vessel.

Vessels embolized with PVA alone tend to recanalize after a few weeks. The particle itself is nonabsorbable, and the extremely irregular surface of each particle creates a high coefficient of friction, which often results in adhesion of the particles proximally to the wall of the vessel. Blood flow is usually eliminated as soon as the procedure has been carried out. However, the thrombus that forms between the particles may eventually recanalize. Neoendothelium covers particles remaining on the surface.[19] Embolization-related complications are thought to be due to an overembolization with small particles, which then block off arterioles, or to an unwanted reflux into healthy branches, when the injection of embolic material is too forceful.

Gelfoam is a sterile sponge material with hemostatic properties. When used as an embolic material, it is completely reabsorbed, usually within a few weeks. Gelfoam can be used as slurry or pledgets, depending on the size of the vessel that has to be occluded. The technical considerations are the same as those for the PVA embolization. The two materials can be used alone or in combination.

11.5.4 Permanent Embolization: Coils, Balloons, and *N*-Butyl Cyanoacrylate

Coils provide quick permanent vessel embolization by a double action: both mechanical and thrombogenic. A vast range of sizes and shapes is available, the choice of which is depending on the injured vessel and on the pathomechanism of the injury. Coils can be used to embolize both terminal branches that bleed and parent vessels like the ICAs and the VAs in the setting of a pseudoaneurysm or an AVF. In the second case, coils have a role in transvenous embolization as well. The optimal deployment of microcoils requires the careful positioning of the microcatheter tip close enough to the bleeding point to avoid the pitfall of proximal ligation with early recanalization from collaterals. However, coils should not exit through the disrupted vessels. If the aim of the procedure is the ICA or VA occlusion, it is mandatory to assess the validity of the collateral circulation to the brain through the communicating vessels before starting the coiling. An occlusion test can be performed using a nondetachable balloon to stop anterograde flow. In the case of a pseudoaneurysm, it is important to analyze the collaterals thoroughly to understand the best position to deploy the coils to close the bleeding spot and to avoid retrograde blood supply by these vessels. The occlusion of a major vessel requires the formation of a dense pack of coils that can be obtained through the positioning of multiple coils, thus making the procedure longer with additional risk of clot migration. In the cerebrovascular trauma setting there is a consistent risk of distal embolization while deploying the coils, especially if there is still some grade of anterograde flow. Stopping the flow using a nondetachable balloon can minimize this risk; the blood stasis will allow the blood between the coils to clot faster, leading to an effective vessel occlusion. This maneuver finds further explanation in the fact that even in the ideal "best packing" situation the coils form at most 35% of the final embolic volume, the rest being filled with clot. Because clotting mechanisms in traumatized patients may not be adequate, stopping the flow may work both as a safety measure against emboli and as an aid to the clotting system.[20] Once coils are placed in the desired position a control run should be performed before final deployment to evaluate the efficacy of the occlusion. Various deploying mechanisms exist, depending on the manufacturer: mechanic, electrical, and hydraulic. To reach a faster and more satisfying occlusion Gelfoam pledgets can be placed against the coil pack.

N-Butyl cyanoacrylate (NBCA) is a liquid embolic agent (also commonly referred as "glue") that solidifies upon contact with blood or saline by binding to hydroxyl ions in ionic solutions. The glue forms a cast of the vessel lumen that immediately obliterates the artery with a complete stop of the blood flow. Even though some recanalization may occur if the injection site is not close enough to the bleeding vessel, this result is almost always considered to be permanent.[21] To occlude a bleeding vessel, a microcatheter should be placed as close as possible to the hemorrhage site, and then be filled with a dextran column to avoid intracatheter polymerization of the glue. The NBCA solution can then be carefully injected under fluoroscopic guidance, until the glue has formed a cast of the vessel distal to the catheter tip. Extra care should be exercised to avoid embolization of unwanted branches. When the liquid solution cannot advance anymore due to polymerization, the catheter should be promptly pulled away to avoid gluing of the tip to the cast with subsequent risk of vessel injury during removal of the catheter. The polymerizing time of the NBCA can be modified by diluting it with various quantities of oil-based contrast agents (ethiodol, lipiodol); this maneuver allows the operators to both make the glue visible under fluoroscopy and to modify the time in which the cast will solidify. More-diluted solutions will advance more before polymerizing and will allow longer and more controlled injection rates, while highly concentrated ones will quickly stop closer to the catheter tip. Choice between various glue dilutions depends on the position of the tip of the microcatheter, the vessel anatomy, the flow rate, and the experience and preferences of the operator. Currently in the United States the use of NBCA is authorized by the Food and Drug Administration only for preoperative embolization of brain arteriovenous malformations,[22] therefore any use in the emergency setting is to be considered off-label. In Europe and Japan this material has been used for more than 25 years to treat various bleeding conditions, both peripheral and neurovascular. In our opinion, this material is ideal for use in the emergency setting of certain ECA traumas because: (1) The preparation and delivery are quicker than for coils, (2) the obliteration of the vessel is permanent with exceedingly rare recanalizations, and (3) the speed of polymerization can be adjusted by diluting the solution using different amounts of oil-based contrast.

Detachable balloons are a third alternative to occlude vessels; however, as most manufacturers have stopped producing them, they will play less of a role in the future.

11.5.5 Vessel Restoration: Stents

Stents can be used when there is the need to maintain or restore vessel patency. Their use allows a reconstructing approach to serious lesions rather than a deconstructive one (i.e., vessel sacrifice) by restoring the vessel anatomy. They can be divided into bare stents and covered stents (stent grafts).

Bare stents are available as self-expanding or balloon-mounted stents. These devices are more flexible and therefore easier to navigate through tortuous vessel anatomies such as those of the ICAs. They find their main applications in the treatment of arterial dissections. Balloon-expandable stents guarantee a more precise stent placement when compared with self-expanding ones. On the other hand, the latter are more compressible and flexible, thus can be preferred in lesions involving lower segments of the cervical ICA. The treatment rationale for stents in the setting of dissections is that the radial force of the stent struts apposes together the intimal layers and maintains vessel patency. This will presumably work better if the stent is very densely woven.

Stent grafts find their use in the treatment of bleeding pseudoaeurysms when vessel sacrifice is not an acceptable option. They are stiffer than bare stents and can be harder to navigate in the ICA.

In the setting of an arterial dissection or of a pseudoaneurysm, the use of stents should be preferred over medical therapy in cases of symptomatic, progressive, or recurrent lesions with poor collateral flow.[23] Whenever possible during the procedure, intravenous heparin should be used to maintain an activated clotting time (ACT) between 250 and 300 seconds. The use of antiplatelet agents is important for long-term patency, especially for covered stents.[24] The complications of stenting are various and include acute thrombosis, distal thromboembolism, arterial spasm, dissection with hemodynamic impact, guidewire perforation, and arterial rupture of the dilatation site in cases of balloon-mounted stents.

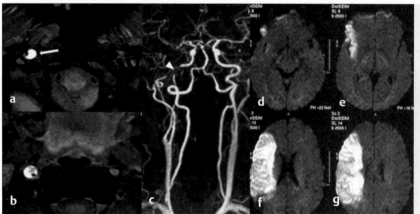

Fig. 11.1 Traumatic internal carotid artery (ICA) dissection with a complete middle cerebral artery (MCA) infarction. (a,b) Magnetic resonance imaging (MRI) demonstrates a crescent-shaped mural hematoma (white arrow) in the vessel wall of the right ICA that is best appreciated on T1 fat-suppressed images. (c) The contrast-enhanced magnetic resonance angiogram (MRA) demonstrates the high-grade stenosis (white arrowhead) that had led to an embolic occlusion of the right MCA as seen on (d-g) diffusion weighted images (DWI).

Overall, endovascular stent placement is the treatment of choice for dissected patients who present acutely with symptomatic hemodynamic compromise. In the setting of a pseudoaneurysm, the sole use of stents instead of vessel occlusion or vessel sacrifice is more controversial: A recent study by Cothren et al has demonstrated that patients who have carotid stents placed for blunt carotid pseudoaneurysms have a 21% complication rate and a documented occlusion rate of 45%. In contrast, patients treated with antithrombotic agents alone had an occlusion rate of 5%.[25]

11.6 Traumatic Arterial Lesions

In this section we focus on the pathological entities resulting from damages to different levels of the arterial wall: dissections, pseudoaneurysms, and AVFs. It is important to remember again that these lesions are dynamic in their natural history and that a lesion involving just one layer of the arterial wall can easily evolve into a pseudoaneurysm or an AVF, manifesting symptoms of these pathologies months or even years after the initial trauma. Vessel transection must be treated with complete occlusion either endovascularly as described above or surgically.

11.6.1 Traumatic Dissections

An arterial dissection is defined as a hematoma within the blood vessel wall that might produce a stenosis of the vessel, a luminal irregularity, and occasionally an aneurysmal dilatation.[26] Most dissections are associated with an intimal defect, if the dissection does not arise from a hemorrhage of the vasa vasorum into the vessel wall. The intimal defect that is associated with the primary injury is most often a tear of the intimal layer that allows propagation of circulating blood into the vessel wall (▶ Fig. 11.1).[27] As in intracranial dissections, different pathomechanisms can be envisioned leading to either hemorrhagic or ischemic symptoms. If blood enters the subintimal space due to a subintimal vessel wall tear it may have different pathologically distinct fates:

1. If the hematoma disrupts the entire vessel wall, a transmural dissection is present: Clinical symptoms will depend on the surroundings of the vessel wall:
   a) An intradural transmural dissection will lead to an SAH.

b) If the transmural dissection occurs in a vessel segment that is surrounded by a venous plexus (i.e., the cavernous sinus [CS] or the vertebral venous plexus) at the atlantal loop, an arteriovenous fistula (AVF) will develop.

c) If the transmural dissection occurs in soft tissues, a pseudoaneurysm (again, one lesion can be derived from a different one and evolve over time) will occur that may lead to mass effect, stenosis, occlusion of the parent vessel, or bleeding.

2. If the dissection remains subintimal, a subadventitial hematoma in the vessel wall will occur. Clinical symptoms will again depend on the fate of this subadventitial hematoma:

a) If there is reopening to the true vessel lumen, the hematoma (having clotted in the false lumen) can be washed out leading to distal emboli, the pathomechanism most commonly seen in adults in extradural ICA dissections (▶ Fig. 11.2).

b) If the hematoma grows inside the vessel wall, the wall itself will get bigger: This can lead to a progressive stenosis of the true lumen (leading to hemodynamic infarctions or embolic events due to critical narrowing and turbulent flow) (▶ Fig. 11.3, ▶ Fig. 11.4, ▶ Fig. 11.5). In intradural arteries, this growing hematoma can lead to occlusion of perforating branches coming off the dissected parent vessel leading to local ischemia.

c) If chronic, the intramural hematoma can organize in the vessel wall, vasa vasorum may sprout into the organizing hematoma and a growing intramural hematoma (due to repetitive dissections) can occur leading to the aspect of a "giant partially thrombosed aneurysm" intracranially.

Consequently, in dissecting diseases symptoms can be related either to mass effect, ischemia, SAH, or in rare cases, in a combination of different presenting symptoms.[28]

Dissections account for the majority of cerebrovascular trauma sequelae. Arterial dissection of the ICA or VA accounts for only 2% of all ischemic strokes. However, in young and middle-aged patients it is an important cause, accounting for 10 to 25% of such cases.

Although delayed cerebral ischemia—due either to distal emboli (predominantly in extradural and only rarely in intradural dissections) or local perforator occlusion (in intradural dissections with mural hematoma)—is the most prevalent clinical presentation, 20 to 33% of patients are clinically

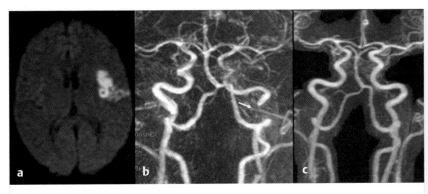

Fig. 11.2 A 41-year-old man presented with a focal deficit 1 week after whiplash trauma. (a) Magnetic resonance imaging (MRI) demonstrated an acute infarction in a middle cerebral artery branch (MCA). (b) The contrast-enhanced magnetic resonance angiogram (MRA) demonstrated a high-grade stenosis of the right internal carotid artery (ICA) related to dissection (white arrow). (c) On follow-up MRA 4 years after the acute trauma,[27] the vessel had repaired itself and there was no longer evidence of a dissection or stenosis despite any surgical or endovascular intervention. This case illustrates that most traumatic dissections regress spontaneously.

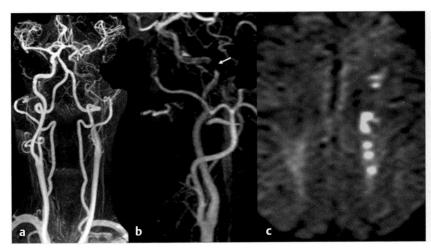

Fig. 11.3 A 54-year-old woman was hospitalized for dissection following whiplash trauma. Despite medical treatment, she developed recurrent symptoms while in the hospital. (a,b) Magnetic resonance angiography demonstrated the dissection of the left internal carotid artery with a high-grade stenosis (white arrow). (c) On diffusion weighted imaging (DWI), watershed ischemia is noted in a pattern typical for hemodynamic infarctions, as the DWI changes are present in the territory in between the lenticulostriate arteries and the deep leptomeningeal perforators.

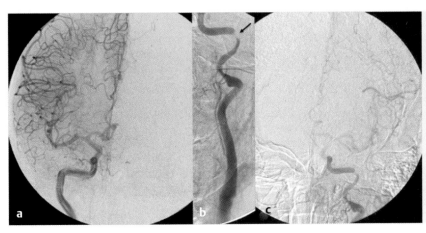

Fig. 11.4 The angiography demonstrates not only insufficient collaterals from the right internal carotid artery (ICA) (a), but also the high-grade stenosis (arrow) related to the previous dissection of the left ICA as it enters the skull base (b). The intracranial circulation is lagging behind the extracranial circulation further substantiating the hemodynamic compromise of the left hemisphere following the dissection (c).

asymptomatic.[29] In the remaining patients, carotodynia, that is neck pain along the course of artery, headaches, or an incomplete Horner syndrome—oculosympathetic paresis with preservation of ipsilateral facial sweating—may be present.[30]

In comparison to spontaneous dissections, where 85% of stenotic lesions improve or resolve on follow-up angiography, traumatic dissections resolve or improve in only 55% of cases, while 25% of stenoses progress to complete occlusion.[31] CTA and MRI might demonstrate the intramural thrombus, the narrowing of the arterial lumen, an intimal flap indicating a true and false lumen and possibly associated distal sequelae like parenchymal changes such as infarction or hemorrhage.

On MRI, the dissection is best visualized in T1 fat-suppressed images as a crescent-shaped hyperintensity in the vessel wall that is due to the methemoglobin in the mural hematoma. Because the bright hematoma can be mistaken for flow in time of flight (TOF) studies, a contrast-enhanced MRA is recommended for an MRI study of the vessels in a dissection. DWI

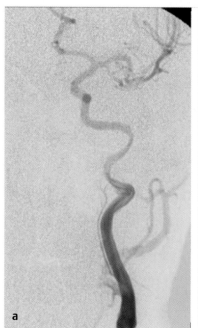 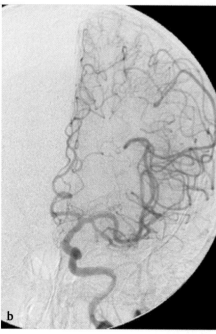

Fig. 11.5 (a,b) Following stent implantation there is reconstitution of the normal blood supply to the left internal carotid artery (ICA). This case illustrates that intervention in traumatic dissections is only necessary if the patient presents with hemodynamic compromise.

and apparent diffusion coefficient (ADC) maps can easily show scattered foci of recent ischemias (hyperintense in DWI and hypointense in ADC), or much less frequently, watershed infarctions due to hemodynamic insufficiency.

On DSA, dissections may present as a luminal stenosis, followed by a tapering of the vessel lumen that might lead to an occlusion of the artery (this is called the flame sign, and is typical for a dissecting process) as a stenosis, which may or may not be followed by an aneurysmal dilatation (string of bead sign) or as an irregularity of the vessel wall.[26] On 3D angiographic images, an intimal flap may be seen. Distal to the lesion, the flow is often slowed, and distal embolic occlusions might be seen.

Intracranial traumatic dissections are rare findings; if present, they typically involve the supraclinoid segment of the ICA and extend to the MCA. Besides ischemia, intracranial dissections can lead to SAHs. Extracranial dissections are far more common. They typically involve both the cervical (C1) and petrous (C2) part of the ICA and spare the bulb.[32] The most common cause for traumatic ICA dissections are motor vehicle accidents that lead either to a hyperextension of the neck associated with contralateral lateral flexion/ rotation (with associated stretching of the ICA across the transverse processes of C2 and C3) or to an abrupt flexion of the ICA between the angle of the mandible and the upper cervical spine (leading to compression of the ICA with subsequent intimal disruption).[33] VA dissections can occur when the head is rotated in extension leading to stretching of the artery between C1 and C2 or when a fracture of the transverse foramen directly results in vessel wall damage.[34,35]

Treatment should primarily aim at prevention of thromboembolic complications and at maintenance of the patency of the stenotic vessel and should be performed with anticoagulation whenever possible.[36,37] Endovascular (stenting) or surgical intervention (bypass graft, thrombectomy, resection of aneurysm or stenoses) should be reserved for those patients that are symptomatic, but

that cannot be managed by anticoagulation given that it may be contraindicated in a trauma patient.[38]

Spontaneous healing of the dissection after trauma in otherwise healthy individuals is the most often observed evolution, presumably because the vessel wall was healthy before the trauma occurred and has therefore maintained its capacity for repair.

The mainstay of endovascular treatment in the symptomatic patients with dissection is vessel reconstruction using stents that may become necessary in the setting of hemodynamic infarctions due to critical hypoperfusion. As described above, deployment of more than one device can be necessary if the dissection involves multiple locations. Whenever the preprocedural cerebral DSA shows embolic occlusion of the MCA, if the symptoms onset is less than 6 hours, mechanical thrombectomy can be attempted as soon as a suitable lumen of the dissected carotid has been restored. We currently utilize Stentriever (Stryker, Inc., Kalamazoo, MI) for this purpose. These devices are resheathable stents specifically designed for mechanical thrombectomy. The supporting system can be constituted by (1) a coaxial system, using an envoy or a balloon-mounted guiding catheter, or (2) by triaxial approach with a shuttle sheath and a distal access catheter. A steerable microwire is gently advanced between the embolus and the arterial wall or through the embolus until the tip is in a thrombus-free segment of the artery. The microcatheter should then be navigated on the wire past the thrombus and the stentretriever system can be delivered through the microcatheter and positioned over the embolus. The unsheathing is made by gently pulling off the microcatheter. The radial force of the stent squeezes the embolus on the arterial wall, immediately restoring some blood flow in the vessel. After some minutes, the thrombus should ideally be trapped in the stent cells: The microcatheter and stent are then pulled away together while suction is applied through the guide catheter to avoid small distal embolizations.

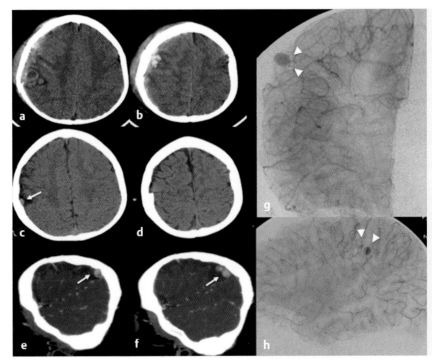

Fig. 11.6 (a,b) This 15-month-old girl presented with a fall resulting in a skull fracture and a contusional hemorrhage. On follow-up 6 months later, a pseudoaneurysm (white arrows) close to the skull fracture was seen on unenhanced computed tomography (CT) (c,d) and computed tomography angiography (CTA) (e,f). Angiography (DSA) (g,h) confirmed the diagnosis of a partially thrombosed traumatic aneurysm (white arrowhead) with slow inflow and outflow. This patient was treated conservatively.

The removed thrombus should be visible between the stent cells. An angiographic assessment of the degree of flow restoration can then be performed. If needed, the procedure can be repeated after careful washing of the stent.

11.6.2 Traumatic Aneurysms

Traumatic aneurysms constitute less than 1% of all intracranial aneurysms; however, the proportion increases up to 20% of all aneurysms in the pediatric population.[39] Their etiology is most often due to penetrating head injury with either complete disruption of the vessel wall or only adventitial damage. In the latter case, the aneurysm can form over a period of years. When the three vessel layers are compromised, active arterial extravasation may occur, or the injury may become contained in the surrounding tissues and result in a pseudoaneurysm. Traumatic aneurysms following blunt or closed head injury can also occur as an evolution of a dissecting lesion. They might present with a wide variety of symptoms (from asymptomatic to death); however, in most instances, the clinical presentation is severe with high rates (up to 50%) of morbidity and mortality for traumatic intracranial aneurysms.[40]

Traumatic extracranial carotid aneurysms may be due to penetrating or blunt trauma. The latter may be caused by rotatory hyperextension, strangulation or fractures of the mandibular angle, whereas extradural carotid aneurysms due to penetrating injuries, which are more common, result typically from stabbing or gunshot wounds.[41] However, these lesions may also be iatrogenic (following endarterectomy, tracheostomy, radical neck dissection, intraoral surgery, biopsy of a middle ear mass in the presence of an intratympanic course of the carotid artery).[42,43,44] Intracranial traumatic aneurysms can be subdivided into three types according to their location:

1. Skullbase, affecting the petrous, cavernous, or supraclinoid tract of the ICA
2. Subcortical, with a peripheral distribution, typically close to the falx or the tentorium, the MCA being the most common location because of the relationship with the pterion, followed by the pericallosal anterior cerebral artery due to its relation with the falx, and the posterior cerebral artery and its relationship with the tentorium
3. Distal cortical (associated with skull fractures and subdural hematomas) (▶ Fig. 11.6)

The intracranial traumatic aneurysm most often encountered is the traumatic aneurysm of the ICA within its cavernous segment (48%), which is typically associated with basal skull fractures. These aneurysms might enlarge and produce a cavernous sinus syndrome with nerve compression, or they might secondarily rupture producing a carotid-cavernous fistula (CCF) or a transdural leakage that will lead to a subarachnoid hemorrhage. The most dangerous form, however, is a medial tear of the ICA with rupture into the sphenoid sinus causing massive and life-threatening epistaxis that cannot be controlled; it requires emergency packing and immediate treatment.[42,45]

On DSA acute traumatic aneurysms can be differentiated from "true" or "classical" aneurysms by the delayed filling and emptying of the traumatic aneurysm, by the location (peripheral and away from branching points), by the irregular contour of the aneurysm, the absence of a neck, and the history of the patient.[46]

Spontaneous regression of the aneurysm is possible, but improbable. A study of 40 patients, who did not receive immediate treatment, revealed that 40% of traumatic ICA aneurysms bled and 21% enlarged.[47]

Treatment strategy should be based on the assumption that the traumatic aneurysm visualized during emergent angiography

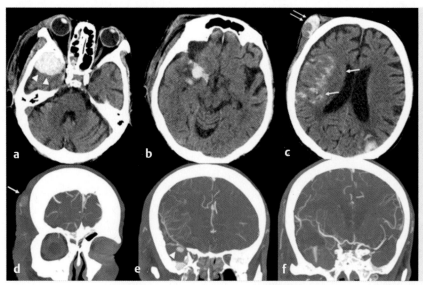

Fig. 11.7 Traumatic pseudoaneurysm. (a–c) The computed tomography (CT) demonstrates acute hemorrhage in multiple compartments including the subarachnoid space (white arrows), the right temporal epidural space (white arrowheads), and the right frontal subgaleal region (thin white double arrows). (d–f) Emergency computed tomography angiography (CTA) at the same time reveals a traumatic pseudoaneurysms indicating acute vessel rupture of the right superficial temporal artery (white arrow) and the right middle meningeal artery (white arrowhead).

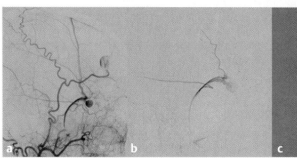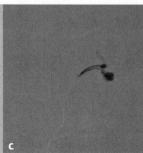

Fig. 11.8 (a,b) Emergency angiography was performed and confirmed two separate traumatic aneurysms that were treated by proximal ligation with *N*-butyl cyanoacrylate (glue). (c) Parent vessel sacrifice is necessary as the aneurysm does not have a wall and the apparent boundaries of the pseudoaneurysm are constituted by the clotted hematoma.

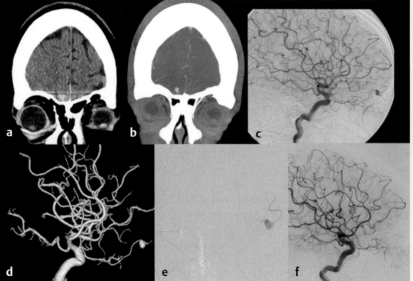

Fig. 11.9 Four weeks following an acute head trauma this patient presented with severe headaches. (a) Computed tomography (CT) and (b) computed tomography angiogram (CTA) revealed a focal right frontal subarachnoid hemorrhage related to a right orbitofrontal artery aneurysm that was supposed to be related to the previous trauma. (c,d) Angiography (DSA) confirmed the presence of a traumatic aneurysm and treatment with parent vessel sacrifice using *N*-butyl cyanoacrylate (glue) was performed (e,f).

is in fact an extravascular pouch that communicates with the intravascular space (▶ Fig. 11.7, ▶ Fig. 11.8).[38] The "walls" of this false aneurysm are constituted by thrombus and extravascular tissues. Superselective catheterization with pressure injection of contrast or embolic material into this false lumen therefore harbors a high risk of rerupture and should be avoided. Because the vessel cannot usually be reconstructed, the goal of treatment

should be an immediate proximal occlusion of the parent artery by embolization. A spasm proximal to the arterial rupture may indirectly point to the leakage site. Vessel sacrifice can be obtained by various means that have been already discussed: coils, glue, particles, or a combination of these methods (▶ Fig. 11.9). In the case of an ICA pseudoaneurysm, collateral circulation should be assessed under flow arrest previous to any

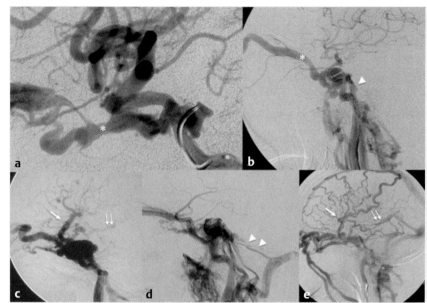

Fig. 11.10 Traumatic (direct) carotid-cavernous fistula (CCF): This picture demonstrates the different outflow routes of direct traumatic CCFs. In the upper row (a,b) the benign CCFs are demonstrated with drainage solely into the ophthalmic veins (a, white asterisk), or into the ophthalmic veins (white asterisk) and the inferior petrosal sinus (b, white arrowhead). In the lower row (c–e), fistulas with cortical venous reflux are demonstrated that may pose a hemorrhagic risk to the patient: Drainage may be directed into the sylvian veins (c and e, white arrows), the superior petrosal sinus and the posterior fossa (d, white arrowheads) or even the hippocampal vein into the basal vein of Rosenthal system (c and e, thin white double arrows).

embolizing maneuver, and a reconstructive approach with a stent graft should be favored if any doubt rises about adequacy of collateral circulation to the brain. Surgical vessel occlusion close to the false aneurysm is also usually adequate to stop the bleeding.

11.6.3 Traumatic Arteriovenous Fistulas

The typical etiology of traumatic AVFs is a skull base fracture; however, iatrogenic fistulas following transsphenoidal surgery might also be encountered.

Posttraumatic AVFs are direct fistulas between an artery as it courses through a venous plexus. They can therefore be present at the cavernous sinus (CS) where the disrupted ICA or its intracavernous branches communicate with the cavernous sinus or as vertebral venous fistulas at the superior third of the extradural vertebral artery as it is surrounded by the venous plexus. The most common traumatic AVFs are CCFs. The mechanism of fistulization is due to tearing of all the wall layers of the ICA, that is fixed within the CS by fibrous trabeculae and small meningeal arteries with subsequent rupture of the ICA or these smaller meningeal arteries into the sinus.[48] Clinical findings are variable and comprise an immediate objective vascular bruit, a pulsating exophthalmos and chemosis (both may occur with some delay), plus variable manifestations of dysfunction of the structures whithin the CS like cranial nerves III, IV, VI, V1, and V2. Ophthalmoplegia is a common finding, which could be due to mass or pulsation effects by the arterialized venous pouches. Blindness related to CCFs always occurs with a delay following secondary glaucoma in which the pathomechanism is related to venous congestion.[49] An immediate blindness must therefore be related to other causes, the most common being traumatic optic avulsion, or more rarely, injury of the ophthalmic artery. Neurologic deficits following venous congestion and subsequent hemorrhagic events are exceedingly rare, but may occur with a delay of several days to months.

If the venous pouches extend beyond the CS into the suprasellar region, rupture may lead to devastating SAH.[50] In cases of massive trauma, the fistula may be associated with additional epistaxis due to a widespread laceration of the ICA with hemorrhage into the ethmoidal cells or sphenoidal sinus. Because the route of venous drainage affects prognosis, it has to be carefully studied. Possible drainage routes are;

1. Anteriorly via the ophthalmic vein into the angular vein and subsequently the facial vein (which is the most often encountered route)
2. Via the inferior petrous sinus into the sigmoid sinus
3. Via the superior petrosal sinus, which usually connects to the transverse-sigmoid sinus, but may also have connections with the posterior fossa veins
4. Via the sphenoparietal sinus into cortical veins further draining into the superior sagittal sinus, or via the basal vein of Rosenthal into the vein of Galen and the straight sinus, respectively. The latter drainage routes present the most dangerous ones because they may result in venous congestion with subsequent hemorrhagic infarction of the posterior fossa (▸ Fig. 11.10).

Traumatic AVF's the VA are 10 times less common than CCF's and are constituted by an abnormal communication between the extracranial VA or its muscular branches and the surrounding venous plexuses.[35]

Clinical symptoms are pulsatile tinnitus or a cervical bruit (present each in 30–40% of patients). Cord or nerve root compression from enlarged venous pouches may lead to symptoms of myelo-radiculopathy or even quadriparesis when severe. Blurred vision is rare, but may be encountered in some patients, and, if present, results from venous hypertension in the posterior cranial fossa and indicates emergency treatment (due to the present danger of hemorrhage subsequent to the venous congestion). In rare instances, reflux into the spinal perimedullary veins will lead to progressive congestive myelopathy. Neck or facial pain and a torticollis may be also be present in some patients. Symptoms of transient ischemic attacks in the posterior circulation, lower cranial nerves deficit and decreased distal pulse of the ipsilateral upper extremity perceived on clinical examination are more likely due to the steal phenomenon of the fistula (▸ Fig. 11.11).[51]

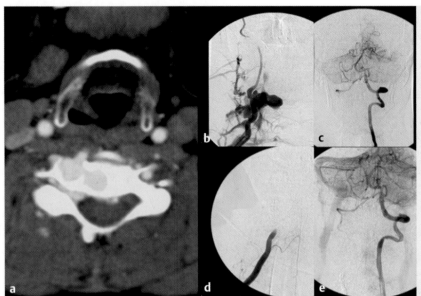

Fig. 11.11 This 50-year-old man presented with a pulse synchronous tinnitus since trauma to the neck many years ago. The symptoms gradually got worse and he presented to the hospital with new right sided C6 nerve compression. (a) Computed tomography (CT) and (b) angiogram (DSA) revealed a right vertebrovenous fistula with a massively dilated venous pouch that presumably lead to compression of the C6 nerve root. There was no significant contribution from the contralateral vertebral artery (VA) and good filling of the entire posterior circulation via the left VA (c), which enabled us to do a parent vessel occlusion of the right VA with coil occlusion of the diseased segment (d,e) and preservation of the anterior spinal artery.

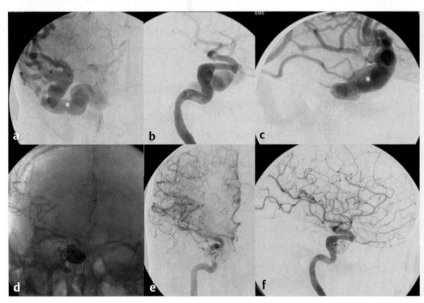

Fig. 11.12 Traumatic carotid-cavernous fistula (CCF) treated with coils. Significant reflux is visualized into the sylvian veins (a–c), white asterisks) in this patient that was subsequently treated with coil occlusion of the CCF. A dense coil mesh was placed into the cavernous sinus via a transarterial approach to occlude the fistulous communication (d–f).

The major pathomechanisms of traumatic AVF's affecting the VA are blunt injury (rotated hyperextension) and penetrating trauma (gunshot wounds, iatrogenic percutaneous punctures, following C-spine surgery). Whereas the latter can appear at any level, the former are typically confined to the C1 to C3 level and must be differentiated from the spontaneous vertebrovenous fistulas (VVFs), that typically demonstrate a segmental involvement and exhibit no history of trauma.[35]

On CT, a skull base fracture may be present that may involve the clivus or the sphenoid bone close to the CS. The combination of severe oronasal bleeding, with air in the carotid canal should alert the treating physician to the presence of a distal internal carotid artery laceration.[52] Diagnostic angiographic workup in traumatic fistulas should include a six-vessel DSA (including both external carotid arteries, both ICA's, and both VA's) to:

1. Visualize the exact site of the fistula (which might only be possible via an indirect filling from the contralateral site)

2. Evaluate the patency of the circle of Willis to determine whether occlusion of the parent artery is possible

3. Assess potential anastomoses (such as present between the ECA and the VA, which might fill the fistula following a too proximal parent artery occlusion)

In cases of VVFs located below the C4 level, injections of the ascending or deep cervical arteries may also help define the fistula location. Three-dimensional angiography is a useful imaging tool for capturing the complex perifistular anatomy.[53]

Endovascular treatment options are manifold and might include endovascular occlusion of the parent artery in patent collaterals using a trapping technique, endovascular occlusion of the fistula site from the arterial site using detachable balloons or coils (▶ Fig. 11.12), endovascular occlusion from the venous side (i.e., coiling of the CS in CCFs). In cases of direct CCF, treatment is therefore directed to the venous side of the fistula. Historically, the most successful and well-established treatment

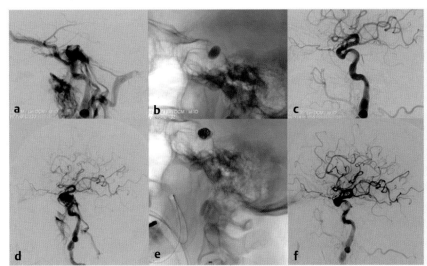

Fig. 11.13 Treatment of this posttraumatic carotid-cavernous fistula (a,b) was first attempted with a balloon that initially led to complete obliteration of the fistula (c). However, on follow-up (d) there was reopening of the fistula, presumably because of deflation of the balloon. Additional coiling (e) was performed that led again to complete and stable obliteration of the fistula (f).

modality involves the placement of a detachable balloon across the CCF, using flow direction from the arterial side. The balloon is then inflated such that it is wedged in the CS against the fistula. The balloon thereby creates a tamponade of the CCF, eliminating flow and permitting healing across the orifice of the fistula (▶ Fig. 11.13). In particularly large CCFs or in fistulas in which the CS is distended, multiple balloons are sometimes needed. The goal is to position the balloons such that the last one placed is wedged against the arterial tear, causing cessation of flow across it. However, even in the case of a direct CCF, it is not always possible to get a balloon to cross the arterial defect to the venous side,[54] in which case coils should be preferred, with or without a balloon-assisted technique. Endovascular vessel wall reconstructing techniques (employing stent grafts) have been reported in case reports; however, their long-term patency is as of yet a matter of debate.[55] If a trapping technique is considered, occlusion of the distal part of the lesion must be performed before the vessel segment proximal to the lesion is occluded to prevent further "steal" phenomenon from the brain circulation.

11.7 Traumatic Venous Lesions

Traumatic venous lesions are often overlooked and may be more common than previously reported. Venous injuries are more common in the setting of penetrating lesions rather than with blunt traumas.[17] Venous injuries can be present in as much as 51% of penetrating injuries to the neck; however, they are more commonly clinically silent if compared with the arterial ones.[8] When an arterial lesion is present as well, an AVF may form. Traumatic thrombosis of veins following penetrating trauma can be due to a tear or laceration of dural sinuses, due to compression of the sinuses secondary to intracranial bleeding or increased pressure or due to an injury to the venous epithelial lining with thrombus formation.[56,57,58] The intramural thrombus might extend, leading to venous hypertension and increased intracranial pressure, and should therefore be suspected if recovery of a cranial trauma is longer than expected, especially if associated signs of increased intracranial pressure are present (headaches, visual disturbances, and

papilledema).[59] Although imaging findings of extensive dural sinus thrombosis on CT, MRI, and DSA are well known, the early findings of traumatic venous lesions might be more subtle. On DSA there might be a delayed arterial transit time or filling of collateral veins that requires the treating physician to make the angiographic run last longer to completely visualize the venous outflow. However, most often traumatic venous lesions can only be suggested due to nonvisualization of the affected structure. Treatment of these lesions should aim at avoiding progression of the thrombus; therefore, dehydration should be avoided and intravenous anticoagulation may be contemplated. The patency of the jugular veins should therefore be assessed before positioning of a jugular line.

References

[1] World Health Organization. The Top 10 Causes of Death. Available at: http://www.who.int/mediacentre/factsheets/fs310/en/index.html. Accessed October 15, 2012

[2] Centers for Disease Control and Prevention. 10 Leading Causes of Death by Age Group, United States - 2010. Available at: http://www.cdc.gov/injury/wisqars/pdf/10LCID_All_Deaths_By_Age_Group_2010-a.pdf. Accessed October 15, 2012

[3] Biffl WL, Moore EE, Ryu RK et al. The unrecognized epidemic of blunt carotid arterial injuries: early diagnosis improves neurologic outcome. Ann Surg 1998; 228: 462–470

[4] Cothren CC, Moore EE, Ray CE et al. Screening for blunt cerebrovascular injuries is cost-effective. Am J Surg 2005; 190: 845–849

[5] Miller PR, Fabian TC, Bee TK et al. Blunt cerebrovascular injuries: diagnosis and treatment. J Trauma 2001; 51: 279–285, discussion 285–286

[6] Nedeltchev K. Baumgartner R. Traumatic cervical artery dissection. In: Baumgartner RW, Bogousslavsky J, Caso V, Paciaroni M, eds. Handbook on Cerebral Artery Dissection. Basel, Switzerland. Karger; 2005: 54–63

[7] Risgaard O, Sugrue M, D'Amours S et al. Blunt cerebrovascular injury: an evaluation from a major trauma centre. ANZ J Surg 2007; 77: 686–689

[8] Steenburg SD, Sliker CW, Shanmuganathan K, Siegel EL. Imaging evaluation of penetrating neck injuries. Radiographics 2010; 30: 869–886

[9] Landreneau RJ, Weigelt JA, Megison SM, Meier DE, Fry WJ. Combined carotid-vertebral arterial trauma. Arch Surg 1992; 127: 301–304

[10] Saletta JD, Lowe RJ, Lim LT, Thornton J, Delk S, Moss GS. Penetrating trauma of the neck. J Trauma 1976; 16: 579–587

[11] Sliker CW. Blunt cerebrovascular injuries: imaging with multidetector CT angiography. Radiographics 2008; 28: 1689–1708, discussion 1709–1710

[12] Feiz-Erfan I, Horn EM, Theodore N et al. Incidence and pattern of direct blunt neurovascular injury associated with trauma to the skull base. J Neurosurg 2007; 107: 364–369

[13] Sung EK, Nadgir RN, Sakai O. Computed tomographic imaging in head and neck trauma: what the radiologist needs to know. Semin Roentgenol 2012; 47: 320–329

[14] Berne JD, Cook A, Rowe SA, Norwood SH. A multivariate logistic regression analysis of risk factors for blunt cerebrovascular injury. J Vasc Surg 2010; 51: 57–64

[15] Biffl WL, Moore EE, Offner PJ, Brega KE, Franciose RJ, Burch JM. Blunt carotid arterial injuries: implications of a new grading scale. J Trauma 1999; 47: 845–853

[16] Kohler R, Vargas MI, Masterson K, Lovblad KO, Pereira VM, Becker MCT. CT and MR angiography features of traumatic vascular injuries of the neck. AJR Am J Roentgenol 2011; 196: W800–9

[17] Stuhlfaut JW, Barest G, Sakai O, Lucey B, Soto JA. Impact of MDCT angiography on the use of catheter angiography for the assessment of cervical arterial injury after blunt or penetrating trauma. AJR Am J Roentgenol 2005; 185: 1063–1068

[18] Geibprasert S, Pongpech S, Armstrong D, Krings T. Dangerous extracranial-intracranial anastomoses and supply to the cranial nerves: vessels the neurointerventionalist needs to know. AJNR Am J Neuroradiol 2009; 30: 1459–1468

[19] Kochan JP. Endovascular therapy. In: Jallo J, Loftus CM, eds. Neurotrauma and Critical Care of .the Brain. New York, NY: Thieme Medical Publishers; 2009:145–148

[20] Radvany MG, Gailloud P. Endovascular management of neurovascular arterial injuries in the face and neck. Semin Intervent Radiol 2010; 27: 44–54

[21] Wikholm G. Occlusion of cerebral arteriovenous malformations with N-butyl cyano-acrylate is permanent. AJNR Am J Neuroradiol 1995; 16: 479–482

[22] Cordis. TRUFILL, Miami Lakes, FL: Cordis. Available at: http://www.access-data.fda.gov/cdrh_docs/pdf/p990040a.pdf. Accessed October 21, 2012

[23] Joo JY, Ahn JY, Chung YS et al. Treatment of intra- and extracranial arterial dissections using stents and embolization. Cardiovasc Intervent Radiol 2005; 28: 595–602

[24] Kadkhodayan Y, Jeck DT, Moran CJ, Derdeyn CP, Cross DT. Angioplasty and stenting in carotid dissection with or without associated pseudoaneurysm. AJNR Am J Neuroradiol 2005; 26: 2328–2335

[25] Cothren CC, Moore EE, Ray CE et al. Carotid artery stents for blunt cerebrovascular injury: risks exceed benefits. Arch Surg 2005; 140: 480–485, discussion 485–486

[26] Zhao WY, Krings T, Alvarez H, Ozanne A, Holmin S, Lasjaunias P. Management of spontaneous haemorrhagic intracranial vertebrobasilar dissection: review of 21 consecutive cases. Acta Neurochir (Wien) 2007; 149: 585–596, discussion 596

[27] Schievink WI. Spontaneous dissection of the carotid and vertebral arteries. N Engl J Med 2001; 344: 898–906

[28] Krings T, Choi IS. The many faces of intracranial arterial dissections. Interv Neuroradiol 2010; 16: 151–160

[29] Scheid R, Zimmer C, Schroeter ML, Ballaschke O, von Cramon DY. The clinical spectrum of blunt cerebrovascular injury. Neurologist 2006; 12: 255–262

[30] Yang ST, Huang YC, Chuang CC, Hsu PW. Traumatic internal carotid artery dissection. J Clin Neurosci 2006; 13: 123–128

[31] Sturzenegger M. Spontaneous internal carotid artery dissection: early diagnosis and management in 44 patients. J Neurol 1995; 242: 231–238

[32] Hart RG, Easton JD. Dissections of cervical and cerebral arteries. Neurol Clin 1983; 1: 155–182

[33] Cothren CC, Moore EE. Blunt cerebrovascular injuries. Clinics (Sao Paulo) 2005; 60: 489–496

[34] Friedman D, Flanders A, Thomas C, Millar W. Vertebral artery injury after acute cervical spine trauma: rate of occurrence as detected by MR angiography and assessment of clinical consequences. AJR Am J Roentgenol 1995; 164: 443–447, discussion 448–449

[35] Golueke P, Sclafani S, Phillips T, Goldstein A, Scalea T, Duncan A. Vertebral artery injury—diagnosis and management. J Trauma 1987; 27: 856–865

[36] Benninger DH, Gandjour J, Georgiadis D, Stöckli E, Arnold M, Baumgartner RW. Benign long-term outcome of conservatively treated cervical aneurysms due to carotid dissection. Neurology 2007; 69: 486–487

[37] Cothren CC, Moore EE, Biffl WL et al. Anticoagulation is the gold standard therapy for blunt carotid injuries to reduce stroke rate. Arch Surg 2004; 139: 540–545, discussion 545–546

[38] Joo JY, Ahn JY, Chung YS et al. Therapeutic endovascular treatments for traumatic carotid artery injuries. J Trauma 2005; 58: 1159–1166

[39] Lasjaunias P, Wuppalapati S, Alvarez H, Rodesch G, Ozanne A. Intracranial aneurysms in children aged under 15 years: review of 59 consecutive children with 75 aneurysms. Childs Nerv Syst 2005; 21: 437–450

[40] Levy ML, Rezai A, Masri LS et al. The significance of subarachnoid hemorrhage after penetrating craniocerebral injury: correlations with angiography and outcome in a civilian population. Neurosurgery 1993; 32: 532–540

[41] Jones RF, Terrell JC, Salyer KE. Penetrating wounds of the neck: an analysis of 274 cases. J Trauma 1967; 7: 228–237

[42] Chambers EF, Rosenbaum AE, Norman D, Newton TH. Traumatic aneurysms of cavernous internal carotid artery with secondary epistaxis. AJNR Am J Neuroradiol 1981; 2: 405–409

[43] Chen D, Concus AP, Halbach VV, Cheung SW. Epistaxis originating from traumatic pseudoaneurysm of the internal carotid artery: diagnosis and endovascular therapy. Laryngoscope 1998; 108: 326–331

[44] Holmes B, Harbaugh RE. Traumatic intracranial aneurysms: a contemporary review. J Trauma 1993; 35: 855–860

[45] Lee JP, Wang AD. Epistaxis due to traumatic intracavernous aneurysm: case report. J Trauma 1990; 30: 619–622

[46] Schuster JM, Santiago P, Elliott JP, Grady MS, Newell DW, Winn HR. Acute traumatic posteroinferior cerebellar artery aneurysms: report of three cases. Neurosurgery 1999; 45: 1465–1467, discussion 1467–1468

[47] Ahmadi J. Vascular lesion resulting from head injury. In: Wilkins RH, Rengachary SS, eds. Neurosurgery. New York, NY: McGraw-Hill;1996: 2821–2840

[48] Love L, Marsan RE. Carotid cavernous fistula. Angiology 1974; 25: 231–236

[49] de Keizer R. Carotid-cavernous and orbital arteriovenous fistulas: ocular features, diagnostic and hemodynamic considerations in relation to visual impairment and morbidity. Orbit 2003; 22: 121–142

[50] Taki W, Nakahara I, Nishi S et al. Pathogenetic and therapeutic considerations of carotid-cavernous sinus fistulas. Acta Neurochir (Wien) 1994; 127: 6–14

[51] Berenstein A, Lasjaunias P,TerBrugge KG. Surgical Neuroangiography 2.1 Clinical and Endovascular Treatment Aspects in Adults. Berlin, Germany: Springer; 2001

[52] Buis DR, Dirven CM, van den Berg R, Manoliu RA, Vandertop WP. Air in the carotid canal as a predictor of distal internal carotid artery laceration. Acta Neurochir (Wien) 2006; 148: 1201–1203, discussion 1203

[53] Kwon BJ, Han MH, Kang HS, Chang KH. Endovascular occlusion of direct carotid cavernous fistula with detachable balloons: usefulness of 3D angiography. Neuroradiology 2005; 47: 271–281

[54] American Society of Interventional and Therapeutic Neuroradiology. Arteriovenous fistulae of the CNS. AJNR Am J Neuroradiol 2001; 22 Suppl: S22–S25

[55] Archondakis E, Pero G, Valvassori L, Boccardi E, Scialfa G. Angiographic follow-up of traumatic carotid cavernous fistulas treated with endovascular stent graft placement. AJNR Am J Neuroradiol 2007; 28: 342–347

[56] Hasso AN, Lasjaunias PL, Thompson JR, Hinshaw DB. Venous occlusions of the cavernous area—a complication of crushing fractures of the sphenoid bone. Radiology 1979; 132: 375–379

[57] Meier U, Gärtner F, Knopf W, Klötzer R, Wolf O. The traumatic dural sinus injury—a clinical study. Acta Neurochir (Wien) 1992; 119: 91–93

[58] Taha JM, Crone KR, Berger TS, Becket WW, Prenger EC. Sigmoid sinus thrombosis after closed head injury in children. Neurosurgery 1993; 32: 541–545, discussion 545–546

[59] Kinal ME. Traumatic thrombosis of dural venous sinuses in closed head injury. J Neurosurg 1967; 27: 142–145

12 Interventional Radiology in Cardiac Trauma

Riyad Karmy-Jones and Eric K. Hoffer

Interventional management of cardiac injuries is extremely rare, and usually is related to coronary artery injuries, which are often managed either surgically or medically, including anticoagulation, depending on the clinical situation.[1]

Injuries after blunt trauma most commonly affect the left anterior descending artery, and can present an acute ischemia or in a delayed fashion with late myocardial infarction, left ventricular aneurysm, and/or septal defects.[2–6] Most commonly, coronary artery occlusion is found, which can be managed by coronary stenting (▶ Fig. 12.1).[4] Non flow limiting dissections may be managed with anticoagulation if there are no contraindications.[7]

Partial occlusions can occur following penetrating (often after repair) and blunt trauma. In some cases these lesions resolve spontaneously.[5]

12.1 Coronary Artery Fistulas

Coronary artery fistulas can also result from blunt and penetrating injury.[8,9] At least half of these originate from the left anterior descending artery. However, the majority of the fistulas drain into the right ventricle.[10] It has been postulated that the majority of fistulas will eventually lead to complications, so when diagnosed, a treatment is indicated.[9] Septal defects are usually managed operatively, but there are reports

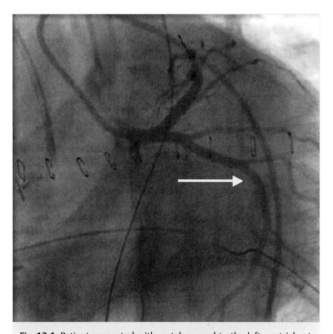

Fig. 12.1 Patient presented with a stab wound to the left ventricle at the junction of the left anterior descending artery (LAD) and second diagonal branch. The injury to the LAD was primarily repaired in conjunction with the myocardial defect, but shortly after, in the intensive care unit, the patient exhibited signs of cardiogenic shock and transesophageal echocardiography suggested apical akinesis, prompting coronary angiography. The arteriogram showed the area of injury slightly narrow, suggesting spasm (arrow), but there was good blood flow and the apical function had returned to normal.

of percutaneous closure devices used in patients who, after emergency open repair, were deemed at high risk for further surgery. They also may be used after blunt trauma for defects presenting in a delayed fashion.[1,11,12,13]

12.2 Missile Embolism

Pulmonary missile embolism is uncommon. The management in asymptomatic patients is unclear. Concerns about complications related to occlusion of major pulmonary artery branches have prompted surgical resection of the affected lobe, or retrieval of the missile by arteriotomy.[14] Kortbeek et al presented a case and reviewed 31 reported cases; they noted that 14 cases were managed conservatively with no complications suggesting that in the absence of complications, or need for thoracotomy for other causes, conservative management can be appropriate.[15] Also, it is unclear that all missile embolisms into the right ventricle require operative removal.[16] On the other hand, the percutaneous removal of bullets is possible.[17,18] Removal can be done via either a transfemoral or transjugular venous approach, depending on the operator's preference. The removal is identical to percutaneous pulmonary embolectomy, and requires a large vascular sheath. Complications of retrieval include arrhythmia, as well as perforation of the pulmonary artery or heart. Therefore, interventional radiologic (IR) retrieval is done in conjunction with a back-up surgical plan.

12.3 Conclusion

Interventional radiologic techniques are gaining increasing support and experience as methods for managing traumatic aortic rupture. Further follow-up data and new graft devices are required before it can be clearly determined or accepted as the first line of treatment in all cases. In other conditions, IR techniques are useful in specific situations after determination by the members of the trauma team.

References

[1] Karmy-Jones R, Jurkovich GJ. Blunt chest trauma. Curr Probl Surg 2004; 41: 211–380

[2] Prêtre R, Kürsteiner K, Khatchatourian G, Faidutti B. Traumatic occlusion of the left anterior descending artery and rupture of the aortic isthmus. J Trauma 1995; 39: 388–390

[3] Gillebert T, van de Werf F, Piessens J, de Geest H. Post-traumatic infarction due to blunt chest trauma. Report of two cases. Acta Cardiol 1980; 35: 445–453

[4] Ginzburg E, Dygert J, Parra-Davila E, Lynn M, Almeida J, Mayor M. Coronary artery stenting for occlusive dissection after blunt chest trauma. J Trauma 1998; 45: 157–161

[5] Gaspard P, Clermont A, Villard J, Amiel M. Non-iatrogenic trauma of the coronary arteries and myocardium: contribution of angiography—report of six cases and literature review. Cardiovasc Intervent Radiol 1983; 6: 20–29

[6] Candell J, Valle V, Payá J, Cortadellas J, Esplugas E, Rius J. Post-traumatic coronary occlusion and early left ventricular aneurysm. Am Heart J 1979; 97: 509–512

[7] Fu M, Wu CJ, Hsieh MJ. Coronary dissection and myocardial infarction following blunt chest trauma. J Formos Med Assoc 1999; 98: 136–140

[8] Williams PD, Mahadevan VS, Clarke B. Traumatic aortic dissection and coronary fistula treated with transcatheter management. Catheter Cardiovasc Interv 2007; 70: 1013–1017

[9] Lowe JE, Adams DH, Cummings RG, Wesly RL, Phillips HR. The natural history and recommended management of patients with traumatic coronary artery fistulas. Ann Thorac Surg 1983; 36: 295–305

[10] Jeganathan R, Irwin G, Johnston PW, Jones JM. Traumatic left anterior descending artery-to-pulmonary artery fistula with delayed pericardial tamponade. Ann Thorac Surg 2007; 84: 276–278

[11] Berry C, Hillis WS, Knight WB. Transcatheter closure of a ventricular septal defect resulting from knife stabbing using the Amplatzer muscular VSD occluder. Catheter Cardiovasc Interv 2006; 68: 153–156

[12] Schwalm S, Hijazi Z, Sugeng L, Lang R. Percutaneous closure of a post-traumatic muscular ventricular septal defect using the Amplatzer duct occluder. J Invasive Cardiol 2005; 17: 100–103

[13] Cowley CG, Shaddy RE. Transcatheter treatment of a large traumatic ventricular septal defect. Catheter Cardiovasc Interv 2004; 61: 144–146

[14] Demirkilic U, Yilmaz AT, Tatar H, Ozturk OY. Bullet embolism to the pulmonary artery. Interact Cardiovasc Thorac Surg 2004; 3: 356–358

[15] Kortbeek JB, Clark JA, Carraway RC. Conservative management of a pulmonary artery bullet embolism: case report and review of the literature. J Trauma 1992; 33: 906–908

[16] Nagy KK, Massad M, Fildes J, Reyes H. Missile embolization revisited: a rationale for selective management. Am Surg 1994; 60: 975–979

[17] O'Neill PJ, Feldman DR, Vujic I, Byrne TK. Trans-jugular extraction of bullet embolus to the heart. Mil Med 1996; 161: 360–361

[18] Best IM. Transfemoral extraction of an intracardiac bullet embolus. Am Surg 2001; 67: 361–363

13 Interventional Radiology in Thoracic Vascular Trauma

Riyad Karmy-Jones and Eric K. Hoffer

13.1 Thoracic Trauma

Thoracic trauma is a significant cause of morbidity and mortality, responsible for up to 25% of blunt trauma fatalities, and plays a significant role in 50% of fatalities. These injuries can be difficult to diagnose and manage, in part because the bony thorax makes access difficult. In addition, in the thorax there are many vital organs that require a variety of different exposures and techniques to repair depending on the specific clinical setting.

Furthermore, thoracotomy, sternotomy, and the repair of intrathoracic injuries are associated with significant morbidity, particularly in patients with multiple organ injury and/or severe physiologic derangement. Interventional radiologic (IR) techniques offer a less disruptive approach to manage acute injuries and complications of trauma. Perhaps an illustrative example of how IR approaches may impact the care of the trauma patient is a recent report of an adolescent with traumatic aortic rupture and coronary-ventricular fistula successfully treated with aortic and coronary stents.[1]

Nevertheless, an image-guided attempt to manage an intrathoracic problem may be risky and delay a definitive procedure, resulting in a worsening clinical situation. Thus, percutaneous interventions must be carefully considered according to the clinical situation, and the management decision should be made by individual or interdisciplinary teams, and have clear understanding of the risks and benefits of alternative therapeutic approaches.

13.1.1 Aortic Rupture

Considering trauma-related mortality, blunt acute traumatic aortic rupture (ATAR) is second only to head injury as the primary cause of death. Despite this, the experience at most centers is relatively limited. One of the largest recent series includes 274 patients admitted to 50 institutions over 2½ years, so the "average" institution would have only 2.2 patients/year.[2]

In practice some trauma centers may manage 8 to 15 patients/year, while the majority may encounter 1 or 2 at most. It is now recognized that the patients can be classified in three categories: (1) those who die at the scene (70–80%); (2) those who present at the emergency room unstable or become unstable (2–5%: mortality of 90–98%), and (3) those who present hemodynamically stable and are diagnosed within 24 hours after the injury (15–25%: mortality of 25%), mainly due to associated injuries.[3] The use of seat belts, air bags, and chest protectors has resulted in an increased number of patients surviving severe motor vehicle and motorcycle crashes with both fewer associated injuries and smaller aortic lesions, resulting in an increased number of patients seen at some centers.[4,5] In addition, other motor safety measures and mainly better and quicker emergency management have been linked with a doubling of prehospital survival.[6] Also, the concept of trauma level I established a few decades ago is an important factor.

The initial and operative management of patients with traumatic aortic rupture is continuously evolving. Early institution of β-blockade in stable patients, as well as the recognition of patients who may benefit from a delayed, rather than an emergent intervention, has increased the margin of safety and has been associated with improved survival.[7,8] Furthermore, modifications in operative techniques, including an increased use of mechanical circulatory support, and modifications in devices that permit much lower doses of heparin reduce (but do not eliminate) the risks of paralysis, end-organ failure, and acute cardiac collapse, and have also been associated with improved outcomes.[9,10,11]

Although operative repair remains the accepted standard of care for most descending thoracic aortic ruptures, there is still the wrong perception that surgery is associated with excessive risk. This may be due to a relative inexperience at most centers, and the desire to operate on patients who could be better managed by delaying a surgical intervention or both. The endovascular repair with thoracic aortic stent grafts (thoracic endovascular aortic repair [TEVAR]) offers an attractive third option, which can avoid the morbidity of a thoracotomy in patients with multiple injuries, with a lower risk of paralysis.[12–17]

At this time, TEVAR is becoming the preferred method of management despite a lack of long-term follow-up durability and continued concerns about complications.[18] The procedure is relatively new so we need years to assess more accurately its role in the management of acute rupture of the thoracic aorta.

13.1.2 Outcomes of Endovascular Stents Utilized in the Trauma Setting

Many published series support that patients who have undergone TEVAR for traumatic aortic disruption have low mortality (the mortality being due to associated injuries) and essentially no risk of postprocedure paralysis. It is important to consider the length of time in which the experience was accrued (as stent-graft technology is continuously improving significantly over the past few years), and recognize the differences between the acute (within 24 hours to 30 days after the injury) versus chronic types and also consider the indications for stent grafting and contraindications to open repair.

We have reviewed 11 series published from 2002 to 2006, including 167 patients, the youngest being 16 years of age.[13,14, 19–28] These series ranged from 5 to 30 patients, over periods ranging from 1 to 7 years. Average follow-up among the 10 series with at least one-year follow-up was 24 months. Virtually all stent grafts were commercially available, although they varied between "dedicated" thoracic stents to a variety of cuff extenders for the main grafts. There were seven (4%) deaths, two procedure related (one collapse and rupture, one stroke). There were type I endoleaks (4.7%), two healed spontaneously, and six required further stenting and/or balloon dilation. There were two iliac arteries ruptured, and three (1.7%) patients of acute stent collapse requiring operative intervention. There were two nonfatal strokes and one brachial artery occlusion requiring thrombectomy. There was no postprocedure paralysis.

Dunham et al noted that in patients with isolated chest injuries, the length of stay in the intensive care unit (ICU) and total hospitalization was as low as 1 and 7 days, respectively.[27] Lin et al summarized 33 studies describing 324 patients managed with TEVAR with follow-up ranging from 6 to 55 months.[29] Technical success was achieved in all but two, and there was only one patient with paraplegia.

Hoofer et al reviewed 50 reports including 722 patients treated with TEVAR. The technical success was 97.1%, and the mortality was 8.1% (1.3% procedure related). Paraplegia occurred in 0.75% and stroke in 0.9%. There were 32 endoleaks (4.6%), three endoleaks associated with mortality, 41% managed endovascularly, and 18% required open repair. Access complications requiring surgical repair occurred in 20 (3%) patients.[30]

These major nonfatal complication rates (excluding endoleak) of 4.3% and mortality of 3.6% justify the excitement of the role of TEVAR in the management of ATAR. Endovascular repair is particularly attractive in patients with associated injuries or comorbid conditions that increase the operative risk for open repair.[31] In addition, endografts may also be used, not as a definitive repair, but in complicated cases as a "bridge" to a definitive treatment in selected patients who are not candidates in the acute phase for either operative repair or medical management.[19]

13.1.3 Comparison between Endovascular and Open Repair

It is difficult to retrospectively compare two techniques not necessarily applied to the same patient population with respect to risk assessment, operative experience, and institutional biases. Each institution center has different patient populations and management strategies making it difficult for broad generalizations based on an individual study. We reviewed eight articles, published between 2004 and 2008 that specifically compared outcomes within their respective institutions between the two approaches.[4,14,20,24,32,33,34,35] One hundred sixty-one patients underwent open repair. There were 24 deaths (14%) and 5 (3%) patients with new postoperative paralysis. One hundred sixty-one patients underwent endovascular repair, with 13 (8%) mortality and no new paralysis/paraplegia. Only one death was procedure—related among the stent-graft group due to acute stent collapse.

Tang and associates presented a meta-analysis comparing the 30-day outcomes between 278 aortic ruptures managed surgically versus 355 managed endovascularly.[36] There were no significant differences in injury severity or age between the groups. The endovascular group had significantly lower mortality (7.6% vs. 15.2%, $p = 0.008$), paraplegia (0% vs. 5.5%, $p < 0.0001$), and stroke (0.81% vs. 5.1%, $p = 0.003$) compared with the open surgical repair cohort.[36]

Hoofer et al performed a meta-analysis of 19 retrospective cohort studies from single institutions comparing 262 endovascular to 376 open repairs.[30] Mortality among the endovascular group was 8.4% and among the open group 20.2% ($p = 0.001$), while paraplegia among the endovascular group was 0.8% versus 5.7% among the open group ($p = 0.01$).

Demetriades et al performed a prospective multicenter study of outcomes of open versus endovascular repair. There were 193 patients, of which 125 (65%) underwent TEVAR. Multivariate analysis identified a significantly lower mortality among TEVAR group (9%) versus OR (16%), $p = 0.001$, but no difference

in paralysis (0.8% TEVAR vs. 2.9% OR, $p = 0.28$). Endoleak occurred in 18 (14%) patients, nine were treated with proximal stent extensions, six were operated on, and three were observed with delayed resolution. There were four (3%) instances of access vessel injury, two (1.6%) strokes, one access site infection and one endograft collapse (resulting in paraplegia).

TEVAR, in the acute setting, results in lower percentages of mortality and paraplegia than with open repair. However, without prospective randomized studies, results are not definitive, given that outcomes depend on the injury severity and initial presentation.[4] In many single cohort studies the time to TEVAR is significantly longer than time to open repair, with potentially significant bias. With good surgical techniques, even though mortality rates depending on associated injuries still range from 8 to 20%, the operative repair is associated with paraplegia in less than 5%.[4,37,38] In addition, there is well-documented long-term follow up on data in open repair. Similar data are still being obtained in the TEVAR population.[39,40]

13.1.4 Endovascular Repair versus Medical Management

A strict "anti-impulse" therapy should be instituted once the diagnosis of aortic rupture is made.[24,41] The "ideal" blood pressure (BP) depends upon the patient's age and presenting BP. Until recently, the goal is a systolic pressure of < 120 mm Hg and/or mean pressure < 60 to 70. More recently, the dictum is "a BP of less than the admission BP" is more appropriate.[3,42] If a strict BP control is implemented in stable patients, the risk of rupture in the first week may be as low as 5% or less.[3] Reports of improved outcomes with both delayed open and endovascular repair, may reflect some selection bias.[24] Reasons for delaying operative intervention include severe head, blunt cardiac, solid organ, and/or acute lung injuries.[10,43] We prefer "serial" surveillance imaging (preferably with computed tomography angiography [CTA]) every 48 hours for 7 to 10 days, to detect changes in size or character of the lesion.[7] Even with carotid BP and heart-rate control, up to 12% of false aneurysms continue to enlarge.[44,45] Although the natural history of pseudoaneurysms appear to follow those of nontraumatic atherosclerotic aneurysms, these lesions should not be ignored; therefore, there should be an early intervention as soon as the patient is medically stable, especially in young patients.

A careful medical control of BP may not be possible in all cases. Many patients require other interventions, and monitoring and controlling BP can be difficult. There are hazards such as renal and splanchnic insufficiency, and secondary brain injury, especially in the setting of increased intracranial pressure.[46] The value of raising cerebral perfusion pressure is controversial as well as assuming that an increased intracranial pressure results in improved cerebral perfusion. There is, on the other hand, general consensus that a "high" pressure is associated with a lower risk of secondary brain injury.[47,48,49,50] Thus, a closed head injury associated with evidence of increased intracranial pressure (by CT and/or intracranial pressure [ICP] monitoring) may actually mandate an operative or endovascular repair.

One significant advantage of the endovascular repair over both the operative and nonoperative management is that after stent placement, in most patients it is possible to allow the BP to normalize, or even increase without the risk of bleeding or rupture of the aortic injury. A note of caution: The risk of rupture, even with serial CTA and careful hemodynamic control, is not zero. Endovascular stenting may be ideal in these patients who cannot undergo an open operative repair because of significant assorted comorbidities.

The extent of the injury also may further the impact of choice between a medical and endovascular management. Minor aortic injuries, involving only small intimal defects, often heal without residual defects.[51,52] On the other hand, even small lesions can rupture if the BP is not controlled.[7] If the BP can be reasonably controlled, and there are no contraindications to medical management, small intimal defects should be managed conservatively with close observation follow-up. Even some small pseudoaneurysms can heal.[7] Thus, while endovascular management appears to be ideal in patients with significant comorbidities and who are considered too high a risk for prolonged medical management, it is unclear that this approach is better than medical management in the above patients with minimal injuries. One simple guideline is if a lesion is too small for open operative repair, it is also too small for endovascular repair.

13.1.5 Current Endografts Available

Some characteristics of an endograft designed for the thoracic aorta as opposed to the abdominal aorta include a long-delivery system to reach the distal arch from the femoral artery, and enough flexibility to accommodate the curvature of the arch. There are variations in the manner of deployment between different types of endografts, also whether the proximal and/or distal end components are bare, whether they contain hooks, and the manner of release from the introducer devices.

In general, there is a shift away from deploying devices in aortic trauma (and type B dissection) that rely on uncovered proximal landing zones because of risks of aortic perforation.[53] A first consideration is that the usual patients sustaining severe chest trauma with aortic rupture are young with a thoracic aortic diameter in the 20-mm range—too small for devices designed for older patients with atherosclerotic aortas.[54] Second, the use of endografts in acute trauma is considered "off-label" by the Food and Drug Administration (FDA) outside of clinical trials. Currently, two devices are approved by the FDA for use in the thoracic aorta, only for atherosclerotic aneurysms.

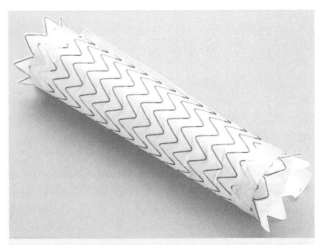

Fig. 13.1 The Gore thoracic aortic graft (TAG; W.L. Gore & Associates, Flagstaff, AZ). (Provided by Gore, Inc.)

There are ongoing high-risk trials to determine and prove the utility of stent grafts in trauma, and endografts used currently in Europe, Canada, and Australia are under evaluation in the United States and will soon be available outside of trials.

The Gore-TAG (W.L. Gore & Associates, Flagstaff, AZ) is made of expanded polytetrafluoroethylene (ePTFE), wrapped in self-expanding Nitinol stents with a sutureless attachment. It is introduced through a 30-cm sheath, the diameter of which varies, depending on the diameter of the graft. The delivery catheter is flexible and 100 cm in length. In appropriately sized patients, the TAG is very easy to introduce due to its flexibility and rapid deployment (▶ Fig. 13.1).[4,29,38,55]

Two other companies, Cook Medical (Bloomington, IN) and Medtronic (Santa Rosa, CA), have also been developing and refining endografts for use in the thoracic aorta. Early experience indicates that they are useful in trauma patients in Europe, Canada, and Australia (▶ Fig. 13.2, ▶ Fig. 13.3).[22,23,27,32,56,57] Medtronic's Valiant thoracic stent graft has been approved by the FDA too. It has a hydrophilic coating to the graft cover to facilitate iliac artery access and stent delivery.

Because of the size constraints in the typical trauma patient, and because the arch is often acutely angled, some groups have used abdominal aortic cuff extenders instead of dedicated thoracic aortic stent grafts.[25,28,58] These are not only smaller, but

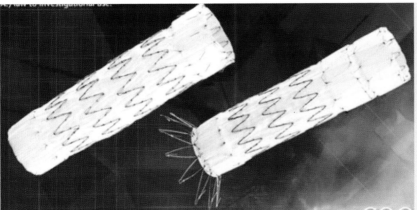

Fig. 13.2 The Cook-Zenith TX2 graft (Cook Medical, Bloomington, IN) with proximal and distal components. (Provided by Cook, Inc.)

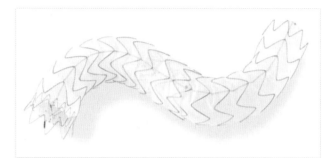

Fig. 13.3 The Valiant thoracic graft (Medtronic, Santa Rosa, CA) with proximal and distal components. (Provided by Medtronic, Inc.)

Table 13.1 Anatomical considerations in thoracic endovascular aortic repair (TEVAR)

Anatomical features to consider	Implications
Diameter of proximal and distal landing zones	Determines size of endograft that can/should be utilized
Distance from lesion to origin of left subclavian artery	Will obtaining an adequate landing zone require coverage of the left subclavian artery?
Distance from lesion to origin of left common carotid artery	If required, is there room to land distal to the origin of the left common carotid artery? Will there be room, if needed, to clamp distal to the origin, or will circulatory arrest be needed, if subsequent operative repair is required?
Degree of curvature across the proximal landing zone	Is there a high likelihood that to avoid malposition along the inner curvature that the graft will have to be placed more proximally?
Quality of the aorta	Is there significant thrombus and/or calcification that would pose a risk of stroke or type I endoleaks?
Quality of access vessels	Is the diameter sufficient to permit the required sheath? Are there more proximal calcifications and/or tortuosity that might prevent safe passage of the sheath?
Distance from proposed access vessel to the lesion	Does the system being used have sufficient length to reach the proposed site?
Length of the injury	If using additional cuffs, how many may be required to ensure fixation?
Vascular anomalies	• Anomalous origin of left vertebral artery? • Patent left internal mammary artery (LIMA) graft? • Aberrant origin of the right subclavian artery? • Other anomalies?

may actually fit the aortic configuration of transected aortas in young patients better, albeit at the expense of needing multiple grafts, of an increased risk of type III endoleaks, and of having to use the shorter delivery system that is designed for the infrarenal aorta.[59] The AneuRx (Medtronic, Santa Rosa, CA) cuff extenders range from 20- to 28-mm diameter, are 4-cm long, and are delivered through a 21-French (F) catheter 59-cm long. The Gore-Excluder aortic cuffs (W.L. Gore & Associates, Flagstaff, AZ) are 3.3-cm long, have diameters of 23, 26, and 28.5 mm, and can be delivered through an 18- or 20-F sheath 61 cm long. Over an 8-year period, we performed 40 TEVAR procedures, 33 with cuff extenders or limbs, one with a Medtronic Talent device, and the remaining six with the Gore-TAG device (▶ Fig. 13.4) (▶ Table 13.1).

13.1.6 Anatomical Considerations

The initial consideration is the diameter of the proximal and distal landing zones, measuring from inner wall to inner wall. The diameter is difficult to measure in the distal arch, so we measure the widest transverse diameter. In young adults the aorta is relatively uniform in diameter through the arch.

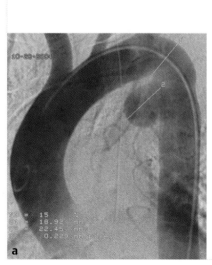

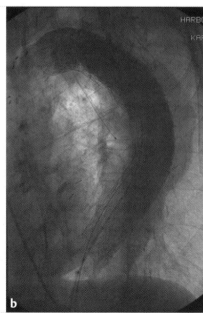

Fig. 13.4 (a) Patient with a traumatic aortic rupture with saccular pseudoaneurysm outpouching. (b) The patient was managed with a TAG. Because of size differential, the patient required a smaller proximal graft with larger distal extension.

Most transections occur distal to the origin of the left subclavian artery, so the next consideration is whether to cover the subclavian artery origin or not, required in up to one-third or more cases.[36,54] Deploying the graft within the distal curve ("gray zone") of the arch may result in partial occlusion of the aorta, increased risk of stent-graft migration and/or collapse (enfolding of the stent-graft), and result in an endoleak.

The proximal landing zone and arch needs to be reviewed for the presence of thrombus and/or calcification. Calcification can elevate a "lip" of endograft, resulting in an endoleak. Significant thrombus increases the risk of distal embolization and stroke.

The length of aorta to be covered requires a minimum of a 2-cm landing zone. If using cuff extenders, usually three are required for stability.[28,59] Sometimes a 2-cm proximal landing zone is not achievable. In a localized lesion of an otherwise normal wall aorta, 5 to 10 mm of apposition provides an adequate seal in the absence of severe angulation.[44,58]

The next consideration is the length of the delivery device. Thoracic endograft delivery systems are long enough to reach the entire aorta from a femoral artery approach, but abdominal aortic cuff extenders are only 61 cm and may not reach from the groin to the arch. Also, the status and diameter of the access arteries and degree of calcification should be determined. Calcifications are better seen with noncontrast images. A noncalcified vessel may tolerate a slightly oversized sheath, but a severely calcified vessel may not accept a sheath that would be predicted to fit based on size criteria alone.

Coverage of the left subclavian artery with subclavian to carotid bypass or transposition raises the question of arm ischemia, vertebral-basilar insufficiency, and/or type II endoleak. In general, critical arm ischemia is rare, affecting less than 2% of patients, and if it occurs can be managed electively in most patients.[13,55,57,60,61] Type II endoleak arising by back flow into the pseudoaneurysm is also uncommon given that most ruptures arise from the inner curve of the aorta. Should type II endoleak occur, or if there is concern prior to the procedure, the left brachial artery can be accessed and once the graft is deployed, the subclavian artery can be occluded with coils or other agents or closed with a peripheral closure device.[62] "Vertebral steal" phenomenon can be addressed electively.[63] Patients with patent left internal mammary artery (LIMA) grafts into the coronary arteries should undergo carotid-subclavian bypass prior to left subclavian coverage.[55,63]

Impeding the flow to the left vertebral artery may pose a risk of posterior cerebral circulatory insufficiency or stroke. Collateral flow from the contralateral vertebral artery maintains flow with a 25 to 48 mm Hg systolic pressure differential.[61,64] However, this may be compromised in cases of a hypoplastic contralateral artery, posteroinferior cerebellar artery termination of the left vertebral reported as 1% incidence and/or concomitant contralateral vertebral artery trauma.

Manninen et al, on a autopsy study of 92 patients, found that covering the left subclavian would put only 5 (5.4%) of patients at risk for posterior stroke due to variation in posterior circulation and right vertebral anatomy.[65]

In our experience, this has never happened in the younger population, but could happen in older patients with diffuse vascular disease. Assessing the cerebral circulation is difficult under emergent conditions. Anatomical assessments can be made by CTA and/or magnetc resonance angiography (MRA) of the head and neck, or cerebral angiography, either prior to stent-graft placement or at the time of the procedure. We have found that transcranial ultrasound (US) Doppler is a useful adjunct. If the basilar artery and the posterior communicating artery can be identified, then flow from both vertebral arteries, the basilar artery, and posterior communicating arteries can be measured, while temporally occluding the origin of the left subclavian artery with an occlusion balloon. Demonstrating intact vertebrobasilar flow after left subclavian artery occlusion precludes the need for prophylactic subclavian artery bypass or transposition of vessels.[64]

Carotid-subclavian bypass is generally well tolerated. However, some have noted an increased stroke risk in patients with atherosclerotic aneurysmal disease.[63,66] This may be related to the increased degree of calcification in the older population, and does not apply to the younger trauma population. Our bias is to try to assess the cerebral circulation the best we can, but if the patient is emergent, and there is no gross evidence of diffuse calcification, we will cover the subclavian artery, if necessary, without waiting for further imaging. If vertebrobasilar or arm ischemia develops, then we treat ischemia electively.

If the proximal landing zone is encroaching upon the origin of the left subclavian artery, but complete coverage is not required, it is possible to access the left brachial artery and leave a wire in the arch, which will allow precise placement of the stent graft and then help stenting of the subclavian artery origin if narrowing occurs.[23]

13.1.7 Femoral, Iliac, and Aortic Access

Access vessel choice depends on the size of the sheath required for the chosen endograft, length of the delivery system, quality and diameter of the pelvic arteries, and clinical setting. Most young trauma patients have normal vasculature, and thus slight mismatch can be tolerated as long as the sheath is advanced easily under fluoroscopy. On the other hand, as we know, a significant number of chest trauma patients are young and therefore have femoral and external iliac arteries smaller than 8 mm in diameter. This makes access with the sheaths required for the dedicated thoracic devices problematic. If there is any concern, a contralateral sheath should be inserted so that a balloon occlusion can be used to occlude the artery in the event of an iliac artery rupture during sheath removal.[34,67] Endografts, such as the TAG, can be advanced without a sheath ("bare back"), but these are not recommended because the graft could easily catch on a plaque, or sharp edge, and deploy prematurely or be damaged. When withdrawing the sheath, particularly if a percutaneous approach has been used, it is critical that the blood pressure be monitored for 2 to 3 minutes because any acute drop indicates an iliac rupture and bleeding. A completion DSA through the sheath or through a contralateral catheter is indicated if there is difficulty during introduction of the sheath.

Retroperitoneal iliac artery surgical exposure may be required when using cuff extenders and the device is not long enough to reach the location of the rupture and/or if the femoral arteries are too small and/or calcified. Obviously, if there is pelvic trauma, approach in the side with the least hematoma is desirable. The common iliac arteries can be accessed directly or a 10-mm silo graft is anastomosed end-to-side. If the pelvis is deep, to avoid a problem with angulation, the silo graft can be tunneled through the lower abdominal soft tissues or, through the femoral canal to the groin. Patients who have had prior aorto-iliac grafts can be challenging because the iliac arteries are often embedded in scar tissue.

The ureter should always be identified and mobilized anteriorly, avoiding dissection on both sides to prevent devascularization. In the majority of cases, the best that can be achieved is that enough dissection of the iliac limb of the graft allows application of a partial occlusion clamp or direct graft puncture. Having completed the procedure, whether anastomosing to graft or native vessel, the conduit is simply truncated and oversewn as a patch. In some circumstances, it may be advisable to convert the conduit to an iliofemoral artery bypass. This allows a relatively easier access route for later percutaneous interventions should the need arise. If the patients have an open abdomen, then a direct infrarenal aortic access can be used.[59] This access would not be a good choice if visceral spillage occurred.

Endovascular stent grafting is a combined procedure between the interventional radiologist and the thoracic cardiovascular surgeon. The room must be designed with this in mind (dedicated room), including sterile setup and laminar air flow. It theoretically can be done in a standard operating suite, using portable C-arm, but the image quality is not ideal. General anesthesia with a single lumen endotracheal tube is sufficient. A right radial arterial catheter for BP monitoring is optimal as the left subclavian artery may be covered or the left brachial artery may be needed for access.

A fluoroscopy check is done to ensure that no tubes, lines, or bony structures obscure the field. We place a 5- or 6-F sheath and multimarker pigtail catheter through the contralateral femoral artery. This allows digital subtraction angiography (DSA) to be done at anytime, even with the nondeployed stent graft in place. It also allows access for an occlusion balloon in the event of iliac artery rupture.

In obese patients, those with a weak pulse or in all patients, US is used to gain entrance into the femoral arteries. Then 5,000 units of heparin are administered. Avoid heparinization if there is concern for bleeding complications.[28]

A 5-F pigtail is advanced over a floppy 3-J wire, and then exchanged for a stiffer wire (Amplatz or Lunderquist). The location of proximal wire is marked on the table to prevent unwanted motion of the wire. The delivery sheath is for the stent graft, advanced under constant fluoroscopy, to the desired position, in the distal aorta. Once the stent graft is in the approximate desired location, the tube is rotated to the ideal angle, and DSA done ideally with respirations suspended.

The ideal angle is decided from the planning CTA, with optimal visualization of the proximal landing zone obtained in a projection orthogonal to the plane of the arch. In a young patient, it is almost a lateral projection. About 40 mL at 20 mL/s of contrast material is adequate for DSA. A "road map" can be obtained and/or the landmarks marked with a felt pen. Then the stent graft is deployed.

We prefer to withdraw the pigtail used for DSA below the stent prior to deployment of the stent. This is an operator preference and no strict rule exists. The deployment is rapid. Hypertension should be avoided. When cuff extenders are used, we prefer adenosine, at least for the first graft, to avoid distal displacement of the graft. When deploying cuffs, in general, we like to start distally because it helps stabilize subsequent insertion of more proximal additional devices.

Once the device(s) is/are deployed, low-pressure balloon (i.e., COVA, others) dilation, starting distally is performed. When using multiple devices, the ballooning should proceed proximally, covering all areas of overlap. When deploying cuffs, the balloons necessarily occlude the aorta, and even the "triple" balloon is deployed across aortic arch in acute proximal hypertension may be noted and the balloon could grab the stent graft.

Ideally, in traumatic rupture of the aorta inflating the balloon can be avoided altogether. If needed, rapid inflation and deflations with one-third contrast and two-thirds saline solution may prevent significant hypertension. Vigorous overdilation should be avoided.

The balloon is withdrawn distal to the stent, always maintaining wire access, and a completion DSA performed. If there are small endoleaks or of there is a lip of graft not being opposed to the inner curvature of the aorta, then repeat balloon dilation should be performed until the graft is attached to the aorta. Sometimes this cannot be achieved, so extending the graft with an additional module (or occasionally to bare uncovered stent) is needed. Large balloons can catch along the edge of the delivery sheath, but a gentle pulling of the balloon and sheath beyond the aortic bifurcation usually allows the balloon catheter to straighten and be removed easily. The sheath is thereafter gently withdrawn to as close to the inguinal ligament as possible (in the patient of femoral access) and a completion pelvic DSA done.

The protocols for follow-up are based on the various clinical trials designed to evaluate thoracic endografting for atherosclerotic aneurysms. Guidelines include CTA at 48 hours, at discharge, and at 1-, 6-, and 12-month intervals, and then annually. These protocols are designed to detect graft collapse, migration or persistent endoleak with aneurismal growth. These guidelines were proposed because in arteriosclerosis the diseased landing zones have a potential for progression in dilation of the thoracic aorta. It is important to think about follow-up with patients with renal insufficiency, because of the contrast material effects on the kidneys. Also, we must consider the large number of studies with high radiation exposures. Patients with renal insufficiency can be followed with intravascular ultrasound, transesophageal echocardiography, MRA, or even CT without contrast material. Our main concern is pseudoaneurysm regression or disappearance or enlargement. A chest radiograph can detect stent deformation or migration.

For patients with aortic transection, we obtain CTA at 48 hours, then in a month, then at one year and thereafter follow with chest radiographs, as needed. It is very important to get follow-up CTA with the same protocols every time: unenhanced, contrast enhanced and delayed images. This is standard procedure in most trauma level I institutions.

We do not use antiplatelet agents after thoracic aortic stent grafting. However, we manage these procedures like any other practice with implanted devices (valve, stents, prostheses, etc.), and recommend antibiotic prophylaxis if any invasive procedure, such as dental work, or other is planned.

13.1.8 Endoleak

Endoleaks are categorized as type I (around the proximal, A, or distal, B, ends of the graft), type II (form an artery feeding into the aneurismal sac), type III (between components), or type IV (failure of graft integrity). Type V, "endotension," is controversial. In the trauma setting, proximal type I and to some degree type II endoleaks are important. Proximal type I occur in 5% of cases. Persistent type I endoleak is associated with a risk of rupture.[56] The predominant mechanism in trauma patients is the combination of a short landing zone and lack of apposition along the inner curvature of the arch.[68] Gentle balloon dilation should be tried first. If not sufficient, extending proximally with another graft is done.[23,69] Type I leaks visualized only on delayed images immediately following deployment may resolve spontaneously following heparin reversal.

We assess these endoleaks at 48 hours with repeat CTA. Blood pressure should be controlled with β-blockade during this period. Proximal type I endoleaks found on follow-up imaging must be managed with repeat interventions, including proximal cuff extenders.[35] Significant leaks at the time of implant, or at follow-up, that do not respond to additional balloon dilation or cuff extension warrant operative repair. In these patients, most type I endoleaks occur within 30 days, but occasionally can be found up to 2 years later, therefore, the need for strict surveillance.[68]

Type II endoleaks should be managed based on whether or not the left subclavian is the source. If it is, coil occlusion of the subclavian, artery, and carotid to subclavian artery bypass with proximal ligation or carotid subclavian artery to carotid artery transposition should be performed. Type II endoleaks secondary to patent bronchial or intercostal arteries are more problematic, but again are less important legions given that there are fewer branches in the proximal descending thoracic aorta. Some believe that these are more benign than in abdominal endografting and that in the majority of patients, they will seal spontaneously.[70] Occasionally, a branch can be catheterized and embolized using microcatheter techniques (▶ Fig. 13.5).

13.1.9 Stent-Graft Collapse

A stent-graft collapse is a catastrophic complication that can occur immediately, within the first 48 hours, or up to 5 months postprocedure.[70–75] This is a combination of graft oversizing and/or a lack of apposition along the inner curve of the aorta. In young patients without calcification, oversizing should be in the 7 to 15% range only rather than the 20% range in atherosclerotic aneurysms.[38,40] In young hyperdynamic pliable aortas, the force of the cardiac ejection that hits the underside of the nonapposed graft can cause infolding and collapse of the graft.[29,73,76] This may lead to immediate aortic occlusion, type I endoleak, and possibly rupture. If this occurs postimplant, the patient will develop signs of acute coarctation, and a rapid onset of paralysis and renal failure. This may not be apparent if the patient is still on the ventilator and sedated.

Prevention includes very accurate sizing, choosing a graft that approximates only a 10% oversizing rather than a 20%. Also, plan pre- and intraoperatively, to avoid landing in the "no man's land" of the aorta. If the proximal portion of the graft is not apposed or at least close to the inner curve of the arch, particularly if there is only a short zone of apposition, perhaps ≤ 50%, the options include extending the graft proximally and/or repeat ballooning.[71] Uncovered metal stents deployed within the stent graft can be used when collapse is acute or delayed.

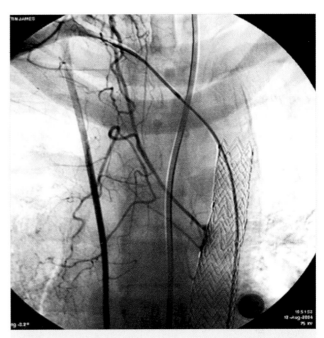

Fig. 13.5 The patient underwent repair of traumatic aortic rupture with an iliac limb from an abdominal aortic stent graft. Persistent opacification suggested a type I endoleak. At angiography, a type II endoleak originating from a thyrocervical to bronchial artery connection was found. This was readily managed by embolization with liquid agents (glues) using a microcatheter technique.

Concerned that uncovered stents may erode over time through the graft fabric or create proximal aortic perforations, there have been numerous anecdotal reports of bare stent extenders used for proximal, partial, or complete collapse with good short-term results. There is growing consensus that cuff extenders, deployed sequentially and thus fit the curvature of the aorta better, may perform better than longer thoracic stent grafts in patients with aortic diameters smaller than 24 mm. At this time, these smaller stent grafts are being developed or available in certain places or manufacturing companies.

If stent-graft collapse occurs postoperatively, it can be detected by plain chest radiography, or noncontrast or contrast-enhanced CT. Immediate intervention is required. In complete collapse, explanting and operative repair is prudent, but ballooning and extending the device with a bare stent can be used with success, and is much easier for the patient.[28] Anecdotally, axillary–femoral–femoral bypass has been used as a temporizing measure, but ultimately the stent must be removed.

13.1.10 Aortic Dissection/Rupture

Rupture can occur at any time. Prevention is strict BP control, particularly during periods or procedures that might acutely elevate the heart rate and/or blood pressure. Great care should be taken to watch the wire advancement. If difficulty negotiating the aortic curvature or narrowing at the injury site is found, a directional catheter such as a vertebral and/or hydrophilic catheter must be used.

There are reports of delayed or immediate rupture after the graft deployment. Endografts with a bare metal proximal extension have been implicated in perforating the aortic wall.[77]

Even covered grafts without this feature have been implicated, if there is poor apposition to the aortic wall with resultant continued motion against the wall of the aorta. All three dedicated thoracic endografts have been implicated in acute or delayed perforation with or without dissection, in the nontrauma experience. As mentioned already, proper graft sizing is essential for good graft-aortic apposition.

Proximal dissection could occur during balloon dilation of the proximal cuff, given the ends of the graft can create a dissection flap that may rapidly progress retrograde. To avoid this, the initial dilation should be as gentle as possible, just enough to document profiling of the balloon along the side of the graft. Dilation should only be done within the graft. Late pseudoaneurysm development is attributed to injury to the aortic wall during stent deployment.[34] Presumably, this is due to a similar mechanism.

13.1.11 Migration

If the proximal landing zone is not long enough, and the aneurysm itself is large, stents can migrate distally. This may be detected on routine chest radiograph, or may present with a new endoleak. In young patients, as the aortic wall grows, an endograft may lose its fixation. In these cases, the options include operative explanting and grafting, or proximal extension with another endograft. Thus, lifelong surveillance is necessary.

13.1.12 Regulatory Issues and Consent Implications

It is important to clarify that the use of endovascular stent grafting for acute traumatic injuries is not approved by the FDA. When discussing the plan with patients or families, approval by the FDA of the graft should be discussed and documented. In particular, the lack of long-term follow-up should be discussed in the context of the long-term efficacy of the open repair, and a clear rationale as to why an endovascular approach is preferred should be explained. Remember that these devices are engineered for a 10-year lifespan. We have no data about longer-term durability. It must be mentioned here that, even if technically, the use of thoracic stent grafting is off-label use; all the above-mentioned concerns are necessary and must be done as suggested. At this time, based on current experience and published evidence and per the guidelines of the Society of Vascular Surgery, it is clear that injuries to the aorta of types A–D are now preferably managed by endovascular grafts rather than open surgery. In this is peculiar situation, because the preference is for endovascular treatment, the grafts are used off-label. Therefore, a change of the approval guidelines needs to be made soon.

13.1.13 The Pediatric and Adolescent Patient

Endovascular aortic stent grafts are not commonly used in pediatric and adolescent patients; they have aortas that are too small for currently available devices.[78] They will grow and the lack of long-term durability is important. The growth of the aorta may predispose to migration or relative coarctation, "pseudocoarctation."[29] Thus, although endovascular approaches may be considered as a bridge to definitive treatment, at this time, surgery is still the standard for children and youth. We have used aortic cuffs and/or abdominal limb extenders as a bridge to definitive treatment in two patients with contraindications to medical therapy with significant ruptures, not candidates for open repair. Thus, TEVAR allowed temporization until elective surgical correction could be performed.

13.1.14 Future Trends

Endograft technology is continuing to evolve. Experience and longer follow-up data are accruing as well. Branched grafts are being designed for both arch and abdominal visceral vessels. Specific for the trauma population, a variety of grafts that are shorter, precurved, and smaller are being developed, which will allow more precise deployment and potentially reduce complication rates. Some of those devices are available, but unfortunately are still being used off-label based on FDA regulation.

13.1.15 Conclusion

Endovascular repair of the traumatically injured thoracic aorta has emerged as an exceptionally promising modality that is typically quicker than open repair, with a reduced risk of paralysis. As a matter of fact, now it is the recommended choice by most professional societies and groups. Undoubtedly, this is going to change. There are a specific set of anatomical criteria that need to be applied, which can be rapidly assessed by CTA. The enthusiasm for endovascular repair must be tempered by the complications and lack of long-term follow-up, particularly in young patients. Thoracic surgeons skilled in open aortic repair must be primarily involved, and take on a leadership role during the planning, deployment, and follow-up of these patients. Familiarity with all of the available devices expands treatment options. As more-specific devices become available, and more follow-up is accrued, the role of endovascular stents will continue to grow. A combined team approach is fostered in our institutions.

13.2 Intrathoracic Great Vessel Injury

Injuries involving the intrathoracic great vessels are often difficult to diagnose, and are associated with other injuries (such as spinal cord) that impact outcome significantly. The incidence varies between autopsy and clinical series, as well as on the mechanisms of injury.[79]

One autopsy study found that the greatest incidence was in pedestrian-struck events (17.6%), as compared with motor vehicle crash fatalities (4.6%).[80] Chen et al studied 166 patients who underwent aortogram for indeterminate mediastinum following blunt trauma.[81] Nine (5%) had branch injuries (total 13 vessels) in seven patients isolated. The arteries used the innominate ($n=4$), left common carotid ($n=4$), left subclavian ($n=3$), internal mammary ($n=1$), and left vertebral arteries ($n=1$). In nine, there was an intimal flap, in the remaining four, a pseudoaneurysm.

Table 13.2 Incidence of thoracic aortic and intrathoracic great vessel injury in patients admitted to Harborview Medical Center 1998–2004

Site of injury	Trauma types	
	Blunt (N = 93)	Penetrating (N = 12)
Ascending/arch of aorta	9	Gunshot 2 stab wound 2
Descending aorta	69	
Innominate	12	Gunshot 2
Left common carotid artery	1	Gunshot 1 stab wound 1
Left subclavian artery	2	Gunshot 3 impalement 1

Ahrar et al reported a similar study in which 24 great vessel injuries were documented in 17 of 89 patients (19%) undergoing aortography. Of those with a great vessel injury, 18% had combined aortic injury as well. In our experience at Harborview Medical Center over a period of 7 years, great vessel injury was most commonly associated with blunt trauma, and unlike other reports, the innominate artery was most frequently involved (▶ Table 13.2).[82] Penetrating injuries are less frequently recorded, perhaps because of higher prehospital mortality.[83]

In the report by Demetriades et al, the incidence of great vessel injury was 5% following gunshot wounds to the chest, and 2% following stab wounds to the chest and neck. Subclavian arterial injuries were associated with a mortality of 65%, suggesting the need to rapidly transport the patient, avoid delays in resuscitation, and do invasive diagnostic tests only in stable patients who are without "hard signs" of injury.[82,83]

13.2.1 Initial Management and Diagnosis

Regarding great vessel injury, it is often difficult to gain exposure and exploration for suspected, but not defined injury. Nevertheless, patients who are unstable and/or who have hard signs of vascular injury (expanding hematoma, ongoing pleural or wound bleeding, and others) should be taken directly to the operating room.[84] In stable patients, CTA has replaced DSA in most cases. Patients with only intimal flaps are candidates for observation, with serial duplex Doppler and/or transcranial Doppler to detect emboli, which would be an indication for more aggressive intervention.[38] Aspirin and other platelet agents are used as per the operator's preference.

13.2.2 Endovascular Repair

Endovascular stent-graft repair has been stimulated by the growing experience in thoracic aortic, cervical, and extremity vascular injuries.[38,85,86,87,88] Endovascular repair is attractive to potentially avoid the morbid large incisions, concerns that hematoma may be disrupted leading to difficult to control hemorrhage, concerns of cerebrovascular complications, as well as potential risk of anticoagulation in patients with significant associated extrathoracic injuries.[89,90,91,92] Patel described six patients with penetrating subclavian injuries treated endovascularly. At mean follow-up of 19 months the stents were patent, although one patient required reintervention for stent

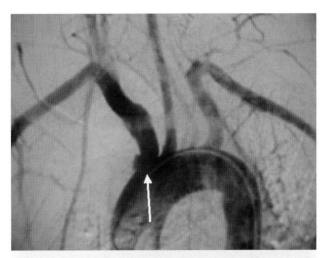

Fig. 13.6 Traumatic rupture of the innominate artery at its origin (arrow). Faintly seen, there is a defect at the origin of the left common carotid artery. At surgery, this was found to be a focal disruption of the vessel also. The patient underwent successful repair with graft of the innominate artery and patch angiography of the common carotid artery lesion without cardiopulmonary bypass. Some origin lesions may be amenable to endovascular approach, but because the injury can extend to the lateral arch, surgery should be performed unless prohibited by comorbid conditions.

fracture.[91] Stent fractures need not be repaired unless there is stenosis or occlusion of the stented artery. Nevertheless, surgical repair has superb results. The mortality or morbidity is related predominantly to associated injuries, particularly to the central nervous system (CNS).[79,93,94,95]

Endovascular approaches should not be considered if there are other suspected injuries, such a tracheobronchial disruption. Specific anatomical considerations must be mentioned. Common origin of the innominate and left common carotid arteries may be present in 11% or more of the general population, but has been documented to be as high as 29% in patients with blunt innominate artery rupture.[93,94] Innominate artery ruptures usually affect the origin of the artery, and occasionally the distal end, near its bifurcation (▶ Fig. 13.6).[81,84,94] Whether a stent graft can reliably exclude an origin rupture is not clear, and distal injuries may require stenting into the right common carotid artery, creating difficulties in getting the correct graft size as well as excluding the right subclavian artery. Stenting the subclavian artery between the first rib and the clavicle should almost never be done; inevitably the graft will collapse and occlude (▶ Fig. 13.7).

If the endovascular approach is the optimal method of treatment, access to either subclavian and/or innominate arteries can be obtained via brachial or femoral approaches. The left common carotid can be accessed by a transfemoral or carotid cut-down approach. If concerns of thrombus could lead to cerebral embolization, distal emboli protection devices are required.

Rarely, an occlusion balloon can be advanced proximal to a site of injury and left in place to provide proximal control. Great caution is needed because of the risk of distal extensive thrombosis, dissection, and/or stroke.[96] Finally, endovascular approaches can be useful in managing electively traumatic arteriovenous fistulas.

The outcomes are not yet documented. At this time, endovascular repairs should be attempted in patients who cannot

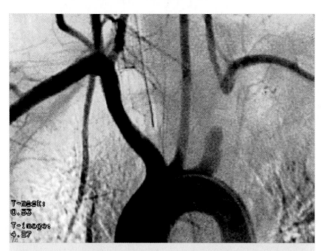

Fig. 13.7 Traumatic left subclavian artery injury. Management by endovascular approach would result in occlusion of the left vertebral artery. At surgery, the artery was found completely disrupted and separated for a distance of several centimeters, but not thrombosed.

tolerate surgical repair and who have suitable anatomy via a team effort by all members of the trauma care team.

13.2.3 Intercostal and Internal Mammary Artery Injury

Hemorrhage secondary to multiple rib fractures following blunt trauma can be controlled using IR approaches.[97] In patients with massive chest wall disruption, often with accompanying diffuse parenchymal injury, "unroofing" the bleed may lead to more massive blood loss and the attendant complications. Embolizing the intercostal artery requires that both ends of the injury be occluded. Each artery injured is identified, and the sites either traversed or controlled via the internal mammary artery, as well as the origin of the intercostal arteries from the aorta.

Our approach is to perform thoracotomy and control the vessels with sutures, clips, etc., and reserve IR approaches for recalcitrant bleeding. Our goal is reducing delay, as well as hopefully reducing the number of arteries that need to be controlled, and in addition, using clips placed at the time of thoracotomy as markers to indicate candidate vessels.[79]

Blunt trauma to the internal mammary arteries is uncommon.[98] Injuries may present as an occlusion, contained hematoma with D-shape collection with the base against the sternum, pseudoaneurysms, or hemothorax.[59,99] Penetrating injuries are more common, but easy to diagnose given that they present with active external and/or intrapleural, hemorrhage. In most cases, bleeding or associated injuries will stimulate operation and subsequent diagnosis, but sometimes the injury is detected at CT or DSA.[98] When localized, these injuries are relatively easy to ligate. However, embolization has been performed in both the acute and chronic situation.[100,101] Whigham et al described 18 patients with blunt and penetrating trauma. Twelve were embolized. One patient had a late rebleed. Two had operations. Four were observed, two of whom developed delayed hemothorax.[100] Embolization requires control from both sides (▶ Fig. 13.8). Thus, the injury site must be traversed or accessed both from the subclavian and the epigastric artery sides. Ideally using microcatheter technology, this can be accomplished with surgery.

For IR management, the origins of the vessels are catheterized with a guiding catheter and a microcatheter advanced through it for embolization with coils or microcoils. When embolizing intercostal arteries, it is critical that the catheter is advanced distal to any spinal arteries to reduce the risk of cord injury. In most cases, in our opinion, these IR techniques should be limited to stable patients or those who have failed operative control.

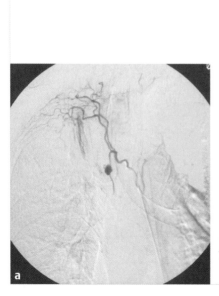
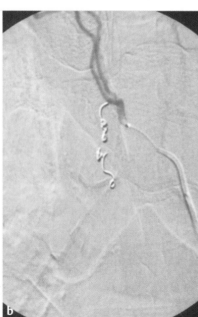

Fig. 13.8 (a) A patient with hemoptysis presenting several days after blunt injury to the chest and pulmonary contusion. Angiography documented a bronchial artery aneurysm, which probably predated the injury. (b) The aneurysm was managed by accessing the origin of the bronchial artery from the arch, and crossing the lesion which allowed embolization with coils, both proximal and distal to the lesion. This is the so-called sandwich technique.

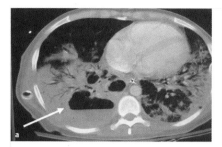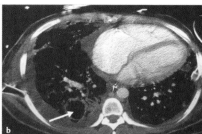

Fig. 13.9 (a) The patient sustained severe blunt trauma and developed necrotizing pneumonia with empyema and a large lung abscess (arrow). Because of her unstable hemodynamic condition and ongoing sepsis requiring vasopressors, as well as significant ventilator requirements, she was managed by computed tomography-guided drainage of empyema with a pigtail catheter and then rigid pleuroscopy. (b) Sepsis rapidly resolved and over the ensuing 2 weeks, the abscess decreased in size, and she was eventually managed with thoracotomy and debridement. She was discharged after a prolonged hospitalization.

13.2.4 Retained Hemothorax and Empyema

Residual hemothorax after chest tube drainage occurs in ~ 5% of cases, but can be as high as 18%.[102,103] Fibrothorax is mentioned as a complication of hemothorax, but rarely occurs without superimposed infection.[27] The primary complication of a retained hemothorax is a secondary empyema. Empyema can be a complication of pneumonia, secondary seeding from other sources of contamination, but in the majority it is attributed to direct seeding of the pleural space at the time of chest tube placement.[104,105] In the trauma patients, the blood acts as a significant source of bacterial nutrition, as well as promoting early and aggressive development of loculations.[2]

The primary management of both hemothorax and empyema is surgical, often using video-assisted thoracoscopy or mini-thoracotomy approaches.[27,106] However, not all patients with hemothorax or pleural effusion following injury need to be treated with a chest tube or operation. Patients who have suffered blunt trauma, who have good pain control, can cough, and ambulate often require no intervention, especially for very small effusions that are presumed to be hemothorax. However, once a tube has been placed, if the hemothorax is still visible, at least on chest radiograph, the risk of infection is significantly higher, and the hemothorax should be aggressively managed, ideally with early thoracoscopy.[107]

Ultrasound and CT can be used for evaluation.[108–112] These may be used to place directed chest tubes, but in the main the tubes are relatively small (up to 24 F) and may not be effective in draining clotted hemothorax or a loculated empyema. Meyer and associates found that thoracoscopy was more effective and resulted in significant cost savings when compared with placing a second chest drainage system in retained hemothorax.[113] Similarly, Wait et al found that compared with thorascopic drainage, the use of lytics to treat posttraumatic empyema was associated with increased cost, length of stay, and had a higher treatment failure rate.[113]

Although the primary therapy for retained hemothorax and/ or empyema is surgical, there is a role for IR management.[114] In our experience, this has been either after a video-assisted thoracoscopic surgery (VATS; in which there is a question of residual pleural infection) or in extremely high-risk patients (although even ventilated patients can be managed with pleuroscopy in many instances).[7] Some patients have deep pockets of residual fluid that would mandate thoracotomy. In most instances, CT-guided drainage is safer, sometimes the patient must be prone for the catheter to reach posterior collections, and in others the scapula or other structures may complete access. Computed tomography, using a marking grid and depth analysis, is relatively safe. Collections that are between the parenchyma and chest wall and accessible can also be drained using US. In general, as large a tube as possible is inserted. Pigtail catheters go up to 16 F in size, but larger tubes can be advanced over a stiff wire as well. Once drains are placed, it is critical to keep drains flushed, connecting a 3-way stopcock and flushing every shift with 5 to 10 cc suffices. Determining when the drain can be removed depends upon the clinical response and repeat CT scanning.

13.2.5 Lung Abscess

Lung abscess can arise originate from a direct complication of penetrating injury, or evolve from pneumatocele, aspiration, ventilator associated pneumonia, postresection, and/or multiple other etiologies.[79] Although the standard therapy includes bronchoscopy, pulmonary toilet, and/or surgical resection, percutaneous drainage can be performed in patients with large, uniloculated collections who are not responding to medical therapy. These can be performed even on patients who are ventilated, and the risk of significant bronchopleural fistula is small. Any attendant empyema can be managed by simple tube thoracostomy or pleuroscopy (▶ Fig. 13.9).[115]

13.2.6 Chylothorax

Primary traumatic chylothorax is uncommon, and the majority of recommendations regarding percutaneous intervention must be adapted from the nontrauma surgical or medical literature. When related to trauma, chylothorax can occur following penetrating injuries to the thoracic inlet, transmediastinal injuries, or blunt trauma.

Of interest, chylothorax is associated with spine fractures in only 20% of patients.[116] Chylothorax can manifest in a delayed fashion with recurrent effusions, as persistent milky pleural output, or rarely as a tension chylothorax.[27] Chylothorax is more commonly seen as a complication following repair of aortic injury or esophageal resection. The diagnosis can be established by documenting triglyceride levels > 110 mg/dL and/or predominant lymphocytes in the effusion. If noted acutely, we must consider the possibility of injuries to adjacent structures, especially the esophagus or aorta. The primary complication is nutritional and immunological compromise.[117] Initial management includes drainage, assuring complete lung expansion (with increased positive end-expiratory pressure in ventilated patients), and parenteral nutritional support. Although low-fat diets reduce the flow of chyle, even oral water has been noted to increase chyle flow. The length of medical therapy trial is not clear, but generally 4 weeks is the maximum duration, depending on the physiological reserves of the patient.[27] A chylothorax noted immediately after operation may be best treated by reoperation and maneuvers described below.

An operation can be performed by thoracoscopy or thoracotomy. The site may be directly visualized, in which case direct ligation with pledgeted sutures and/or glue application may be performed. Localization can be improved by feeding the patient dairy cream prior to operation. "Mass" ligation at the level of the diaphragm on the right can resolve both right and left leaks. Caution: the duct and surrounding tissue can be very friable; thus ligation can lead to a new site of leaks. In addition, collaterals that bypass the site of ligation may exist. We have found that a critical component is to ensure complete decortication (to allow lung expansion), pleural abrasion or decortication, and if in doubt, to continue ventilation for 24 hours to assist full lung expansion.[118] A strict nothing-by-mouth (NPO) status for 7 days is a must.[27] If no leak is documented, and collaterals are noted to drain into the venous system, medical management has a higher success rate.[117] With parenteral nutrition and strict NPO, an almost immediate cessation of chyle flow is a good prognostic sign that supports medical management. Octreotide has been used as an adjunct.[119,120]

If the duct can be identified, then transabdominal embolization with coils or microcoils has been successful. A persistent space (especially after pneumonectomy), widespread disruption (after esophagectomy for example), or persistent high output with medical therapy, is associated with high failure rates so an earlier intervention is warranted.

Ultimately, an operation should be considered if the leak persists after 2 weeks, and certainly by four weeks, if the patient is deteriorating immunologically or nutrionally, and clearly if there is another indication for operation. Patients who present in a delayed fashion are managed similarly. We believe that, if after one week of optimal medical therapy the patient continues to drain more than 1500 mL/24 h and/or is clearly closing ground nutritionally, in most cases we would try thoracic duct or cystema chyle embolization and if this is not possible or is unsuccessful, then perform open ligation.

Interventional radiologic approaches are image-directed catheter placement to help "seal the space," lymphangiogram, and, rarely percutaneous occlusion.[121] Lymphangiography (either by CT, nuclear studies, or lymphangiogram) may be helpful in determining the sites of leak, presence of collaterals, and volume of the leak, all of which may predict success or failure of medical therapy.[121] If the retroperitoneal lymphatic ducts can be visualized and transabdominal catheterization is possible, the duct can be occluded by either embolization or glue or onyx injections. About two-thirds or more patients can be successfully treated.[121, 122,123,124,125,126,127,128] Furthermore, IR approaches should be reserved for patients who fail surgical management, or who are deemed too high a risk for operation.

13.2.7 Pericardial Effusion

Pericardial tamponade commonly presents as an acute surgical event that requires immediate operative management. Sometimes, the effusion may develop subacutely or be a consequence of pericarditits either from a missed small penetrating injury, following surgery, or as a blunt cardiac injury.[54,129,130,131] Pericardial drainage under US can be an effective temporizing or therapeutic procedure depending upon the circumstances.[132,133] Acutely realizing that surgery will be required, patients with pericardial tamponade are at risk of cardiac decompensation during intubation. Therefore, placing a pericardial drain can permit safer induction of anesthesia, as long as it is understood that surgery is still needed. A simple approach is a subxiphoid or anterior approach using a central catheter kit. In more chronic situations, using a pigtail catheter is optimal for drainage.

13.2.8 Conclusion

Interventional radiologic techniques are gaining increasing support and experience as methods for the management of traumatic aortic rupture. Further follow-up data and new graft devices are required before it can be clearly determined or accepted as the first line of treatment in all patients. In other setting conditions, IR techniques are useful in specific situations after determination by the members of the trauma team.

References

[1] Williams PD, Mahadevan VS, Clarke B. Traumatic aortic dissection and coronary fistula treated with transcatheter management. Catheter Cardiovasc Interv 2007; 70: 1013–1017

[2] Fabian TC, Richardson JD, Croce MA et al. Prospective study of blunt aortic injury: Multicenter Trial of the American Association for the Surgery of Trauma. J Trauma 1997; 42: 374–380, discussion 380–383

[3] Mattox KL, Wall MJ. Historical review of blunt injury to the thoracic aorta. Chest Surg Clin N Am 2000; 10: 167–182, x

[4] Cook J, Salerno C, Krishnadasan B, Nicholls S, Meissner M, Karmy-Jones R. The effect of changing presentation and management on the outcome of blunt rupture of the thoracic aorta. J Thorac Cardiovasc Surg 2006; 131: 594–600

[5] Arajärvi E, Santavirta S. Chest injuries sustained in severe traffic accidents by seatbelt wearers. J Trauma 1989; 29: 37–41

[6] Siegel JH, Smith JA, Siddiqi SQ. Change in velocity and energy dissipation on impact in motor vehicle crashes as a function of the direction of crash: key factors in the production of thoracic aortic injuries, their pattern of associated injuries and patient survival. A Crash Injury Research Engineering Network (CIREN) study. J Trauma 2004; 57: 760–777, discussion 777–778

[7] Holmes JH, Bloch RD, Hall RA, Carter YM, Karmy-Jones RC. Natural history of traumatic rupture of the thoracic aorta managed nonoperatively: a longitudinal analysis. Ann Thorac Surg 2002; 73: 1149–1154

[8] Pate JW, Gavant ML, Weiman DS, Fabian TC. Traumatic rupture of the aortic isthmus: program of selective management. World J Surg 1999; 23: 59–63

[9] Miller PR, Kortesis BG, McLaughlin CA et al. Complex blunt aortic injury or repair: beneficial effects of cardiopulmonary bypass use. Ann Surg 2003; 237: 877–883, discussion 883–884

[10] Karmy-Jones R, Carter YM, Nathens A et al. Impact of presenting physiology and associated injuries on outcome following traumatic rupture of the thoracic aorta. Am Surg 2001; 67: 61–66

[11] Forbes AD, Ashbaugh DG. Mechanical circulatory support during repair of thoracic aortic injuries improves morbidity and prevents spinal cord injury. Arch Surg 1994; 129: 494–497, discussion 497–498

[12] Fujikawa T, Yukioka T, Ishimaru S et al. Endovascular stent grafting for the treatment of blunt thoracic aortic injury. J Trauma 2001; 50: 223–229

[13] Lawlor DK, Ott M, Forbes TL, Kribs S, Harris KA, DeRose G. Endovascular management of traumatic thoracic aortic injuries. Can J Surg 2005; 48: 293–297

[14] Lebl DR, Dicker RA, Spain DA, Brundage SI. Dramatic shift in the primary management of traumatic thoracic aortic rupture. Arch Surg 2006; 141: 177–180

[15] Kühne CA, Ruchholtz S, Voggenreiter G et al. AG Polytrauma DGU. [Traumatic aortic injuries in severely injured patients] Unfallchirurg 2005; 108: 279–287

[16] Uzieblo M, Sanchez LA, Rubin BG et al. Endovascular repair of traumatic descending thoracic aortic disruptions: should endovascular therapy become the gold standard? Vasc Endovascular Surg 2004; 38: 331–337

[17] Sayed S, Thompson MM. Endovascular repair of the descending thoracic aorta: evidence for the change in clinical practice. Vascular 2005; 13: 148–157

[18] Demetriades D, Velmahos GC, Scalea TM et al. American Association for the Surgery of Trauma Thoracic Aortic Injury Study Group. Operative repair or endovascular stent graft in blunt traumatic thoracic aortic injuries: results of an American Association for the Surgery of Trauma Multicenter Study. J Trauma 2008; 64: 561–570, discussion 570–571

[19] Wellons ED, Milner R, Solis M, Levitt A, Rosenthal D. Stent-graft repair of traumatic thoracic aortic disruptions. J Vasc Surg 2004; 40: 1095–1100

[20] Andrassy J, Weidenhagen R, Meimarakis G, Lauterjung L, Jauch KW, Kopp R. Stent versus open surgery for acute and chronic traumatic injury of the thoracic aorta: a single-center experience. J Trauma 2006; 60: 765–771, discussion 771–772

[21] Thompson CS, Rodriguez JA, Ramaiah VG et al. Acute traumatic rupture of the thoracic aorta treated with endoluminal stent grafts. J Trauma 2002; 52: 1173–1177

[22] Orford VP, Atkinson NR, Thomson K et al. Blunt traumatic aortic transection: the endovascular experience. Ann Thorac Surg 2003; 75: 106–111, discussion 111–112

[23] Neuhauser B, Czermak B, Jaschke W, Waldenberger P, Fraedrich G, Perkmann R. Stent-graft repair for acute traumatic thoracic aortic rupture. Am Surg 2004; 70: 1039–1044

[24] Rousseau H, Dambrin C, Marcheix B et al. Acute traumatic aortic rupture: a comparison of surgical and stent-graft repair. J Thorac Cardiovasc Surg 2005; 129: 1050–1055

[25] Peterson BG, Matsumura JS, Morasch MD, West MA, Eskandari MK. Percutaneous endovascular repair of blunt thoracic aortic transection. J Trauma 2005; 59: 1062–1065

[26] Marty-Ané CH, Berthet JP, Branchereau P, Mary H, Alric P. Endovascular repair for acute traumatic rupture of the thoracic aorta. Ann Thorac Surg 2003; 75: 1803–1807

[27] Dunham MB, Zygun D, Petrasek P, Kortbeek JB, Karmy-Jones R, Moore RD. Endovascular stent grafts for acute blunt aortic injury. J Trauma 2004; 56: 1173–1178

[28] Tehrani HY, Peterson BG, Katariya K et al. Endovascular repair of thoracic aortic tears. Ann Thorac Surg 2006; 82: 873–877, discussion 877–878

[29] Lin PH, Huynh TT, Coselli JS, Mattox KL. Endovascular repair of traumatic thoracic aortic injuries. Endovascular Today 2007; 6: 56–66

[30] Hoffer E, Forauer AR, Silas AM, Gemery JM. Endovascular stent-graft or open surgical repair for blunt thoracic aortic trauma: systematic review. J Vasc Interv Radiol 2008 Aug; 19: 1153–1164

[31] Kasirajan K, Heffernan D, Langsfeld M. Acute thoracic aortic trauma: a comparison of endoluminal stent grafts with open repair and nonoperative management. Ann Vasc Surg 2003; 17: 589–595

[32] Amabile P, Collart F, Gariboldi V, Rollet G, Bartoli JM, Piquet P. Surgical versus endovascular treatment of traumatic thoracic aortic rupture. J Vasc Surg 2004; 40: 873–879

[33] Akowuah E, Baumbach A, Wilde P, Angelini G, Bryan AJ. Emergency repair of traumatic aortic rupture: endovascular versus conventional open repair. J Thorac Cardiovasc Surg 2007; 134: 897–901

[34] Buz S, Zipfel B, Mulahasanovic S, Pasic M, Weng Y, Hetzer R. Conventional surgical repair and endovascular treatment of acute traumatic aortic rupture. Eur J Cardiothorac Surg 2008; 33: 143–149

[35] Kokotsakis J, Kaskarelis I, Misthos P et al. Endovascular versus open repair for blunt thoracic aortic injury: short-term results. Ann Thorac Surg 2007; 84: 1965–1970

[36] Tang GL, Tehrani HY, Usman A et al. Reduced mortality, paraplegia, and stroke with stent graft repair of blunt aortic transections: A modern meta-analysis. J Vasc Surg 2007

[37] von Oppell UO, Dunne TT, De Groot MK, Zilla P. Traumatic aortic rupture: twenty-year metaanalysis of mortality and risk of paraplegia. Ann Thorac Surg 1994; 58: 585–593

[38] Starnes BW, Arthurs ZM. Endovascular management of vascular trauma. Perspect Vasc Surg Endovasc Ther 2006; 18: 114–129

[39] Pedro Bonamigo T, Luis Lucas M, Carlos Felicetti J, da Cunha Sales M. [Traumatic rupture of the thoracic aorta: long-term results] Rev Port Cir Cardiotorac Vasc 2007; 14: 25–31

[40] Svensson LG, Kouchoukos NT, Miller DC et al. Society of Thoracic Surgeons Endovascular Surgery Task Force. Expert consensus document on the treatment of descending thoracic aortic disease using endovascular stent-grafts. Ann Thorac Surg 2008; 85 Suppl: S1–S41

[41] Fabian TC, Davis KA, Gavant ML et al. Prospective study of blunt aortic injury: helical CT is diagnostic and antihypertensive therapy reduces rupture. Ann Surg 1998; 227: 666–676, discussion 676–677

[42] Feliciano DV. Trauma to the aorta and major vessels. Chest Surg Clin N Am 1997; 7: 305–323

[43] Maggisano R, Nathens A, Alexandrova NA et al. Traumatic rupture of the thoracic aorta: should one always operate immediately? Ann Vasc Surg 1995; 9: 44–52

[44] Pacini D, Angeli E, Fattori R et al. Traumatic rupture of the thoracic aorta: ten years of delayed management. J Thorac Cardiovasc Surg 2005; 129: 880–884

[45] Richeux L, Dambrin C, Marcheix B et al. [Towards a new management of acute traumatic aortic ruptures] J Radiol 2004; 85: 101–106

[46] Mattison R, Hamilton IN, Ciraulo DL, Richart CM. Stent-graft repair of acute traumatic thoracic aortic transection with intentional occlusion of the left subclavian artery: case report. J Trauma 2001; 51: 326–328

[47] Myburgh JA. Driving cerebral perfusion pressure with pressors: how, which, when? Crit Care Resusc 2005; 7: 200–205

[48] Pace MC, Cicciarella G, Barbato E et al. Severe traumatic brain injury: management and prognosis. Minerva Anestesiol 2006; 72: 235–242

[49] Kinoshita K, Sakurai A, Utagawa A et al. Importance of cerebral perfusion pressure management using cerebrospinal drainage in severe traumatic brain injury. Acta Neurochir Suppl (Wien) 2006; 96: 37–39

[50] Czosnyka M, Hutchinson PJ, Balestreri M, Hiler M, Smielewski P, Pickard JD. Monitoring and interpretation of intracranial pressure after head injury. Acta Neurochir Suppl (Wien) 2006; 96: 114–118

[51] Kepros J, Angood P, Jaffe CC, Rabinovici R. Aortic intimal injuries from blunt trauma: resolution profile in nonoperative management. J Trauma 2002; 52: 475–478

[52] Fisher RG, Oria RA, Mattox KL, Whigham CJ, Pickard LR. Conservative management of aortic lacerations due to blunt trauma. J Trauma 1990; 30: 1562–1566

[53] Malina M, Brunkwall J, Ivancev K et al. Late aortic arch perforation by graft-anchoring stent: complication of endovascular thoracic aneurysm exclusion. J Endovasc Surg 1998; 5: 274–277

[54] Borsa JJ, Hoffer EK, Karmy-Jones R et al. Angiographic description of blunt traumatic injuries to the thoracic aorta with specific relevance to endograft repair. J Endovasc Ther 2002; 9 Suppl 2: II84–II91

[55] Wheatley GH, Gurbuz AT, Rodriguez-Lopez JA et al. Midterm outcome in 158 consecutive Gore TAG thoracic endoprostheses: single center experience. Ann Thorac Surg 2006; 81: 1570–1577, discussion 1577

[56] Fattori R, Nienaber CA, Rousseau H et al. Talent Thoracic Retrospective Registry. Results of endovascular repair of the thoracic aorta with the Talent thoracic stent graft: the Talent Thoracic Retrospective Registry. J Thorac Cardiovasc Surg 2006; 132: 332–339

[57] Scheinert D, Krankenberg H, Schmidt A et al. Endoluminal stent-graft placement for acute rupture of the descending thoracic aorta. Eur Heart J 2004; 25: 694–700

[58] Hoffer EK, Karmy-Jones R, Bloch RD et al. Treatment of acute thoracic aortic injury with commercially available abdominal aortic stent-grafts. J Vasc Interv Radiol 2002; 13: 1037–1041

[59] Cheng SG, Glickerman DJ, Karmy-Jones R, Borsa JJ. Traumatic sternomanubrial dislocation with associated bilateral internal mammary artery occlusion. AJR Am J Roentgenol 2003; 180: 810

[60] Fattori R, Napoli G, Lovato L et al. Indications for, timing of, and results of catheter-based treatment of traumatic injury to the aorta. AJR Am J Roentgenol 2002; 179: 603–609

[61] Görich J, Asquan Y, Seifarth H et al. Initial experience with intentional stent-graft coverage of the subclavian artery during endovascular thoracic aortic repairs. J Endovasc Ther 2002; 9 Suppl 2: II39–II43

[62] Hoppe H, Hohenwalter EJ, Kaufman JA, Petersen B. Percutaneous treatment of aberrant right subclavian artery aneurysm with use of the Amplatzer septal occluder. J Vasc Interv Radiol 2006; 17: 889–894

[63] Peterson BG, Eskandari MK, Gleason TG, Morasch MD. Utility of left subclavian artery revascularization in association with endoluminal repair of acute and chronic thoracic aortic pathology. J Vasc Surg 2006; 43: 433–439

[64] Rehders TC, Petzsch M, Ince H et al. Intentional occlusion of the left subclavian artery during stent-graft implantation in the thoracic aorta: risk and relevance. J Endovasc Ther 2004; 11: 659–666

[65] Manninen H, Tulla H, Vanninen R, Ronkainen A. Endangered cerebral blood supply after closure of left subclavian artery: postmortem and clinical imaging studies. Ann Thorac Surg 2008; 85: 120–125

[66] Appoo JJ, Moser WG, Fairman RM et al. Thoracic aortic stent grafting: improving results with newer generation investigational devices. J Thorac Cardiovasc Surg 2006; 131: 1087–1094

[67] Reed AB, Thompson JK, Crafton CJ, Delvecchio C, Giglia JS. Timing of endovascular repair of blunt traumatic thoracic aortic transections. J Vasc Surg 2006; 43: 684–688

[68] Steingruber IE, Czermak BV, Chemelli A et al. Placement of endovascular stent-grafts for emergency repair of acute traumatic aortic rupture: a single-centre experience. Eur Radiol 2007; 17: 1727–1737

[69] Orend KH, Scharrer-Pamler R, Kapfer X, Liewald F, Görich J, Sunder-Plassmann L. [Endoluminal stent-assisted management of acute traumatic aortic rupture] Chirurg 2002; 73: 595–600

[70] Mertens R, Valdés F, Krämer A et al. [Endovascular treatment of descending thoracic aorta aneurysm] Rev Med Chil 2003; 131: 617–622

[71] Idu MM, Reekers JA, Balm R, Ponsen KJ, de Mol BA, Legemate DA. Collapse of a stent-graft following treatment of a traumatic thoracic aortic rupture. J Endovasc Ther 2005; 12: 503–507

[72] Mestres G, Maeso J, Fernandez V, Matas M. Symptomatic collapse of a thoracic aorta endoprosthesis. J Vasc Surg 2006; 43: 1270–1273

[73] Muhs BE, Balm R, White GH, Verhagen HJ. Anatomic factors associated with acute endograft collapse after Gore TAG treatment of thoracic aortic dissection or traumatic rupture. J Vasc Surg 2007; 45: 655–661

[74] Steinbauer MG, Stehr A, Pfister K et al. Endovascular repair of proximal endograft collapse after treatment for thoracic aortic disease. J Vasc Surg 2006; 43: 609–612

[75] Go MR, Barbato JE, Dillavou ED et al. Thoracic endovascular aortic repair for traumatic aortic transection. J Vasc Surg 2007; 46: 928–933

[76] Muhs BE, Vincken KL, van Prehn J et al. Dynamic cine-CT angiography for the evaluation of the thoracic aorta; insight in dynamic changes with implications for thoracic endograft treatment. Eur J Vasc Endovasc Surg 2006; 32: 532–536

[77] D'Ancona G, Bauset R, Normand JP, Turcotte R, Dagenais F. Endovascular stent-graft repair of a complicated penetrating ulcer of the descending thoracic aorta: a word of caution. J Endovasc Ther 2003; 10: 928–931

[78] Milas ZL, Milner R, Chaikoff E, Wulkan M, Ricketts R. Endograft stenting in the adolescent population for traumatic aortic injuries. J Pediatr Surg 2006; 41: e27–e30

[79] Karmy-Jones R, Jurkovich GJ. Blunt chest trauma. Curr Probl Surg 2004; 41: 211–380

[80] Dosios TJ, Salemis N, Angouras D, Nonas E. Blunt and penetrating trauma of the thoracic aorta and aortic arch branches: an autopsy study. J Trauma 2000; 49: 696–703

[81] Chen MY, Regan JD, D'Amore MJ, Routh WD, Meredith JW, Dyer RB. Role of angiography in the detection of aortic branch vessel injury after blunt thoracic trauma. J Trauma 2001; 51: 1166–1171, discussion 1172

[82] Weaver FA, Suda RW, Stiles GM, Yellin AE. Injuries to the ascending aorta, aortic arch and great vessels. Surg Gynecol Obstet 1989; 169: 27–31

[83] Demetriades D. Penetrating injuries to the thoracic great vessels. J Card Surg 1997; 12 Suppl: 173–179, discussion 179–180

[84] Karmy-Jones R, DuBose R, King S. Traumatic rupture of the innominate artery. Eur J Cardiothorac Surg 2003; 23: 782–787

[85] White R, Krajcer Z, Johnson M, Williams D, Bacharach M, O'Malley E. Results of a multicenter trial for the treatment of traumatic vascular injury with a covered stent. J Trauma 2006; 60: 1189–1195, discussion 1195–1196

[86] Berne JD, Reuland KR, Villarreal DH, McGovern TM, Rowe SA, Norwood SH. Internal carotid artery stenting for blunt carotid artery injuries with an associated pseudoaneurysm. J Trauma 2008; 64: 398–405

[87] Chandler TA, Fishwick G, Bell PR. Endovascular repair of a traumatic innominate artery aneurysm. Eur J Vasc Endovasc Surg 1999; 18: 80–82

[88] Joo JY, Ahn JY, Chung YS et al. Therapeutic endovascular treatments for traumatic carotid artery injuries. J Trauma 2005; 58: 1159–1166

[89] Mertens R, Valdés F, Kramer A, Mariné L, Vergara J, Valdebenito M. [Traumatic pseudoaneurysms of aortic arch branches: endovascular treatment. Report of 3 cases] Rev Med Chil 2002; 130: 1027–1032

[90] McArthur CS, Marin ML. Endovascular therapy for the treatment of arterial trauma. Mt Sinai J Med 2004; 71: 4–11

[91] Patel AV, Marin ML, Veith FJ, Kerr A, Sanchez LA. Endovascular graft repair of penetrating subclavian artery injuries. J Endovasc Surg 1996; 3: 382–388

[92] Marin ML, Veith FJ, Panetta TF et al. Transluminally placed endovascular stented graft repair for arterial trauma. J Vasc Surg 1994; 20: 466–472, discussion 472–473

[93] Johnston RH Jr Wall MJ Jr Mattox KL. Innominate artery trauma: a thirty-year experience. J Vasc Surg 1993; 17: 134–139, discussion 139–140

[94] Graham JM, Feliciano DV, Mattox KL, Beall AC. Innominate vascular injury. J Trauma 1982; 22: 647–655

[95] Weiman DS, McCoy DW, Haan CK, Pate JW, Fabian TC. Blunt injuries of the brachiocephalic artery. Am Surg 1998; 64: 383–387

[96] Desai M, Baxter AB, Karmy-Jones R, Borsa JJ. Potentially life-saving role for temporary endovascular balloon occlusion in atypical mediastinal hematoma. AJR Am J Roentgenol 2002; 178: 1180

[97] Carrillo EH, Heniford BT, Senler SO, Dykes JR, Maniscalco SP, Richardson JD. Embolization therapy as an alternative to thoracotomy in vascular injuries of the chest wall. Am Surg 1998; 64: 1142–1148

[98] Madoff DC, Brathwaite CE, Manzione JV et al. Coexistent rupture of the proximal right subclavian and internal mammary arteries after blunt chest trauma. J Trauma 2000; 48: 521–524

[99] Mohlala ML, Vanker EA, Ballaram RS. Internal mammary artery haematoma. S Afr J Surg 1989; 27: 136–138

[100] Whigham CJ, Fisher RG, Goodman CJ, Dodds CA, Trinh CC. Traumatic injury of the internal mammary artery: embolization versus surgical and nonoperative management. Emerg Radiol 2002; 9: 201–207

[101] Kawamura S, Nishimaki H, Takigawa M et al. Internal mammary artery injury after blunt chest trauma treated with transcatheter arterial embolization. J Trauma 2006; 61: 1536–1539

[102] Luchette FA, Barrie PS, Oswanski MF et al. Eastern Association for Trauma. Practice management guidelines for prophylactic antibiotic use in tube thoracostomy for traumatic hemopneumothorax: the EAST Practice Management Guidelines Work Group. J Trauma 2000; 48: 753–757

[103] Maxwell RA, Campbell DJ, Fabian TC et al. Use of presumptive antibiotics following tube thoracostomy for traumatic hemopneumothorax in the prevention of empyema and pneumonia—a multi-center trial. J Trauma 2004; 57: 742–748, discussion 748–749

[104] Aguilar MM, Battistella FD, Owings JT, Su T. Posttraumatic empyema. Risk factor analysis. Arch Surg 1997; 132: 647–650, discussion 650–651

[105] Richardson JD, Carrillo E. Thoracic infection after trauma. Chest Surg Clin N Am 1997; 7: 401–427

[106] Coselli JS, Mattox KL, Beall AC. Reevaluation of early evacuation of clotted hemothorax. Am J Surg 1984; 148: 786–790

[107] Eddy AC, Misbach GA, Luna GK. Traumatic rupture of the thoracic aorta in the pediatric patient. Pediatr Emerg Care 1989; 5: 228–230

[108] Abboud PA, Kendall J. Emergency department ultrasound for hemothorax after blunt traumatic injury. J Emerg Med 2003; 25: 181–184

[109] Brooks A, Davies B, Smethhurst M, Connolly J. Emergency ultrasound in the acute assessment of haemothorax. Emerg Med J 2004; 21: 44–46

[110] Bruckner BA, DiBardino DJ, Cumbie TC et al. Critical evaluation of chest computed tomography scans for blunt descending thoracic aortic injury. Ann Thorac Surg 2006; 81: 1339–1346

[111] Sisley AC, Rozycki GS, Ballard RB, Namias N, Salomone JP, Feliciano DV. Rapid detection of traumatic effusion using surgeon-performed ultrasonography. J Trauma 1998; 44: 291–296, discussion 296–297

[112] Velmahos GC, Demetriades D, Chan L et al. Predicting the need for thoracoscopic evacuation of residual traumatic hemothorax: chest radiograph is insufficient. J Trauma 1999; 46: 65–70

[113] Meyer DM, Jessen ME, Wait MA, Estrera AS. Early evacuation of traumatic retained hemothoraces using thoracoscopy: a prospective, randomized trial. Ann Thorac Surg 1997; 64: 1396–1400, discussion 1400–1401

[114] Mandal AK, Thadepalli H, Mandal AK, Chettipalli U. Posttraumatic empyema thoracis: a 24-year experience at a major trauma center. J Trauma 1997; 43: 764–771

[115] Karmy-Jones R, Vallieres E, Harrington R. Surgical management of necrotizing pneumonia. Clin Pulm Med 2003; 10: 17–25

[116] Ikonomidis JS, Boulanger BR, Brenneman FD. Chylothorax after blunt chest trauma: a report of 2 cases. Can J Surg 1997; 40: 135–138

[117] Vallières E, Karmy-Jones R, Wood DE. Early complications. Chylothorax. Chest Surg Clin N Am 1999; 9: 609–616, ixix

[118] Ragosta KG, Alfieris G. Chylothorax: a novel therapy. Crit Care Med 2000; 28: 1208–1209

[119] Kalomenidis I. Octreotide and chylothorax. Curr Opin Pulm Med 2006; 12: 264–267

[120] Rosti L, Bini RM, Chessa M, Butera G, Drago M, Carminati M. The effectiveness of octreotide in the treatment of post-operative chylothorax. Eur J Pediatr 2002; 161: 149–150

[121] Boffa DJ, Sands MJ, Rice TW et al. A critical evaluation of a percutaneous diagnostic and treatment strategy for chylothorax after thoracic surgery. Eur J Cardiothorac Surg 2008; 33: 435–439

[122] Eicken A, Genz T, Wild F, Balling G, Schreiber C, Hess J. Resolution of persistent late postoperative chylothorax after coil occlusion of aortopulmonary collaterals. Int J Cardiol 2007; 115: e80–e82

[123] Patel N, Lewandowski RJ, Bove M, Nemcek AA, Salem R. Thoracic duct embolization: a new treatment for massive leak after neck dissection. Laryngoscope 2008; 118: 680–683

[124] Cope C. Management of chylothorax via percutaneous embolization. Curr Opin Pulm Med 2004; 10: 311–314

[125] Cope C, Salem R, Kaiser LR. Management of chylothorax by percutaneous catheterization and embolization of the thoracic duct: prospective trial. J Vasc Interv Radiol 1999; 10: 1248–1254

[126] Hoffer EK, Bloch RD, Mulligan MS, Borsa JJ, Fontaine AB. Treatment of chylothorax: percutaneous catheterization and embolization of the thoracic duct. AJR Am J Roentgenol 2001; 176: 1040–1042

[127] Schild H, Hirner A. Percutaneous translymphatic thoracic duct embolization for treatment of chylothorax. Rofo 2001; 173: 580–582

[128] Cope C, Kaiser LR. Management of unremitting chylothorax by percutaneous embolization and blockage of retroperitoneal lymphatic vessels in 42 patients. J Vasc Interv Radiol 2002; 13: 1139–1148

[129] DuBose RA, Karmy-Jones R. Delayed diagnosis and management of an "occult" stab wound to the heart. Am Surg 2005; 71: 879–881

[130] Bellanger D, Nikas DJ, Freeman JE, Izenberg S. Delayed posttraumatic tamponade. South Med J 1996; 89: 1197–1199

[131] Tabatznik B, Isaacs JP. Postpericardiotomy syndrome following traumatic hemopericardium. Am J Cardiol 1961; 7: 83–96

[132] Seferović PM, Ristić AD, Imazio M et al. Management strategies in pericardial emergencies. Herz 2006; 31: 891–900

[133] Graham CA, Latif Z, Muriithi EW, Belcher PR, Ireland AJ. Acute traumatic cardiac tamponade treated solely by percutaneous pericardial drainage. Injury 1998; 29: 473–474

14 Interventional Radiology in Abdominal Trauma: Surgery versus Interventional Radiology

Thomas M. Scalea and John Henry Adamski II

The evolution of interventional radiographic (IR) techniques has added to the surgeon's diagnostic and therapeutic armamentarium. For instance, plain film radiography was once used to identify a widened mediastinum or intra-abdominal free air. This has essentially been replaced by computed tomography (CT). Further advances in CT technology now allows for both characterization of solid organ injuries, as well as identification of intraparenchymal vascular injuries.

Most recently, identification of injuries to specific blood vessels is possible. This increase in diagnostic sophistication and advances in technology has created a situation where radiologic intervention can treat some of these injuries forging a true partnership between the IR and trauma surgeons. Thus, the question of nonoperative versus surgical management has become now more correctly a discussion of deciding between simple observations versus catheter-based IR or surgical therapy or combination.

Prior to 1960, laparotomy was needed for the diagnosis and management of all abdominal injuries, particularly penetrating injuries to the torso. As a direct extension of wartime policies, it was assumed that penetrating trauma was associated with a high incidence of visceral injuries that carried a high morbidity, and mortality if surgical intervention was delayed.[1,2,3] Moreover, it was accepted that surgery did not add to the hospital length of stay or to the incidence of complications.[4] Thus, it seemed rational for trauma and other surgeons to perform surgical exploration as a diagnostic test in blunt trauma because intra-abdominal injuries were difficult to assess without a direct observation of the organs or tissues.[5]

Because all therapy was surgical, the only important issue was to determine the presence of injury. Injury mechanism, clinical exam, and hemodynamic instability were used to determine the need for an operation. Hemodynamic instability and/or a transient response to fluid resuscitation were considered as evidence of an ongoing hemorrhage prompting exploration.[6,7]

In 1960, Shaftan advocated a selective management of patients with abdominal trauma to limit the number of unnecessary surgeries and its complications.[8] This approach involved using ancillary tests, and particularly good surgical judgment to treat patients following blunt trauma. In the 1970s, the paradigm shifted from operative management led by pediatric surgeons who adopted a practice of nonoperative management for spleen and liver injuries.[9,10] Initially, the methods and diagnostic tests that were used to determine suitability for nonoperative management included serial physical exams and radionuclide scans.

The first commercially viable CT scanner was invented by Sir Godfrey Houndsfield in 1967 in the United Kingdom. Allan McLeod Cormack simultaneously invented a similar technology in the United States.[11] Clinicians were then able to characterize organ specific injuries. Subsequently, grading systems developed that classified injuries by severity. Computed tomography also allowed identification and quantification of hemoperitoneum. Injuries contained within the parenchyma and injuries to multiple organs could also be identified. This resulted in a more careful planning; therefore, a nonoperative management of blunt solid organ injuries evolved into the standard of care in adults, as well as in children.[12]

As time progressed, newer generations of CT scanners provided better resolution of the injury characteristics. Lastly, helical CT scanning now allows for the identification of intraparenchymal vascular injuries. Most recently, CT angiography (CTA) has allowed for further refinements of the vascular anatomy and even better and specific characterization of vascular injuries.

Transcatheter embolization in pelvic trauma was first described in 1972 by Margulies et al.[13] In 1985, Panetta et al published one of the first series demonstrating real success in controlling pelvic fracture bleeding with embolization.[14] Thus, we now had another tool to obtain hemostasis other than direct surgical exploration and ligation of the injured vessels, or removal of the injured organs; thereby avoiding an operation.

Thereafter, embolization techniques have continued to evolve. Embolization can be performed with different materials such as stainless steel coils or particulate Gelfoam (Pfizer, New York, NY). Either can be sized to occlude injured blood vessels at a desired location. Embolization can be performed more proximally, which is technically simpler, but cuts blood flow to a wider area of tissue. Conversely, more selective embolization is technically more challenging, but occludes only the injured blood vessel.[4]

Embolization can be performed as a primary hemostatic maneuver, such as when it is used for an isolated solid organ injury in a hemodynamically stable patient. It can also be combined as part of the resuscitation process to avoid a surgical exploration that may be difficult and even less likely to be successful, such as in pelvic fracture bleeding. Finally, it can be performed as adjunctive hemostasis combined with surgery, such as part of damage control for severe liver trauma.

The wise use of IR requires careful consideration of its advantages and disadvantages. Angiography is often somewhat time-consuming. Mobilization of the IR team can take up to hours, particularly on evenings and weekends when those resources may not be physically present in the hospital. Thus, surgical therapy is usually preferred in hemodynamically labile patients. We do not recommend angiography or IR in unstable patients.

It is always possible to directly visualize injured organs or blood vessels at laparotomy. Apparent injuries can be expeditiously repaired with standard surgical techniques. However, angiography gives a better assessment of injuries deep in the parenchyma of solid organs, such as liver and spleen. Thus, the discussion involves using the techniques most suitable for the particular set of injuries taken in consideration of the patient's hemodynamic status.

14.1 Spleen

The management of splenic injuries is continuously evolving. Up until the late 1960s, virtually all splenic injuries were treated with splenorrhaphy or splenectomy. Conventional knowledge dictated that the injured spleen could not repair by itself; therefore, all injuries required some form of surgical therapy. The decision for laparotomy was usually made by either physical examination or diagnostic peritoneal lavage; therefore, the diagnosis of splenic injury was more often made at exploratory laparotomy.

In 1968, Upadhyaya and Simpson demonstrated the safety and efficacy of nonoperative management of blunt splenic trauma in children.[10] Also, the rate of overwhelming postsplenectomy infection was found to be much more common in children than in adults, and carried a substantial morbidity and mortality.[15] Thus, splenic salvage became a high priority.

Thereafter, more data became available that demonstrated the successful nonoperative management of pediatric splenic injuries between 70% and 95% of times.[6–22] Moreover, numerous authors demonstrated that in children, splenic injuries managed nonoperatively required fewer blood transfusions, had shorter hospital lengths of stay, and decreased morbidity and mortality.[23,24] Pediatric and trauma surgeons began managing the vast majority of children with blunt splenic injury nonoperatively, including blood transfusions to avoid laparotomy and splenectomy.

On the other hand, nonoperative management in adults took longer to be established. Adult surgeons cited concerns such as differences in the splenic capsule in adults versus children, believing that nonoperative therapy would fail more often. In addition, there was no clear algorithm for observations of adults with splenic injuries.

In general, patients are kept nothing by mouth (NPO), at bed rest, and have serial hematocrits and physical exams to determine if the nonoperative management continued to be wise. Yet, these are very nonspecific and even today; practice varies greatly from institution to institution. For instance, it is unclear how long to observe a patient. It was also unclear how long patients should be kept in bed, recognizing that immobility put the patients at risk for deep vein thrombosis. It is also unclear how much a drop in hemaglobin (Hgb) could be due to other injuries or hemodilution, and how much drop in Hgb and hematocrit (Hct) should prompt laparotomy. Early on, concerns about the consequences of failed nonoperative therapy prompted some authors to restrict this to patients with relatively low-grade injuries and operate those with grade III, IV, and V injuries.[16,19,25,26] Smith et al also suggested nonoperative management only in patients under the age of 55 years.[27]

As nonoperative therapy became preferred for hemodynamically stable patients, data from both adult and pediatric literature demonstrated that CT grade injury alone did not indicate the need for operation.[28,29] More data emerged demonstrating that patients older than 55 could safely be treated nonoperatively.[30,31] The degree of hemoperitoneum or presence of contrast extravasation or active bleeding on CT scan, or the lack of hemodynamically responsive fluid administration seemed more relevant in predicting the failure of nonoperative management.[16,32–36] Peitzman et al published one of the largest series of nonoperative management of splenic injury in a multi-institutional study of the Eastern Association for the Surgery of Trauma.[35] They retrospectively reviewed 1,600 patients, including hemodynamic on presentation, grade of injury, and degree of hemoperitoneum, all factors independently predicted the

failure of nonoperative management. The overall failure in this study was 11.8%.

In 1995, Sclafani et al published the first series using embolization as treatment to extend nonoperative management techniques in blunt splenic trauma.[37] In this series, all patients with CT diagnosed splenic injuries underwent diagnostic arteriography. Patients without intraparenchymal vascular injuries were observed. Those with diagnosed vascular injuries underwent proximal embolization with coils. The thought was that the proximal embolization would drop the perfusion blood pressure of the spleen, allowing for spontaneous hemostasis. Splenic viability was preserved by collateral flow through the short gastric gastroepiploic and pancreatic branches. They reported 98.5% splenic salvage, which are still the best results to date in the literature. However, the study was done at Kings County Hospital, an inner-city hospital in the middle of Brooklyn, New York, and did not have a large percentage of high-grade splenic injuries.

Haan et al reported on the use of superselective embolization in a series in which angiography was used as a screening for all patients with blunt splenic injuries.[30] Only the injured vessels are embolized using a combination of microcoils and Gelfoam. The potential advantage is that perfusion to the rest of the spleen remains normal. In contrast, proximal embolization renders the entire spleen somewhat ischemic. This series had a larger percentage of high-grade injuries.[30] The splenic salvage rate dropped to 93%. In addition, ~ 10% of the patients required repeat embolization to achieve these results.

In 1998, Davis et al also demonstrated improved success in the nonoperative management in blunt splenic injuries with embolization.[38] However, angiography was performed only in patients with pseudoaneurysms demonstrated by helical CT scanning. In this study, CT scans were repeated in all patients with splenic injuries. Interestingly, 80% of the pseudoaneurysms were not identified on the initial CT scan, but were found 3 days later on repeat CT scans. This suggests that some injuries may be small or not erodent due to vasospasm at the time of presentation. Thereafter, the lesions are erodent several days later. Presumably, the pseudoaneurysm can also continue to enlarge and produce blood loss if untreated. This may explain the decreased success rate, given that some vascular injuries may have been missed.

Subsequent data from Haan et al demonstrated an increase in incidence of vascular injuries with increasing splenic grade.[30,31,39] These studies also demonstrated a significantly better outcome in grades II, III, and IV splenic injuries when embolization techniques were used. Similar salvage rates were demonstrated with a more restrictive protocol, while angiography was only used for high-grade injuries or those with evidence of vascular injuries on CT (pseudoaneurysm, arteriovenous fistula [AVF], or contrast-material extravasation).[31,40] Finally, superselective embolization may fail more often than proximal embolization, thus it has been abandoned by some.[31]

The mean time to failure of nonoperative management in these series was approximately 3 days. However, recent data from Savage et al have demonstrated that there is approximately a 1% incidence of late failure of nonoperative management of splenic injury, defined as failure after discharge.[41] In addition, there is approximately a 20% complication rate of proximal embolization. Although this is largely asymptomatic, relatively minor splenic infarction, the failure rate of embolization in grade IV injuries is still ~ 25%, so patients with higher-grade injuries that are embolized still require ongoing evaluation.[31,39] A few patients develop symptomatic splenic infarction and/or splenic abscess eventually requiring splenectomy.[30,39]

Moreover, some patients are not good candidates for nonoperative management, including embolization. Hemodynamically unstable patients are best served by exploration, splenorrhaphy, or splenectomy. It is important to remember that splenectomy is curative in virtually 100% of patients and overwhelming postsplenectomy infection is very rare in adults. Thus, all nonoperative management techniques must be compared against this gold standard. Hagiwara et al have extended the used of splenic artery embolization, with good results in hemodynamically unstable patients who transiently responded to an initial 2-L bolus of intravenous (IV) fluids.[42,43] In their institution, the patients can be in the angiography suite in 30 minutes, even at night or on weekends. This is not possible in most U.S. trauma centers. Also, nonoperative management should be undertaken with care in neurologically impaired patients given that the failure of nonoperative management may be difficult to assess. However, data demonstrate that embolization can be safe in those with neurologic injuries.[44,45]

It seems clear that stable patients with blunt splenic injuries can be managed nonoperatively. Embolization can extend the role of nonoperative management. Yet, in patients who are labile or in institutions where embolization is not readily available or where it requires prolonged time to mobilize a team (> 90 min), consideration should be given to laparotomy, particularly in high-grade injuries. At our institution, where embolization is the standard of care, splenic injuries are managed with primary laparotomy in approximately one-third of the cases.[30, 31,39,40] Obviously, no patient should be harmed by the physicians trying to salvage a spleen, particularly when an operation cures the problem.

14.2 Liver

With the success of the nonoperative management of splenic injuries in children, it was not surprising that pediatric surgeons pioneered similar management in liver trauma. Oldham et al successfully applied the nonoperative management in 92% of 53 children with blunt liver injuries.[46] Also surgeons attending adults documented spontaneous hemostasis in 60 to 80% of liver injuries at the time of laparotomy.[39,47,48]

Pachter et al demonstrated successful outcomes in low-grade liver injuries with moderate hemoperitoneum when managed nonoperatively.[6,7,49] In fact, 98% of patients who were admitted with the intent to treat nonoperatively were successfully observed.[7] Virtually, all low-grade injuries were observed. Approximately two-thirds of complications occurred in the 14% of patients with high-grade injuries. Others confirmed similar findings in grades III and IV injuries.[50,51,52] Across all injuries grades, the nonoperative management was successful 60 to 89% of the time.[50,53–57]

In contrast to splenic injuries, embolization for liver injuries only modestly improves overall nonoperative outcome.[58] This may be because observation alone is so successful. Embolization has proven valuable when active contrast-material extravasation or pseudoaneurysms are seen on admission CT scans of

hemodynamically stable patients and transient responders.[57,59, 60,61,62] Embolization may prevent progression of arterial injuries and delayed hemodynamic compromise when done early. Higher-grade injuries tend to be combined arterial and venous or extension of injuries into one or more major hepatic veins, and thus make laparotomy necessary more often.[34,58,63] Unlike splenic trauma, where high-grade injuries often have vascular injuries, even if they are not seen on initial CT, it is not clear that angiography in all patients with high-grade liver injuries is needed.

The indications for operation in liver injuries are similar to that for splenic trauma. However, the combined efforts of surgery and IR are becoming more common for the definitive treatment of high-grade injuries. Although splenectomy can cure a splenic injury, major hepatic resection is much more morbid and is a huge surgical challenge. A hemodynamically unstable patient may be best treated with emergent exploration and liver packing to control hemorrhage. Even severe arterial or venous injuries may not be identified or repaired at the initial surgery without complex liver resections, systemic bypass, and potential disruption of a retrocaval hematoma. Therefore, a temporary operative hemorrhage control with techniques such as packing can serve as a bridge to angiographic identification of associated vascular injuries and embolization for definitive hemostasis. Likewise, complications of liver injury management such as hemobilia, biloma, liver abscess, and delayed bleeding may be managed with IR techniques. The diagnoses are often made by CT scanning. Embolization can control pseudoaneurysms and promote hemostasis. Similarly, percutaneous drainage can control bile leaks as well as infection (abscess) or other collections.

Although embolization can be lifesaving after major hepatic injury, recent data from our institution have demonstrated that major hepatic necrosis is a common complication after embolization for high-grade liver injuries.[64] Hepatic viability is maintained because of its dual blood supply. However, injuries, especially when combined with packing, may occlude the central venous supply within the liver. Hepatic arterial occlusion by embolization can then produce hepatic ischemia and/or necrosis given that collateral arterial circulation does not exist as in the spleen. This confounding complication must be considered when dealing with IR control as a means of treating liver injuries.

14.3 Kidney

Unlike the spleen and liver, the kidneys are relatively well protected by their anatomical location in the retroperitoneum. The Gerota fascia also provides an envelope of tissue to tamponade bleeding when it occurs. Swiersie recognized these anatomical benefits and the potential application of nonoperative management 64 years ago.[65]

In the 1980s, it was found that CT scanning accurately identified vascular injuries, parenchymal lacerations, perirenal hematomas, and urine extravasations.[66,67,68] Numerous studies then recognized blunt renal trauma as commonly being relatively minor, but having associated intraperitoneal injuries 20 to 90% of the time.[66,69,70,71,72] In contrast, penetrating injuries to the anterior abdomen were recognized as a significant cause of high-grade renal injuries.[73,74,75,76]

Nonoperative management has evolved for the treatment of patients with blunt renal trauma. Although the initial studies dealt only with low-grade injuries, many groups have shown improved outcomes for the nonoperative management of even higher-grade injuries. A meta-analysis of 324 grade IV renal injuries showed successful management of 90% of patients with observation. Moreover, nephrectomy was limited to only 4.6% of those injured kidneys.[77,78] Likewise, Altman et al successfully treated 50% of 13 grade V injuries without surgery.[79] In the past, nephrectomy rates were higher in patients who were surgically explored instead of clinically observed (35% vs. 12.6%).[80] Most recently, Moudouni's group showed a sixfold decrease in nephrectomy with implementation of a protocol using nonoperative management for kidney injuries.[47,48]

Similar to nonoperative management of spleen injuries, embolization is a useful adjunct in management of grade III–V renal injuries and in those patients who present hemodynamically compromised, but respond to initial resuscitation.[61] Interventional techniques are also valuable in managing complications of renal trauma. Percutaneous nephrostomy, percutaneous drainage of an abscess or urinoma, or other fluid collections, embolization of AVF and pseudoaneurysms, as well as selective embolization of segmental or smaller arteries are common strategies for the nonoperative approach to blunt and isolated penetrating renal trauma.[81–85]

Despite these advances, persistent hemorrhages from the kidney, pulsatile perirenal hematomas, and renal pedicle avulsions remain indications for surgical exploration. Ureteral and renal pelvic injuries associated with urinary extravasation and nonviable parenchyma are relative indications for surgery, but may be repaired in a delayed fashion.[77,78] The management of renal artery occlusion or thrombosis remains controversial. Warm renal ischemia time less than 2 hours is generally considered an indication for arterial reconstruction.[86,87,88,89] Unfortunately, the diagnosis is seldom made within 2 hours and outcomes tend to be poor.[86] On the other hand, patients with a single functional kidney, bilateral renovascular injuries, or a nontrauma diseased kidney are more appropriately treated with surgical intervention. In the future, it is hoped that advances in IR will almost certainly improve care for these injuries by means of endovascular stenting and angioplasty. This has been reported in the treatment of small intimal arterial flaps.

14.4 Missed Injuries

The nonoperative management of injuries to the spleen, liver, and kidneys is gaining favor among trauma and other surgeons in the recent decades. However, some questions about missed injuries and resultant complications remain. Studies prior to CT reported associated intra-abdominal injury rates of 3 to 13% in blunt liver or spleen trauma.[89,90] Consequently, many surgeons believed that the nonoperative management of solid-organ injuries would be associated with an increased in evidence of missed injuries and ultimately increased morbidity.

The limitations of detecting hollow viscus and mesenteric injuries on earlier CT scan compounded these concerns. The results of the early literature for CT's ability to detect organ injury varied greatly among institutions.[91] Separate articles by Guarino et al and Sherck et al labeled CT scanning as unreliable in identifying small bowel injuries.[92,93,94] In contrast, Janzen et al and Malhoutra

et al reported reliable accuracy for both mesenteric and bowel injuries with advancements in CT technology.[95,96] This was echoed by Hagiwara's 99.9% accuracy for identifying small bowel injuries within the mesentery in > 8,000 CT scans.[97]

Most recently, Velmahos' prospective study of the nonoperative management of spleen, liver, and renal injuries demonstrated less than 1% missed small bowel injuries using CT scans.[98] Likewise, a multicenter study of 275,000 patients from the Eastern Association for the Surgery of Trauma showed an incidence of 0.3% of bowel injuries from blunt abdominal trauma.[99] Nevertheless, there is increasing incidence of hollow viscera injuries in patients with increasing numbers of injured solid organs.[100]

Miller et al showed a higher incidence of bowel injuries (11%) and pancreatic injuries (7%) in blunt liver trauma managed nonoperatively.[84] In the same study, there was no difference in incidence of diaphragm and bladder injuries associated with either blunt liver or blunt spleen trauma.[101] Conversely, the overall associated injuries were higher in the blunt liver injury group. These findings are not surprising considering the amount of energy transfer needed to injure a liver rather than a spleen. Therefore, the surgeons who favor the nonoperative management of blunt solid organ injuries must consider the potentially associated undiagnosed hollow visceral injuries.

14.5 Penetrating Abdominal Trauma

A logical extension of the successful nonoperative management of blunt abdominal trauma has contributed to focus the discussion of the role of CT and embolization techniques in the management of penetrating abdominal trauma as well. Routine laparotomy was introduced by the U.S. Army in 1915 as a result of the high mortality associated with penetrating injuries during the World War I.[4] Surgeons then applied this dictum to the management of civilian penetrating trauma. This philosophy was first challenged by Shaftan who advocated a trained surgical judgment instead of a mandatory exploratory laparotomy for the management of penetrating trauma.[8] Ancillary adjuncts such as deep peritoneal lavage and local wound exploration were incorporated to improve the successful outcomes from the nonoperative management.

Recently, Demetriades et al showed that ~ 50% of stab wounds to the anterior abdomen and ~ 85% of stab wounds to the back (posterior abdomen) could be managed nonoperatively in hemodynamically stable patients.[102,103] The same group reported the successful management of stab wounds to isolated intraperitoneal organs, same as the liver.[104] Subsequently, others have applied this approach to civilian gunshot wounds of the abdomen. In 1994, Renz and Feliciano documented the successful nonoperative management of 13 patients with gunshot wounds to the liver diagnosed by CT.[105] Chmielewski et al, Demetriades et al, and Ginzburg et al reported similar findings.[106–110]

Moreover, the successful nonoperative management of penetrating injury to the kidney has also been reported.[111,112] Most recently, Demetriades et al prospectively studied 152 patients with 185 penetrating solid-organ injuries. Forty-three patients with various solid-organ injuries did not require immediate operation and were treated nonoperatively without complication;

35% had grade III to V injuries. Embolization was successful as an adjunct in the management of four penetrating liver injuries.[113]

In a retrospective study of 792 patients (of 1,856) with abdominal gunshot wounds, Velmahos et al showed a 4% delayed laparotomy rate, 0.3% complication rate, and 38% rate of successful nonoperative management. It was estimated that 47% of unnecessary surgical explorations would have been performed. The nonoperative management decreased hospital charges by approximately $10 million over 8 years.[114]

In 1997, Velmahos et al also showed the benefits of embolization as an adjunct to control bleeding after penetrating abdominal trauma.[115] The authors mentioned embolization as a means to (1) stop bleeding not producing hemodynamic instability or other clinical signs mandating surgery, (2) stop bleeding not controlled by surgical exploration, and (3) stop delayed postoperative bleeding or bleeding secondary to complications.[115,116]

Also, the triple-contrast CT scanning can be used to evaluate penetrating injuries to the flank and back after a negative physical exam and peritoneal lavage was reported in 1986.[117] Thereafter, it has been used as a single diagnostic study in patients with anterior abdominal penetrations without a diagnostic peritoneal lavage. Furthermore, triple-contrast CT scanning after penetrating abdominal trauma has been advocated as a means to selectively manage patients nonoperatively.[118] In 2001, Shanmuganathan et al showed a successful nonoperative management of 67 of 69 hemodynamically stable patients with penetrating torso trauma who had a negative triple-contrast CT scan.[119,120] Chiu et al and Munera et al prospectively reported 95% and 96% accuracy in predicting the need for laparotomy with triple-contrast CT evaluation of stable patients, respectively.[121,122] Moreover, Chui et al demonstrated that the number of entrance wounds did not dictate the need for laparotomy. Despite these encouraging outcomes, selective nonoperative management of penetrating abdominal injuries is only limited to a few institutions with special expertise in trauma, where close monitoring, advanced resources, and clinical experience allow this management strategy safely.

The benefits of the nonoperative management of penetrating trauma seem similar to that for blunt abdominal trauma. In contrast, peritoneal violation from penetrating trauma is associated with a higher incidence of injury severity and complications.[1,123] Moreover, because hollow visceral injuries are the most common injuries after penetrating trauma and the ability of CT scan to identify small bowel injuries remains controversial, many surgeons remain skeptical of the nonoperative management of penetrating trauma. Without adequate experience, sophisticated diagnostic imaging capabilities and trained personnel, this reluctance is understandable.

The principles of when to operate are the same for both blunt and penetrating trauma: Patients who are hemodynamically unstable or have evidence of gastrointestinal contamination belong in the operating room. The risks of the nonoperative management must now be weighed against its benefits. Obviously, these risk-benefit ratios are patient, institution, and surgeon specific.

14.6 Conclusion

The management of blunt and penetrating abdominal trauma has dramatically evolved during the past 30 years. Although

operative therapy has been the foundation for the care of the injured patients in the past, advancements in CT scanning and IR techniques have permitted the widespread use of nonoperative management as the standard of care for blunt abdominal trauma. Further, the nonoperative management has expanded for penetrating abdominal trauma as well. Although various algorithms exist for the management of solid-organ injuries, the main question to be answered in the decision process must be what will benefit the patient most. The decision not to operate is multifaceted and influenced by many factors, such as injury severity, hemodynamic stability, concomitant injuries, physician preference, and available institutional resources.

Our goal in writing this chapter is to provide a good framework to understanding the effectiveness of the nonoperative management of solid-organ injury, particularly when alternative therapies such as embolization are available. A good surgical judgment must be applied without prejudices. However, some generalizations can be made. In hemodynamic instability and solid-organ injury, surgical exploration is the therapy of choice. In high-grade liver injuries this may be augmented by embolization to achieve hemostasis. In hemodynamically stable patients, the nonoperative management is the standard of care for grade I–III blunt solid organ injuries regardless of age, extra-abdominal injuries, and mental status. In higher injury grades and/or in the presence of a contrast material "blush," active extravasation, or vascular disruption, on angiography and/or CT scan, embolization improves successful nonoperative outcomes. Even if the incidence of a missed intestinal injury is low, the surgeon must be diligent in monitoring for clinical signs of such.

A careful observation and close monitoring are essential requirements for nonoperative management. The surgeons must be ready to operate immediately if the patient deteriorates. The operating room must be always ready. Furthermore, application of these principles to the penetrating injuries, or transient hemodynamically stable patients, with blunt trauma is recommended, only on protocol and in institutions with expert knowledge and immediately available surgeons and interventional radiologists. Although considered "conservative management" by some, it is evident that the nonoperative management of solid organ injuries is labor intensive and involves the mutual cooperation between interventional radiologists, surgeons, trauma surgeons, and others. Continued advances in technology and improved experience with the nonoperative therapy will only challenge current limitations and promote better applicability in the trauma community.

References

[1] Moore EE, Marx JA. Penetrating abdominal wounds. Rationale for exploratory laparotomy. JAMA 1985; 253: 2705–2708

[2] Moore EE, Moore JB, Van Duzer-Moore S, Thompson JS. Mandatory laparotomy for gunshot wounds penetrating the abdomen. Am J Surg 1980; 140: 847–851

[3] Nance FC, Cohn I. Surgical judgment in the management of stab wounds of the abdomen: A retrospective and prospective analysis based on a study of 600 stabbed patients. Ann Surg 1969; 170: 569–580

[4] Beekley AC, Blackbourne LH, Sebesta JA, McMullin N, Mullenix PS, Holcomb JB 31st Combat Support Hospital Research Group. Selective nonoperative management of penetrating torso injury from combat fragmentation wounds. J Trauma 2008; 64 Suppl: S108–S116, discussion S116–S117

[5] Goan YG, Huang MS, Lin JM. Nonoperative management for extensive hepatic and splenic injuries with significant hemoperitoneum in adults. J Trauma 1998; 45: 360–364, discussion 365

[6] Pachter HL, Hofstetter SR. The current status of nonoperative management of adult blunt hepatic injuries. Am J Surg 1995; 169: 442–454

[7] Pachter HL, Knudson MM, Esrig B et al. Status of nonoperative management of blunt hepatic injuries in 1995: a multicenter experience with 404 patients. J Trauma 1996; 40: 31–38

[8] Shaftan GW. Indications for operation in abdominal trauma. Am J Surg 1960; 99: 657–664

[9] Stylianos S. Compliance with evidence-based guidelines in children with isolated spleen or liver injury: a prospective study. J Pediatr Surg 2002; 37: 453–456

[10] Upadhyaya P, Simpson JS. Splenic trauma in children. Surg Gynecol Obstet 1968; 126: 781–790

[11] Caroline R. Obituary – Sir Godfrey Hounsfield BMJ 2004; 329: 687

[12] Yanar H, Ertekin C, Taviloglu K, Kabay B, Bakkaloglu H, Guloglu R. Nonoperative treatment of multiple intra-abdominal solid organ injury after blunt abdominal trauma. J Trauma 2008; 64: 943–948

[13] Margolies MN, Ring EJ, Waltman AC, Kerr WS, Baum S. Arteriography in the management of hemorrhage from pelvic fractures. N Engl J Med 1972; 287: 317–321

[14] Panetta T, Sclafani SJ, Goldstein AS, Phillips TF, Shaftan GW. Percutaneous transcatheter embolization for massive bleeding from pelvic fractures. J Trauma 1985; 25: 1021–1029

[15] Holdsworth RJ, Irving AD, Cuschieri A. Postsplenectomy sepsis and its mortality rate: actual versus perceived risks. Br J Surg 1991; 78: 1031–1038

[16] Buntain WL, Gould HR, Maull KI. Predictability of splenic salvage by computed tomography. J Trauma 1988; 28: 24–34

[17] Buntain WL, Gould HR. Splenic trauma in children and techniques of splenic salvage. World J Surg 1985; 9: 449–454

[18] Buntain WL, Lynn HB. Splenorrhaphy: changing concepts for the traumatized spleen. Surgery 1979; 86: 748–760

[19] Cogbill TH, Moore EE, Jurkovich GJ et al. Nonoperative management of blunt splenic trauma: a multicenter experience. J Trauma 1989; 29: 1312–1317

[20] Schwab CW. Selection of nonoperative management candidates. World J Surg 2001; 25: 1389–1392

[21] Tom WW, Howells GA, Bree RL, Schwab R, Lucas RJ. A nonoperative approach to the adult ruptured spleen sustained from blunt trauma. Am Surg 1985; 51: 367–371

[22] Wesson DE, Filler RM, Ein SH, Shandling B, Simpson JS, Stephens CA. Ruptured spleen—when to operate? J Pediatr Surg 1981; 16: 324–326

[23] Francke EL, Neu HC. Postsplenectomy infection. Surg Clin North Am 1981; 61: 135–155

[24] Potoka DA, Schall LC, Ford HR. Risk factors for splenectomy in children with blunt splenic trauma. J Pediatr Surg 2002; 37: 294–299

[25] Pachter HL, Guth AA, Hofstetter SR, Spencer FC. Changing patterns in the management of splenic trauma: the impact of nonoperative management. Ann Surg 1998; 227: 708–717, discussion 717–719

[26] Scatamacchia SA, Raptopoulos V, Fink MP, Silva WE. Splenic trauma in adults: impact of CT grading on management. Radiology 1989; 171: 725–729

[27] Smith JS, Wengrovitz MA, DeLong BS. Prospective validation of criteria, including age, for safe, nonsurgical management of the ruptured spleen. J Trauma 1992; 33: 363–368, discussion 368–369

[28] Knudson MM, Maull KI. Nonoperative management of solid organ injuries. Past, present, and future. Surg Clin North Am 1999; 79: 1357–1371

[29] Powell M, Courcoulas A, Gardner M et al. Management of blunt splenic trauma: significant differences between adults and children. Surgery 1997; 2: 654–660

[30] Haan JM, Biffl W, Knudson MM et al. Western Trauma Association Multi-Institutional Trials Committee. Splenic embolization revisited: a multicenter review. J Trauma 2004; 56: 542–547

[31] Haan JM, Bochicchio GV, Kramer N, Scalea TM. Nonoperative management of blunt splenic injury: a 5-year experience. J Trauma 2005; 58: 492–498

[32] Galvan DA, Peitzman AB. Failure of nonoperative management of abdominal solid organ injuries. Curr Opin Crit Care 2006; 12: 590–594

[33] Nance ML, Mahboubi S, Wickstrom M, Prendergast F, Stafford PW. Pattern of abdominal free fluid following isolated blunt spleen or liver injury in the pediatric patient. J Trauma 2002; 52: 85–87

[34] Pal JD, Victorino GP. Defining the role of computed tomography in blunt abdominal trauma: use in the hemodynamically stable patient with a depressed level of consciousness. Arch Surg 2002; 137: 1029–1032, discussion 1032–1033

[35] Peitzman AB, Heil B, Rivera L et al. Blunt splenic injury in adults: Multi institutional Study of the Eastern Association for the Surgery of Trauma. J Trauma 2000; 49: 177–187, discussion 187–189

[36] Schurr MJ, Fabian TC, Gavant M et al. Management of blunt splenic trauma: computed tomographic contrast blush predicts failure of nonoperative management. J Trauma 1995; 39: 507–512, discussion 512–513

[37] Sclafani SJ, Shaftan GW, Scalea TM et al. Nonoperative salvage of computed tomography-diagnosed splenic injuries: utilization of angiography for triage and embolization for hemostasis. J Trauma 1995; 39: 818–825, discussion 826–827

[38] Davis KA, Fabian TC, Croce MA et al. Improved success in nonoperative management of blunt splenic injuries: embolization of splenic artery pseudoaneurysms. J Trauma 1998; 44: 1008–1013, discussion 1013–1015

[39] Haan J, Scott J, Boyd-Kranis RL, Ho S, Kramer M, Scalea TM. Admission angiography for blunt splenic injury: advantages and pitfalls. J Trauma 2001; 51: 1161–1165

[40] Haan JM, Ilahi ON, Kramer M, Scalea TM, Myers J. Protocol-driven nonoperative management in patients with blunt splenic trauma and minimal associated injury decreases length of stay. J Trauma 2003; 55: 317–321, discussion 321–322

[41] Savage SA, Zarzaur BL, Magnotti LJ et al. The evolution of blunt splenic injury: resolution and progression. J Trauma 2008; 64: 1085–1091, discussion 1091–1092

[42] Hagiwara A, Minakawa K, Fukushima H, Murata A, Masuda H, Shimazaki S. Predictors of death in patients with life-threatening pelvic hemorrhage after successful transcatheter arterial embolization. J Trauma 2003; 55: 696–703

[43] Hagiwara A, Yukioka T, Ohta S, Nitatori T, Matsuda H, Shimazaki S. Nonsurgical management of patients with blunt splenic injury: efficacy of transcatheter arterial embolization. AJR Am J Roentgenol 1996; 167: 159–166

[44] Archer LP, Rogers FB, Shackford SR. Selective nonoperative management of liver and spleen injuries in neurologically impaired adult patients. Arch Surg 1996; 131: 309–315

[45] Shapiro MB, Nance ML, Schiller HJ, Hoff WS, Kauder DR, Schwab CW. Nonoperative management of solid abdominal organ injuries from blunt trauma: impact of neurologic impairment. Am Surg 2001; 67: 793–796

[46] Oldham KT, Guice KS, Ryckman F, Kaufman RA, Martin LW, Noseworthy J. Blunt liver injury in childhood: evolution of therapy and current perspective. Surgery 1986; 100: 542–549

[47] Moudouni SM, Patard JJ, Manunta A, Guiraud P, Guille F, Lobel B. A conservative approach to major blunt renal lacerations with urinary extravasation and devitalized renal segments. BJU Int 2001; 87: 290–294

[48] Moudouni SM, Hadj Slimen M, Manunta A et al. Management of major blunt renal lacerations: is a nonoperative approach indicated? Eur Urol 2001; 40: 409–414

[49] Pachter HL, Spencer FC, Hofstetter SR, Liang HG, Coppa GF. Significant trends in the treatment of hepatic trauma. Experience with 411 injuries. Ann Surg 1992; 215: 492–500, discussion 500–502

[50] Croce MA, Fabian TC, Menke PG et al. Nonoperative management of blunt hepatic trauma is the treatment of choice for hemodynamically stable patients. Results of a prospective trial. Ann Surg 1995; 221: 744–753, discussion 753–755

[51] Malhotra AK, Fabian TC, Croce MA et al. Blunt hepatic injury: a paradigm shift from operative to nonoperative management in the 1990s. Ann Surg 2000; 231: 804–813

[52] Mirvis SE, Whitley NO, Vainwright JR, Gens DR. Blunt hepatic trauma in adults: CT-based classification and correlation with prognosis and treatment. Radiology 1989; 171: 27–32

[53] Boone DC, Federle M, Billiar TR, Udekwu AO, Peitzman AB. Evolution of management of major hepatic trauma: identification of patterns of injury. J Trauma 1995; 39: 344–350

[54] Delius RE, Frankel W, Coran AG. A comparison between operative and nonoperative management of blunt injuries to the liver and spleen in adult and pediatric patients. Surgery 1989; 106: 788–792, discussion 792–793

[55] Meyer AA, Crass RA, Lim RC, Jeffrey RB, Federle MP, Trunkey DD. Selective nonoperative management of blunt liver injury using computed tomography. Arch Surg 1985; 120: 550–554

[56] Moore EE. Edgar J. Poth Lecture. Critical decisions in the management of hepatic trauma. Am J Surg 1984; 148: 712–716

[57] David Richardson J, Franklin GA, Lukan JK et al. Evolution in the management of hepatic trauma: a 25-year perspective. Ann Surg 2000; 232: 324–330

[58] Poletti PA, Mirvis SE, Shanmuganathan K, Killeen KL, Coldwell D. CT criteria for management of blunt liver trauma: correlation with angiographic and surgical findings. Radiology 2000; 216: 418–427

[59] Denton JR, Moore EE, Coldwell DM. Multimodality treatment for grade V hepatic injuries: perihepatic packing, arterial embolization, and venous stenting. J Trauma 1997; 42: 964–967, discussion 967–968

[60] Fang JF, Chen RJ, Wong YC et al. Pooling of contrast material on computed tomography mandates aggressive management of blunt hepatic injury. Am J Surg 1998; 176: 315–319

[61] Hagiwara A, Yukioka T, Ohta S et al. Nonsurgical management of patients with blunt hepatic injury: efficacy of transcatheter arterial embolization. AJR Am J Roentgenol 1997; 169: 1151–1156

[62] Hagiwara A, Murata A, Matsuda T, Matsuda H, Shimazaki S. The efficacy and limitations of transarterial embolization for severe hepatic injury. J Trauma 2002; 52: 1091–1096

[63] Velmahos GC, Toutouzas K, Radin R et al. High success with nonoperative management of blunt hepatic trauma: the liver is a sturdy organ. Arch Surg 2003; 138: 475–480, discussion 480–481

[64] Dabbs DN, Stein DM, Scalea TM. Major hepatic necrosis: a common complication after angioembolization for treatment of high-grade liver injuries. J Trauma 2009; 66: 621–627, discussion 627–629

[65] Swiersie AK. Experiences and lessons of emergency urological surgery in war. J Urol 1947; 47: 938–944

[66] Bretan PN, McAninch JW, Federle MP, Jeffrey RB. Computerized tomographic staging of renal trauma: 85 consecutive cases. J Urol 1986; 136: 561–565

[67] McAninch JW, Carroll PR. Renal trauma: kidney preservation through improved vascular control-a refined approach. J Trauma 1982; 22: 285–290

[68] Sagalowsky AI, McConnell JD, Peters PC. Renal trauma requiring surgery: an analysis of 185 cases. J Trauma 1983; 23: 128–131

[69] Cass AS, Cass BP. Immediate surgical management of severe renal injuries in multiple-injured patients. Urology 1983; 21: 140–145

[70] Mee SL, McAninch JW, Robinson AL, Auerbach PS, Carroll PR. Radiographic assessment of renal trauma: a 10-year prospective study of patient selection. J Urol 1989; 141: 1095–1098

[71] Mendez R. Renal trauma. J Urol 1977; 118: 698–703

[72] Nicolaisen GS, McAninch JW, Marshall GA, Bluth RF, Carroll PR. Renal trauma: re-evaluation of the indications for radiographic assessment. J Urol 1985; 133: 183–187

[73] Eastham JA, Wilson TG, Ahlering TE. Urological evaluation and management of renal-proximity stab wounds. J Urol 1993; 150: 1771–1773

[74] Heyns CF, de Klerk DP, de Kock ML. Stab wounds associated with hematuria—a review of 67 cases. J Urol 1983; 130: 228–231

[75] Heyns CF, Van Vollenhoven P. Selective surgical management of renal stab wounds. Br J Urol 1992; 69: 351–357

[76] McAninch JW, Carroll PR, Armenakas NA, Lee P. Renal gunshot wounds: methods of salvage and reconstruction. J Trauma 1993; 35: 279–283, discussion 283–284

[77] Santucci RA, Fisher MB. The literature increasingly supports expectant (conservative) management of renal trauma—a systematic review. J Trauma 2005; 59: 493–503

[78] Santucci RA, McAninch JW, Safir M, Mario LA, Service S, Segal MR. Validation of the American Association for the Surgery of Trauma organ injury severity scale for the kidney. J Trauma 2001; 50: 195–200

[79] Altman AL, Haas C, Dinchman KH, Spirnak JP. Selective nonoperative management of blunt grade 5 renal injury. J Urol 2000; 164: 27–30, discussion 30–31

[80] Bergren CT, Chan FN, Bodzin JH. Intravenous pyelogram results in association with renal pathology and therapy in trauma patients. J Trauma 1987; 27: 515–518

[81] Broghammer JA, Fisher MB, Santucci RA. Conservative management of renal trauma: a review. Urology 2007; 70: 623–629

[82] Knudson MM, Harrison PB, Hoyt DB et al. Outcome after major renovascular injuries: a Western trauma association multicenter report. J Trauma 2000; 49: 1116–1122

[83] Mansi MK, Alkhudair WK. Conservative management with percutaneous intervention of major blunt renal injuries. Am J Emerg Med 1997; 15: 633–637

[84] Santucci RA, Wessells H, Bartsch G et al. Evaluation and management of renal injuries: consensus statement of the renal trauma subcommittee. BJU Int 2004; 93: 937–954

[85] Velmahos GC, Demetriades D, Cornwell EE et al. Selective management of renal gunshot wounds. Br J Surg 1998; 85: 1121–1124

[86] Glenski WJ, Husmann DA. Traumatic renal artery thrombosis: Management and long-term follow up. J Urol 1995; 153: 316–321

[87] Haas CA, Spirnak JP. Traumatic renal artery occlusion: a review of the literature. Tech Urol 1998; 4: 1–11

[88] Haas CA, Dinchman KH, Nasrallah PF, Spirnak JP. Traumatic renal artery occlusion: a 15-year review. J Trauma 1998; 45: 557–561

[89] Turner WW, Snyder WH, Fry WJ. Mortality and renal salvage after renovascular trauma. A review of 94 patients treated in a 20 year period. Am J Surg 1983; 146: 848–851

[90] Buckman RF, Piano G, Dunham CM, Soutter I, Ramzy A, Militello PR. Major bowel and diaphragmatic injuries associated with blunt spleen or liver rupture. J Trauma 1988; 28: 1317–1321

[91] Killeen KL, Shanmuganathan K, Poletti PA, Cooper C, Mirvis SE. Helical computed tomography of bowel and mesenteric injuries. J Trauma 2001; 51: 26–36

[92] Guarino J, Hassett JM, Luchette FA. Small bowel injuries: mechanisms, patterns, and outcome. J Trauma 1995; 39: 1076–1080

[93] Sherck J, Shatney C, Sensaki K, Selivanov V. The accuracy of computed tomography in the diagnosis of blunt small-bowel perforation. Am J Surg 1994; 168: 670–675

[94] Sherck JP, Oakes DD. Intestinal injuries missed by computed tomography. J Trauma 1990; 30: 1–5, discussion 5–7

[95] Janzen DL, Zwirewich CV, Breen DJ, Nagy A. Diagnostic accuracy of helical CT for detection of blunt bowel and mesenteric injuries. Clin Radiol 1998; 53: 193–197

[96] Malhotra AK, Fabian TC, Katsis SB, Gavant ML, Croce MA. Blunt bowel and mesenteric injuries: the role of screening computed tomography. J Trauma 2000; 48: 991–998, discussion 998–1000

[97] Hagiwara A, Yukioka T, Satou M et al. Early diagnosis of small intestine rupture from blunt abdominal trauma using computed tomography: significance of the streaky density within the mesentery. J Trauma 1995; 38: 630–633

[98] Velmahos GC, Toutouzas KG, Radin R, Chan L, Demetriades D. Nonoperative treatment of blunt injury to solid abdominal organs: a prospective study. Arch Surg 2003; 138: 844–851

[99] Watts DD, Fakhry SM EAST Multi-Institutional Hollow Viscus Injury Research Group. Incidence of hollow viscus injury in blunt trauma: an analysis from 275,557 trauma admissions from the East multi-institutional trial. J Trauma 2003; 54: 289–294

[100] Nance ML, Peden GW, Shapiro MB, Kauder DR, Rotondo MF, Schwab CW. Solid viscus injury predicts major hollow viscus injury in blunt abdominal trauma. J Trauma 1997; 43: 618–622, discussion 622–623

[101] Miller PR, Croce MA, Bee TK, Malhotra AK, Fabian TC. Associated injuries in blunt solid organ trauma: implications for missed injury in nonoperative management. J Trauma 2002; 53: 238–242, discussion 242–244

[102] Demetriades D, Rabinowitz B. Indications for operation in abdominal stab wounds. A prospective study of 651 patients. Ann Surg 1987; 205: 129–132

[103] Demetriades D, Rabinowitz B, Sofianos C et al. The management of penetrating injuries of the back. A prospective study of 230 patients. Ann Surg 1988; 207: 72–74

[104] Demetriades D, Rabinowitz B, Sofianos C. Non-operative management of penetrating liver injuries: a prospective study. Br J Surg 1986; 73: 736–737

[105] Renz BM, Feliciano DV. Gunshot wounds to the liver. A prospective study of selective nonoperative management. J Med Assoc Ga 1995; 84: 275–277

[106] Chmielewski GW, Nicholas JM, Dulchavsky SA, Diebel LN. Nonoperative management of gunshot wounds of the abdomen. Am Surg 1995; 61: 665–668

[107] Demetriades D, Gomez H, Chahwan S et al. Gunshot injuries to the liver: the role of selective nonoperative management. J Am Coll Surg 1999; 188: 343–348

[108] Demetriades D, Velmahos G, Cornwell E et al. Selective nonoperative management of gunshot wounds of the anterior abdomen. Arch Surg 1997; 132: 178–183

[109] Demetriades D, Velmahos G. Technology-driven triage of abdominal trauma: the emerging era of nonoperative management. Annu Rev Med 2003; 54: 1–15

[110] Ginzburg E, Carrillo EH, Kopelman T et al. The role of computed tomography in selective management of gunshot wounds to the abdomen and flank. J Trauma 1998; 45: 1005–1009

[111] Armenakas NA, Duckett CP, McAninch JW. Indication for non-operative management of renal stab wounds. J Urol 1994; 161: 768–771

[112] Wessells H, McAninch JW, Meyer A, Bruce J. Criteria for nonoperative treatment of significant penetrating renal lacerations. J Urol 1997; 157: 24–27

[113] Demetriades D, Hadjizacharia P, Constantinou C et al. Selective nonoperative management of penetrating abdominal solid organ injuries. Ann Surg 2006; 244: 620–628

[114] Velmahos GC, Demetriades D, Toutouzas KG et al. Selective nonoperative management in 1,856 patients with abdominal gunshot wounds: should routine laparotomy still be the standard of care? Ann Surg 2001; 234: 395–402, discussion 402–403

[115] Velmahos GC, Demetriades D, Foianini E et al. A selective approach to the management of gunshot wounds to the back. Am J Surg 1997; 174: 342–346

[116] Velmahos GC, Demetriades D, Chahwan S et al. Angiographic embolization for arrest of bleeding after penetrating trauma to the abdomen. Am J Surg 1999; 178: 367–373

[117] Phillips TF, Sclafani SJA, Goldstein AS, Scalea TM, Panetta T, Shaftan G. Use of the contrast-enhanced CT enema in the management of penetrating trauma to the flank and back. J Trauma 1986; 26: 593–601

[118] Velmahos GC, Constantinou C, Tillou A, Brown CV, Salim A, Demetriades D. Abdominal computed tomographic scan for patients with gunshot wounds to the abdomen selected for nonoperative management. J Trauma 2005; 59: 1155–1160, discussion 1160–1161

[119] Shanmuganathan K, Mirvis SE, Chiu WC, Killeen KL, Scalea TM. Triple-contrast helical CT in penetrating torso trauma: a prospective study to determine peritoneal violation and the need for laparotomy. AJR Am J Roentgenol 2001; 177: 1247–1256

[120] Shanmuganathan K, Mirvis SE, Chiu WC, Killeen KL, Hogan GJ, Scalea TM. Penetrating torso trauma: triple-contrast helical CT in peritoneal violation and organ injury—a prospective study in 200 patients. Radiology 2004; 231: 775–784

[121] Chiu WC, Shanmuganathan K, Mirvis SE, Scalea TM. Determining the need for laparotomy in penetrating torso trauma: a prospective study using triple-contrast enhanced abdominopelvic computed tomography. J Trauma 2001; 51: 860–868, discussion 868–869

[122] Múnera F, Morales C, Soto JA et al. Gunshot wounds of abdomen: evaluation of stable patients with triple-contrast helical CT. Radiology 2004; 231: 399–405

[123] Moore EE, Shackford SR, Pachter HL et al. Organ injury scaling: spleen, liver, and kidney. J Trauma 1989; 29: 1664–1666

15 Interventional Radiology in Abdominal Trauma: Spleen

James M. Haan

The spleen is the most commonly injured intra-abdominal organ in trauma. Due to the high nonoperative mortality rates, splenectomy was the treatment of choice in the early 1900s. In 1919 Bullock recognized the overwhelming postsplenectomy sepsis, an uncommon, but often lethal condition. This led to the concept of surgical splenic conservation using splenorrhaphy or partial splenectomy in the 1950s. In 1968 nonoperative management for splenic injury in children was first described. In the 1980s this expanded nonoperative management of splenic injuries in children was the standard of care, even if the patients required transfusion. The success of these nonoperative algorithms later led to the common nonoperative management of hemodynamically stable adult patients with blunt splenic injury. Nonoperative management of splenic injury has now become the standard of care in hemodynamically stable adult patients with blunt splenic trauma.[1–19] Many trauma level I centers and others use splenic arteriography and embolization of vascular injuries as an adjunct to improve the success rate of nonoperatively managed splenic injuries.[1–19]

15.1 Population

Determining the optimal therapy for the trauma patient with splenic rupture remains a topic of debate. The simple observation of hemodynamically stable patients with low-grade injuries is widely accepted. Also, nearly all authors agree that hemodynamically unstable patients require immediate operative rather than interventional radiologic (IR) management. The optimal management is less clear for other groups of patients. Risk factors for nonoperative failure include evidence of vascular injury, the American Association for the Surgery of Trauma (AAST) Organ Injury Grade (OIG) three or above, or large hemoperitoneum on abdominal multidetector computed tomography (MDCT). Transfusion requirements, additional

abdominal injuries, and age greater than 55 years are also often cited as mandating surgery due to increased failure rates. Additional concerns include associated severe neurologic injury given that hypotensive episodes will double neurologic mortality. The discussion splits from those advocating early surgery, from those who recommend IR embolization as a nonoperative adjunct.

15.2 Injury Severity

The Organ Injury Scaling Committee of the American Association for the Surgery of Trauma has described a grading system based on the anatomic disruption as seen on multiplanar abdominal CT (▶ Fig. 15.1). Higher grades correlate with increasing anatomic splenic injury. Although there is some predictive value in this system (i.e., increasing injury grades have increasing nonoperative failure rates), this scale is limited because it does not take into account evidence of vascular injury, degree of hemoperitoneum, and the patient's clinical situation.

15.3 Diagnosis

Multidetector CT plays a very important role in the detection and characterization of splenic injuries. It is highly accurate and can detect splenic vascular lesions, the presence of which is a predictor of failure of nonoperative management. The recent availability of MDCT in most trauma level I centers in the United States has led to increased detection and diagnostic accuracy of patients with splenic injury. The ability to produce high-resolution axial images obtained with no motion, as well as isotropic multiplanar (3D) reformatted images and maximum-intensity projection (MIP) images, has helped to increase the diagnostic confidence of the radiologist and clinicians as well.[1–7]

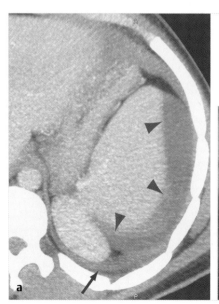
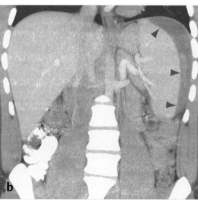

Fig. 15.1 Subcapsular hematoma in a male admitted following blunt force trauma. (a) Axial and (b) coronal images show a mixed attenuation subcapsular hematoma (arrowheads). Intraperitoneal blood (arrow) is seen posterior to the spleen.

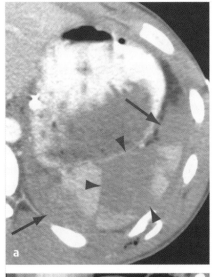

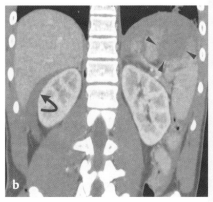

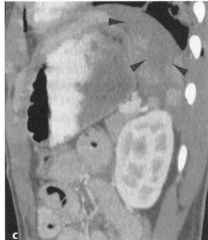

Fig. 15.2 Splenic hematoma in a male involved in a motor vehicle collision. (a) Axial, (b) coronal, and (c) sagittal reformatted images show free intraperitoneal blood in the hepatorenal fossa (curved arrow) and adjacent to the spleen (arrows). An irregular mixed attenuation area (arrowheads) seen within the spleen represents a hematoma.

15.3.1 Whole-Body MDCT Technique

The majority of the patients admitted to the University of Maryland Shock Trauma Center (UMSTC) have multisystem injuries. The abdomen is assessed as part of a total-body CT (TBCT) in which scans are obtained from the vertex of the head to the symphysis pubis after administration of oral and intravenous (IV) contrast material.

Despite controversies over the use of oral contrast material in this setting, studies have shown an extremely low risk of aspiration.[5,8,9] A total of 600 mL of 2% sodium diatrizoate (hypaque sodium; Amersham Health, Princeton, NJ) is administered orally 30 minutes before and immediately before the scan. Oral contrast material is routinely administered, either orally or, if the patient is unable to drink the contrast material, through a nasogastric tube.

Two MDCT scanners (16- and 64-slice) are available adjacent to the admitting area for trauma patients at our institution. Delayed images are routinely obtained in the "portal" venous phase on the 64-slice scanner and at 2 to 3 minutes following injection of IV contrast in the excretory phase on the 16-slice scanner.

MDCT Findings of Splenic Injuries

Multidetector CT is highly accurate (98%) in diagnosing splenic injuries.[1,4,6,10,11,12] The main or commonly seen types of splenic injury include hematoma, laceration, active hemorrhage, post-traumatic splenic infarct, shattered spleen, and vascular injuries, including pseudoaneurysms and arteriovenous fistulas (AVFs).

Splenic hematomas may be intraparenchymal or subcapsular. Single or multiple hematomas may occur after blunt trauma. On unenhanced MDCT subcapsular hematomas are hyperdense relative to normal splenic parenchyma. On contrast-enhanced CT subcapsular hematomas are typically low attenuation collections of blood between the splenic capsule and the enhancing splenic parenchyma (▶ Fig. 15.1). Subcapsular hematomas often compress the underlying splenic parenchyma and this CT finding helps to differentiate true subcapsular hematomas from small collections of blood or fluid in the perisplenic space. Uncomplicated subcapsular hematomas typically resolve within 4 to 6 weeks. The attenuation values of the subcapsular hematoma usually decreases with the age of the lesion, unless there is recurrent hemorrhage. On contrast-enhanced MDCT, acute hematomas appear as irregular high or low attenuation areas within the splenic parenchyma (▶ Fig. 15.2).

Acute splenic lacerations have sharp or jagged margins and appear as linear or branching low attenuation areas on contrast-enhanced CT (▶ Fig. 15.3). As time goes by, the margins of these splenic lacerations and hematomas become less well

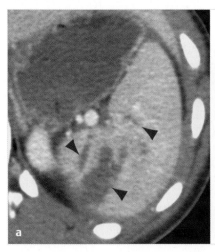
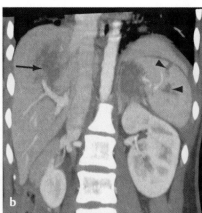

Fig. 15.3 Splenic laceration in a male. (a) Axial and (b) coronal images show multiple irregular linear low attenuation areas (arrow) representing splenic lacerations. Low attenuation area in the region of hilum of liver represents a hematoma.

defined and the lesions decrease in size until the areas become isodense with normal splenic parenchyma. Enlargement or extension of the lesions on follow-up CT should raise the possibility of injury progression, warranting close clinical follow-up, repeated follow-up CT, or arteriography. Complete healing by CT appearance may take weeks to months usually depending on the initial size of the injury.

Splenic clefts or lobulations can mimic lacerations on CT, but typically these have smooth or rounded edges without adjacent free intraperitoneal fluid. On delayed images lacerations will "fill-in" while the clefts will persist.

15.4 Active Hemorrhage

The significant difference between the attenuation values of extravasated contrast material (range, 85–350 Hounsfield units [HU], mean, 132 HU) and hematoma (range, 40–70 HU, mean, 51 HU) is helpful in differentiating active bleeding from clotted blood.[13,14] On contrast-enhanced MDCT active hemorrhage in the spleen is seen as an irregular or linear area of contrast extravasation (▶ Fig. 15.4), similar in attenuation to contrast material in adjacent vessels. Active splenic hemorrhage may be seen within the splenic parenchyma, subcapsular space, or intraperitoneally (▶ Fig. 15.4). Ongoing hemorrhage during scanning may be found as an increase in the amount of IV contrast material extravasated on images obtained in the identical anatomical region in the delayed phases (▶ Fig. 15.4). Occasionally, an active bleeding may be seen only on delayed images on MDCT. This may be related to the very short scanning time required with protocols used with the newest 64 detector scanners that cover a large anatomical region per gantry rotation. It is always very important to carefully review images obtained in the identical anatomical regions during the different phases together, side-by-side, to accurately diagnose a subtle active bleeding.

15.5 Vascular Injuries

Posttraumatic splenic vascular injuries include pseudoaneurysms (▶ Fig. 15.5) and AVFs (▶ Fig. 15.6). These lesions may have a similar appearance on MDCT and can be clearly differentiated on

splenic DSA. Pseudoaneurysms and AVFs of the spleen appear as well-circumscribed focal areas of increased attenuation on contrast-enhanced MDCT and are often surrounded by low-attenuation areas. The attenuation values of these lesions are typically within 10 HU of the adjacent contrast-enhanced artery. On delayed images, these lesions wash out and become minimally hyperdense or isodense compared with normal splenic parenchyma. This helps to differentiate splenic vascular injuries from areas of active bleeding.

A retrospective study by Anderson et al[6] reported, using similar criteria that delayed phase imaging was useful to differentiate splenic active bleeding ($n = 9$) or vascular injury ($n = 10$) in 19 patients. The authors measured the change in the size and attenuation values of the high attenuation splenic lesions in both phases of imaging. On delayed imaging active bleeding increased in size, or the lesions measured more than 10 HU of that of the aorta, whereas vascular lesions were stable or decreased in size and the attenuation values were within 10 HU of that of the aorta.

A posttraumatic pseudoaneurysm is formed by an injury to the arterial wall. The defect in the wall allows a small amount of blood to track into the injured vessels. This blood is retained by the adventitia, and the surrounding perivascular tissues form the wall of the pseudoaneurysm. Arteriovenous fistulas may develop in the immediate posttraumatic period, as a result of injury to both the artery and adjacent vein. On contrast-enhanced CT, these AVFs may have the same imaging characteristics of pseudoaneurysms and can be differentiated only on splenic angiography. Sometimes a clear differentiation is possible if one has a high degree of suspicion.

Although the natural history of both these lesions is not clearly understood, the major potential complication of all visceral pseudoaneurysms (including splenic) is rupture, with a rate reported of 3 to 46%.[15] Their presence, therefore, represents a predictor for failed nonsurgical management. Schurr et al[16] reported the presence of "vascular blush" in a significantly higher number of patients who failed nonoperative management, than in patients successfully managed nonoperatively (67% and 6%, respectively; $p = 0.0001$). Gavant et al[12] reported failure of nonsurgical management in 11 (15%) of 72 patients with blunt splenic injury. Well-defined splenic vascular injuries were noted on helical CT in nine (82%) of these 11 patients.

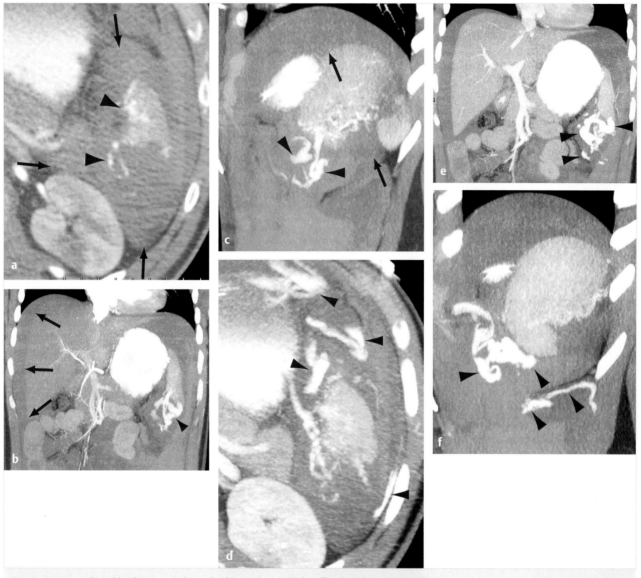

Fig. 15.4 Active splenic bleeding in a male involved in a motor vehicle collision. Maximum intensity projection (MIP) (a) axial, (b), sagittal and (c) coronal reformatted images obtained during the midarterial phase demonstrates active bleeding (arrowheads) from the spleen into the peritoneum. Delayed maximum intensity projection (MIP) (d) coronal (e), axial and (f) sagittal reformatted images obtained in a similar anatomical location during the portal venous phase demonstrate increase in the amount of active peritoneal bleeding.

The ability to scan during peak contrast enhancement in the mid or late arterial phase on MDCT or portal venous phase on CT scanners and obtain delayed images during the portal venous phases is helpful to differentiate active bleeding from vascular injuries (▶ Fig. 15.4, ▶ Fig. 15.5, ▶ Fig. 15.6). A prospective study performed at the UMSTC reported that MDCT showed an overall sensitivity of 76%, specificity of 90%, and an accuracy of 83% in diagnosing active bleeding and vascular injury using surgery and splenic arteriography as the reference standard.[1]

Some studies have reported that it is important to differentiate active splenic bleeding from vascular injury.[1,6] A far larger proportion of patients with active bleeding (unlike vascular injury) continues to bleed and require splenectomy or embolization for hemodynamic instability ($p < 0.0001$).[1] In our experience, 50% of these patients required surgery while awaiting angiography. In those who remained stable, however, success was greater than 90%. This has led to a recommendation that active bleeding injuries be treated surgically, unless the patient is hemodynamically stable and the IR team is immediately available. In most trauma level I centers, the IR team is or must be ready in 30 minutes or less. This is a relatively standard rule in most academic centers. The majority of patients with posttraumatic splenic vascular injury remains stable following MDCT and is successfully treated with splenic artery embolization.

15.6 Technique

Expeditious splenic embolization in coordination with the trauma team is paramount to success. Embolization requires close monitoring and resuscitation by the trauma team,

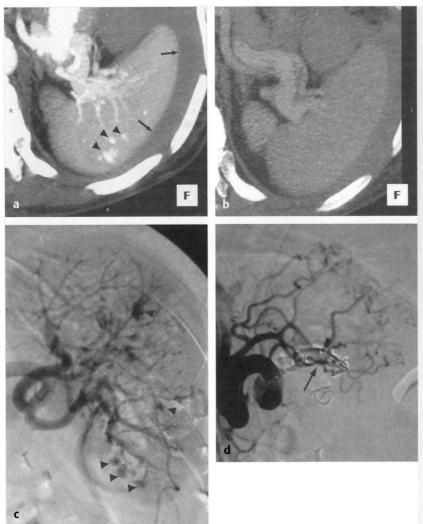

Fig. 15.5 Posttraumatic vascular injury. (a) Axial maximum intensity projection (MIP) image demonstrates multiple vascular injuries (arrowheads) and a large amount of perisplenic blood (arrows). (b) Axial MIP image shows wash out of contrast material from the vascular lesions and the lesions are similar in attenuation to splenic parenchyma. (c) Splenic arteriogram shows multiple splenic pseudoaneurysms (arrowheads) throughout the spleen. (d) Postembolization of the main splenic artery—no splenic pseudoaneurysms are seen.

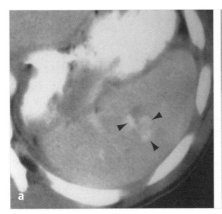
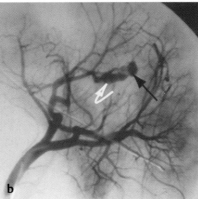

Fig. 15.6 Posttraumatic splenic arteriovenous fistula. (a) Axial image shows multiple vascular lesions (arrowheads) in the spleen. (b) Splenic arteriogram shows a splenic arteriovenous fistula (arrow). A large draining vein (curved arrow) is also seen. (Used with permission from Shanmuganathan K, Mirvis SE, Boyd-Kranis R, et al. Nonsurgical management of blunt splenic injury: use of CT criteria to select patients for splenic arteriography and potential endovascular therapy. Radiology 2000 Oct;217(1):75–82.)

combined with embolization during the early injury window to avoid deterioration of the patients and the need for emergency surgery while the patients await injury hemostasis.

Celiac angiography can be performed first, then with advancement of the catheter into the proximal splenic artery. Anteroposterior and oblique views are obtained to determine areas of bleeding. Two different types of embolization are available: central or peripheric. For central embolization, the optimal catheter placement, to avoid embolizing collaterals, is the main splenic artery. More advanced guide wire/microcatheter technology may be needed if a superselective technique is desired. The two main approaches, as mentioned, are proximal and distal embolization. Combined embolization can be performed in isolated instances of diffuse splenic injury combined

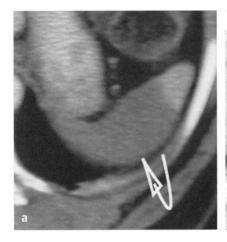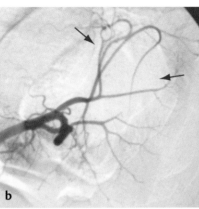

Fig. 15.7 Splenic infarct in a patient admitted following blunt force trauma. (a) Axial image shows a well-demarcated wedge-shaped low-attenuation area (curved arrow) in the posterior aspect of the spleen. (b) Splenic arteriogram shows lack of splenic artery branches in the mid and upper aspect of the spleen corresponding to the low attenuation area seen on computed tomography. (Used with permission from Shanmuganathan K. Imaging of abdominal trauma. In Mirvis SE, Shanmuganathan K, eds. Imaging in Trauma and Critical Care. Philadelphia, PA: Elsevier;2003:417.)

with a rapid peripheral bleeding vessel, but complication rates are much higher in these circumstances and should only be used on a case by case basis.

Main or proximal embolization was popularized by Scalfani and Scalea in the early 1990s. Different types of coils are placed in the proximal splenic artery while leaving the distal artery open to pancreatic and short gastric collateral blood flow. The decrease in the arterial pressure-head allows the injured vessels to clot while the organ is perfused by the lower pressure collateral system. Initially, large coils can be injected to allow nesting of multiple smaller coils to occlude flow. Ideally, this should be proximal to the dorsal pancreatic artery origin to maintain the collateral flow to the distal splenic artery. This is important given that the inferior pole of the spleen often may not remain viable if only short gastric vessels are patent. Advantages to this technique are ease and speed of embolization and a lower infarction rate in comparison to superselective techniques. This also has decreased costs because of shorter angiography suite duration and a lower utilization of specialized catheters and equipment. Another advantage in children is the decreased radiation exposure to the patient in central versus peripheral embolization. Although a trend toward improved splenic salvage was seen in our experience, this did not achieve statistical significance and has not been examined in other studies.

Superselective or distal embolization is used as the standard of care in many institutions. In some cases this is due to massive bleeding from a peripheral branch. However, the most frequent reason cited is to maintain immunocompetence of the injured spleen. The theory is that a limited infarct from the distal embolization ensures splenic function similar to splenorrhaphy if at least one-third of the organ remains. Immunocompetence differences following main or distal embolization have yet to be proven and no recommendations can be made based on current data. What is clear is that in cases of AVFs, superselective embolization is the only option. Failure rates exceed 50% if main artery embolization is used. Additionally, Gelfoam® pledgets recanalize in weeks or months. Therefore, theoretically, the AVF would recur upon recanalization.

15.7 Results

Success rates for splenic embolization vary from a low 89% to a high 97%. These rates vary based on institution screening

criteria, severity of splenic injuries, experience of the operators, and other factors.

15.8 Complications

Posttraumatic splenic infarct is a rare complication in 1.4% of patients with blunt splenic injury.[17] The segmental infarct typically involves 25 to 50% of the splenic parenchyma. The appearance on contrast-enhanced MDCT is a wedge-shaped area of decreased enhancement, with a well-defined margin, demarcating the infarct from the normal parenchyma. On delayed imaging, the infarct remains unchanged in size and enhancement.

The exact mechanism of splenic infarction after blunt trauma is not known. The typical angiographic findings of splenic infarction support an abrupt mechanical stretching of the splenic artery branches within the parenchyma at the moment of impact. This is likely to result in a focal intimal tear leading to thrombosis. The size of the infarct may vary depending on the amount of collateral flow to the spleen. Fortunately, the majority of splenic infarcts heal spontaneously without complications.[17] On follow-up MDCT, the majority of infarcts decrease in size or remain unchanged. Rare complications include delayed new areas of infarction, abscess formation, and delayed splenic rupture associated with a high rate of morbidity and mortality.[17]

In general, complications after splenic artery embolization are relatively common, seen in up to 32% of patients.[18] The majority of patients will have a low-grade fever and left-upper-quadrant pain and may require analgesics to relieve symptoms. Major complications occur in 19% of patients, and minor complications in 23% of patients.[18] Complications include hemorrhage, infarction, abscess formation, missed injuries, iatrogenic vascular injury, and coil migration.

Infarction occurs in 100% of patients after distal embolization and 63% of patients after proximal main artery embolization.[19] Infarcts after distal embolization occur just distal to the site of embolization and tend to be large (▶ Fig. 15.7). After proximal embolization, infarcts tend to be multiple, smaller, and located in the periphery of the splenic parenchyma (▶ Fig. 15.8). Most infarcts will decrease in size or remain unchanged and resolve without any sequelae.[19]

At UMSTC, the authors have observed development of persistent (▶ Fig. 15.9) or new splenic pseudoaneurysms following

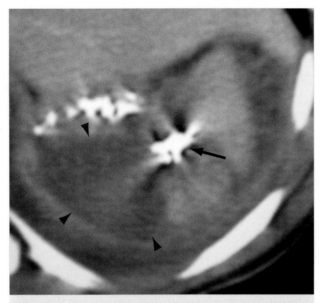

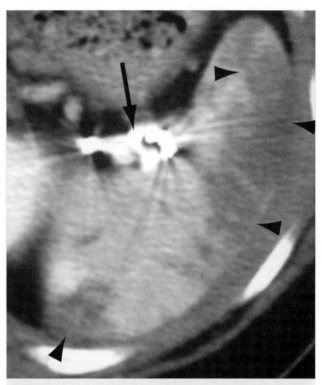

Fig. 15.8 Splenic infarct following distal embolization. Axial computed tomography image shows a large wedge-shaped area of infarction (arrowheads) distal to the embolization coil (arrow) seen within the splenic parenchyma.

Fig. 15.9 Infarction following main splenic artery embolization. Axial computed tomography (CT) image shows embolization coils (arrow) within the distal main splenic artery. Multiple small peripheral low attenuation lesions (arrowheads) represent areas of infarction.

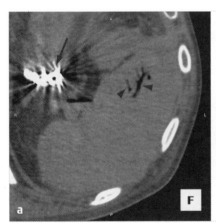

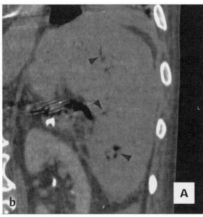

Fig. 15.10 Splenic necrosis following embolization. (a) Axial and (b) coronal reformatted images show embolization coils within the main splenic artery. The branching pattern of air (arrowheads) seen within the splenic parenchyma is concerning for necrosis.

main splenic artery embolization on follow-up MDCT. A study to determine the outcome and need for further management of these patients by Haan et al[2] was published. Splenic artery embolization was performed in 33% (130 of 400 patients) of hemodynamically stable patients with blunt splenic injury. Among the splenic artery embolization group, 32 (25%) of the patients had pseudoaneurysms (27 persistent and 5 new pseudoaneurysms) on follow-up MDCT. The nonoperative success rate and splenic salvage rate in patients with persistent pseudoaneurysms were 91% and 94%, respectively. The majority of these pseudoaneurysms resolved on follow-up imaging and did

well without the need for any additional intervention. We currently discharge these patients on hospital day 3 with precautions and without any further imaging.

Splenic gas may be seen within the parenchyma after embolization. A few bubbles of air may be introduced during the procedure. However, the presence of a branching pattern of air bubbles (▶ Fig. 15.10) within the parenchyma, air fluid levels within the subcapsular space, perisplenic pneumoperitoneum, or an increase in the amount of parenchymal air on follow-up MDCT may be cause of more concern. These findings may represent abscess formation or splenic necrosis.

References

[1] Marmery H, Shanmuganathan K, Mirvis SE et al. Correlation of multidetector CT findings with splenic arteriography and surgery: prospective study in 392 patients. J Am Coll Surg 2008; 206: 685–693

[2] Haan JM, Marmery H, Shanmuganathan K, Mirvis SE, Scalea TM. Experience with splenic main coil embolization and significance of new or persistent pseudoaneurym: reembolize, operate, or observe. J Trauma 2007; 63: 615–619

[3] Marmery H, Shanmuganathan K. Multidetector-row computed tomography imaging of splenic trauma. Semin Ultrasound CT MR 2006; 27: 404–419

[4] Miller LA, Shanmuganathan K. Multidetector CT evaluation of abdominal trauma. Radiol Clin North Am 2005; 43: 1079–1095, viii

[5] Federle MP, Yagan N, Peitzman AB, Krugh J. Abdominal trauma: use of oral contrast material for CT is safe. Radiology 1997; 205: 91–93

[6] Anderson SW, Varghese JC, Lucey BC, Burke PA, Hirsch EF, Soto JA. Blunt splenic trauma: delayed-phase CT for differentiation of active hemorrhage from contained vascular injury in patients. Radiology 2007; 243: 88–95

[7] Becker CD, Spring P, Glättli A, Schweizer W. Blunt splenic trauma in adults: can CT findings be used to determine the need for surgery? AJR Am J Roentgenol 1994; 162: 343–347

[8] Nastanski F, Cohen A, Lush SP, DiStante A, Theuer CP. The role of oral contrast administration immediately prior to the computed tomographic evaluation of the blunt trauma victim. Injury 2001; 32: 545–549

[9] Federle MP, Peitzman A, Krugh J. Use of oral contrast material in abdominal trauma CT scans: is it dangerous? J Trauma 1995; 38: 51–53

[10] Wing VW, Federle MP, Morris JA, Jeffrey RB, Bluth R. The clinical impact of CT for blunt abdominal trauma. AJR Am J Roentgenol 1985; 145: 1191–1194

[11] Davis KA, Fabian TC, Croce MA et al. Improved success in nonoperative management of blunt splenic injuries: embolization of splenic artery pseudoaneurysms. J Trauma 1998; 44: 1008–1013, discussion 1013–1015

[12] Gavant ML, Schurr M, Flick PA, Croce MA, Fabian TC, Gold RE. Predicting clinical outcome of nonsurgical management of blunt splenic injury: using CT to reveal abnormalities of splenic vasculature. AJR Am J Roentgenol 1997; 168: 207–212

[13] Jeffrey RB, Cardoza JD, Olcott EW. Detection of active intraabdominal arterial hemorrhage: value of dynamic contrast-enhanced CT. AJR Am J Roentgenol 1991; 156: 725–729

[14] Shanmuganathan K, Mirvis SE, Sover ER. Value of contrast-enhanced CT in detecting active hemorrhage in patients with blunt abdominal or pelvic trauma. AJR Am J Roentgenol 1993; 161: 65–69

[15] Smith JA, Macleish DG, Collier NA. Aneurysms of the visceral arteries. Aust N Z J Surg 1989; 59: 329–334

[16] Schurr MJ, Fabian TC, Gavant M et al. Management of blunt splenic trauma: computed tomographic contrast blush predicts failure of nonoperative management. J Trauma 1995; 39: 507–512, discussion 512–513

[17] Miller LA, Mirvis SE, Shanmuganathan K, Ohson AS. CT diagnosis of splenic infarction in blunt trauma: imaging features, clinical significance and complications. Clin Radiol 2004; 59: 342–348

[18] Haan JM, Biffl WB, Knudson MM et al. Western Trauma Association Multi-Institutional Trials Committee. Splenic embolization revisited: a multicenter review. J Trauma 2004; 56: 542–547

[19] Killeen KL, Shanmuganathan K, Boyd-Kranis R, Scalea TM, Mirvis SE. CT findings after embolization for blunt splenic trauma. J Vasc Interv Radiol 2001; 12: 209–214

16 Interventional Radiology in Abdominal Trauma: Liver

Charles A. Ehlenberger, Jaime Tisnado, and Jamie Tisnado

16.1 Introduction

Traumatic liver injury and how to treat it is an age-old problem. Descriptions of liver injuries can be found in Greek and Roman mythology.[1] Today the problem still exists. However, over the past three decades the management of liver and splenic trauma has undergone significant changes, a paradigm shift.[1,2,3,4]

The major change has been a shift from operative to nonoperative management of blunt hepatic trauma in such a way that nearly 80% of blunt hepatic injuries are now treated nonoperatively.[1,2,3,5,6,7] This is a major change because previously only ~30% were managed nonoperatively given the operative repair was the standard of care for both blunt and penetrating liver injury.

The surgeons' decisions were heavily based on hemodynamic stability of the patient. Stable patients after blunt trauma are managed nonoperatively after a computed tomography (CT) scan.[8] On the other hand, penetrating liver injuries are still mostly managed with emergent laparotomy, even if some studies have demonstrated the successful nonsurgical management of penetrating liver injuries.[9] Currently, the mortality for severe and complex injuries has been dramatically reduced.[1,2,5,10,11] The benefits of the conservative, nonoperative management include significantly decreased mortality rates, and also abdominal complications and blood transfusion requirements as well.[4]

These dramatic changes in the way that liver injuries are handled are due to marked improvements in diagnostic imaging (ultrasound [US] and CT), the widespread availability and performance of angiography and embolization, the use of noninvasive techniques for the management of complications, and an improved understanding of the natural history of liver injuries. Also marked improvements in surgical techniques have contributed to such good outcomes.

The exponential increase in the speed, accuracy, and widespread use of CT in trauma patients has greatly contributed to the aforementioned changes in management. Computed tomography defines pathologic anatomy, grades injury severity, quantifies hemoperitoneum, demonstrates the site(s) of active bleeding, and identifies associated injuries. Computed tomography is > 90% sensitive and > 90% specific for detecting liver and other abdominal organ injuries.[5,8] Multidetector CT scanners can easily differentiate between active ongoing bleeding and clotted blood and help the trauma team in deciding whether to send the patient to the operating room (OR) or to the interventional radiology (IR) suite or to simply observe the patient closely in a very conservative no-operational or interventional manner.

The other and arguably more important, from our perspective, contribution of radiology to the management of liver trauma is the ready availability and widespread management by the interventional radiologist with arterial embolization. Arterial embolization was described as early as the mid- to late-1970s for control of pelvic arterial hemorrhage.[12] With the development of catheters, microcatheters, wires, and different embolic agents, arterial bleeding now can rapidly be controlled from a percutaneous approach in up to 90% or more of cases.[2,4]

Interventional radiologic embolization can be performed either as a definitive procedure or as an adjunct to surgery.[10,12,13] The effectiveness and availability of IR in a 24/7 schedule allows for surgical management as a staged damage control procedure with an initial liver packing or suturing to control bleeding, followed by IR to control inaccessible, residual, or recurrent bleeding (▶ Fig. 16.1).[2,11]

Furthermore, IR has an essential role in the management of eventual complications of liver injuries. About half of the patients with a major hepatic trauma eventually develop trauma-related complications: IR is indispensable and the ideal method of choice in the care and management of most or all of these complications.[10] Some of these complications are delayed or recurrent hemorrhage; biliary complications such as biliary leaks, bilomas, hemobilia, etc.; also hepatic necrosis; hepatic abscess; other fluid collections in the liver; aneurysms and pseudoaneurysms, AVFs; and other less common complications.

16.2 Grading of Liver Injuries

Liver injuries on CT are graded according to the American Association for the Surgery of Trauma (AAST) organ injury scale (▶ Table 16.1). The scale is a formal grading system to anatomically describe the injuries and the assigned grade is based upon the most accurate assessment by CT, surgery, or autopsy. There are shortcomings to this grading system, as in other grading scales or systems, in that it does not determine the need for operative intervention. There may be major discrepancies between CT grading and the operative grading and it does not emphasize the presence or absence of active arterial bleeding at the time of the examination.[5,6,14]

16.3 Computed Tomography Findings

The main findings on CT include lacerations, subcapsular hematomas, parenchymal hematomas, contusions, active hemorrhage, hemoperitoneum, pseudoaneurysms, AVF, juxtahepatic venous injuries, periportal low attenuation areas, and a "flat" inferior vena cava (IVC), usually indicating hypovolemia.[15]

Lacerations are the most common parenchymal injuries. They are shown on CT as irregular linear or branching low-attenuation areas that can be superficial (< 3 cm) or deep (> 3 cm). Lacerations that extend to the porta hepatis are often associated with bile duct injuries and are most prone to complications ▶ Fig. 16.2).

Hematomas and contusions on CT are low-density areas with poorly defined and irregular margins. Acute hematomas are hyperdense (40–60 Hounsfield units [HU]) to normal liver parenchyma. Subcapsular hematomas are ellipsoid collections of variable density causing compression of the liver parenchyma.

Hemoperitoneum (blood in the peritoneal space) can be differentiated from other fluid collections by its density on CT. Clotted blood measures between 45 to 70 HU and unclotted

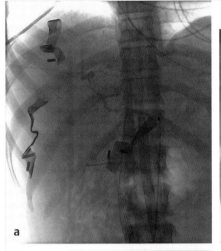
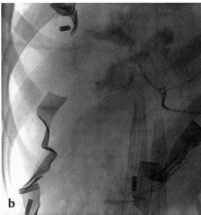

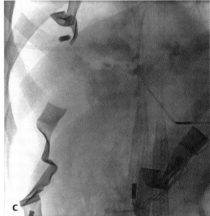

Fig. 16.1 Massive bleeding in the liver after severe blunt trauma to the abdomen and attempted surgical management with packing and suturing. (a,b) A selective hepatic arteriogram shows massive continued bleeding in the right lobe and center of liver. (c) After embolization with stainless steel coils of the entire right hepatic artery, there is no longer active bleeding. The hepatic arteries can be embolized with impunity, provided the portal vein is patent and no history of liver surgery is disclosed.

extravascular blood usually measures between 30 to 45 HU.[5,6] Computed tomography is great for assessment of the age of the hematoma as well. (▶ Fig. 16.3)

Active hemorrhage is identified as extravasation of contrast material, measuring between 91 to 247 HU (▶ Fig. 16.1, ▶ Fig. 16.3).[5,6] The extravasation may be free into the peritoneum or localized in a hematoma or pseudoaneurysm. Usually, the hemorrhage is arterial in origin, but also may be venous due to portal venous or hepatic venous sources. It is important to

mention that the absence of contrast material extravasation, besides the other CT findings of liver injury, does not exclude an active hemorrhage, which may have temporarily stopped. Rebleeding may occur as blood pressure is restored and vasoconstriction decreased with resuscitation; also there may be autologous lysis of clot.

Pseudoaneurysms, more common in penetrating trauma, often present as late complications as a relatively well-circumscribed collection of extravascular contrast material adjacent to an artery with varying degrees of surrounding clotted blood. Pseudoaneurysms are an important finding given that they can rupture and form an AVF and/or bile duct fistulas resulting in hemobilia and/or gastrointestinal (GI) bleeding.[5,6,10,12,14]

Major hepatic venous injuries should be suspected if lacerations or hematomas extend into major hepatic veins or the IVC.[5,6,14] These venous injuries can be severe and life threatening. At surgery, major hemorrhage can occur when the liver is mobilized in the presence of a major hepatic venous injury. In addition, these injuries are indirect indicators of active arterial bleeding. An IVC is termed "flattened" when the anteroposterior diameter of the IVC is about one-fourth of the transverse diameter when measured below the entrance of the renal veins, indicating hypovolemia and/or shock.[5,6,14]

Periportal low attenuation areas or edema have many causes. In proximity to a laceration or hematoma it may be due to blood tracking along the periportal tissues. This may also be caused by

Table 16.1 American Association for the Surgery of Trauma Liver Injury Scale

Grade	Features
I	Capsular avulsion Superficial laceration < 1 cm deep Subcapsular hematoma < 1 cm
II	Laceration 1–3 cm Subcapsular hematoma 1–3 cm
III	Laceration > 3 cm deep Central/subcapsular hematoma > 3 cm
IV	Central/subcapsular hematoma > 10 cm Lobar tissue destruction or devascularization
V	Bilobar tissue destruction or devascularization

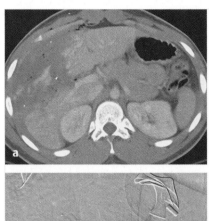

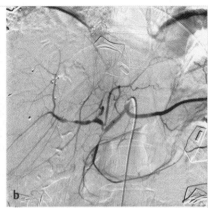

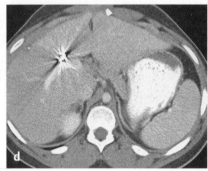

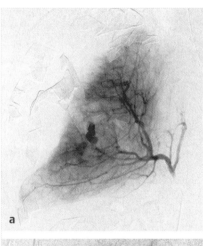

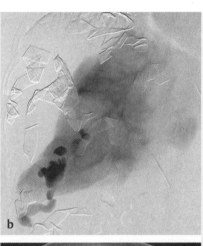

Fig. 16.2 The patient went to laparotomy for attempts at controlling hemorrhage. Thereafter, the patient came to the angiographic laboratory. (a) Extreme distortion of the liver parenchyma in this patient who sustained severe blunt trauma to abdomen. Grade IV liver lacerations are obvious in the computed tomography (CT) scan. (b) Celiac arteriogram as a "mapping" prior to embolization demonstrates diffuse and generalized spasm of hepatic arterial branches. Almost complete absence of lumen of proper and right hepatic arteries is noted. Complete transection of the right hepatic artery required occlusion. (c) After coil embolization of the right hepatic artery, no active extravasation is seen. The patient eventually did well and recovered. (d) Follow-up CT scan shows almost "normal" liver. The coils are causing some artifacts. Remarkable recovery is expected after complete embolization of liver parenchyma in patients with no liver disease besides the traumatic injuries because the liver has dual supply by hepatic arteries (20–25%) and portal vein (75–80%).

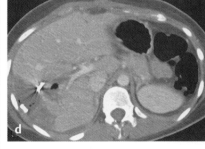

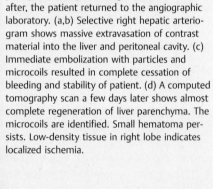

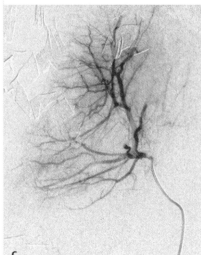

Fig. 16.3 A man sustained severe abdominal trauma in a car accident. Massive hepatic injuries prompted attempts at surgical control. Thereafter, the patient returned to the angiographic laboratory. (a,b) Selective right hepatic arteriogram shows massive extravasation of contrast material into the liver and peritoneal cavity. (c) Immediate embolization with particles and microcoils resulted in complete cessation of bleeding and stability of patient. (d) A computed tomography scan a few days later shows almost complete regeneration of liver parenchyma. The microcoils are identified. Small hematoma persists. Low-density tissue in right lobe indicates localized ischemia.

distension of the periportal lymphatics due to elevated venous pressures. There are also numerous other nontraumatic causes of this finding. Therefore, it is not specific for liver trauma.[5,6,14]

The management of the patient with traumatic liver injury begins in the trauma bay under the astute eyes of the trauma surgeon. Resuscitation begins with blood products and/or crystalloids and assessment of the hemodynamic condition of the victim. Hemodynamic stability is the only determining factor for nonoperative management.[2,4,5,6,11] The unstable patient that does not respond to resuscitative measures has "bought a ticket to the OR" whether the liver injury is blunt or penetrating. Penetrating trauma victims may not need operative management if they are stable and have no peritoneal signs, have a negative focused assessment with ultrasound for trauma (FAST) or CT .

A few of the shortcomings of the AAST Organ Injury Scale have been briefly described above. Attempts have been made to create a CT-based trauma classification system to guide management.[3,5,6] In an early attempt, Mirvis et al developed a CT-based classification system that was unable to predict the need for operative management.[16] Another study found that the CT findings of intraperitoneal contrast material extravasation and hemoperitoneum in the six abdominal compartments (bilateral subphrenic, Morrison pouch, right and left paracolic gutters, pouch of Douglas, and interloop spaces) were the most important independent risk factors in predicting the need for operative management.

If the CT findings do not warrant surgery, however subjective this decision may be, the next choice to make is whether a visit to IR is warranted. In the hemodynamically stable patients, indications for angiography include active contrast material extravasation on CT, decreasing Hb levels, and high grade (IV or V) liver injuries.[4,6] It has been advocated by some authors that all stable patients with high-grade (IV or V) liver injuries should undergo angiography.[4,11]

Those patients undergoing angiography for blunt hepatic trauma have a 20 × greater need for embolization when there are CT findings of active contrast extravasation versus those without this finding.[16] Alternatively, some studies have suggested that intraparenchymal contrast material pooling on CT can be managed with close observation. Angiography may be needed if there is a drop in hematocrit or increased transfusion requirements.[17]

Delay of angiography and embolization in favor of conservative management can result in increased transfusion requirements and the development of liver fluid collections. Conversely, angiography and embolization are not risk-free or noninvasive procedures, and are associated with serious consequences and complications.[10,12,18,19] Some of the complications are major hepatic necrosis, biliary complications such as biliary leaks, gallbladder necrosis, biliary stricture, abscess or other fluid collections, cholecystitis, aneurysms and pseudoaneurysms, contrast-induced nephropathy, AVFs, and complications of angiography at the access site.

16.4 Hepatic Angiography and Embolization

Hepatic angiography with embolization is beneficial in both blunt and penetrating liver trauma, and for those patients managed operatively and nonoperatively. There is a high (near 100%) success rate in controlling arterial hemorrhage with embolization. The identification of the location of injury and the site(s) of bleeding can be done with CT and this information should be used to plan the procedure and thereby reduce the exposure to radiation, and limit the volume of contrast material used. Computed tomography can noninvasively identify aberrant arterial anatomy that may be the source(s) of bleeding. It is imperative that the CT images be thoroughly reviewed by the interventional radiologist and all members of the trauma team (▶ Fig. 16.2, ▶ Fig. 16.3, ▶ Fig. 16.4)

An understanding of the vascular anatomy of the liver and some of the liver's unique characteristics is important prior to angiography. The classic anatomy indicates that the celiac axis arises from the aorta and branches into splenic, common hepatic, and left gastric arteries (▶ Fig. 16.2). The common hepatic continues into the gastroduodenal and proper hepatic arteries and the proper hepatic artery branches into the left and right hepatic arteries. However, this classic anatomy occurs only in ~ 55% or less of people.[20] The most common variant is a replaced or accessory right hepatic artery originating from the superior mesenteric artery, occurring in 10 to 20% of the people. Somewhat less common is a replaced or accessory left hepatic artery arising from the left gastric artery, the so-called left gastric–left hepatic trunk.

The liver receives a dual blood supply from the hepatic artery and portal vein in a roughly 25 to 30% and 70 to 75% contribution, respectively. This unique feature makes the liver remarkably tolerant to arterial embolization procedures. In reality, one can embolize completely the arterial supply to the liver with near impunity, provided no preexisting vascular or other pathology exists. However, the bile ducts are largely supplied by the hepatic arteries; therefore, arterial embolization may result in bile duct wall necrosis with subsequent bile leakage.[12,19,20]

Prior to the procedure pertinent laboratory values should be checked. Platelets ideally need to be > 50,000 and international normalized ratio (INR) < 1.5. However, in emergent situations deficiencies in coagulation parameters can be corrected with blood products. Coagulation parameters are important because many of the embolic agents require a functioning coagulation cascade to be effective.[20] The creatinine and estimated glomerular filtration rate (GFR) are important parameters to assess the risk of contrast-induced nephropathy. With a decreased GFR the patient can be given intravenous (IV) fluids with sodium bicarbonate to "protect" renal function and the operator should use the minimum volume of contrast material in the procedure. Other measures, like the use of Mucomyst (Bristol-Myers Squibb Co., New York, NY) have not been shown to reduce the risk of contrast-induced nephropathy. Liver enzymes and bilirubin may also be useful. An elevated bilirubin may be indicative of preexisting liver disease and may be predictive of an increased likelihood of complications after embolization.[21,22]

Access would normally be obtained in the common femoral artery. We routinely place a 5-French (F) sheath because multiple catheter exchanges may be necessary. However, the sheath can be withheld and the catheter placed directly in the vessel if there is concern for postprocedure bleeding. An aortogram is not needed given that the source of bleeding may often be determined on CT or from the surgeon's report. This saves on contrast given the patient may have already received up to

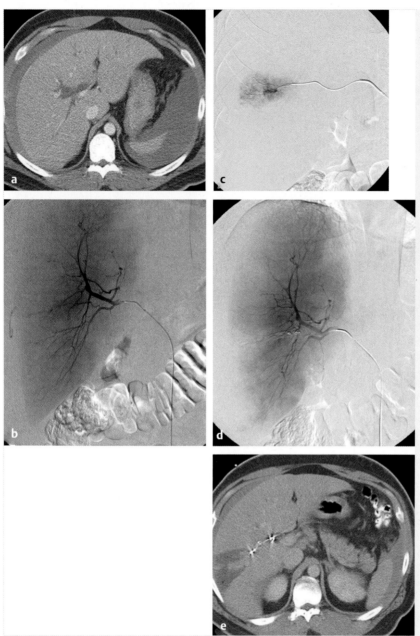

Fig. 16.4 A young patient with acute intra-abdominal bleeding after blunt trauma to the abdomen. (a) A computed tomography (CT) scan shows a large liver subcapsular hematoma and massive bleeding around the spleen. (b) Selective right hepatic arteriogram demonstrates active subcapsular bleeding in the midportion of the liver. (c) Superselective embolization with a coaxial system using a 5-French catheter and a microcatheter advanced well into the bleeding branch. (d) After microcoil embolization, there is no longer active bleeding and patency of almost all the hepatic artery branches. (e) Postembolization CT scan shows a small wedge-shaped defect in the right lobe of the liver.

150 mL of contrast material for CT. An aortogram may be necessary to locate bleeding from an accessory vessel like an inferior phrenic artery, but this is so rare that only mention is made here (▶ Fig. 16.4).

A 5-F RC-2 catheter is very effective for catheterizing the celiac axis. Alternately, a Simmons-1 catheter can be used. The only drawback with this catheter is the added step of forming the catheter. The celiac axis is usually found around the T12 level. Then a celiac arteriogram is performed for anatomy and to potentially identify the sources of bleeding. The arteries are usually small, constricted, and spastic due to hypotension and depleted intravascular volume. Vasospasm while advancing guidewires and catheters is rather common so a gentle technique with wire and catheter manipulation is recommended. Frequently, a microcatheter is advanced through the larger catheter to enable as selective an embolization as possible.

If a source of bleeding is not identified despite selective catheterization of branches, there are several possibilities. If no acute bleeding was noted on CT then there may, indeed, be no bleeding or there may be an accessory or replaced artery that is the source of the bleed. The most common accessory hepatic arteries arise from the superior mesenteric artery and the left gastric arteries.[20] Rarely, bleeding may be from the inferior phrenic artery and an aortogram may be needed to identify this culprit. Finally, if the IR suite has the appropriate equipment, cone beam CT may be of benefit in identifying the vessel that is bleeding.

Cone beam CT, also referred to as C-arm CT, is a helpful technique where the C-arm is rotated around the patient as the X-rays are emitted in a conical distribution. The setup, scanning, and image reconstruction time adds 5 to 10 minutes to the procedure. The technique is used successfully in identifying feeding arteries in transarterial chemoembolization (TACE) procedures

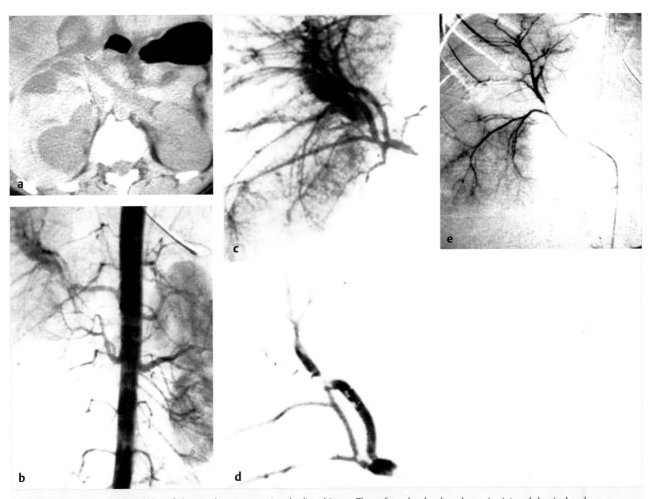

Fig. 16.5 A teen-aged girl with liver failure underwent transjugular liver biopsy. Thereafter, she developed massive intra-abdominal and retroperitoneal hematoma. Her hematocrit fell precipitously. (a) Computed tomography scan shows a right renal and retroperitoneal bleeding. (b) Emergency arteriography was then performed. The abdominal aortogram shows a large hepatic artery to portal vein arteriovenous fistula (AVF). (c) Selective arteriography shows the arterioportal AVF more clearly. (d) Superselective embolization of the hepatic artery branch supplying the AVF was easily done with a coaxial system using a 4-French catheter and a microcatheter. (e) Arteriogram after embolization shows successful occlusion of AVF.

and is more sensitive and specific than conventional digital subtraction angiography (DSA).[23,24] An additional 10 to 20 mL of contrast material is necessary for the procedure, depending on the vessel where the catheter tip is. This technique is especially useful in a patient that went directly to the OR and subsequently to the IR suite for embolization without ever having noninvasive imaging: US, CT, magnetic resonance imaging (MRI).

In general it is best to embolize as selectively as possible to decrease the risk of liver ischemia and to preserve patent arterial branches, which are important for the resorption of local contusion and hematoma.[18,25] The embolic agents we prefer are Gelfoam (Pfizer, New York, NY) mixed into slurry and microcoils. Other liquid agents, such as *N*-butyl cyanoacrylate and ethylene alcohol copolymer/Onyx, are available.[25] However, these agents are expensive, require significantly more time to set up than Gelfoam and coils, and have their own inherent risks and precautions. In general, these agents are not used for trauma embolization in our institution (▶ Fig. 16.5).

There is always a possibility of revascularization of the injured segment from distal branches, so ideally embolization should be done distal and proximal to the lesion.[26] This is

frequently not possible so we inject Gelfoam slurry for distal embolization and embolize proximally with microcoils and Gelfoam particles, a technique referred to as the "sandwich" technique (▶ Fig. 16.6,▶ Fig. 16.7,▶ Fig. 16.8).

An injury to the common or proper hepatic arteries can be embolized proximally and distally by the so-called sandwich technique; however, in these cases a covered stent deployment may be beneficial, if technically possible, to spare the arterial supply to the liver.[25] Ideally, embolization of the right hepatic artery should be done distal to the origin of the cystic artery to avoid the potential serious complications of cholecystitis, gallbladder rupture, and/or gallbladder infarction.[10,26]

It is obvious that angiography and embolization are not without risk (see above). As the grade of hepatic injury increases, so does the rate of complications with embolization.[10,19,25] One study has demonstrated an overall postembolization complication rate of 60% in treated grade III and higher injuries. Major hepatic necrosis occurred in roughly 40% of these patients and was more common in patients with higher grade of injury in penetrating trauma, and in those that had undergone operative management prior to embolization. Furthermore, the more

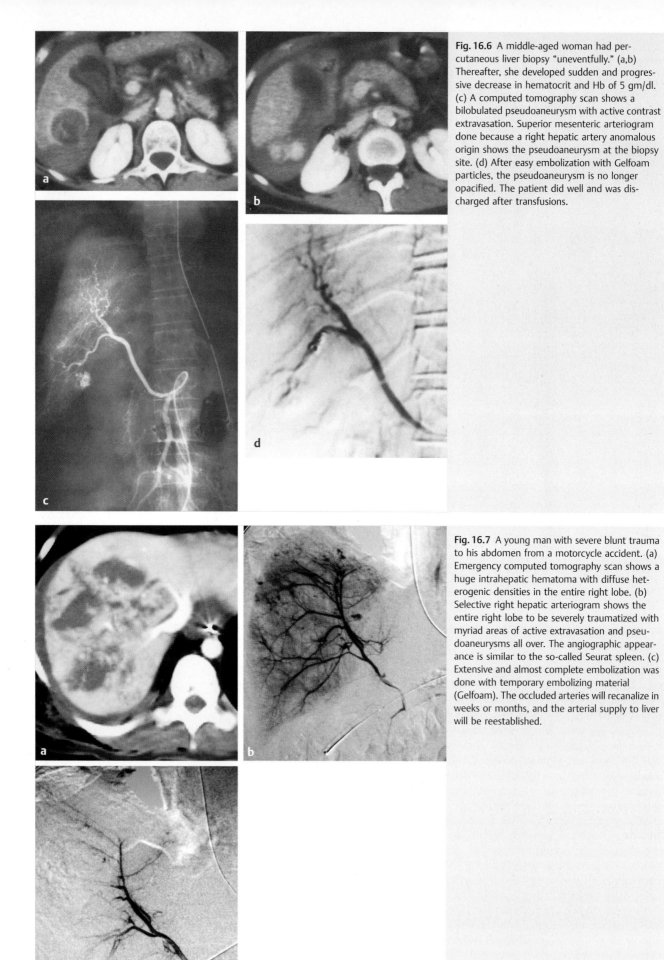

Fig. 16.6 A middle-aged woman had percutaneous liver biopsy "uneventfully." (a,b) Thereafter, she developed sudden and progressive decrease in hematocrit and Hb of 5 gm/dl. (c) A computed tomography scan shows a bilobulated pseudoaneurysm with active contrast extravasation. Superior mesenteric arteriogram done because a right hepatic artery anomalous origin shows the pseudoaneurysm at the biopsy site. (d) After easy embolization with Gelfoam particles, the pseudoaneurysm is no longer opacified. The patient did well and was discharged after transfusions.

Fig. 16.7 A young man with severe blunt trauma to his abdomen from a motorcycle accident. (a) Emergency computed tomography scan shows a huge intrahepatic hematoma with diffuse heterogenic densities in the entire right lobe. (b) Selective right hepatic arteriogram shows the entire right lobe to be severely traumatized with myriad areas of active extravasation and pseudoaneurysms all over. The angiographic appearance is similar to the so-called Seurat spleen. (c) Extensive and almost complete embolization was done with temporary embolizing material (Gelfoam). The occluded arteries will recanalize in weeks or months, and the arterial supply to liver will be reestablished.

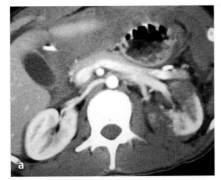

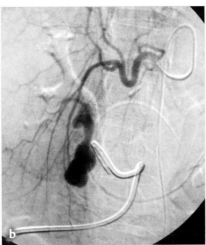

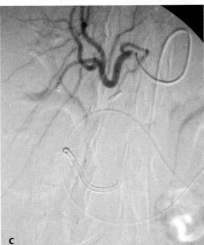

Fig. 16.8 A middle-aged woman underwent cholecystectomy followed by intra-abdominal bleeding and dropping hematocrit. (a) Computed tomography scan shows intra-abdominal bleeding and left renal infarctions. (b) Selective right hepatic arteriogram shows a large pseudoaneurysm from one of the right hepatic branches. The patient was hemodynamically unstable. (c) After selective embolization with particles of different size, the pseudoaneurysm is no longer seen. The patient became stable.

proximal the embolization or embolization of multiple foci also increased the risks. Necrosis can be suspected when the patients have fever, leukocytosis, and elevated lactate, bilirubin, and liver enzymes. Hepatic resection and debridement and/or multiple drainage procedures may be needed. Interestingly, the mortality from liver injury does not increase even if the patients develop major hepatic necrosis.[4,10,19]

16.5 IR Management of Liver Injury Complications

Interventional radiology also has a significant role in the management of complications related to the liver injury itself, as well as the surgical and postembolization complications.[1,2,3,5,10,11,12,14,19,26] With the increase in the nonoperative management of liver trauma there has been a concomitant increase in posttraumatic complications. Up to 25% of nonoperatively treated liver trauma patients require some intervention for complications.[2,5,10] The general rate of complications in major hepatic trauma is around 50%.[10] The panoply of complications that can occur in this setting include delayed hemorrhage, pseudoaneurysm, hemobilia, biloma, bile leak and bile peritonitis, abscess, abdominal compartment syndrome, hepatic necrosis, gallbladder necrosis and perforation, and cholecystitis, among others. [1,2,5,7,11]

16.5.1 Hemorrhage

Delayed hemorrhage can occur after embolization, surgical intervention, and as a direct complication of the injury.

Postsurgical hemorrhage may result after the packing material is removed, as part of a staged laparotomy.[11] A delayed hemorrhage after embolization often is a result of retrograde filling of a distal branch of an occluded vessel. A delayed hemorrhage from whatever source is amenable to repeat arterial embolization successfully.

16.5.2 Biliary Complications

Biliary complications in nonoperatively managed patients are common and reported in ~ 20%.[2] Distal bile leaks are frequently transient with no clinical sequelae. More proximal leaks may result in bilomas or bile peritonitis.[5,14] Bilomas can be identified easily with CT and US and are amenable to percutaneous drainage with either modality.[1,2,5,11,14] Bile peritonitis can be suspected clinically with fever, abdominal pain and tenderness, and leucocytosis. On CT imaging it will appear as increasing amounts of low attenuation fluid with enhancement and thickening of the peritoneum. If a bile leak is suspected, hepatobiliary scintigraphy (HIDA scan) is a useful imaging tool.[27] Bile leaks may require percutaneous biliary stenting and drainage if this cannot be done through endoscopic retrograde cholangiopancreatography (ERCP). Significant leaks have a protracted course and may require a month or more of percutaneous drainage(▶ Fig. 16.8).[10]

16.5.3 Hemobilia

Hemobilia is a rarer biliary complication. This was first described in 1654 by Francis Glisson, a 17th century English

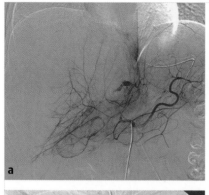

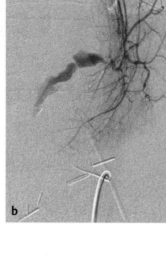

Fig. 16.9 (a,b) Massive active bleeding in the center of the liver after severe blunt abdominal trauma. (c) After selective embolization, there is no longer intrahepatic parenchymal bleeding.

physician who is also credited with the "discovery" of rickets.[12] It is due to the intrahepatic communication of a blood vessel, almost always arterial, and the biliary tree. The most common cause is iatrogenic following liver biopsy.[28] The incidence following trauma is low, around 3%.[2,28] It can produce abdominal pain, GI bleeding, and jaundice, if the bile ducts become obstructed by clot and debris. The clinical presentation may be immediate or delayed. Late presentation may be due to a hematoma or bilhemia that impairs liver healing, resulting in necrosis of the surrounding liver parenchyma and erosion into the bile ducts. Alternatively, a pseudoaneurysm may erode and rupture into an adjacent bile duct. The ideal treatment is with selective embolization of the offending vessel.[2,28]

16.5.4 Bilhemia

An even more esoteric biliary complication is bilhemia.[29] This consists of a fistula between a bile duct and a hepatic vein with subsequent flow of bile into the vascular system. This would present with elevated serum bilirubin and jaundice. Treatment consists of common bile duct stenting, which inverts the pressure between the bile ducts and suprahepatic veins and directs biliary flow away from the vein. Direct occlusion of the fistula via ERCP or angiography may also be possible. Interestingly, this entity is not seen in intubated patients.[1,29]

16.5.5 Pseudoaneurysms

Posttraumatic hepatic artery pseudoaneurysms are relatively rare with an occurrence of ~ 1%. They can occur immediately at the time of injury or be a delayed complication. They are also secondary to iatrogenic injuries after percutaneous and even transjugular liver biopsy. They are usually asymptomatic and discovered incidentally at follow-up CT or US. If symptomatic, they could present with abdominal pain, hematemesis, anemia, hypovolemia, and/or jaundice.[31] Potential serious complications include rupture with hemorrhage, fistula formation in the duodenum producing GI bleeding, and hemobilia if it decompresses into the biliary tree. It is its propensity to rupture that demands prompt therapy, once discovered (▶ Fig. 16.8 ▶ Fig. 16.9).[5,14,27,30,31]

Pseudoaneurysms can be treated radiologically with coil embolization, intravascular stent placement, and/or percutaneous thrombin injection. When embolizing with intravascular coils, it is important to embolize proximal and distal to the neck of the aneurysm to avoid retrograde filling of the sac (sandwich technique). Covered stent deployment across the neck of the pseudoaneurysm can spare embolization of the vessel. Noncovered stents can also be used, but will not necessarily thrombose the aneurysm. In this case a catheter or microcatheter can be introduced through the stent interstices and coils, Thrombin, or glues (cyanoacrylate) can be introduced to thrombose the pseudoaneurysm sac. A percutaneous approach can also be used if the pseudoaneurysm can be identified with US. Under US guidance, thrombin can be injected into the pseudoaneurysm in the same manner that femoral artery puncture pseudoaneurysms are treated.[5,31] Percutaneous thrombin injection however carries the risk of distal or peripheral embolization, particularly if the pseudoaneurysm neck is wide (▶ Fig. 16.10).

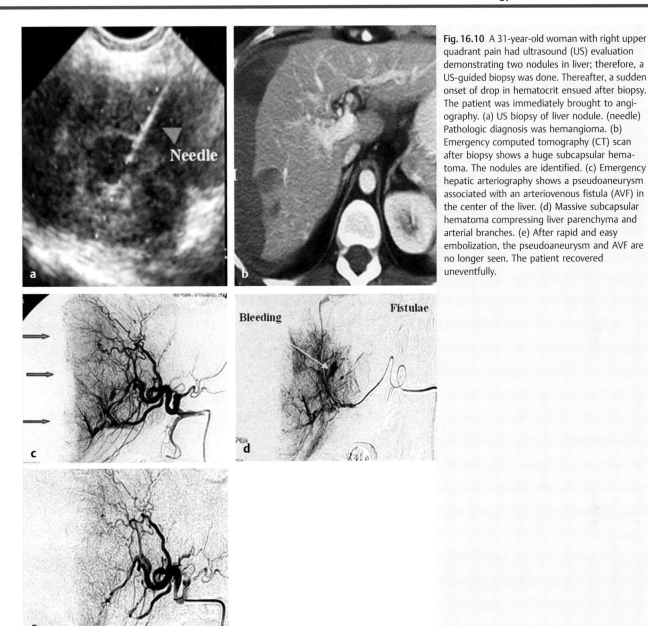

Fig. 16.10 A 31-year-old woman with right upper quadrant pain had ultrasound (US) evaluation demonstrating two nodules in liver; therefore, a US-guided biopsy was done. Thereafter, a sudden onset of drop in hematocrit ensued after biopsy. The patient was immediately brought to angiography. (a) US biopsy of liver nodule. (needle) Pathologic diagnosis was hemangioma. (b) Emergency computed tomography (CT) scan after biopsy shows a huge subcapsular hematoma. The nodules are identified. (c) Emergency hepatic arteriography shows a pseudoaneurysm associated with an arteriovenous fistula (AVF) in the center of the liver. (d) Massive subcapsular hematoma compressing liver parenchyma and arterial branches. (e) After rapid and easy embolization, the pseudoaneurysm and AVF are no longer seen. The patient recovered uneventfully.

16.5.6 Arteriovenous Fistula

Posttraumatic AVFs can occur between a hepatic artery and a hepatic vein or between a hepatic artery and a portal vein.[8,32,33] Hepatoportal AVFs are rare; clinically they present with postprandial pain, diarrhea, ascites, and bleeding varices.[32,33,34]

Approximately half of traumatic hepatoportal AVFs occur at the time of the injury and the other half due to a delayed rupture of a pseudoaneurysm. The symptoms are a result of portal hypertension due to the increased portal blood flow in the presence of normal portal vascular resistance. These lesions can be imaged with US and contrast-enhanced CT. On CT, hepatoportal AVFs appear as early enhancement of peripheral portal vein branches and transient wedge-shaped enhancement of a segment of liver parenchyma in the arterial phase.[35] The usual management consists of observation, surgery, and/or endovascular embolization. The supplying branch of the hepatic artery

can be embolized or a covered stent placed across the fistula. Observation would only be recommended in cases of small, intraparenchymal fistulas, as these may regress spontaneously (▶ Fig. 16.5).[32,33,35]

16.6 Conclusion

Hepatic arterial injuries commonly result from interpersonal violence and motor vehicle accidents. The liver is frequently injured, and the spleen is also commonly traumatized. CT scan is the primary evaluation of these patients (▶ Fig. 16.11)

The management of liver injuries has evolved dramatically, from surgery to a combined approach of surgery, IR, and observation. Interventional radiology is used as much as possible to avoid more complicated and risky surgery that may put the patient at more risk.

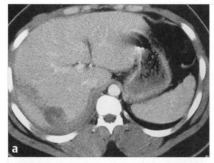
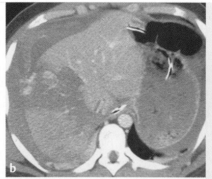
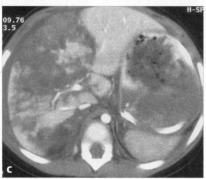
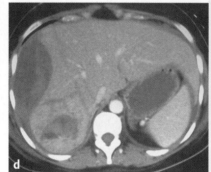

Fig. 16.11 Computed Tomography (CT) scan of different grades of liver injury. (a) Intraparenchymal hematoma with minimal amount of perihepatic fluid (blood). (b) Fracture of the right lobe of the liver with large amount of perihepatic blood and "blush" within the parenchyma, suggesting active bleeding. (c) Massive destruction of the right lobe of liver with multiple sites of bleeding. (d) Subcapsular hematoma of the right lobe of the liver (note compression of the adjacent liver tissue) and intraparenchymal hematoma at the lower portion of the right lobe.

References

[1] Lee SK, Carrillo EH. Advances and changes in the management of liver injuries. Am Surg 2007; 73: 201–206

[2] Piper GL, Peitzman AB. Current management of hepatic trauma. Surg Clin North Am 2010; 90: 775–785

[3] MacLean AA, Durso A, Cohn SM, Cameron J, Munera F. A clinically relevant liver injury grading system by CT, preliminary report. Emerg Radiol 2005; 12: 34–37

[4] Misselbeck TS, Teicher EJ, Cipolle MD et al. Hepatic angioembolization in trauma patients: indications and complications. J Trauma 2009; 67: 769–773

[5] Yoon W, Jeong YY, Kim JK et al. CT in blunt liver trauma. Radiographics 2005; 25: 87–104

[6] Fang JF, Wong YC, Lin BC, Hsu YP, Chen MF. The CT risk factors for the need of operative treatment in initially hemodynamically stable patients after blunt hepatic trauma. J Trauma 2006; 61: 547–553, discussion 553–554

[7] David Richardson J, Franklin GA, Lukan JK et al. Evolution in the management of hepatic trauma: a 25-year perspective. Ann Surg 2000; 232: 324–330

[8] Romano L, Giovine S, Guidi G, Tortora G, Cinque T, Romano S. Hepatic trauma: CT findings and considerations based on our experience in emergency diagnostic imaging. Eur J Radiol 2004; 50: 59–66

[9] Gonullu D, Koksoy FN, Ilgun S, Demiray O, Yucel O, Yucel T. Treatment of penetrating hepatic injuries: a retrospective analysis of 50 patients. Eur Surg Res 2009; 42: 174–180

[10] Mohr AM, Lavery RF, Barone A et al. Angiographic embolization for liver injuries: low mortality, high morbidity. J Trauma 2003; 55: 1077–1081, discussion 1081–1082

[11] Sriussadaporn S, Pak-art R, Tharavej C, Sirichindakul B, Chiamananthapong S. A multidisciplinary approach in the management of hepatic injuries. Injury 2002; 33: 309–315

[12] Petroianu A. Arterial embolization for hemorrhage caused by hepatic arterial injury. Dig Dis Sci 2007; 52: 2478–2481

[13] Lin BC, Wong YC, Lim KE, Fang JF, Hsu YP, Kang SC. Management of ongoing arterial haemorrhage after damage control laparotomy: optimal timing and efficacy of transarterial embolisation. Injury 2010; 41: 44–49

[14] Taourel P, Vernhet H, Suau A, Granier C, Lopez FM, Aufort S. Vascular emergencies in liver trauma. Eur J Radiol 2007; 64: 73–82

[15] Liu PP, Chen CL, Cheng YF et al. Use of a refined operative strategy in combination with the multidisciplinary approach to manage blunt juxtahepatic venous injuries. J Trauma 2005; 59: 940–945

[16] Mirvis SE, Whitley NO, Vainwright JR, Gens DR. Blunt hepatic trauma in adults: CT-based classification and correlation with prognosis and treatment. Radiology 1989; 171: 27–32

[17] Kozar RA, Moore FA, Moore EE et al. Western Trauma Association critical decisions in trauma: nonoperative management of adult blunt hepatic trauma. J Trauma 2009; 67: 1144–1148, discussion 1148–1149

[18] Monnin V, Sengel C, Thony F et al. Place of arterial embolization in severe blunt hepatic trauma: a multidisciplinary approach. Cardiovasc Intervent Radiol 2008; 31: 875–882

[19] Dabbs DN, Stein DM, Scalea TM. Major hepatic necrosis: a common complication after angioembolization for treatment of high-grade liver injuries. J Trauma 2009; 66: 621–627, discussion 627–629

[20] Hiatt JR, Gabbay J, Busuttil RW. Surgical anatomy of the hepatic arteries in 1000 cases. Ann Surg 1994; 220: 50–52

[21] Tan KK, Bang SL, Vijayan A, Chiu MT. Hepatic enzymes have a role in the diagnosis of hepatic injury after blunt abdominal trauma. Injury 2009; 40: 978–983

[22] Seamon MJ, Franco MJ, Stawicki SP et al. Do chronic liver disease scoring systems predict outcomes in trauma patients with liver disease? A comparison of MELD and CTP. J Trauma 2010; 69: 568–573

[23] Kakeda S, Korogi Y, Ohnari N et al. Usefulness of cone-beam volume CT with flat panel detectors in conjunction with catheter angiography for transcatheter arterial embolization. J Vasc Interv Radiol 2007; 18: 1508–1516

[24] Iwazawa J, Ohue S, Mitani T et al. Identifying feeding arteries during TACE of hepatic tumors: comparison of C-arm CT and digital subtraction angiography. AJR Am J Roentgenol 2009; 192: 1057–1063

[25] Lopera JE. Embolization in trauma: principles and techniques. Semin Intervent Radiol 2010; 27: 14–28

[26] Carrafiello G, Laganà D, Dizonno M, Cotta E, Ianniello A, Fugazzola C. Emergency percutaneous treatment in iatrogenic hepatic arterial injuries. Emerg Radiol 2008; 15: 249–254

[27] Fleming KW, Lucey BC, Soto JA, Oates ME. Posttraumatic bile leaks: role of diagnostic imaging and impact on patient outcome. Emerg Radiol 2006; 12: 103–107

[28] Schouten van der Velden AP, de Ruijter WM, Janssen CM, Schultze Kool LJ, Tan EC. Hemobilia as a late complication after blunt abdominal trauma: a case report and review of the literature. J Emerg Med 2010; 39: 592–595

[29] Struyven J, Cremer M, Pirson P, Jeanty P, Jeanmart J. Posttraumatic bilhe-mia: diagnosis and catheter therapy. AJR Am J Roentgenol 1982; 138: 746–747

[30] Ahmed A, Samuels SL, Keeffe EB, Cheung RC. Delayed fatal hemorrhage from pseudoaneurysm of the hepatic artery after percutaneous liver biopsy. Am J Gastroenterol 2001; 96: 233–237

[31] Francisco LE, Asunción LC, Antonio CA, Ricardo RC, Manuel RP, Caridad MH. Post-traumatic hepatic artery pseudoaneurysm treated with endovascular embolization and thrombin injection. World J Hepatol 2010; 2: 87–90

[32] Taourel P, Perney P, Bouvier Y et al. Angiographic embolization of intrahepatic arterioportal fistula. Eur Radiol 1996; 6: 510–513

[33] Tarazov PG. Intrahepatic arterioportal fistulae: role of transcatheter emboli-zation. Cardiovasc Intervent Radiol 1993; 16: 368–373

[34] Quiroga S, Sebastià MC, Moreiras M, Pallisa E, Rius JM, Alvarez-Castells A. Intrahepatic arterioportal shunt: helical CT findings. Eur Radiol 1999; 9: 1126–1130

[35] Ibn Majdoub Hassani K, Mohsine R, Belkouchi A, Bensaid Y. Post-traumatic arteriovenous fistula of the hepatic pedicle. J Visc Surg 2010; 147: e333–e336

17 Interventional Radiology in Abdominal Trauma: Vessels

Christopher J. Dente, David V. Feliciano, and Chad G. Ball

The management of injuries to the major retroperitoneal and portal vessels is a significant challenge to the trauma surgeon as many patients with such injuries present with signs of severe hemorrhagic shock. Classic operative management includes complete exploration with formal proximal and distal control of the injured vessels, followed by temporary intraluminal shunting, primary repair, reanastomosis or insertion of an interposition graft. These options remain appropriate for the vast majority of patients. In the past several decades, however, catheter-based techniques have been used occasionally as an adjunct in the care of these patients. This has been especially true in the management of injuries to vessels within solid organs such as the liver and the spleen, but the occasional patient with true abdominal vascular injury may benefit from the application of one or more of these techniques. Specifically, catheter-based techniques may be useful in patients who present acutely with vascular thrombosis rather than hemorrhage, and in addition, in patients who present with a delayed diagnosis of a vascular injury in the presence of a hostile abdomen. In this chapter, we will summarize the current literature on the use of catheter-based therapy in patients with true abdominal vascular injuries. The management of injuries to solid organs and of bleeding associated with pelvic fractures is covered elsewhere in the text.

17.1 Epidemiology

Abdominal vascular injury is rare in military conflicts because of the significant destructive power of military weapons. DeBakey and Simeone documented only 49 abdominal arterial injuries out of the 2,471 arterial injuries they described in World War II.[1] Similarly, abdominal vascular injuries only accounted for 2.3% and 2.9% of vascular injuries documented in the Korean and Vietnam wars, respectively.[2,3]

A large civilian series revealed a much different incidence of abdominal vascular injury. A 30-year review of vascular injuries treated at Ben Taub General Hospital in Houston documented that 33.8% of 5,760 cardiovascular injuries occurred in the abdomen.[4] Even with the recent decrease in the volume of penetrating trauma in some centers, many patients with abdominal vascular injuries continue to be treated. For example, there were 302 patients with 238 abdominal arterial and 266 abdominal venous injuries who underwent operative repair at the Los Angeles County Hospital (University of Southern California) from 1992 to 1997.[5] Similarly, there were 300 patients with 205 abdominal arterial and 284 abdominal venous injuries who underwent operative repair at the Grady Memorial Hospital (Emory University) from 1989 to 1998.[6]

At present, the incidence of injury to major abdominal vessels in patients sustaining blunt abdominal trauma is estimated to approximately 5 to 10%.[7,8] This is compared with patients with penetrating stab wounds to the abdomen, who sustain a major abdominal vascular injury ~ 10% of the time[9] and patients with gunshot wounds to the abdomen, who have injury to a major vessel 20 to 25% of the time.[10]

17.2 Definitions

The major sites of hemorrhage in patients sustaining blunt or penetrating abdominal trauma are the viscera, the mesentery, or the major abdominal vessels. Although any vessel in the abdomen can bleed, the term *abdominal vascular injury* generally refers to injury to major intraperitoneal or retroperitoneal vessels and may be classified as follows (with accompanying vessels):

- Zone 1: Midline retroperitoneum, supramesocolic
  - Suprarenal abdominal aorta, celiac axis, proximal superior mesenteric artery, proximal renal artery, and superior mesenteric vein
- Zone 1: Midline retroperitoneum, inframesocolic
  - Infrarenal abdominal aorta, infrahepatic inferior vena cava
- Zone 2: Upper lateral retroperitoneum
  - Renal artery, renal vein
- Zone 3: Pelvic retroperitoneum
  - Iliac artery, iliac vein
  - Portal-retrohepatic area
  - Portal vein, hepatic artery, retrohepatic vena cava

The magnitude of abdominal vascular injury is best described using the Organ Injury Scale of the American Association for the Surgery of Trauma (AAST).[5]

17.3 Pathophysiology

17.3.1 Blunt Injuries

Rapid deceleration in motor vehicle crashes may cause two different types of vascular injury in the abdomen. The first is avulsion of small branches from major vessels. A common example of this is the avulsion of intestinal branches from either the proximal or distal superior mesenteric artery at sites of fixation. A second type of vascular problem seen with deceleration injury is an intimal tear with secondary thrombosis of the lumen, such as seen in patients with renal artery thrombosis, or a full-thickness tear with a secondary pseudoaneurysm of the renal artery.[11,12,13]

Crush injuries to the abdomen, such as a lap seat belt or a posterior blow to the spine also may cause two different types of vascular injury. The first is an intimal tear or flap with secondary thrombosis of a vessel such as the superior mesenteric artery,[14] infrarenal abdominal aorta,[15,16] or iliac artery.[17,18] The "seat-belt aorta" is a classic example of an injury resulting from this mechanism.[15,19,20,21] Direct blows can also completely disrupt more anterior vessels, such as the left renal vein over the aorta[22] or the superior mesenteric artery or vein at the base of the mesentery,[23] leading to massive intraperitoneal hemorrhage, or even partly disrupt the infrarenal abdominal aorta, leading to a false aneurysm.[24,25]

17.3.2 Penetrating Injuries

Penetrating injuries, in contrast, create the same types of abdominal vascular injuries as seen in the vessels of the extremities, producing blast effects with intimal flaps and secondary thrombosis, lateral-wall defects with free-bleeding or pulsatile hematomas (early false aneurysms), or complete transection with either free bleeding or thrombosis.[26] On rare occasions, a penetrating injury may produce an arteriovenous fistula (AVF) involving the portal vein and hepatic artery, renal vessels, or iliac vessels.

Iatrogenic injuries to major abdominal vessels are an uncommon, but persistent problem. Reported iatrogenic causes of abdominal vascular injury have included diagnostic procedures (angiography, cardiac catheterization, laparoscopy), abdominal operations (pelvic and retroperitoneal procedures), spinal operations (removal of a herniated disk), and adjuncts to cardiac surgery (cardiopulmonary bypass, intra-aortic balloon assist).[27,28,29]

17.4 Role of Interventional Radiology

17.4.1 Intra-Abdominal Aorta

Patients with injury to the intra-abdominal aorta, especially after penetrating trauma, often present with hemorrhagic shock and free intraperitoneal hemorrhage. Alternatively, they may present acutely or in a delayed fashion with thrombotic sequelae. First described by Campbell in 1969,[30] seat-belt aorta describes acute aortic occlusion related to lap-belt injuries. These injuries may present acutely with signs of acute arterial insufficiency or they may present chronically with abdominal pain, claudication, and a decrease in peripheral pulses. In the past, the most common method of definitive management was insertion of an interposition prosthetic graft, although some injuries have been managed with endarterectomy and intimal suture. Others have recommended extra-anatomic bypass, especially in the face of concomitant injury to a hollow viscus.[31] In the past 15 years, endovascular techniques have also been described to address thrombotic complications of aortic injury in both the acute and chronic setting.

In 1997, Vernhet et al[32] described the management of three patients with acute infrarenal aortic dissection after trauma with percutaneous placement of a stent. These patients presented without obvious hemorrhagic shock and had varying degrees of arterial insufficiency. All were managed successfully in the early postinjury period with wallstents (Schneider wallstent; Schneider Stent Division, Pfizer, Minneapolis, MN) used to cover their intimal injuries, obliterate the dissections and restore perfusion. At 6-month to 2-year follow-up, no complications were noted.[32] Other groups have presented similar case reports and case series, with successful use of stents to restore perfusion after blunt aortic injury.[33,34]

In recent years, stent grafts have also been used to manage aortic trauma in both the acute setting and in more chronic situations, especially in patients with missed injuries and "hostile" abdomens. In 1997, a German group first reported the use of a self-expanding covered stent (Corvita S.A., Belgium) in a patient with a delayed presentation of aortic trauma after a motorcycle crash. The multiple-injured patient developed hemorrhagic shock 6 days after a laparotomy in which injuries to the small bowel, colon, liver, and spleen were managed. A computed tomography (CT) scan revealed a retroperitoneal hematoma, and an aortogram revealed hemorrhage from the infrarenal aorta into the retroperitoneum. The patient was managed with the emergent placement of a 28-mm endograft placed transfemorally. A wallstent was used proximally to ensure fixation due to the oversizing of the graft. After a 24-month follow-up, no graft-related complications were noted.[35]

More recently, Yeh et al[36] reported the use of a Zenith stent graft (Cook Group Inc, Bloomington, IN) in a patient 2 weeks after laparotomy for multiple gunshot wounds to the torso. This patient presented with abrupt onset of hemorrhage and hemodynamic instability in the face of matted viscera and a hostile abdomen. Attempts at open repair failed, and the patient was packed and brought to the interventional radiology (IR) suite where the stent graft was placed with successful cessation of hemorrhage. This patient survived a prolonged hospital course and was noted to have no aortic complications at a one-year follow-up. In 2005, Tucker et al[37] reported on a patient with a delayed diagnosis of a supraceliac aorta-inferior vena cava fistula managed with an AneuRx device (Medtronic, Minneapolis, MN) at 29 days postinjury. That same year, Waldrop et al[38] described another traumatic aortocaval fistula managed successfully with the same device in a patient diagnosed 18 days after injury. Finally, in a less acute setting, Teruya et al[39] reported the successful use of a 22-mm AneuRx device to relieve symptoms of hip and buttock claudication in a 26-year-old patient with documented infrarenal aortic stenosis 6 months after a motor vehicle collision.

Although the data on the use of interventional techniques in aortic injuries is clearly preliminary, with most reports involving isolated patients or small groups of patients, the IR or endovascular surgeon can clearly assist in managing several subsets of patients with aortic injuries, that is those who present acutely with dissections and thrombotic sequelae, those with missed injuries who present chronically with ischemic symptoms, and those who present subacutely with delayed hemorrhagic or pseudoaneurysmal complications in the presence of a hostile abdomen (▶ Fig. 17.1).

17.4.2 Inferior Vena Cava

Injuries to the inferior vena cava are generally the result of penetrating trauma and have been managed with many techniques including ligation in the infrarenal inferior vena cava. The practice of ligation in the damage control setting is surprisingly well-tolerated with few long-term sequelae if certain precautions are observed in the perioperative period. The first of these is to measure the pressures in the anterior compartments of the legs and to perform bilateral below-knee four-compartment fasciotomies at the first operation if the pressure is 30 to 35 mm Hg, depending on the patient's hemodynamic status. Bilateral thigh fasciotomies may be necessary as well within the first 48 hours after ligation. The second is to maintain circulating volume in the postoperative period through infusion of appropriate fluids. The third is to apply elastic compression wraps to both lower extremities and keep them continuously elevated for ~ 5 to 7 days after the operation. Patients should wear the wraps when they start to ambulate as well. If there is some residual edema, even with the wraps in place at the time of hospital discharge, the patient should be fitted with full-length, custom-made support hose. Although the majority of patients in the authors'

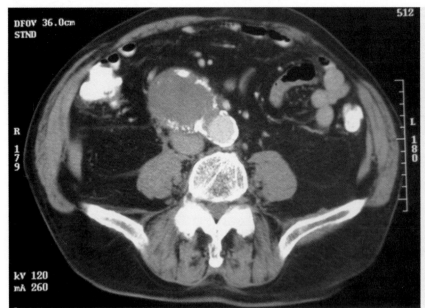

Fig. 17.1 Aortic pseudoaneurysm diagnosed 2 months after a motor vehicle collision. The patient's initial injury complex included a seatbelt sign. The pseudoaneurysm was repaired with an endostent. (Reprinted with permission from Dr. Mark T. Nutley, Assistant Professor, Department of Surgery and Interventional Radiology, Laval University and Dr. Randy D. Moore, Assistant Professor, Department of Vascular Surgery, University of Calgary)

experience will have no or minimal long-term edema, there have been occasional reports of severe edema in the postoperative period, which has required later interposition grafting.

In the last few years, several reports have described the use of IR techniques to assist in the management of these complex injuries. Castelli et al[40] reported on a patient who presented with hemorrhagic shock 4 hours after a motor vehicle collision. Computed tomography angiography (CTA) revealed an injury to the vena cava at the confluence of the iliac veins. In the IR suite, a Gore Excluder stent graft was used (W.L. Gore, Flagstaff, AZ) to control hemorrhage from the injury. The duration of the procedure was 9 minutes. Unfortunately, the patient died of a severe traumatic brain injury on posttrauma day 2. Two other case reports describe a similar management technique.[41,42] Clearly, in the right institution, the technology is available to perform these procedures expeditiously, and this technique may benefit a small group of patients. One concern over placing stent grafts in the venous system is a question of durability and the ability to administer postoperative anticoagulation. Stent grafts are felt to be highly thrombogenic in the first month, and it is unknown whether their insertion in major venous structures will require routine postoperative anticoagulation. This may limit the use of this technique in the multiply-injured patient.

17.4.3 Celiac Axis

Injury to the main celiac axis is rare. One of the largest series in the literature, reported by Asensio et al[43] described only 13 patients with this injury. Penetrating injuries were the cause in 12 patients, and overall mortality was 62%. Eleven patients were treated with ligation and 1 with primary repair, with the final patient exsanguinating prior to therapy. Of the five survivors, four had undergone ligation. All deaths occurred in the operating room. This group also performed an extensive literature review and could only document 33 previously reported cases, all the result of penetrating trauma. Furthermore, they could find no survivor treated with any sort of complex repair.[43]

While there are no reports of the use of endovascular techniques for an injury to this vessel, several authors have reported the use of endovascular techniques in the management of spontaneous celiac dissections and aneurysms.[44] Whether this can be extrapolated to the trauma patient, most of whom are younger, healthier and with longer life expectancy, is unknown.

Branches of the celiac axis may be amenable to endovascular techniques (▶ Fig. 17.2). Splenic and hepatic artery injuries are covered elsewhere in this text. Successful embolization of a left gastric artery pseudoaneurysm after blunt abdominal trauma has been reported.[45]

17.4.4 Superior Mesenteric Artery

Injury to the superior mesenteric artery is fortunately rare, with most cases being the result of penetrating trauma. In 1972, Fullen et al[46] described an anatomical classification of injury that continues to be used today. Fullen zone I injuries occur beneath the pancreas and are very difficult to access without division of the overlying pancreatic parenchyma. Fullen zone II injuries occur just below the pancreas, at the base of the transverse mesocolon. Fullen zone III injuries are those beyond the middle colic branch, and zone IV occur at the level of the enteric branches. Even in the modern trauma center, mortality rates range from 40 to 50% after this uncommon injury, with patients sustaining Fullen zone I or II injuries faring even less well. Because most of these patients present with severe shock and because there is concomitant need to evaluate intestinal viability, endovascular management of traumatic injuries to the superior mesenteric artery has not been described and is likely unwise. This remains fundamentally different from patients with intestinal angina secondary to stenosis of their superior mesenteric artery (▶ Fig. 17.2, ▶ Fig. 17.3).

17.4.5 Renal Arteries

Renovascular injuries are difficult to manage operatively, especially when the renal artery is involved. It is an extraordinarily

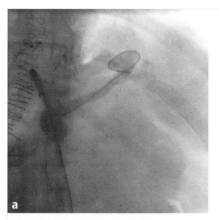

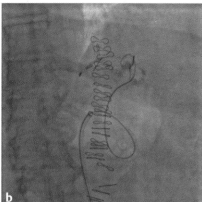

Fig. 17.2 (a) Celiac axis aneurysm extending into the proximal splenic artery after a motor vehicle collision. (b) The injury was treated with a covered stent. (c) Post deployment.

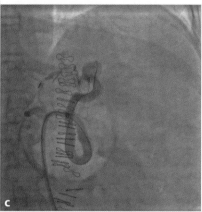

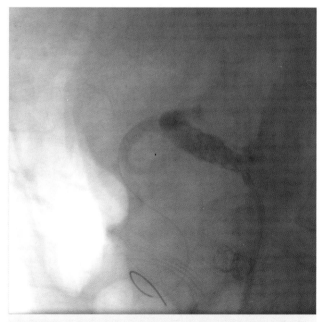

Fig. 17.3 Treatment of superior mesenteric artery stenosis with an expandable metal stent. (Reprinted with permission from Dr. Mark T. Nutley, Assistant Professor, Department of Surgery and Interventional Radiology, Laval University)

small vessel that is deeply embedded in the retroperitoneum. Standard operative techniques for repair, including lateral arteriorrhaphy and end-to-end anastomosis have been used with some success, although more complex repairs with interposition grafts have waned in popularity due to the poor function of most of the kidneys salvaged with this method.

Diagnosis of patients with blunt injury to the renal artery is more difficult than in those patients with penetrating mechanisms. Intimal tears in the renal arteries may result from deceleration in motor vehicle crashes, automobile–pedestrian accidents, and falls from heights. These usually lead to secondary thrombosis of the vessel and complaints of upper abdominal and flank pain as previously noted. One older literature review noted that only 30% of patients with intimal tears in the renal arteries had gross hematuria, 43% had microscopic hematuria, and 27% had no blood in the urine.[47] Hence, the diagnosis may be missed, because a CT scan may not be performed expeditiously in a stable patient with normal abdominal examination.

If a CT scan documents occlusion of a renal artery (▶ Fig. 17.4), the surgeon must decide on the need for intervention. The time interval from the episode of trauma appears to be the most critical factor in saving the affected kidney. In one study, there was an 80% chance of restoring some renal function at 12 hours, but this dropped to 57% at 18 hours after the onset of occlusion.[47] In a recent series, only two of five kidneys were salvaged after attempted revascularization, with one early salvage requiring a late nephrectomy at 6 months for severe hypertension, leading to a long-term salvage rate of only one kidney (20%). Of interest, only three of seven patients not undergoing revascularization required late nephrectomy.[13]

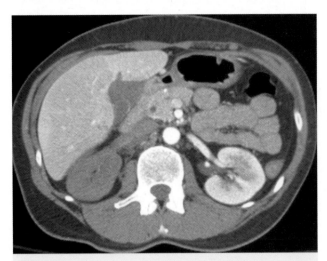

Fig. 17.4 Occlusion of the right renal artery following a motor vehicle collision.

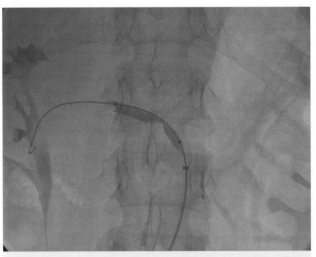

Fig. 17.5 Balloon dilatation of a stenosed renal artery following a remote renal artery repair for blunt trauma. (Reprinted with permission from Dr. Mark T. Nutley, Assistant Professor, Department of Surgery and Interventional Radiology, Laval University)

Because of the relatively poor function of kidneys revascularized with open surgery, multiple authors have described endovascular management of injuries to the renal vasculature. Renal arteries and major branches have been embolized back into the 1980s with good renal preservation. For example, Sclafani et al[48] reported on eight patients with renal injuries that were treated with angiographic embolization. The injuries were the result of stab wounds in five patients, blunt trauma in two patients, and a gunshot wound in one patient. Angiographic findings included two pseudoaneurysms, two AVF, two arteriocalyceal fistulas, and one renal artery-pleural fistula. Of interest, seven of eight patients had successful procedures, and all seven had preservation of the kidney, with one nephrectomy performed for persistent hematuria. A more recent study revealed renal vascular injury in eight patients, of which seven were successfully treated with angiographic embolization, obviating the need for open surgery. At discharge, all survivors had normal renal function (serum creatinine 0.6–1.3 mg/dL) and all patients were normotensive.[49] Thus, in the hemodynamically normal patient, transcatheter embolization has been used successfully to manage a variety of renovascular injuries and allow for organ preservation.

In more recent years, with improving technology, there has been an increased interest in preserving blood flow to the renal parenchyma with the use of expandable stents rather than transcatheter embolization. In 1994, Whigham et al[50] used a Palmaz stent (Johnson & Johnson Interventional Systems, Warren, NJ) to successfully obliterate an intimal defect in the right renal artery of a patient who had fallen 30 feet. The defect was located 2 cm from the ostium and the patient had preserved renal function and resolution of his hematuria. He was noted to have peripheral renal infarcts on a CT scan done 11 days after injury, although his urine output and renal function appeared normal. The patient was treated with aspirin postprocedure, but no long-term follow-up was reported.

A Palmaz stent was also used by Lee et al[51] to manage a 22-year-old man with a right renal artery intimal flap after a fall with preservation of renal function and no early complications.

More recently, Villas et al[52] reported on a patient managed with a wallstent after sustaining a large right renal artery intimal flap after a fall. The patient maintained normal renal function and blood pressure during her early postprocedure course and was discharged without complication.

Balloon angioplasty is also a viable option for patients who return with stenosed renal arteries following previous renal artery repairs (▶ Fig. 17.5). This technique allows dilation of the vessel and return of blood flow.

In summary, because of the poor renal salvage rates after blunt occlusion of the renal artery discussed above, there is decreasing interest in surgical revascularization especially after a delayed diagnosis or in a patient with a unilateral injury. Some of these patients may be candidates for interventional procedures in an effort to preserve renal parenchymal function. Obviously, patients with bilateral renal artery injuries or those with injuries to a solitary kidney should be treated aggressively to prevent the need for chronic hemodialysis. In addition, prolonged follow-up is appropriate for all patients with renal artery injuries, given that some will develop hypertension.[13]

17.4.6 Iliac Arteries

Hemorrhage, in the pelvic retroperitoneum, is notoriously difficult to manage operatively, especially in a male patient. The majority of injuries to the iliac vessels reported in a major series are the result of penetrating trauma. It is of interest, however, that major blunt abdominal trauma or pelvic fractures, particularly of the open type, have become a more frequent cause of occlusion or laceration of the iliac arteries than previously noted (▶ Fig. 17.6).[17,18,19]

Penetrating injuries to the common or external iliac artery require restoration of flow to the extremity and should be repaired or temporarily shunted at operation, if at all possible (▶ Fig. 17.7). The use of endovascular techniques in this location has been reported as well. Ligation of either vessel in the hypotensive patient will lead to progressive ischemia of the lower extremity and the need for a high above-knee amputation or a

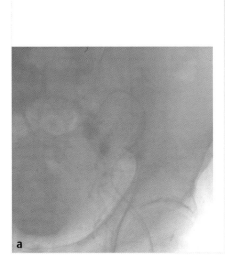
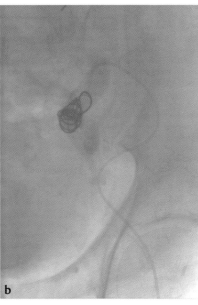

Fig. 17.6 (a) Angiographic embolization of a bleeding internal iliac artery after a motor vehicle collision. (b) Coil deployment. (Reprinted with permission from Dr. Mark T. Nutley, Assistant Professor, Department of Surgery and Interventional Radiology, Laval University)

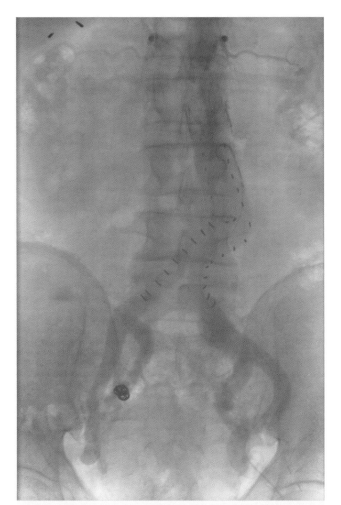

Fig. 17.7 Acute aortic injury extending into the iliac artery treated with an endovascular bifricated stent graft. Concurrent hemorrhage from the right internal iliac artery was arrested with embolization. (Reprinted with permission from Dr. Mark T. Nutley, Assistant Professor, Department of Surgery and Interventional Radiology, Laval University)

hip disarticulation in the later postoperative course. In fact, ligation of these vessels in World War II led to amputation rates of ~ 50%. Furthermore, in a large review by Burch et al[53] in the 1980s, mortality associated with this technique was 90%. In recent years, the insertion of temporary intraluminal shunts has been used in unstable patients, while options in the more stable patient include the following: lateral arteriorrhaphy, completion of a partial transection and end-to-end anastomosis, resection of the injured area and insertion of a saphenous vein or polytetrafluoroethylene (PTFE) graft, mobilization of the ipsilateral internal iliac artery to serve as a replacement for the external iliac artery, or transposition of one iliac artery to the side of the contralateral iliac artery for wounds at the bifurcation. Many of these techniques are difficult, and extensive injuries to the common or external iliac artery in the presence of significant enteric or fecal contamination in the pelvis remain a serious problem for the trauma surgeon. Both end-to-end repairs and vascular conduits in this location have been followed by the development of a postoperative pseudoaneurysm and even blowouts secondary to pelvic infection from the original intestinal contamination. In such a situation, extra-anatomical bypass has been performed traditionally, although endovascular techniques may provide an alternative modality for management.

Blunt trauma to the iliac arteries is much less common because they are protected by the bony pelvis and lie deep in the retroperitoneum. These injuries may be the result of direct compressing forces of the artery against the bony pelvis or the result of a shearing injury causing an intimal flap. Some patients have also been noted to have significant atherosclerotic disease at the site of injury; therefore, plaque rupture may play a role in this injury complex. In a review of such injuries, Lyden et al[54] reported that 12 were the result of motor vehicle collisions, seven occurred after crush injury and three others were the result of two falls and one motorcycle collision. Multiple management paradigms have been used in this rare injury complex including interventional techniques. These seem especially appropriate given the patients generally present with thrombotic manifestations and not active hemorrhage and may have concomitant enteric contamination.

One of the earliest descriptions of endovascular management of traumatic aortoiliac disease was reported by Parodi in 1993.[55] Building on his experience with stent-graft management of aortic aneurysmal disease, the management of arteriovenous fistulas in the iliac system was described in seven patients with up to 14-month follow-up and 100% technical success. In this study, PTFE grafts combined with Palmaz stents were used to repair the injured arterial wall under fluoroscopic guidance.[55]

In more recent years, several authors have reported on the use of stent grafts in traumatic iliac thrombosis. In 1997, Lyden et al[54] used a 10 × 60 mm Smart Stent (Cordis Endovascular, Miami, FL) to manage a common iliac artery dissection and thrombosis after a motor vehicle collision. They were able to restore flow within 4 hours of injury, and while the patient had an excellent short-term result, he expired on hospital day 6 with a severe traumatic brain injury. Marin et al[56] also successfully managed several traumatic vascular injuries with stent grafts, including one injury to the common iliac artery, with patency documented at 2 months.

One of the largest series of nonthoracic vascular injuries managed with covered stents in the literature was published in 2006.[57] In this multicenter trial, 62 patients were managed with wallgraft endoprosthesis grafts over 6 years. This included 33 patients with injuries to the iliac vessels, most of which were iatrogenic in nature, and included 27 perforations, 4 arteriovenous fistulas, 1 pseudoaneurysm, and 1 dissection. Technical success, as defined by total postprocedure exclusion, was achieved in all but one patient with an iliac injury and primary patency at one year was 76% for these patients. Adverse events occurred early in 14% of patients, mostly related to puncture site complications, and a late adverse event occurred in another 6.5% of patients with one systemic infection, one occlusion and three stenoses of the repair. All-cause mortality was 6.5% in the early postprocedure period and 17.7% in later follow-up. None of the deaths was thought to be the result of the stent graft.[57]

Therefore, in reviewing the literature on interventional techniques as a mode of therapy in traumatic iliac vascular injuries, one comes to the conclusion that improving technology and techniques may have an expanding role in the management of such injuries in the future. Unfortunately, long-term follow-up data are nonexistent; therefore, it is unknown whether endovascular prosthesis will be subject to the same risk of contamination and failure that has been seen with prosthetic material placed surgically.

17.4.7 Lumbar Arteries

A lumbar artery pseudoaneurysm is a known sequela of penetrating retroperitoneal trauma. Such an injury may present as a pulsatile mass in the back with an audible bruit or palpable thrill. It may also present as unexplained back pain related to compression of a lumbar nerve root. As the diagnosis is often delayed, endovascular management is preferred with embolization being a well-described therapy.[58,59] Embolization should be performed as close as possible to the neck of the aneurysm to avoid backfilling of the aneurysm from collaterals, as well as to avoid occlusion of the collateral circulation to the spinal cord. Pseudoaneurysm occlusion may also be performed by a direct

posterior percuateneous approach under angiographic and CT guidance.[60]

17.5 Special Issues

17.5.1 Remote Aortic Occlusion

Patients with abdominal vascular injury often present in extremis, which may preclude management of the injury by percutaneous techniques. In the past, some groups have advocated thoracotomy to obtain proximal aortic control in the chest prior to laparotomy.[61] This technique has the disadvantage of opening another body cavity and does not prevent exsanguination from backbleeding in the abdomen while the thoracotomy is performed. In the past decade, remote aortic occlusion via a percutaneous approach has been described by multiple authors. This technique was actually used as far back as the Korean War in three soldiers who presented in hemorrhagic shock from penetrating truncal trauma.[62] In more recent years, it has been described for use in patients with ruptured abdominal aortic aneurysms from both a femoral and a brachial approach, with experienced centers quoting balloon placement in 5 minutes or less.[63] This technique may have some applicability, in experienced hands, in trauma patients with suspected major vascular injury and may have less morbidity than a thoracotomy; however, experience remains preliminary. To prevent any delays, an insititution should have immediate endovascular capability in the operating room (OR) with a fluoroscopic C-arm and have physicians and support staff who are well versed in the technique. Lacking this, standard maneuvers should be performed to obtain proximal control of the aorta in the abdomen either involving a formal left medial visceral rotation or immediate control of the supraceliac aorta at the hiatus via the midline.

17.6 Technical Issues

Although a thorough review of the technical aspects of abdominal aortography and interventional techniques is beyond the purview of this chapter, some comments regarding emergent use of interventional procedures in this critically ill population are warranted.

An institution interested in having an interventionalist participate in the care of the critically injured patient should, at a minimum, have the following: an endovascular team immediately available, an OR with full radiographic capabilities (fixed installation or mobile C-arm), and a full complement of guidewires, catheters, balloons, self-expanding and balloon-expandable stents and multiple sizes and configurations of stent grafts.[64] The team should include an endovascular surgeon or interventional radiologist and include nurses and technologists familiar with the equipment and techniques. Experienced endovascular colleagues are particularly crucial in treating long-term complications (▶ Fig. 17.8), as well as advanced maneuvers (▶ Fig. 17.9). The OR should have advanced fluoroscopy capabilities and the means to perform power injection of contrast.

17.7 Iatrogenic Injuries

Interventional techniques are often very useful in the management of iatrogenic injuries to the major abdominal vessels.

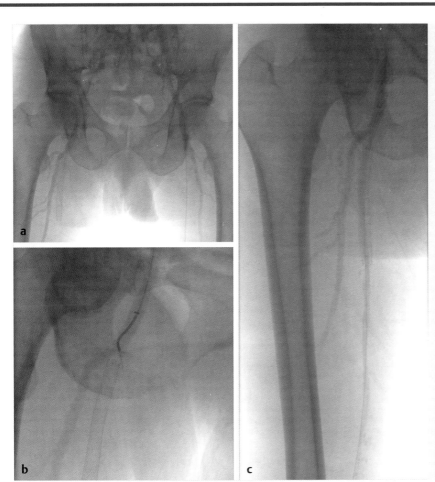

Fig. 17.8 Recanulation and angioplasty of an occluded superficial femoral artery stent initially placed after a motor vehicle collision. (a) Occluded superficial femoral artery. (b) Stent deploymenet. (c) Post deployment. (Reprinted with permission from Dr. Mark T. Nutley, Assistant Professor, Department of Surgery and Interventional Radiology, Laval University)

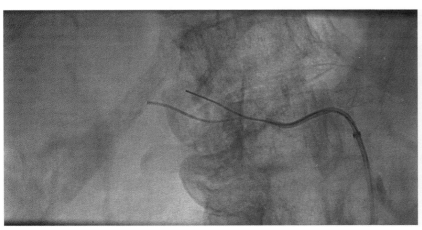

Fig. 17.9 Double-wire technique used to protect arterial branches distal to a balloon angioplasty or stent.

Several large series have been published in recent years, documenting the management of patients with a wide variety of complications. In 2003, Batlacioglu et al[65] reported on 17 patients who underwent stent-graft repair of iatrogenic vascular lesions, several of which involved the aortoiliac system. Injuries included eight AVF, six pseudoaneurysms, and one rupture. Technical success was achieved in all patients, and at a mean 8-month follow-up, no stent-graft related complications were noted. More recently, Makar et al[66] reported on the endovascular management of a patient where massive bleeding was encountered during a hip arthroplasty. Initial tamponade was achieved with a Sengstaken-Blakemore tube placed into the depths of the wound, and the patient was transferred to the IR suite and an angiogram revealed an injury to the external iliac artery which was successfully managed with a Jostent (Abbott Laboratories, Abbott Park, IL). Normal perfusion was restored to the extremity with no further bleeding during the hospital stay.

Thus, an immediately available endovascular surgeon or experienced interventional radiologist may be able to assist in the management of iatrogenic abdominal vascular complications and preclude the need for an additional operative procedure.

17.8 Conclusion

Abdominal vascular injuries are commonly seen in patients with penetrating wounds to the abdomen. Various blunt mechanisms, however, may also be the cause, and symptoms of a major vascular injury may occur in a delayed fashion. Contained injuries to the major abdominal vasculature, after penetrating trauma, may also be missed at the initial laparotomy. Although the majority of patients will present with exsanguinating hemorrhage and are best treated with expeditious laparotomy and formal vascular exploration and repair, a smaller subset of patients may present with injuries amenable to interventional techniques. They generally present with thrombotic manifestations of injury or with contained injuries or possibly in a delayed fashion in the presence a hostile abdomen. With the appropriate institutional support, the experienced endovascular surgeon or interventional radiologist may be a tremendous asset in the care of these patients. Using these concepts, certain critically ill patients with major abdominal vascular injuries can be salvaged without operation.

References

[1] Debakey ME, Simeone FA. Battle injuries of the arteries in World War II: An analysis of 2,471 cases. Ann Surg 1946; 123: 534–579

[2] Hughes CW. Arterial repair during the Korean war. Ann Surg 1958; 147: 555–561

[3] Rich NM, Baugh JH, Hughes CW. Acute arterial injuries in Vietnam: 1,000 cases. J Trauma 1970; 10: 359–369

[4] Mattox KL, Feliciano DV, Burch J, Beall AC, Jordan GL, De Bakey ME. Five thousand seven hundred sixty cardiovascular injuries in 4459 patients. Epidemiologic evolution 1958 to 1987. Ann Surg 1989; 209: 698–705, discussion 706–707

[5] Asensio JA, Chahwan S, Hanpeter D et al. Operative management and outcome of 302 abdominal vascular injuries. Am J Surg 2000; 180: 528–533, discussion 533–534

[6] Davis TP, Feliciano DV, Rozycki GS et al. Results with abdominal vascular trauma in the modern era. Am Surg 2001; 67: 565–570, discussion 570–571

[7] Fischer RP, Miller-Crotchett P, Reed RL. Gastrointestinal disruption: the hazard of nonoperative management in adults with blunt abdominal injury. J Trauma 1988; 28: 1445–1449

[8] Cox EF. Blunt abdominal trauma. A 5-year analysis of 870 patients requiring celiotomy. Ann Surg 1984; 199: 467–474

[9] Rapaport A, Feliciano DV, Mattox KL. An epidemiologic profile of urban trauma in America—Houston style. Tex Med 1982; 78: 44–50

[10] Feliciano DV, Burch JM, Spjut-Patrinely V, Mattox KL, Jordan GL. Abdominal gunshot wounds. An urban trauma center's experience with 300 consecutive patients. Ann Surg 1988; 208: 362–370

[11] Swana HS, Cohn SM, Burns GA, Egglin TK. Renal artery pseudoaneurysm after blunt abdominal trauma: case report and literature review. J Trauma 1996; 40: 459–461

[12] Jebara VA, El Rassi I, Achouh PE, Chelala D, Tabet G, Karam B. Renal artery pseudoaneurysm after blunt abdominal trauma. J Vasc Surg 1998; 27: 362–365

[13] Haas CA, Dinchman KH, Nasrallah PF, Spirnak JP. Traumatic renal artery occlusion: a 15-year review. J Trauma 1998; 45: 557–561

[14] Pezzella AT, Griffen WO, Ernst CB. Superior mesenteric artery injury following blunt abdominal trauma: case report with successful primary repair. J Trauma 1978; 18: 472–474

[15] Michaels AJ, Gerndt SJ, Taheri PA et al. Blunt force injury of the abdominal aorta. J Trauma 1996; 41: 105–109

[16] Siavelis HA, Mansour MA. Aortoiliac dissection after blunt abdominal trauma: case report. J Trauma 1997; 43: 862–864

[17] Nitecki S, Karmeli R, Ben-Arieh Y, Schramek A, Torem S. Seatbelt injury to the common iliac artery: report of two cases and review of the literature. J Trauma 1992; 33: 935–938

[18] Buscaglia LC, Matolo N, Macbeth A. Common iliac artery injury from blunt trauma: case reports. J Trauma 1989; 29: 697–699

[19] Roth SM, Wheeler JR, Gregory RT et al. Blunt injury of the abdominal aorta: a review. J Trauma 1997; 42: 748–755

[20] Dajee H, Richardson IW, Iype MO. Seat belt aorta: acute dissection and thrombosis of the abdominal aorta. Surgery 1979; 85: 263–267

[21] Warrian RK, Shoenut JP, Iannicello CM, Sharma GP, Trenholm BG. Seatbelt injury to the abdominal aorta. J Trauma 1988; 28: 1505–1507

[22] Feliciano DV. Abdominal vascular injuries. Surg Clin North Am 1988; 68: 741–755

[23] Courcy PA, Brotman S, Oster-Granite ML, Soderstrom CA, Siegel JH, Cowley RA. Superior mesenteric artery and vein injuries from blunt abdominal trauma. J Trauma 1984; 24: 843–845

[24] Matsubara J, Seko T, Ohta T, Shionoya S, Ban I. Traumatic aneurysm of the abdominal aorta with acute thrombosis of bilateral iliac arteries. Arch Surg 1983; 118: 1337–1339

[25] Bass A, Papa M, Morag B, Adar R. Aortic false aneurysm following blunt trauma of the abdomen. J Trauma 1983; 23: 1072–1073

[26] Feliciano DV. Pitfalls in the management of peripheral vascular injuries. Probl Gen Surg 1986; 3: 101–104

[27] Rich NM, Hobson RW, Fedde CW. Vascular trauma secondary to diagnostic and therapeutic procedures. Am J Surg 1974; 128: 715–721

[28] McDonald PT, Rich NM, Collins GJ, Andersen CA, Kozloff L. Vascular trauma secondary to diagnostic and therapeutic procedures: laparoscopy. Am J Surg 1978; 135: 651–655

[29] Kozloff L, Rich NM, Brott WH et al. Vascular trauma secondary to diagnostic and therapeutic procedures: cardiopulmonary bypass and intraaortic balloon assist. Am J Surg 1980; 140: 302–305

[30] Campbell DK, Austin RF. Acute occlusion of the infrarenal aorta from blunt trauma. Radiology 1969; 92: 123–124

[31] Randhawa MPS, Menzoian JO. Seat belt aorta. Ann Vasc Surg 1990; 4: 370–377

[32] Vernhet H, Marty-Ané CH, Lesnik A et al. Dissection of the abdominal aorta in blunt trauma: management by percutaneous stent placement. Cardiovasc Intervent Radiol 1997; 20: 473–476

[33] Berthet JP, Marty-Ané CH, Veerapen R, Picard E, Mary H, Alric P. Dissection of the abdominal aorta in blunt trauma: Endovascular or conventional surgical management? J Vasc Surg 2003; 38: 997–1003, discussion 1004

[34] Picard E, Marty-Ané CH, Vernhet H et al. Endovascular management of traumatic infrarenal abdominal aortic dissection. Ann Vasc Surg 1998; 12: 515–521

[35] Scharrer-Pamler R, Görich J, Orend KH, Sokiranski R, Sunder-Plassmann L. Emergent endoluminal repair of delayed abdominal aortic rupture after blunt trauma. J Endovasc Surg 1998; 5: 134–137

[36] Yeh MW, Horn JK, Schecter WP, Chuter TAM, Lane JS. Endovascular repair of an actively hemorrhaging gunshot injury to the abdominal aorta. J Vasc Surg 2005; 42: 1007–1009

[37] Tucker S, Rowe VL, Rao R, Hood DB, Harrell D, Weaver FA. Treatment options for traumatic pseudoaneurysms of the paravisceral abdominal aorta. Ann Vasc Surg 2005; 19: 613–618

[38] Waldrop JL, Dart BW, Barker DE. Endovascular stent graft treatment of a traumatic aortocaval fistula. Ann Vasc Surg 2005; 19: 562–565

[39] Teruya TH, Bianchi C, Abou-Zamzam AM, Ballard JL. Endovascular treatment of a blunt traumatic abdominal aortic injury with a commercially available stent graft. Ann Vasc Surg 2005; 19: 474–478

[40] Castelli P, Caronno R, Piffaretti G, Tozzi M. Emergency endovascular repair for traumatic injury of the inferior vena cava. Eur J Cardiothorac Surg 2005; 28: 906–908

[41] Erzurum VZ, Shoup M, Borge M, Kalman PG, Rodriguez H, Silver GM. Inferior vena cava endograft to control surgically inaccessible hemorrhage. J Vasc Surg 2003; 38: 1437–1439

[42] Watarida S, Nishi T, Furukawa A et al. Fenestrated stent-graft for traumatic juxtahepatic inferior vena cava injury. J Endovasc Ther 2002; 9: 134–137

[43] Asensio JA, Petrone P, Kimbrell B, Kuncir E. Lessons learned in the management of thirteen celiac axis injuries. South Med J 2005; 98: 462–466

[44] Sachdev U, Baril DT, Ellozy SH et al. Management of aneurysms involving branches of the celiac and superior mesenteric arteries: a comparison of surgical and endovascular therapy. J Vasc Surg 2006; 44: 718–724

[45] Varela JE, Salzman SL, Owens C, Doherty JC, Fishman D, Merlotti G. Angiographic embolization of a left gastric artery pseudoaneurysm after blunt abdominal trauma. J Trauma 2006; 60: 1350–1352

[46] Fullen WD, Hunt J, Altemeier WA. The clinical spectrum of penetrating injury to the superior mesenteric arterial circulation. J Trauma 1972; 12: 656–664

[47] Maggio AJ, Brosman S. Renal artery trauma. Urology 1978; 11: 125–130

[48] Sclafani SJA, Becker JA. Interventional radiology in the treatment of retroperitoneal trauma. Urol Radiol 1985; 7: 219–230

[49] Hagiwara A, Sakaki S, Goto H et al. The role of interventional radiology in the management of blunt renal injury: a practical protocol. J Trauma 2001; 51: 526–531

[50] Whigham CJ, Bodenhamer JR, Miller JK. Use of the Palmaz stent in primary treatment of renal artery intimal injury secondary to blunt trauma. J Vasc Interv Radiol 1995; 6: 175–178

[51] Lee JT, White RA. Endovascular management of blunt traumatic renal artery dissection. J Endovasc Ther 2002; 9: 354–358

[52] Villas PA, Cohen G, Putnam SG, Goldberg A, Ball D. Wallstent placement in a renal artery after blunt abdominal trauma. J Trauma 1999; 46: 1137–1139

[53] Burch JM, Richardson RJ, Martin RR, Mattox KL. Penetrating iliac vascular injuries: recent experience with 233 consecutive patients. J Trauma 1990; 30: 1450–1459

[54] Lyden SP, Srivastava SD, Waldman DL, Green RM. Common iliac artery dissection after blunt trauma: case report of endovascular repair and literature review. J Trauma 2001; 50: 339–342

[55] Parodi JC, Barone HD, Schonholz C. Transfemoral endovascular treatment of aortoiliac aneurysms and arteriovenous fistulas with stented Dacron grafts. In: Vejth FJ, ed. Current Critical Problems in Vascular Surgery. St. Louis, MO: Quality Medical Publishing; 1993:264

[56] Marin ML, Veith FJ, Panetta TF et al. Transluminally placed endovascular stented graft repair for arterial trauma. J Vasc Surg 1994; 20: 466–472, discussion 472–473

[57] White R, Krajcer Z, Johnson M, Williams D, Bacharach M, O'Malley E. Results of a multicenter trial for the treatment of traumatic vascular injury with a covered stent. J Trauma 2006; 60: 1189–1195, discussion 1195–1196

[58] Silberzweig JE. Ruptured lumbar artery pseudoaneurysm: a diagnostic dilemma in retroperitoneal hemorrhage after abdominal trauma. J Trauma 1999; 46: 531–532

[59] Sclafani SJ, Florence LO, Phillips TF et al. Lumbar arterial injury: radiologic diagnosis and management. Radiology 1987; 165: 709–714

[60] Goffette PP, Laterre PF. Traumatic injuries: imaging and intervention in post-traumatic complications (delayed intervention). Eur Radiol 2002; 12: 994–1021

[61] Ledgerwood AM, Kazmers M, Lucas CE. The role of thoracic aortic occlusion for massive hemoperitoneum. J Trauma 1976; 16: 610–615

[62] Hughes CW. Use of an intra-aortic balloon catheter tamponade for controlling intra-abdominal hemorrhage in man. Surgery 1954; 36: 65–68

[63] Arthurs ZM, Sohn VY, Starnes BW. Ruptured abdominal aortic aneurysms: remote aortic occlusion for the general surgeon. Surg Clin North Am 2007; 87: 1035–1045, viii

[64] Moore RD, Villalba L, Petrasek PF, Samis G, Ball CG, Motamedi M. Endovascular treatment for aortic disease: is a surgical environment necessary? J Vasc Surg 2005; 42: 645–649, discussion 649

[65] Baltacioğlu F, Cimşit NC, Cil B, Cekirge S, Ispir S. Endovascular stent-graft applications in latrogenic vascular injuries. Cardiovasc Intervent Radiol 2003; 26: 434–439

[66] Makar RR, Salem A, McGee H, Campbell D, Bateson P. Endovascular treatment of bleeding external iliac artery pseudo-aneurysm following control of haemorrhage with Sengstaken tube during revision of total hip arthroplasty. Ann R Coll Surg Engl 2007; 89: 1–4

18 Interventional Radiology in Pelvic Trauma

Malcolm K. Sydnor, Daniel J. Komorowski, and Mark M. Levy

Complicated pelvic fractures carry a high mortality, ranging from 6 to 18%, usually secondary to severe hemorrhage.[1] Although the mortality rate is less than 5% for hemodynamically stable patients, it has been reported around 38% for hypotensive patients.[2] Bleeding may originate from arteries, veins, cancellous bone, or crushed soft tissue. With the exception of arterial hemorrhage, all of these sources can be controlled with fracture stabilization by external fixation devices.

Hemodynamic resuscitation in the intensive care unit (ICU) is not a viable option because these patients will become hypercoagulable and continue to bleed. Surgical treatment for exsanguinating pelvic bleeding has not been widely accepted for multiple reasons: Opening the pelvis will release the tamponade on the retroperitoneal hematoma and may cause uncontrollable venous hemorrhage, bleeding vessels are difficult to find and control, and internal iliac artery proximal ligation will not be effective due to the rich supply of pelvic collaterals.

Pelvic packing after external fixation is often employed when severe pelvic bleeding is found, particularly after exploratory laparotomy to treat concomitant intra-abdominal injuries. Pelvic arterial angiography and embolization was first described in 1972 by Margolies et al[3] when autologous blood clot was used to successfully treat active arterial bleeding in the internal iliac arteries. The primary embolic agents for trauma injuries now in use are Gelfoam (Pfizer, New York, NY) pledgets and platinum or stainless steel coils and microcoils. With the development of microcatheter technology, a wide variety of pelvic and other arterial injuries can be rapidly and successfully treated with selective and superselective angiographic techniques.

18.1 Pelvic Fractures

Lateral compression fractures occur in 65% of cases and are usually stable without significant ligamentous injury. These fractures tend to decrease the volume of the pelvis and only require angiography in 1% of cases.[4] Anteroposterior, and particularly vertical shear and combined injuries more often result in ligamentous injury and increased pelvic volume. A 3-cm diastasis of the pubic symphysis doubles the volume of the pelvis to 8 liters.[5] These injuries require angiography in up to 20% of cases.[4] Overall, between 5 and 15% of patients with pelvic fractures will require angiographic intervention.[5,6,7,8,9]

18.2 Triage

Despite fracture classification, studies have shown that fracture pattern does not always correlate with the need for arterial embolization,[10] clinical conditions remain the most important determinant and many of these patients rapidly develop a bleeding diathesis due to massive transfusions and hypothermia. It is important to aggressively treat the coagulopathy and hypothermia and maintain blood pressure with vasopressors, but not to volume overload with crystalloid/colloid infusion because this can lead to increased bleeding by disrupting fresh clot and cause other problems.[11]

External fixation is also very important to stabilize ligamentous injury and to decrease the pelvic volume. Pelvic binders and sheets can provide circumferential compression in the prehospital setting. In multiple studies, standard anterior external fixation has been shown to provide benefit in patients with hemodynamically unstable pelvic fractures. In patients with significant posterior disruption, the use of a posteriorly applied C-clamp (usually under fluoroscopic guidance) can provide stabilization.[12]

About 31% of these patients have an associated intra-abdominal injury[13] and most stable patients undergo a computed tomography (CT) scan. For visualization of pelvic bleeding (based on active extravasation or a large retroperitoneal hematoma) with single-channel helical CT scanners, the reported sensitivity and specificity are 90% and 98%, respectively. With multichannel detector CT,[14,15] these numbers are higher. Patients with CT scans suspicious for active pelvic bleeding should undergo emergent angiography and patients with pelvic fractures and negative CT scan who have a persistent transfusion requirement of greater than 4 to 6 U in 24 hours should also undergo angiography.[5,6,7,16]

Hemodynamically unstable patients with mechanically unstable pelvic fractures and negative abdominal sonogram or supraumbilical diagnostic peritoneal lavage (DPL) will often undergo external fixation and then proceed to angiography. The exception to this is the patient who is rapidly deteriorating despite resuscitation. These patients may be taken to the operating room (OR) depending on the time it takes to have the interventional radiology (IR) team in place. During this scenario, the IR team should be ready to receive the patient back from the OR.

Patients with pelvic hemorrhage and concomitant positive sonogram or DPL will often be taken to the OR for exploratory laparotomy to treat the unknown intra-abdominal injury, which may be assumed to be more life threatening. This may increase the retroperitoneal bleed by partially releasing the tamponade.[17] In this circumstance, the IR team should be ready to receive the patient from the OR. Alternatively, and depending on the clinical scenario, the patient with polytrauma can be brought to the IR suite first for extensive angiographic evaluation and treatment of an abdominal injury in conjunction with the pelvic injury.

These are decisions made by the trauma surgeons based on the independent circumstances of each patient including patient condition, extent of injuries, and immediate availability of the IR team. A patient with pelvic bleeding should never be considered "too unstable" to go to the IR suite. Every effort possible should be made to make sure the IR suite has the entire necessary inventory to take care of the decompensating trauma patient.

18.3 Pelvic Arteriography

As the patient is transferred to the IR suite, the IR should review all of the imaging findings to determine, in conjunction with the trauma team, whether additional angiographic evaluation

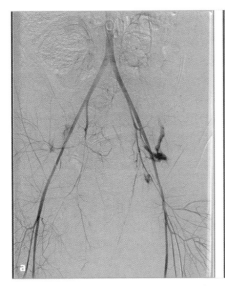
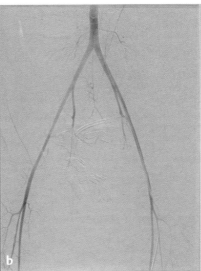

Fig. 18.1 (a) An unstable 17-year-old girl status post motor vehicle accident. Digital subtraction angiography demonstrates diffuse vaso-constriction and multiple areas of extravasation from both internal iliac arteries. (b) There is resolution of contrast extravasation after selective bilateral Gelfoam embolization using a 4-French Cobra catheter.

iswarranted. No time should be wasted as the unstable patient is transferred to the angiography table; if not already done, pelvic external fixation can be performed at this point under fluoroscopy.

The common femoral artery is the preferred access site. There is often a femoral arterial line in place which can also be rewired for a larger sheath to save time and prevent further needle sticks in coagulopathic patients. A 6-French (F) sheath is often necessary to work with a 5-F catheter system while measuring continuous intra-arterial pressures through the sheath. Occasionally, due to extreme pelvic and/or femoral injuries, a brachial access may be necessary. Rarely, in elderly patients with severe atherosclerotic disease, it may be necessary to access both femoral arteries rather than negotiate a tortuous aortic bifurcation. Whatever the access site, sheaths should always be placed to allow for security of the vascular access and rapid catheter exchanges. This is standard practice in most institutions.

Once the access site has been established, a 5-F pigtail catheter is advanced into the distal abdominal aorta and pelvic angiography is performed in at least the anteroposterior (AP) projection with prolonged filming and contrast injections of ~ 8 mL per second for a total of 32 mL. This allows for an anatomical overview and severe pelvic extravasation may be visualized to direct the next catheterization to the site of most significant injury.

A negative aortogram does not exclude injury; both internal iliac arteries as well as both external iliac arteries should be catheterized. The internal iliac arteries are often best catheterized with a Cobra 2 catheter over an angled-tip hydrophilic glide wire. Prolonged filming and injection rates of around 5 to 8 mL per second for a total of 20 to 30 mL are utilized. Sometimes a 4-F glide catheter will help to catheterize diminutive internal iliac arteries in patients with diffuse vasoconstriction (▶ Fig. 18.1). Microcatheters are used routinely if needed.

The most commonly injured vessels in order of frequency (in our experience) are the superior gluteal, internal pudendal, obturator, inferior gluteal, lateral sacral, iliolumbar, external iliac, deep circumflex iliac, and inferior epigastric arteries.[4]

During DSA, care should be taken not to confuse bowel gas, ureteral peristalsis, normal uterine blush, or the bulbospongiosal stain at the base of the penis for arterial injury. The spectrum of traumatic arterial injury includes transection, intimal disruption, pseudoaneurysm, or arteriovenous fistula. Respectively, these injuries may be identified angiographically as active extravasation of contrast or staining, vascular irregularity, abrupt vessel cutoff, or early venous filling. Abrupt vessel cutoff is often difficult to distinguish from spasm. This can be treated with empiric embolization or close observation, depending on the hemodynamic status of the patient.

18.4 Pelvic Arterial Embolization

The interventional radiologist should be constantly aware of the hemodynamic status of the patient by direct communication with the IR nurses. If there are multiple areas of injury or midline bleeding in the unstable patient, rapid Gelfoam embolization of both internal iliac arteries should be performed (▶ Fig. 18.2). If the patient is relatively stable and only one or a few areas of injury are visualized, more elegant embolization with a 4-F or microcatheter system could be performed, given that there is some time for such management.

The ideal embolic agent should be matched to medium-sized arteries and resorb with time. The suitable agent is Gelfoam, which can be rapidly prepared by cutting into small pledgets, soaking in contrast, and injecting through a 1-cc syringe. For larger vascular injuries or arteriovenous fistula (AVF), platinum or stainless steal coils can be deployed with precision (▶ Fig. 18.3). The use of Gelfoam powder or other particulate embolic agents should be avoided because they are far more likely to cause tissue ischemia. Occasionally, there may also be a need for balloon occlusion catheters and covered stents, particularly with penetrant injuries to the external iliac artery, common femoral artery, or superficial femoral artery and extravasation of contrast and/or pseudoaneurysms (▶ Fig. 18.4).

Complications of pelvic embolization include those that are access-site related as well as nontarget embolization and tissue

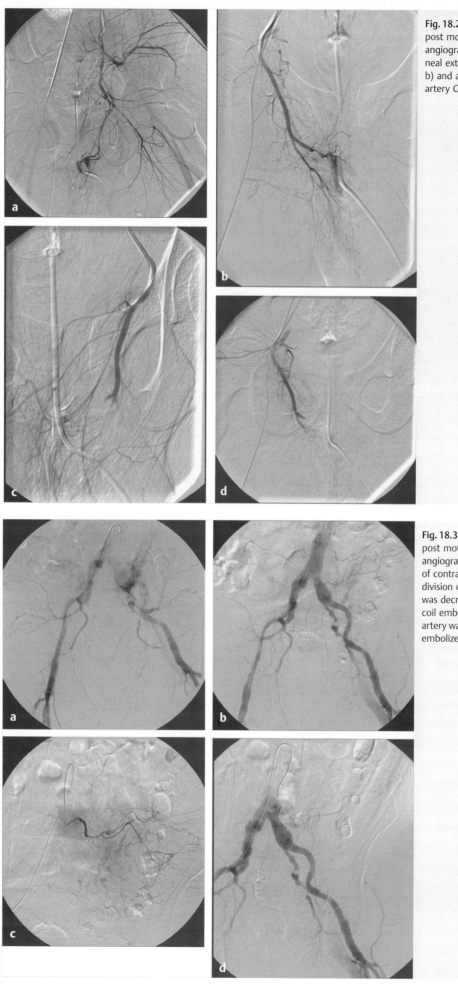

Fig. 18.2 An unstable 42-year-old man status post motor vehicle accident. Digital subtraction angiography demonstrates active midline perineal extravasation of contrast material before (a, b) and after (c,d) bilateral internal pudendal artery Gelfoam embolization.

Fig. 18.3 (a) An unstable 72-year-old man status post motor vehicle accident. Digital subtraction angiography demonstrates massive extravasation of contrast material from the proximal posterior division of the left internal iliac artery. (b) There was decreased, but residual extravasation after coil embolization. The fourth left-sided lumbar artery was also (c) selectively catheterized and (d) embolized with Gelfoam.

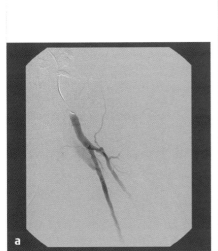

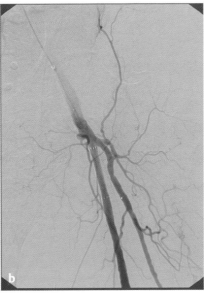

Fig. 18.4 The same patient as ▶ Fig. 18.3 had (a) early filling of the left femoral vein secondary to an arteriovenous fistula, which was (b) successfully excluded with a covered stent in the proximal superficial femoral artery.

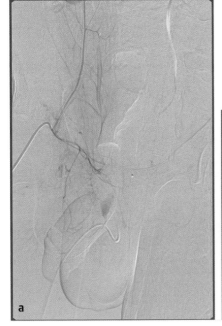

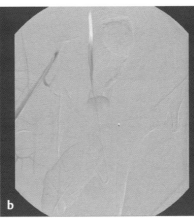

Fig. 18.5 A 54-year-old man has persistent hemodynamic instability after bilateral internal iliac artery embolization. (a) Digital subtraction angiography of the right external iliac artery demonstrates extravasation from a branch of the right inferior epigastric artery. (b) The stump of the inferior epigastric artery is visualized following Gelfoam embolization.

necrosis. Inadvertent reflux of Gelfoam into the profunda femoris artery or other muscular branches will most likely be clinically silent. However, significant Gelfoam embolization down the leg is likely to cause an ischemic limb. This complication can often be treated in the angiography suite with suction embolectomy, Fogarty balloon embolectomy, or others.

Tissue ischemia becomes a concern when both internal iliac arteries are embolized. Although Velmahos et al[18] published a series of 30 bilateral internal iliac artery embolizations with no such complications, Suzuki et al[18] more recently reported 12 cases of gluteal necrosis in a series of 165 bilateral internal iliac embolizations. At least six of these did not have gluteal injuries on admission and therefore were attributed to the embolization and three of these six patients died due to sepsis. Long-term follow-up after bilateral pelvic embolization has not been reported. While these potential complications are concerning, the risks are outweighed by the alternative of continued extravasation with subsequent exsanguination and eventually death.

After embolization, the hemodynamic status of the patient often dramatically improves. Repeat views should then be obtained with the same catheterization level and image obliquity in which the injury was seen prior to treatment. In addition, a pelvic flush arteriogram from the distal abdominal aorta should be performed to ensure adequate treatment and to evaluate for other injuries or collateral filling of the same site of injury. Special attention should be paid to the external iliac artery injection as frequently pelvic collaterals including replaced obturator branches often originate from the inferior epigastric artery (▶ Fig. 18.5). Midline bleeding sites can originate from both internal iliac arteries, as well as external iliac branches. The source of a lateral pelvic bleed may be from a lumbar, iliac circumflex, profunda femoris, or other branches.[4]

Upon examination of the five most recent series[18,19,20,21,22] of pelvic embolizations for trauma (ranging between 15 to 65 patients each pelvic embolizations), there were a 152 pelvic embolizations performed with technical success in 147 cases (97%). Mortality ranged from 14 to 46% and most deaths were attributable to concomitant injuries other than the pelvic bleed. There were three (2%) reported angiographic complications in these series. Only a small percentage of these patients underwent external pelvic fixation prior to angiography.

18.5 Conclusion

The treatment for acute hemorrhage after an unstable pelvic fracture involves close coordination between the trauma, orthopedic, vascular, and IR services and includes control of hypotension and coagulopathy, pelvic stabilization, and percutaneous pelvic arterial embolization. When pelvic hemorrhage is the main issue, the faster the patient can be mobilized to the IR suite for embolization the better, regardless of stability. When the patient is taken to the OR for a concomitant intra-abdominal injury, the IR team should be ready to receive the patient back from the OR for subsequent pelvic embolization. The role of IR for the treatment of concomitant abdominal organ injury continues to evolve and depends in part on how fast the IR team can be mobilized.

References

[1] Mucha P, Welch TJ. Hemorrhage in major pelvic fractures. Surg Clin North Am 1988; 68: 757–773

[2] Naam NH, Brown WH, Hurd R, Burdge RE, Kaminski DL. Major pelvic fractures. Arch Surg 1983; 118: 610–616

[3] Margolies MN, Ring EJ, Waltman AC, Kerr WS, Baum S. Arteriography in the management of hemorrhage from pelvic fractures. N Engl J Med 1972; 287: 317–321

[4] Kaufman JA. Abdominal aorta and iliac arteries. In: The Requisites: Vascular and Interventional Radiology. Philadelphia, PA: Mosby; 2004:246–285

[5] Agnew SG. Hemodynamically unstable pelvic fractures. Orthop Clin North Am 1994; 25: 715–721

[6] Kaufman JA, Waltman AC. Angiographic management of hemorrhage in pelvic fractures. In: Abrams' Angiography Interventional Radiology. 2nd ed. Philadelphia, PA: Lippincott Williams & Wilkins; 2005:1004–1018

[7] Ben-Menachem Y, Coldwell DM, Young JWR, Burgess AR. Hemorrhage associated with pelvic fractures: causes, diagnosis, and emergent management. AJR Am J Roentgenol 1991; 157: 1005–1014

[8] Cryer HM, Miller FB, Evers BM, Rouben LR, Seligson DL. Pelvic fracture classification: correlation with hemorrhage. J Trauma 1988; 28: 973–980

[9] Burgess AR, Eastridge BJ, Young JWR et al. Pelvic ring disruptions: effective classification system and treatment protocols. J Trauma 1990; 30: 848–856

[10] Sarin EL, Moore JB, Moore EE et al. Pelvic fracture pattern does not always predict the need for urgent embolization. J Trauma 2005; 58: 973–977

[11] Stern SA, Wang X, Mertz M et al. Under-resuscitation of near-lethal uncontrolled hemorrhage: effects on mortality and end-organ function at 72 hours. Shock 2001; 15: 16–23

[12] Hak DJ, Smith WR, Suzuki T. Management of hemorrhage in life-threatening pelvic fracture. J Am Acad Orthop Surg 2009; 17: 447–457

[13] Demetriades D, Karaiskakis M, Toutouzas K, Alo K, Velmahos G, Chan L. Pelvic fractures: epidemiology and predictors of associated abdominal injuries and outcomes. J Am Coll Surg 2002; 195: 1–10

[14] Pereira SJ, O'Brien DP, Luchette FA et al. Dynamic helical computed tomography scan accurately detects hemorrhage in patients with pelvic fracture. Surgery 2000; 128: 678–685

[15] Stephen DJ, Kreder HJ, Day AC et al. Early detection of arterial bleeding in acute pelvic trauma. J Trauma 1999; 47: 638–642

[16] Panetta T, Sclafani SJ, Goldstein AS, Phillips TF, Shaftan GW. Percutaneous transcatheter embolization for massive bleeding from pelvic fractures. J Trauma 1985; 25: 1021–1029

[17] Hagiwara A, Murata A, Matsuda T, Matsuda H, Shimazaki S. The usefulness of transcatheter arterial embolization for patients with blunt polytrauma showing transient response to fluid resuscitation. J Trauma 2004; 57: 271–276, discussion 276–277

[18] Velmahos GC, Chahwan S, Hanks SE et al. Angiographic embolization of bilateral internal iliac arteries to control life-threatening hemorrhage after blunt trauma to the pelvis. Am Surg 2000; 66: 858–862

[19] Agolini SF, Shah K, Jaffe J, Newcomb J, Rhodes M, Reed JF. Arterial embolization is a rapid and effective technique for controlling pelvic fracture hemorrhage. J Trauma 1997; 43: 395–399

[20] Wong YC, Wang LJ, Ng CJ, Tseng IC, See LC. Mortality after successful transcatheter arterial embolization in patients with unstable pelvic fractures: rate of blood transfusion as a predictive factor. J Trauma 2000; 49: 71–75

[21] Velmahos GC, Toutouzas KG, Vassiliu P et al. A prospective study on the safety and efficacy of angiographic embolization for pelvic and visceral injuries. J Trauma 2002; 53: 303–308, discussion 308

[22] Fangio P, Asehnoune K, Edouard A, Smail N, Benhamou D. Early embolization and vasopressor administration for management of life-threatening hemorrhage from pelvic fracture. J Trauma 2005; 58: 978–984, discussion 984

19 Interventional Radiology in Obstetric and Gynecologic Trauma

Uma R. Prasad and Jaime Tisnado

Recent advances in interventional radiologic (IR) procedures have facilitated a nonsurgical approach to most bleeding of obstetric and gynecologic origin, sparing the patient a hysterectomy in many instances. In the current chapter, we describe these indications and techniques, emphasizing a combined team approach.

19.1 Vascular Anatomy

The abdominal aorta bifurcates into the two common iliac arteries. They course downward and laterally, and divide into the external iliac and internal iliac arteries. The external iliac arteries continue into the common femoral arteries and supply the lower extremities. The internal iliac arteries supply the internal organs and walls of the pelvis.

The arterial supply to the uterus is primarily through the uterine arteries, which reach the uterus at the level of the cervix and lower uterine segment. Uterine venous channels follow a course similar to that of the arteries. The bladder is supplied by visceral branches arising from the internal iliac arteries. The prostate in men is supplied by numerous small branches from the internal iliac arteries as well. The ovaries are supplied by the ovarian arteries; branches of aorta on the right side, and the renal artery on the left side. The sigmoid colon and rectum are supplied by branches of the inferior mesenteric artery and internal iliac arteries.

In general the internal iliac arteries supply all the gynecologic organs and pelvic walls by their two divisions, anterior and posterior. The veins follow similar courses to the arteries and form the internal iliac veins that join the external iliac veins and join the common iliac veins, which in turn join together to form the inferior vena cava (IVC).

19.2 Embolization of Obstetric and Gynecologic Trauma

Transcatheter arterial embolization is a highly effective technique for controlling obstetric and gynecologic hemorrhage. Its advantages include low complications, avoidance of surgical risks and general anesthesia, and preservation of fertility in young women. Complications of arterial embolization in this setting are uncommon.

The procedures are as follows: Using the Seldinger technique through one common femoral artery, an initial pelvic arteriogram is performed, followed by selective bilateral internal iliac arteriography and uterine arteriography, if needed. Embolic particles are carefully injected into the uterine artery until stasis of flow is confirmed. An internal iliac arteriography is repeated to exclude the possibility of additional feeding arteries, which may become apparent only after the major feeding artery is occluded. The contralateral internal iliac artery, uterine artery, and branches are then examined in the same manner.

Embolization of both bleeding arteries is necessary because of the possibility of cross-filling. If arterial bleeding does not stop after embolization, other arteries, such as the ovarian, inferior epigastric, or middle sacral arteries, should be examined.

For general gynecologic trauma management, various embolization materials are used including Gelfoam (Pfizer, New York, NY), coils, detachable balloons, thrombin, and polyvinyl alcohol. Most iatrogenic gynecologic vascular abnormalities can be safely and effectively treated by embolization with pledgets of absorbable Gelfoam. The few weeks duration of the occlusion is sufficient to stop hemorrhage while still permitting slow development of collateral vessels. For occlusion of the proximal vessels in cases of pseudoaneurysms arising from larger branches or AVF of traumatic origin, metallic coils are preferred because the risk of shunting of particulate embolic material into the systemic circulation or into the pseudoaneurysm, is avoided. In young women after embolization of the pelvic arteries, preservation of fertility is possible because of the temporary nature of the occlusion and the presence of numerous collaterals. Therefore, transcatheter arterial embolization is the therapy of choice in women with iatrogenic vascular abnormalities, preserving reproductive capacity.

Uterine curettage or gynecologic surgical trauma can cause uterine vascular abnormalities. The usual workup, in cases of pseudoaneurysm, includes color and duplex ultrasound (US), which shows a blood-filled cystic structure with swirling arterial flow. In cases of arteriovenous malformation (AVM) and arterial venous fistula (AVF) of traumatic origin, color Doppler US shows an intense tangle of vessels, whereas duplex US shows low-resistance, high-velocity arterial flow. If an AVM is combined with a pseudoaneurysm, the findings of both AVM and pseudoaneurysm are present. Color and Doppler US is the ideal modality for detection and diagnosis of these conditions and follow-up of patients after therapeutic embolization, because embolization is a safe and effective method of treating these conditions. Surgery with its attendant complications is avoided.

Pelvic bleeding due to trauma and tumors, and iatrogenic causes, is a major challenge for the trauma team. The patients can lose large amounts of blood, either internally or externally. The presence of hematomas can be further complicated by eventual superimposed infections. Patients on chemotherapy and/or radiation therapy can have vascular changes that may cause a continuous loss of blood. Some of these can be readily managed using embolization with permanent agents.

Obstetric postpartum hemorrhage is a common cause of maternal morbidity and mortality. Percutaneous embolization techniques are ideal for the treatment of selected cases of post-cesarean bleeding, vaginal wall injuries and hematomas, cervical ectopic pregnancy, different causes of postpartum bleeding, and the so-called placenta accreta.

Some special cases of complicated pregnancy with abnormal placental implantation are being managed with placement of balloon occlusion catheters and embolization of the internal iliac arteries prior to, or during, the cesarean section or hysterectomy, resulting in a remarkable reduction in intraoperative blood loss. Surgical options such as ligation of the internal iliac arteries are limited in these complicated but rare situations. Even exploratory laparotomy can be detrimental because the tamponade effect on the hematoma is lost.

With improvements in US technique, the diagnosis of some potential high-risk conditions for postpartum hemorrhage, such as placenta accreta and variations, can be made prenatally. The patient can then be prepared in the immediate predelivery or C-section period with prophylactic placement of balloon occlusion catheters. The benefit is a potential avoidance of hysterectomy in young women who desire future pregnancies.

Transcatheter arterial embolization is highly effective in controlling acute and chronic vaginal bleeding in a wide variety of obstetric and gynecologic disorders. Benefits include low complication rates, fertility preservation in young women of childbearing age and shorter hospitalization times. The procedure is cost effective as well. The problems associated with surgery are avoided.

Some indications for pelvic embolotherapy, types of embolotherapy, technical considerations, success rates, causes of failure, complications, and outcome will be discussed below.

19.2.1 Coagulopathy

Selective transcatheter uterine artery embolization may be used to control life-threatening pelvic hemorrhage unresponsive to "traditional" local measures. For example, Von Willebrand disease is an uncommon inherited bleeding disorder caused by quantitative or qualitative defects of Von Willebrand factor, which may lead to postpartum bleeding problems. In such patients, persistent postpartum hemorrhage may be treated effectively by transcatheter arterial embolization of both internal iliac arteries. Selective embolization of the uterine arteries is another option.

19.3 Gynecologic Abnormalities

Menstrual irregularities are the most common cause of abnormal vaginal bleeding in adolescence and are responsible for ~ 50% of gynecologic visits in this age group. Most abnormal bleeding in adolescents is caused by immaturity of the hypothalamic–pituitary–ovarian axis resulting in anovulation or oligoovulation due to the noncyclic release of follicle stimulating hormone and luteinizing hormone during adolescence. On occasion acute menorrhagia may occur due to pregnancy and related complications, such as threatened abortion, incomplete or complete abortion, ectopic pregnancy, and postabortal trophoblastic disease.

Vaginal ulcerations and objects introduced into the vagina occasionally cause irregular bleeding as well. Tumors such as clear cell adenocarcinoma of the vagina and sarcoma botryoides may present as metrorrhagia also. These etiologic factors are responsible in ~ 5% of adolescent girls who complain of irregular vaginal bleeding. Conservative treatment may be helpful. However, if the bleeding continues or does not improve, arteriography of both internal iliac arteries and branches is indicated. Sometimes, arteriography can identify a single bleeding artery as the cause and can facilitate superselective embolization of the bleeding sites with particles like Gelfoam, polyvinyl alcohol (PVA), embospheres, or even platinum microcoils.

19.4 Postpartum Hemorrhage

Obstetric hemorrhage is one of the most common and feared potential causes of maternal mortality and morbidity. Post C-section bleeding, vaginal wall hematoma, cervical ectopic pregnancies, postpartum bleeding, and pelvic trauma, due to direct or indirect injuries can cause significant bleeding and can be successfully treated with transcatheter embolization (▶ Fig. 19.1, ▶ Fig. 19.2). Embolization controls active severe obstetric bleeding and has the great advantage of preserving fertility. The success rate of embolization in patients with normal clotting parameters is reportedly > 90%.

Complications of transcatheter embolization are low. However, in addition to the usual complications of angiography, embolization may result in pelvic infection (pelvic abscess), and very rarely, bladder gangrene. The post embolization syndrome, a self-limited condition of nausea and vomiting, cramps, fever, elevated WBC, and pain from tissue necrosis and/or vascular thrombosis is rather common and not a true complication. The treatment is symptomatic.

19.5 Uterine Vascular Abnormalities

19.5.1 Placenta Accreta and Variations

The incidence of placenta accreta is variable, with rates reported in the literature ranging from less than 1:700,000 to 1:500 pregnancies. Although this incidence is relatively low, the associated maternal and perinatal mortality rates are as high as 10%.

Placenta accreta in general is the abnormal penetration of the placenta into the underlying uterine wall, which may result in severe postpartum hemorrhage. We include here different variations of placental penetration. Invasion of the placental villi into the myometrium is called placenta accreta. Penetration of the villi through the myometrium is termed placenta increta, and invasion of the villi through the serosa is termed placenta percreta. For our brief discussion all variations are considered together as the IR management is similar, if not identical.

Risk factors for placenta accreta include placenta previa, previous C-section deliveries, multiparity, advanced maternal age, and prior dilation and curettage. Antepartum diagnosis is very important to allow time for the health care team to prepare for the potentially lethal complications associated with abnormal placentation. Because placenta accreta is not always diagnosed early, a conservative treatment includes dilation and curettage and subsequent arterial embolization.

Traditionally, the gynecologic treatment of placenta accreta, increta, and percreta has involved C-section, followed by hysterectomy. Intraoperative bleeding has been and is a major complication at the time of hysterectomy. This bleeding is treated by bilateral internal iliac and/or uterine artery ligation. However, because of the extensive collateral circulation in the pelvis, an adequate control of bleeding may be achieved in only less than 50% of patients. In women with placenta percreta with invasion of adjacent tissues and organs including the bladder, the bleeding may be profuse, so even surgery is associated with a high morbidity and mortality rate.

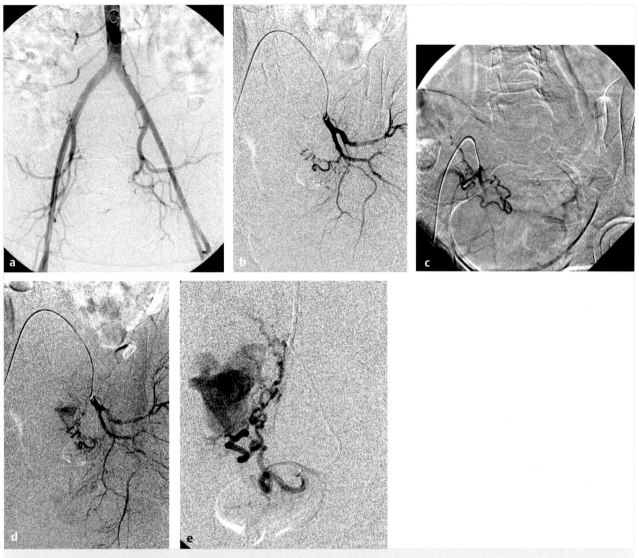

Fig. 19.1 A young woman developed massive postpartum vaginal bleeding. The patient was brought to the angiography suite for pelvic arteriography and embolization. (a–c) Pelvic arteriography and left selective internal iliac arteriography shows active bleeding from left internal iliac artery branches. (d,e) Superselective bilateral uterine arteriography demonstrates massive bleeding from the left uterine artery. Both uterine arteries were successfully embolized with Gelfoam particles and polyvinyl alcohol. The patient recovered.

Management

The current management of these three different types of placental penetration is the temporary placement of occlusive balloon catheters in both internal iliac arteries from a contralateral femoral artery approach before C-section delivery. Of course, a combined effort between gynecologists, surgeons, interventional radiologists, and others is a must for success.

Preoperative internal iliac artery balloon occlusion placement is a safe and easy technique that significantly reduces or eliminates intraoperative blood loss and transfusion requirements in these women. Prior to the procedure, a complete discussion between gynecologists, interventional radiologists, and other physicians involved is important. The patient and families should be informed of the risks, benefits, and alternatives of the procedure.

Technique

Using the Seldinger technique, both common femoral arteries are punctured, vascular sheaths inserted, and both internal iliac arteries selectively catheterized from a contralateral approach. Then two 7-French (F) balloon occlusion catheters are inserted. Arteriography is done to confirm catheter placement. With balloon catheters secured in place, the patients are transferred to the operating room for C-section delivery. The balloons can be inflated at the exact time of delivery to achieve hemostasis. The balloons are deflated and removed when no longer needed. One great advantage of the management is that it limits blood loss, and minimizes the risk of transfusion reactions and blood-borne diseases such as hepatitis C and/or human immuno-deficiency virus (HIV).

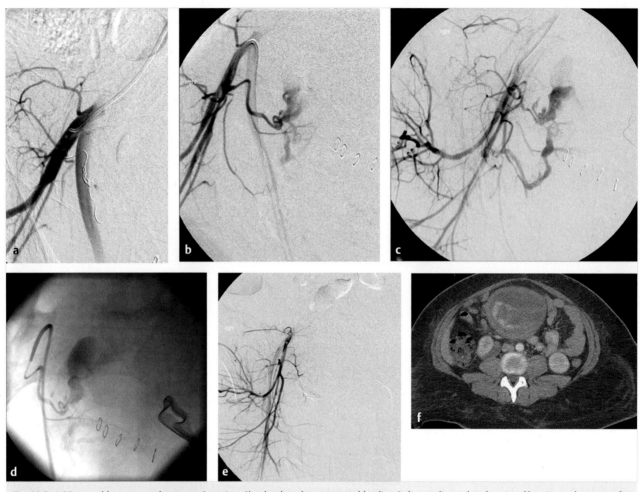

Fig. 19.2 A 27-year-old woman underwent a C-section. She developed postpartum bleeding 3 days earlier and underwent *dilatation and curettage* for suspected retained products of conception. Presented to the emergency room with recurrent vaginal bleeding and dropping hematocrit. (a) An emergency pelvic computed tomography scan shows a large mass in the pelvis with nonhomogeneous densities indicating acute and subacute ongoing hemorrhage. (b-d) Selective right internal iliac and uterine arteriography shows massive active extravasation of contrast material in the pelvis. (e, f) Successful embolization with embospheres and microcoils. Bleeding no longers demonstrated. The patient recovered.

The temporary occlusion of the internal iliac arteries does not affect the blood flow to the uterus because of the rich supply of collaterals, especially in these women of childbearing age. For optimal outcome, a team approach to patient care and timely action by the interventional radiologists are essential. The interventional radiologists, as always, must be available 24/7.

19.6 Gynecologic Bleeding

Some or most episodes of pelvic bleedings of gynecologic origin are usually managed surgically. Uterine packing is done frequently and successfully. On occasion, some traumatic and other bleeding episodes do not stop with packing. An alternative to uterine packing is the use of uterine tamponade balloons. Some have described the use of the Sengstaken-Blakemore tube, used for the treatment of gastrointestinal (GI) bleeding varices, to be inserted in the uterine cavity for tamponade of certain unusual cases of uterine bleeding.[1,2] In most women, bleeding stops after placement and inflation of the tube. A recently approved tube is the SOS Bakri tamponade

balloon (Cook Urological, Spencer, IN) for temporary control or reduction of hemorrhage. It has a filling capacity of 500 mL and strength to withstand a pressure of 300 mm Hg. This device can be placed to stabilize bleeding in certain patients, and transcatheter embolization can then be performed. This combined approach is highly successful in controlling hemorrhage.

In pregnant women who are bleeding it is very important to ensure minimal fetal radiation exposure during the procedures, using appropriate shielding and intermittent low-dose fluoroscopy. This is a general principle applied in all conditions when a fetus is in the uterus and any radiologic study needs to be done.

19.6.1 Uterine Vascular Abnormalities

Uterine curettage, surgical trauma, or other iatrogenic procedure complications can result in uterine vascular abnormalities, such as pseudoaneurysms, AVFs, and/or rupture of arteries and veins. Recognition of the cause of hemorrhage is important because they can be managed safely and effectively with embolization rather than further uterine curettage, which may worsen the situation and perpetuate massive uterine bleeding.

Ultrasonography (US) is the initial imaging study used for the evaluation of abnormal uterine bleeding. Color and duplex Doppler US detects and diagnoses most of these vascular abnormalities, and helps to differentiate vascular abnormalities that require embolization, from nonvascular abnormalities that require different management.

In pseudoaneurysms, color and duplex Doppler US shows a blood-filled cystic structure with swirling arterial flow. In AVFs and AVMs, color and duplex Doppler US show an intense vascular tangle, with low-resistance, high-velocity arterial flow. Some AVFs and AVMs are combined with pseudoaneurysms as well, so the US demonstrates combinations of findings of both lesions.

Transcatheter embolization is the therapy of choice for most of these acquired lesions, with the advantage of maintaining reproductive capacity. Evaluation by color and duplex Doppler US of any abnormal uterine bleeding must be done to identify and characterize the lesions that may be amenable to IR management by embolization.[3,4]

Color Doppler US shows a circular pattern of blood flow signals in the outer myometrium from the arcuate arteries and venous plexus and a radial pattern of blood flow signals in the middle and the inner myometrium from the radial and spiral arteries and accompanying veins.[4]

19.6.2 Postcurettage Bleeding

Hemorrhage is one of the main complications of uterine curettage and/or pelvic surgery, developing in up to 5% of abortion procedures.[5,6] Intractable hemorrhage, refractory to conservative measures, may be due to uterine arterial injuries. In a recent report, 3 out of 14 patients had an intractable delayed postpartum hemorrhage from uterine vascular abnormalities.[7]

Some lesions include pseudoaneurysms, acquired AVFs, AVMs, and direct vessel rupture.[1,2,7–14] These lesions may be causes of massive uterine bleeding and may be aggravated by further dilatation and curettage (D&C). These lesions are different from the common causes of excessive uterine bleeding, which responds to D&C.[10] In the past, in the event of failure of conservative local measures, the patients went to the operating room (OR) for surgical treatment consisting of bilateral internal iliac artery ligation and/or even total hysterectomy. (▶ Fig. 19.1, ▶ Fig. 19.2)

Until relatively recently, some of these lesions were overlooked due to lack of diagnostic imaging.[15,16] Consequently, neither surgery nor IR could be done. An increasing awareness of these entities coupled with the more widespread use of noninvasive imaging (US, CT, magnetic resonance imaging [MRI]) allows detection of uterine vascular abnormalities with increased frequency. In a recent report of 24 cases of iatrogenic uterine arterial injuries, there were seven pseudoaneurysms, nine "acquired" AVMs and AVFs, six "combined" AVMs and pseudoaneurysms, and two uterine arterial ruptures. All women were in the reproductive age (21–39 years old) with intractable vaginal bleeding. Twenty-one patients had a D&C (1–5 D&C procedures per patient), two had a C-section, and one had a traumatic delivery. Because these otherwise asymptomatic women had abnormal bleeding shortly after the procedures, a causal link was suspected. All patients underwent

transabdominal and endovaginal gray-scale, color Doppler, and duplex Doppler US followed by angiography and embolization (one embolization in 22 women and two embolizations in two women). Hysterectomy was performed in two women with pseudoaneurysms and failed embolization. All patients, except the two who had hysterectomy, underwent Doppler US immediately after embolization, and then at 3-month intervals for 1-year and yearly for up to 3 years. No recurrence was detected at follow-up US.

Pseudoaneurysms usually result from an inadequate sealing of a laceration or puncture of the arterial wall during surgery or penetrating trauma. Blood dissects into the tissues around the damaged artery and forms a perfused sac that communicates with the arterial lumen. A D&C, C-section, or other operations on the uterus may be the cause.[1,2,7,8,9]

Duplex Doppler US shows turbulent arterial flow, high-velocity, and high-resistance arterial flow within the sac, depending on the variable degree of turbulence. Angiography clearly demonstrates one or more pseudoaneurysms supplied by one or more feeding arteries. In general, urgent intervention is required because pseudoaneurysms are at risk of expanding and/or rupturing. Therefore, embolization is the management of choice.[1,2,7,8,9]

Furthermore, retained villi are abundant within a pseudoaneurysm; a rapid recruitment of collateral vessels following embolization may occur and result in recanalization of the pseudoaneurysm. Particular attention to the serum beta-human chorionic gonadotropin (β-HCG) is needed. Methotrexate therapy or a retrial of D&C immediately after embolization may decrease recanalization of pseudoaneurysms or other vascular lesions.[17,18]

Another cause of embolization failure is the inadequate embolization of a pseudoaneurysm supplied by extrauterine arteries, such as the internal pudendal, ovarian, inferior epigastric, or contralateral uterine arteries.[7,8,17] A careful search for other feeding arteries is recommended. Sometimes a simultaneous cross-filling of the sac by two or more arteries is found. Ultrasound cannot demonstrate retained villi or extrauterine feeding arteries. Perhaps MRI has a role in such cases.

19.7 Arteriovenous Malformation and Arteriovenous Fistula

Arteriovenous malformations are congenital vascular lesions characterized by multiple communications of varying sizes between arteries and veins in the vicinity. An AVF is an abnormal direct passage between an artery and an adjoining vein.[19] Traditionally, uterine AVMs have been classified as congenital or acquired.[12] Congenital uterine AVMs result from an abnormality in the embryologic development of primitive vascular structures, which result in multiple abnormal communications between arteries and veins.[12] Acquired uterine AVMs are in reality multiple small AVFs between intramural arterial branches and the myometrium venous plexus, and appear as vascular tangles, mimicking congenital AVMs. An acquired pelvic AVF is an abnormal direct passage between an artery and an adjoining vein without a network of abnormal vessels, potentially arising outside the uterus.[20,21]

Although endometrial carcinoma, cervical carcinoma, gestational trophoblastic disease, and maternal diethylstilbestrol exposure have been implicated,[10,] acquired uterine AVMs are traumatic given that there is usually a history of D&C, uterine surgery, or trauma to the uterus.[10,11,12]

Because of different structural characteristics, acquired AVMs are easier to treat with embolization than congenital AVMs. The patient clinical history and the angiographic findings are helpful in differentiating between acquired and congenital AVMs. The pattern of bleeding is intermittent and torrential, suggestive of arterial hemorrhage.[21] Uterine bleeding is thought to occur when vessels are exposed from sloughing of the endometrium, iatrogenically during D&C, or spontaneously during menses.[12] Angiography usually shows a complex tangle of vessels supplied by enlarged feeding arteries, in association with early venous drainage, and stasis of contrast medium within the abnormal vasculature and the blood supply and collateral flow. Embolization is then done as necessary.

Embolization is the therapy of choice, and has the important advantage of retaining reproductive capacity of the women.[15-] Both uterine arteries must be embolized because of the constant occurrence of cross-filling, which may not be evident at the time of the initial embolization.[8,21] Doppler US is the method of choice for follow-up after treatment and should be obtained every 3 months for the first year.

Embolization is a highly effective technique for controlling acute and chronic genital bleeding in a wide variety of obstetric and gynecologic disorders, especially in a trauma setting. Here we must comment that old ORs are not equipped with high-resolution angiographic equipment for selective and superselective embolization. New IR suites are now designed to meet size requirements, infection control guidelines, and air circulation standards found in the conventional OR. Anesthesiology and neonatology teams with appropriate equipment need to be present. Therefore, the IR management of pelvic bleeding of gynecologic origin is now preferred.

On occasion, perforation during instrumentation of the uterus can result in severe bleeding and massive blood loss. The bleeding is usually arterial, but sometimes can be venous as well. Rupture of an arterial branch can result in a rapid bleeding because the uterus is a very vascular organ, especially in young women. Some patients go to the OR for a surgical procedure that may result in iatrogenic bleeding. Thereafter, the patients must be brought to the IR suite for management of severe bleeding. Therefore, the IR suite should always be ready for patients incompletely managed in the OR, and/or when complications have occurred.

Therefore, the contribution of the IR team in the management of trauma of gynecologic origin is by different steps or situations. Sometimes, the patients go to the IR suite directly from the scene of an accident, or as soon as a bleeding source has been evaluated by noninvasive methods. Sometimes, the patients go directly to the OR for surgical management and subsequently brought to the IR suite from the OR in the course of their management, when some iatrogenic or spontaneous complication may have occurred.

19.8 Conclusion

Pelvic bleeding of obstetric and gynecologic origin is rather more frequently seen in this era of aggressive and "defensive" medical care and interpersonal violence of our society.

Traditionally, most of these episodes of bleeding of variable amount and frequency were managed exclusively by surgical means, often resulting in hysterectomy.

With the explosive advances in IR procedures, most bleeding of obstetric and gynecologic origin is now managed by IR, avoiding the serious complications of surgery and preserving the uterus in most women who are young and of child-bearing age.

References

[1] Chow TW, Nwosc EC, Gould DA, Richmond DH. Pregnancy following successful embolization of a uterine vascular malformation. Br J Obstet Gynaecol 1995; 102: 166–168

[2] Poppe W, Van Assche FA, Wilms G, Favril A, Baert A. Pregnancy after transcatheter embolization of a uterine arteriovenous malformation. Am J Obstet Gynecol 1987; 156: 1179–1180

[3] Ojala K, Perälä J, Kariniemi J, Ranta P, Raudaskoski T, Tekay A. Arterial embolization and prophylactic catheterization for the treatment for severe obstetric hemorrhage. Acta Obstet Gynecol Scand 2005; 84: 1075–1080

[4] Fuller AJ, Carvalho B, Brummel C, Riley ET. Epidural anesthesia for elective cesarean delivery with intraoperative arterial occlusion balloon catheter placement. Anesth Analg 2006; 102: 585–587

[5] Ornan D, White R, Pollak J, Tal M. Pelvic embolization for intractable postpartum hemorrhage: long-term follow-up and implications for fertility. Obstet Gynecol 2003; 102: 904–910

[6] Wang H, Garmel S. Successful term pregnancy after bilateral uterine artery embolization for postpartum hemorrhage. Obstet Gynecol 2003; 102: 603–604

[7] Pelage JP, Le Dref O, Jacob D, Soyer P, Herbreteau D, Rymer R. Selective arterial embolization of the uterine arteries in the management of intractable postpartum hemorrhage. Acta Obstet Gynecol Scand 1999; 78: 698–703

[8] Vedantham S, Goodwin SC, McLucas B, Mohr G. Uterine artery embolization: an underused method of controlling pelvic hemorrhage. Am J Obstet Gynecol 1997; 176: 938–948

[9] McIvor J, Cameron EW. Pregnancy after uterine artery embolization to control haemorrhage from gestational trophoblastic tumour. Br J Radiol 1996; 69: 624–629

[10] Vedantham S, Goodwin SC, McLucas B, Mohr G. Uterine artery embolization: an underused method of controlling pelvic hemorrhage. Am J Obstet Gynecol 1997; 176: 938–948

[11] Vashisht A, Smith JR, Thorpe-Beeston G, McCall J. Pregnancy subsequent to uterine artery embolization. Fertil Steril 2001; 75: 1246–1248

[12] Pron G, Bennett J, Common A et al. Ontario UFE Collaborative Group. Technical results and effects of operator experience on uterine artery embolization for fibroids: the Ontario Uterine Fibroid Embolization Trial. J Vasc Interv Radiol 2003; 14: 545–554

[13] Miller DA, Chollet JA, Goodwin TM. Clinical risk factors for placenta previa-placenta accreta. Am J Obstet Gynecol 1997; 177: 210–214

[14] Read JA, Cotton DB, Miller FC. Placenta accreta: changing clinical aspects and outcome. Obstet Gynecol 1980; 56: 31–34

[15] Clark SL, Koonings PP, Phelan JP. Placenta previa/accreta and prior cesarean section. Obstet Gynecol 1985; 66: 89–92

[16] McIvor J, Cameron EW. Pregnancy after uterine artery embolization to control haemorrhage from gestational trophoblastic tumour. Br J Radiol 1996; 69: 624–629

[17] Chow TW, Nwosc EC, Gould DA, Richmond DH. Pregnancy following successful embolization of a uterine vascular malformation. Br J Obstet Gynaecol 1995; 102: 166–168

[18] Poppe W, Van Assche FA, Wilms G, Favril A, Baert A. Pregnancy after transcatheter embolization of a uterine arteriovenous malformation. Am J Obstet Gynecol 1987; 156: 1179–1180

[19] Frates MC, Benson CB, Doubilet PM , et al. Cervical ectopic pregnancy: results of conservative treatment. Radiology 1994; 191: 773–775

[20] Wang H, Garmel S. Successful term pregnancy after bilateral uterine artery embolization for postpartum hemorrhage. Obstet Gynecol 2003; 102: 603–604

[21] Ornan D, White R, Pollak J, Tal M. Pelvic embolization for intractable postpartum hemorrhage: long-term follow-up and implications for fertility. Obstet Gynecol 2003; 102: 904–910

20 Interventional Radiology in Genitourinary Trauma

Jaime Tisnado, Shima Goswami, Daniel J. Komorowski, Marco A. Amendola, and Rao Ivatury

20.1 Genitourinary Trauma

About 28 million patients pass through the doors of emergency departments in the United States each year for trauma-related injuries. Because 10% of all those cases involve the genitourinary (GU) system, these organs must be carefully examined with a high degree of suspicion for injuries.[1]

Within the GU tract, each different organ has its own potential for injuries and an individual approach to diagnosis and treatment. In this chapter, we will discuss injuries to seven different organs: kidneys, bladder, ureter, urethra, penis, testicles/scrotum, and female genitalia, addressing each organ's anatomical features and the diagnosis of injuries, followed by some interventional radiologic (IR) protocols for the management of these injuries.

20.1.1 Kidneys

Blunt and penetrating injuries are the most common cause of significant trauma to the abdomen. The kidneys are the third most frequently injured abdominal organ (after the spleen and liver), representing ~ 8 to 10% of those injuries.[2,3] Typically renal injuries are broken down into blunt and penetrating, with the vast majority belonging to the former group, which also includes decelerating injuries.

Blunt trauma to the kidneys can be further stratified into a five-part classification system as outlined by the Organ Injury Scaling (OIS) Committee of the American Association for the Surgery of Trauma (AAST) depending on the severity of the injury (1 = least severe; 5 = most severe).[4]

Grade 1 includes renal contusion without a parenchymal laceration and a nonexpanding hematoma. This is the most common, accounting for 64 to 81% of renal injuries.[5]

Grade 2 includes superficial lacerations < 1 cm deep (thus not involving the collecting system) and a nonexpanding hematoma. These first two groups (1 and 2) are considered mild injuries that require conservative management alone, and usually do not need IR management and/or follow-up.

Grade 3 includes lacerations > 1 cm deep that still do not extend into the collecting system and a nonexpanding perinephric hematoma. If these patients are hemodynamically stable and show no devascularized fragments, they may not require follow-up imaging either.

Grade 4 consists of lacerations that extend into the collecting system and the main and segmental renal vessels. These injuries require follow-up computed tomography (CT) at 36 to 72 hours to monitor extravasation of contrast via the collecting system. Typically, urine extravasation is self-limiting and will resolve spontaneously during this time frame, so an expectant management is appropriate. However, if urine leaks persist, catheter drainage is preferred or surgical repair, if antegrade urine flow is impaired. Localized urine leaks (urinomas) are managed readily with percutaneous drainage by the interventional radiologist.

Grade 5 includes a shattered kidney with or without dispersion of the portions, avulsion, laceration, or thrombosis of the main renal vessels, and ureteropelvic junction (UPJ) avulsion. This is the most severe category and requires mandatory angiography. Surgical intervention, often a nephrectomy, is the standard of care, if there is injury to the renal pedicle, avulsion, or a shattered kidney. Detecting contrast material in the ureter distal to the UPJ helps to differentiate a laceration from avulsion, which may be managed differently. If findings on CT or intravenous urography (IVU) are equivocal, occasionally retrograde pyelography may help in the evaluation.[3]

Penetrating trauma results from gunshot, stabbings, and shrapnel wounds. Usually, all victims with renal injuries secondary to anterior gunshot wounds have had associated intra-abdominal injuries at surgery. On the other hand, only half of patients with posterior or flank stab wounds have associated intra-abdominal injuries.[6]

It is routine for us to obtain a contrast-enhanced CT in stab wounds limited to the flank/back to assess the extent of the injuries and prevent surgical exploration. Interventional radiology can manage those patients.

Deep lacerations may be associated with delayed hemorrhage between 2 days and 5 weeks later, particularly after stab wounds; likely because of pseudoaneurysm or arterial venous fistula (AVF) formation. These lesions are well managed with IR techniques.[8]

An interesting and rare complication from missile wounds is a delayed ureteral obstruction caused by migration of missile into the collecting system after a long latent period. This is known as "buckshot colic" and resolves spontaneously. However, if the projectile is a bullet or a shrapnel fragment, this is known as "bullet colic" or "birdshot calculus" and requires surgery to remove the obstruction.[3]

Furthermore, some victims require more aggressive procedures. This group includes patients with a solitary kidney, and perhaps a "horseshoe" kidney. It is critical to preserve the functioning kidney. In patients with a solitary kidney, IR management with selective embolization is necessary.[8] Patients with chronic hydronephrosis, renal carcinoma, renal malformations, and renal transplants require special management as well.

Some preexisting abnormalities that may increase the risk of injury (more in children than in adults), include disruption of the renal pelvis or UPJ in patients with hydronephrosis, an extrarenal pelvis, intracystic hemorrhage or rupture of a renal cyst with or without communication with the collecting system, rupture of a tumor, lacerations of poorly protected ectopic or horseshoe kidneys, and lacerations of infected kidneys.[3]

Imaging Evaluation

Computed tomography with early and delayed phases is the gold-standard imaging for assessing renal injury in blunt trauma. Computed tomography determines the degree of injury (trivial managed conservatively, or severe requiring intervention; either IR or surgery). Computed tomography provides accurate evaluation of renal lacerations, the presence and location of hematomas with or without active arterial extravasation, and outlines devascularized segments of renal parenchyma.[8]

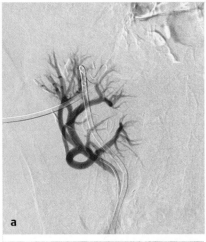

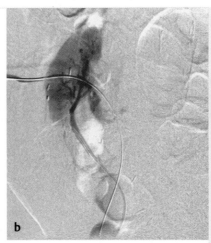

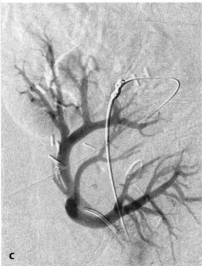

Fig. 20.1 This patient with a renal transplant had placement of a percutaneous nephrostomy tube for drainage of hydronephrosis. Thereafter, he presented with gross hematuria. Therefore, arteriography was done. (a) Selective transplant arteriogram shows no evidence of bleeding or extravasation. The percutaneous nephrostomy (PCN) tube is in place. (b) The PCN tube was removed over a guidewire. Repeat arteriogram shows significant extravasation of contrast in center of kidney and renal pelvis. (c) The bleeding branch was selectively catheterized and embolized with microcoils. Arteriogram after embolization shows no longer bleeding. The PCN tube was thereafter reinserted. Tamponade by drainage tubes may obscure sites of active bleeding. Therefore, the tubes must be removed over a wire if one suspects continued bleeding despite negative arteriogram.

Other studies are not routinely used. Intravenous urography can be used for gross assessment of renal function and to evaluate the uninjured kidney in hemodynamically unstable patients. Ultrasonography is useful for detecting hemoperitoneum, but is inferior to CT for evaluating the renal parenchyma. Nuclear scintigraphy may help to determine the presence of a functioning kidney in patients with contraindication or allergies to iodinated contrast material or as a follow-up after repair of renovascular trauma. Magnetic resonance imaging (MRI) can also be used in instances of iodinated contrast material contraindications. Furthermore, MRI with gadolinium enhancement can be useful in search of urinary extravasation.

Angiography

Angiography is of great importance in the evaluation of renal trauma. Here we discuss in detail the indications, contraindications, findings, and its role in treatment.

There are four major indications for endovascular management of renal injuries.

The first is recurrent hemodynamic lability despite resuscitation or > 4 units of packed red blood cell (PRBC) transfusion requirements in 24 hours and CT findings demonstrating a fractured kidney, a large subcapsular hematoma, or active extravasation.

This indication is illustrated by a patient with a renal transplant, who had placement of a percutaneous nephrostomy tube for drainage of hydronephrosis. Thereafter, he presented with gross hematuria. Arteriography was performed. Selective transplant arteriogram (▶ Fig. 20.1a) showed no evidence of bleeding or extravasation. The percutaneous nephrostomy (PCN) tube seemed to be in place. The PCN tube was removed over a guidewire. A repeat arteriogram (▶ Fig. 20.1b) showed a significant extravasation of contrast in center of kidney and renal pelvis. The bleeding branch was selectively catheterized and embolized with microcoils (▶ Fig. 20.1c). Arteriogram after embolization showed control of bleeding. The PCN tube was thereafter reinserted. This case also illustrates how tamponade by drainage tubes may obscure sites of active bleeding.

Severe blunt abdominal trauma can cause retroperitoneal hemorrhage with or without injury to the kidney. Inverventional Radiology is especially valuable to determine the source and also intervene therapeutically. An example is illustrated in ▶ Fig. 20.2. An adolescent boy suffered severe blunt trauma to his back and developed backache, tachycardia, and hypotension. Abdominal CT scan (▶ Fig. 20.2a) showed a huge retroperitoneal hematoma on the right side displacing the kidney. Intraparenchymal bleeding and foci of active extravasation in the kidney were also evident (▶ Fig. 20.2b). Right renal arteriogram

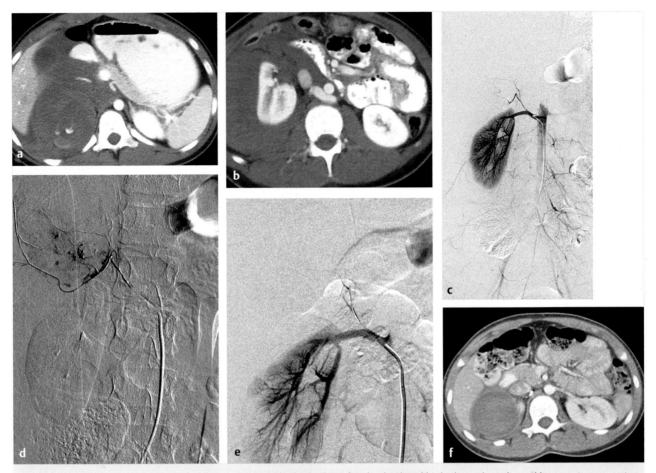

Fig. 20.2 An adolescent boy suffered severe blunt trauma to his back. Thereafter, he developed backache, tachycardia, and hypotension prompting clinical evaluation. (a) Abdominal CT scan shows a huge retroperitoneal hematoma on the right side pushing, compressing and displacing the kidney. Large renal intraparenchymal bleeding is also evident. (b) Intrarenal bleeding was suspected. There are also foci of active extravasation. (c) Right renal arteriogram shows normal kidney and no lesion to suggest cause of hemorrhage. The kidney is displaced downward and active bleeding was suspected in the adrenal region. There is enlargement of inferior adrenal arteries. (d) Selective inferior adrenal arteriogram demonstrated numerous sites of acute arterial extravasation of contrast material. (e) After embolization, no longer bleeding. The child recovered and went home. No other management was needed. The embolization was done with Gelfoam slurry and platinum microcoils. (f) Follow-up CT scan 2 weeks later showed resolving right renal, adrenal, and retroperitoneal hematoma.

(► Fig. 20.2c) showed no lesions to suggest a cause of hemorrhage. The kidney was displaced downward and active bleeding was suspected in the adrenal region. Selective inferior adrenal arteriogram (► Fig. 20.2d) demonstrated numerous sites of acute arterial extravasation of contrast material. These were embolized with platinum microcoils and Gelfoam slurry, successfully controlling the bleeding points (► Fig. 20.2e). A follow-up CT scan 2 weeks later (► Fig. 20.2f) showed resolving right renal adrenal and retroperitoneal hematoma.

Large perinephric hematomas may also be a result of penetrating trauma to the flank or back. In stable patients, these will be demostrated by a CT scan and further delineation of the source of bleeding, whether renal or extra-renal, can be determined by selective arteriography. An example is a middle-aged man who was stabbed in the back during an altercation. He presented to the emergency department with back pain and dropping hemaglobin and hematocrit. Computed tomography (► Fig. 20.3a,b) showed a massive retroperitoneal hemorrhage with active bleeding. Aortography (► Fig. 20.3c,d) showed normal kidneys, but a transection of the left fourth lumbar artery

with a large pseudoaneurysm. The fourth lumbar artery was superselectively catheterized with a microcatheter and the artery was embolized proximal and distal to the pseudoaneurysm using the so-called sandwich technique.

These considerations are illustrated by a 10-year-old girl, who presented with severe abdominal pain after a go-kart injury sustaining blunt abdominal and back trauma. Ultrasound (US) examination of the left kidney (► Fig. 20.4a) demonstrated a marked hydronephrosis of the left kidney. Computed tomography, reformatted in axial and coronal planes (► Fig. 20.4b,c) revealed an undiagnosed left ureteropelvic junction obstruction. Delayed images (► Fig. 20.4d) demonstrated rupture of the renal pelvis with extravasation of urine. She underwent an emergent percutaneous nephrostomy (PCN) placement for decompression, followed by an elective pyeloplasty after discharge. She is currently doing well.

Absence of visualization of the kidney on contrast-enhanced CT should suggest a revovascular injury and prompt renal arteriography, as shown in ► Fig. 20.5. This patient was involved in a car crash with severe blunt trauma to back. Abdominal

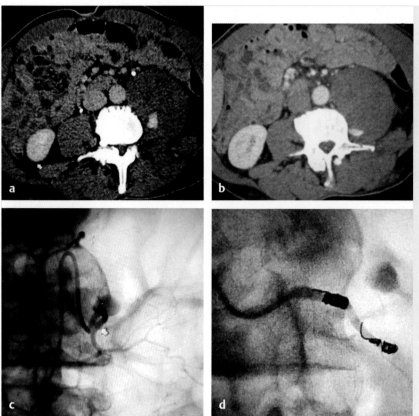

Fig. 20.3 This middle-aged man was stabbed in the back during an altercation. Thereafter, he presented to the emergency room with back pain and dropping hemaglobin and hematocrit. (a,b) Computed tomography showed a massive retroperitoneal hemorrhage with active bleeding. (c,d) Arteriography was performed. Transsection of the left fourth lumbar artery with a large pseudoaneurysm was found. The fourth lumbar artery was superselectively catheterized with a microcatheter and the artery embolized distally and proximally to the pseudoaneurysm using the so-called sandwich technique.

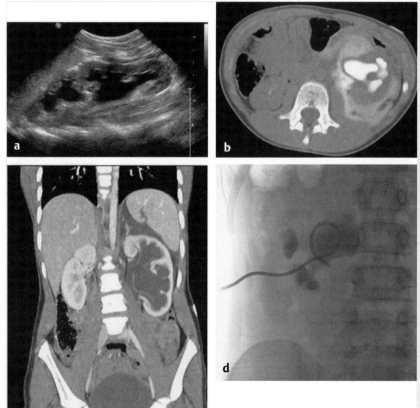

Fig. 20.4 This 10-year-old girl presented with severe abdominal pain after a go-kart injury sustaining blunt abdominal and back trauma. (a) Ultrasound (US) examination of the left kidney demonstrates marked hydronephrosis (b,c) Computed tomography in axial and coronal reformatted revealed an undiagnosed left ureteropelvic junction obstruction. Delayed images demonstrated rupture of the renal pelvis with extravasation of urine. (d) She underwent emergent percutaneous nephrostomy (PCN) placement for decompression and to promote healing, followed by an elective pyeloplasty after discharge. She is currently doing well and followed by urology with serial US exams.

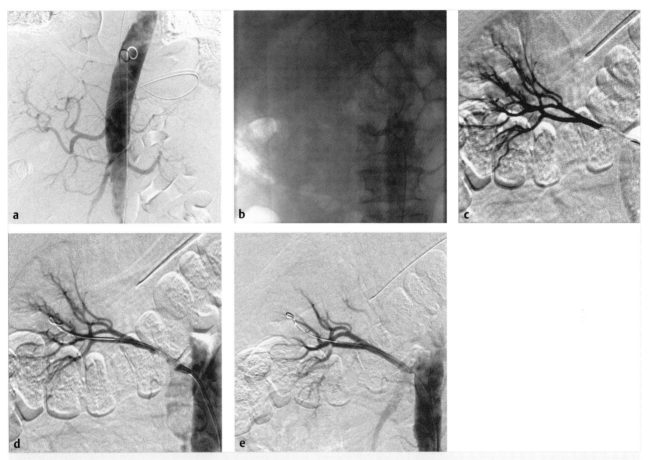

Fig. 20.5 A patient involved in a car accident with severe blunt trauma to back. (a) Abdominal aortogram shows absence of opacification of right renal artery. (b) Selective right renal arteriogram shows complete occlusion of the right renal artery. (c) The occluded artery was carefully traversed with a glidewire. (d) Then a glide catheter was used to advance a 0.14-inch wire into distal portion of segmental branch. (e) Poststenting arteriogram shows excellent reconstitution of renal artery lumen, previously occluded. Adequate opacification of most branches is evident.

aortogram (▶ Fig. 20.5a) showed absence of opacification of right renal artery. Selective right renal arteriogram (▶ Fig. 20.5b) confirmed complete occlusion of the right renal artery. The occluded artery was carefully traversed with a guide wire (▶ Fig. 20.5c), and a glide catheter was used to advance a 0.14-inch wire into distal portion of segmental branch (▶ Fig. 20.5d). Post-stenting arteriogram showed excellent reconstitution of renal artery lumen and adequate opacification of most branches (▶ Fig. 20.5e).

Interventional Radiology is also helpful in dealing with delayed complications after renal trauma. A 14-year-old boy was transferred from an outside hospital with a devascularized right kidney following prolonged hospitalization after falling from a tree. His clinical course and ultrasound-guided aspiration of the renal parenchyma suggested a renal abscess with Gram-negative rods. Abdominal aortogram (▶ Fig. 20.6a,b) showed a significant irregularity of the right renal artery with minimal perfusion of the renal parenchyma. Selective renal arteriogram (▶ Fig. 20.6c) showed almost complete occlusion of main artery. Only a sliver of renal cortex in the upper pole showed perfusion. Enlarged adrenal and capsular collateral arteries were present in an attempt to perfuse the ischemic kidney. The right renal artery was subsequently embolized

(▶ Fig. 20.6d) with multiple platinum microcoils. Subsequent surgical nephrectomy was rather easy and bloodless.

The expanding role of IR in renal trauma is illustrated by another patient, an elderly woman who fell on her back sustaining severe trauma to the left side. Computed tomography in axial and coronal views (▶ Fig. 20.7a,b) showed a large subcapsular hematoma compressing the kidney parenchyma medially and an extensive retroperitoneal hematoma. Coronal reformat (▶ Fig. 20.7c) confirmed the huge retroperitoneal hematoma, pushing the kidney upward and compressing it. A selective renal arteriogram (▶ Fig. 20.7d) showed bleeding from one of the segmental arteries to the midportion of the kidney. The bleeding branch was easily catheterized with a microcatheter (▶ Fig. 20.7e) and embolized with platinum microcoils. The patient recovered fully.

A third indication for endovascular intervention is an abdominal bruit or thrill, which would suggest an arterio-venous fistula (AVF). A middle-aged patient underwent biopsy of a renal transplant and subsequently developed gross hematuria. Color duplex Doppler exam of the transplanted kidney (▶ Fig. 20.8a, b) showed an AVF in the center of the kidney. Selective renal arteriogram (▶ Fig. 20.8c) showed early filling of renal veins indicative of an AVF. After coil embolization of the feeding artery (▶ Fig. 20.8d), the AVF was controlled.

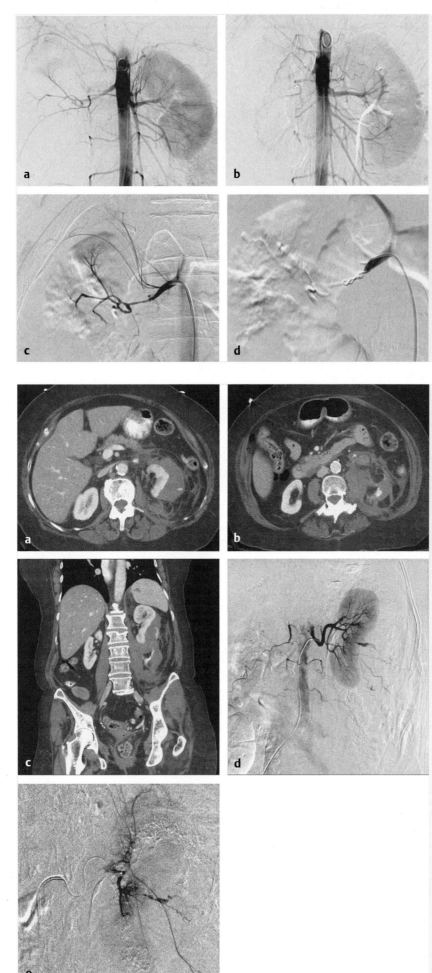

Fig. 20.6 A 14-year-old boy was transferred from an outside hospital with a devascularized right kidney following prolonged hospitalization after falling from a tree. Ultrasound-guided aspiration of the renal parenchyma yielded. Gram-negative rods, indicating a developing abscess. (a,b) Abdominal aortogram confirmed significant irregularity of the right renal artery with minimal perfusion of the renal parenchyma. (c) Selective renal arteriogram shows almost complete occlusion of main artery with only tiny cortex perfused in the upper pole. Enlarged adrenal and capsular arteries are present in an attempt to perfuse ischemic kidney. (d) The right renal artery was subsequently embolized with multiple platinum microcoils prior to surgical nephrectomy. The operation was rather easy and bloodless. The child recovered.

Fig. 20.7 An elderly woman fell on her back sustaining severe trauma to the left side. (a,b) Computed tomography in axial and coronal shows a large subcapsular hematoma compressing the kidney parenchyma medially. Extensive retroperitoneal hematoma is evident. (c) Coronal reformat shows the huge retroperitoneal hematoma. The kidney is pushed upward and compressed. (d) The patient underwent interventional radiology (IR) management of traumatic lesion. A selective L RA shows bleeding from one of the segmental arteries to the midportion of the kidney. A large subcapsular and retroperitoneal hematoma is evident. (e) The bleeding branch was easily catheterized with a microcatheter and embolized with platinum microcoils. The patient recovered fully.

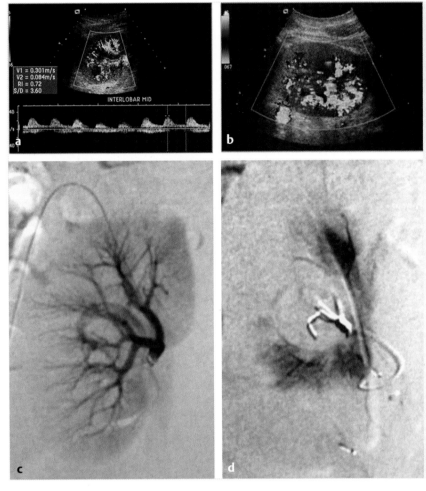

Fig. 20.8 A middle-aged patient underwent biopsy of a renal transplant in the right lower abdomen. The patient developed gross hematuria. (a,b) Color duplex Doppler exam of the transplanted kidney showed an arterial venous fistula (AVF) in the center of the kidney. (c) Selective renal arteriogram showed early filling of renal veins indicative of an AVF. (d) After coil embolization of the feeding artery, there is a zone of kidney devascularized.

A similar case of successful embolization of traumatic AVF secondary to renal biopsy is illustrated in ▶ Fig. 20.9. AVF may also result from blunt abdominal trauma and present in a delayed fashion. As an example, ▶ Fig. 20.10 illustrates the case of a middle-aged man evaluated for a loud bruit in the right flank, with a remote history of blunt trauma. A coronal postgadolinium magnetic resonance angiogram (▶ Fig. 20.10a) demonstrated a large enhanced renal vein associated with simultaneous enhancement of the proximal inferior vena cava (IVC). The distal IVC was not enhanced, suggesting a AVF in the right kidney. An abdominal aortogram (▶ Fig. 20.10b) prior to embolization demonstrated the huge AVF.

Almost complete preservation of renal parenchyma was accomplished in these patients, a particularly important outcome for many of them, already in renal failure or insufficiency.

Lastly, in unrelenting gross hematuria and/or severe unremitting urinary colic suggests an arteriocalyceal fistula that requires IR management.[2]

Interventional radiology is of limited value when there is intraperitoneal involvement, requiring surgical intervention. However, if the injury is limited to the retroperitoneum, embolization can decrease the risk for nephrectomy, especially in iatrogenic vascular injury following a renal biopsy or a nephrostomy.

For both blunt and penetrating trauma, there are absolute and relative contraindications to endovascular management:

(1) an intractable hemodynamic lability not responsive to resuscitation, and (2) CT evidence of intraperitoneal injury (e.g., pancreatic laceration, spillage of urine, etc.) are absolute contraindications. Both of these require emergent laparotomy. A relative contraindication to endovascular intervention is pregnancy.[2]

When there is suspicion of injury to the main renal artery, an aortogram and selective renal arteriography are needed. An arteriogram in multiple projections must be done to detect subtle abnormalities.

Angiographic findings include extravasation, occlusion, AVF, arteriocalyceal fistula, intimal tear, and pseudoaneurysm. Each abnormality requires a specific endovascular management. Dissections, lacerations, or extravasation from the main renal artery, require placement of covered stents provided the lesion can be crossed safely to preserve flow to the kidney.

In very rare instances of occlusions of the main renal artery, if the procedure can be performed within 6 hours of the onset of organ ischemia, low dose intra-arterial tissue plasminogen activator (tPA) can be infused with extreme care to prevent thrombosis.

If there is intraparenchymal hemorrhage or pseudoaneurysm, embolization with Gelfoam (Pfizer, New York, NY), particulates, or coils is done. The goal is to preserve the maximum amount of renal tissue. Therefore, we prefer coils; however,

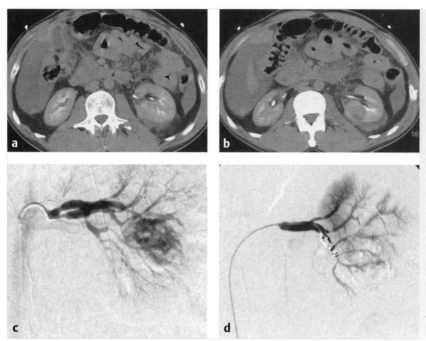

Fig. 20.9 Successful embolization of traumatic arterial venous fistula (AVF) secondary to biopsy of the left kidney. (a,b) An abdominal computed tomography scan with intravenous contrast material shows an enhancing lesion with active extravasation and subcapsular bleeding in the left kidney. Fluid around the liver is evident. (c) Selective renal arteriogram shows a large hypervascular lesion associated with early filling of veins indicative of an AVF secondary to the biopsy. (d) Superselective catheterization was done with a coaxial system and a microcatheter. Many platinum microcoils were deposited in the offending branch with immediate control of the large AVF.

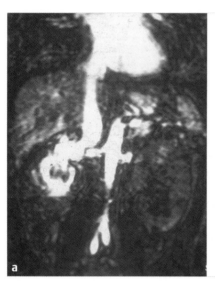

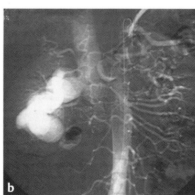

Fig. 20.10 A middle-aged man evaluated for a loud bruit in the right flank. He sustained severe blunt trauma in the past. (a) A coronal postgadolinium magnetic resonance angiogram demonstrates a large enhanced renal vein associated with simultaneous enhancement of the proximal inferior vena cava (IVC). The distal IVC is not enhanced. This indicates an arterial venous fistula (AVF) in the right kidney. (b) An abdominal aortogram prior to embolization more clearly demonstrates the huge AVF at better advantage. Almost complete preservation of renal parenchyma is accomplished in these patients who require biopsy of kidney given that they present with renal failure or insufficiency in the first place.

much of this will depend on the level of expertise in superselective catheterization. In cases of intraparenchymal fistulas, we must embolize the vessel proximal to the site of injury with microcoils. Arteriovenous fistulas are much easier to visualize than arteriocalyceal fistulas because contrast excretes into the collecting system in the latter. One helpful imaging finding of an arteriocalyceal fistula is an early opacification of a calyx. We must remember here that renal arteries are "end arteries" so all interventions must be done keeping this important anatomical feature in mind.

This is illustrated by the case of a middle-aged woman with remote history of trauma to the back, who presented with left back pain. A computed tomography scan (▶ Fig. 20.11a) showed a huge low density unenhancing mass in the left kidney with a rim of calcification. An abdominal aortogram (▶ Fig. 20.11b)

demonstrated a huge lesion with heterogeneous filling with contrast material, typical of a pseudoaneurysm. Embolization of this traumatic pseudoaneurysm was done with a large amount of coils to almost fill the sac (▶ Fig. 20.11c). Angiogram after embolization (▶ Fig. 20.11d) showed preservation of kidney parenchyma in both upper and lower poles with the central pseudoaneurysm obliterated with coils. The patient went home after procedure.

20.1.2 Bladder

Urinary bladder trauma can be blunt or penetrating, with 67 to 86% being blunt.[8] It is a very important distinction to remember that, anatomically, part of the bladder is intraperitoneal and part is extraperitoneal.[8,9] Approximately 80% of all bladder

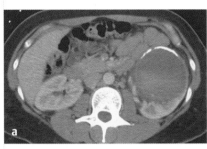

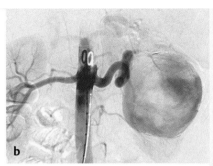

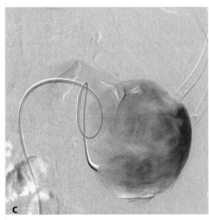

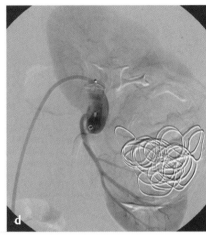

Fig. 20.11 A middle-aged woman with remote history of trauma to back presented with left back pain. (a) A computed tomography scan shows a huge low density unenhancing mass in the left kidney with a rim of calcification. (b) An abdominal aortogram shows the huge lesion with heterogeneous filling with contrast material. (c) Embolization of this huge traumatic pseudoaneurysm was done with a large amount of coils to almost fill the sac. (d) Angiogram after embolization shows preservation of kidney parenchyma in both upper and lower poles with the central pseudoaneurysm full of coils The patient went home after procedure.

ruptures are extraperitoneal. Distinguishing between these two types is essential for diagnosis and treatment.[10] Moreover, in approximately 5% of cases, there is both intraperitoneal and extraperitoneal rupture.

To illustrate, the bladder system can be considered as a storage balloon. Only two things can result from applying pressure to a balloon: Essentially it will either "bend," stretch, and get bruised; or burst. It is important to think of it in this manner, to understand why distended bladders are much more prone to injuries than collapsed bladders.

The common cause of blunt trauma to the bladder is motor vehicle crashes (particularly with inappropriately placed lower seatbelt across the waist), falls, crush injuries, and blows to the lower abdomen. About 80% of blunt bladder injuries are seen in conjunction with pelvic fractures.[5] Ruptures to the bladder routinely occur in alcoholic patients involved in car accidents with pelvic trauma, when their bladder is full. Given that the urinary bladder traverses the peritoneal border, classification is made into the following four categories; contusion, intraperitoneal rupture, extraperitoneal rupture, and penetrating trauma.[9] This system is logical from an imaging point of view, though is not the only one. The Organ Injury Scale (OIS) of the American Association for the Surgery of Trauma (AAST) is a five-point scale, but for the sake of simplicity and consistency, in this chapter we use the four-tier system.

Imaging Evaluation

A trauma victim with gross hematuria and a pelvic fracture requires immediate cystography; either under fluoroscopic or CT guidance. Relative indications for imaging of bladder trauma include gross hematuria without pelvic fracture, microhematuria

with pelvic fracture, and/or isolated microhematuria. Both "conventional" cystography (fluoroscopically-guided) and CT cystography have similar sensitivity and specificity in detecting and characterizing bladder injuries.[5] Regardless of which method is chosen, it is essential that the bladder be filled with at least 250 cc of contrast material to categorically exclude the possibility of bladder rupture.[10]

During conventional cystography, any contrast material outside the bladder indicates rupture. If it remains confined to the pelvis, an *extraperitoneal* leak exists, whereas if the contrast material outlines bowel loops, extends into the paracolic gutters, and spreads diffusely into the peritoneal cavity, an *intraperitoneal* leak exists. It is critical that fluoroscopic images are obtained during maximal filling as well as after drainage of contrast, because ~ 10% of ruptures can only be detected postdrainage.[5]

During CT cystography, we must remember that a rupture can be missed if CT images are taken during passive filling of the bladder by excreted contrast material. Contrast must be actively instilled into the bladder prior to scanning for accurate results. No postdrainage imaging is required. In extraperitoneal injuries, contrast may be confined to the pelvis and demonstrate a "molar-tooth" appearance of extravasation, or it may extend into the Retzius space, anterior abdominal wall, thigh, and/or scrotum. Similar to conventional cystography, intraperitoneal ruptures will demonstrate contrast outlining the bowel and diffusely through the mesenteric folds.

Management

A contusion is a bladder wall bruise, but not a rupture (i.e., purely a mucosal injury) and cannot be detected by imaging. A contusion is the mildest form of injury and is treated with a simple large bore Foley catheter to ensure that blood clots pass through the system easily and do not cause obstruction.

An intraperitoneal rupture occurs when there is a blow/compression to the lower abdomen causing a sudden rise in intraluminal pressure of the bladder and rupture of the dome, which is covered by peritoneum. All intraperitoneal ruptures require surgical repair, particularly to avoid the risk of peritonitis with urine leakage. Thereafter, a catheter should be placed and remain for at least 2 weeks to ensure bladder rest.

The exact mechanism for extraperitoneal rupture is unclear, but it is often associated with pelvic fractures. These ruptures are further classified into simple or complex. Contrast material is confined to the pelvic extraperitoneal space in the former, while it can spread diffusely into various other extraperitoneal structures in the latter. Most patients with extraperitoneal rupture can be managed conservatively, with large-bore catheter placement for a minimum of 10 days. Catheters should not be removed until there is radiographic confirmation that the leak has resolved. However, if the bladder neck is involved, bony fragments are present in the bladder wall, or there is bony entrapment of the bladder wall, surgical exploration is warranted.

Lastly, injuries due to penetrating trauma, secondary to gunshot, stabbing, or shrapnel, always require emergent surgical exploration, repair, and catheter placement for 2 weeks or so, to ensure bladder rest.

20.1.3 Ureters

Ureteral injuries comprise only 1% of all GU trauma. The ureters are often spared because of their small size, mobility, and protected location. About 75% of all ureteral injuries are iatrogenic in nature, with most (75%) of those related to gynecologic procedures, generally affecting the lower-third (pelvic portion) of the ureter. The remainder of injuries is due to "civil" trauma, with the majority occurring from blunt versus penetrating forces. Blunt trauma is usually the result of a deceleration injury resulting in UPJ injury.[8]

The OIS Committee of the AAST has a five-point grade system to break down ureteral injuries, summarized as the following:
- 1 = hematoma
- 2 and 3 = lacerations
  - involving < 50% (2) and > 50% (3) of the circumference
- respectively, and 4 and 5 = complete tears
  - with < 2 cm of devascularization (4) and > 2 cm of devascularization (5)

However, this grading is unlikely to be of radiologic benefit given that the degree of accuracy in detecting the depth of laceration is extremely limited. Therefore, from a radiologic standpoint, it is enough to classify the injury as either a laceration or a transection, or as the case may be, a stricture or a fistula.

Imaging

The two best imaging modalities for the detection of ureteral injuries are IVU and contrast-enhanced CT (CECT) with delayed phases. The "conventional" retrograde urography can be helpful if findings on the main two examinations are equivocal and the patient is hemodynamically stable. Findings in the studies of

choice to suggest ureteral injury include contrast material extravasation and/or obstruction. Contrast material passing into the distal ureter suggests a laceration, while absence of contrast in the distal ureter suggests a transection. Fistulas can be detected on all studies, even if extremely subtle. Furthermore, CECT provides additional information about the presence of urinary ascites, urinomas, and other fluid collections.

Iatrogenic injuries not detected at the time of the injury can be evaluated with either technique. When a UPJ injury is suspected, CECT during the excretory phase is a reliable method. In immediate penetrating trauma, preoperative imaging is not needed and the patient is taken immediately to the operating room. However, missile paths in proximity to the ureters may cause significant soft tissue damage and delayed presentation of a true ureteral injury. In this case, IVU or CECT with delayed phases must be performed.

Interventional Radiology

The role of the interventional radiologist is very important in ureteral injuries predominantly providing two procedures; percutaneous nephrostomy (PCN) and/or ureteral/nephroureteral stent placements. Percutaneous nephrostomy decompression results in a significantly decreased need for reoperation and decreased morbidity. In acute trauma, PCN can also serve as a bridge to surgery in the management of urinary fistulas, urinomas, and urinary ascites.

In renal transplant patients with posttransplant ureteral leaks, fistulas, strictures, and obstructions, PCN decompression is invaluable when a retrograde ureteral access is difficult or impossible. Although it is understood that a surgical repair might be ultimately necessary, those patients who undergo PCN decompression first have an 87% success rate versus a 13% success rate in those patients without initial decompression; thus PCN optimizes the patient and improves the chances of maintaining a viable renal transplant.[11] In our experience, we must do everything possible to salvage a kidney due to the critical shortage of organs in the United States and the world.

20.1.4 Urethra

Urethral injuries are far more common in men than in women because of the differences in their anatomical structure. Women are protected from urethral injuries because their urethras are short and not firmly attached to the pubic bones. Typically, urethral injuries in women are seen only in association with vaginal and/or rectal injuries. Male urethras on the other hand, are long and fixed to the bones, making them more prone to injury. An important distinction is whether it is the anterior or posterior urethra in a man that is injured because it will help to guide management.

The anterior male urethra is composed of the penile and bulbous portions and is contained completely in the corpus spongiosum, except the proximal 2 cm of the bulbous portion (i.e., the pars nuda). A direct blow to the perineum, such as in a straddle injury, will compress the urethra and corpus spongiosum between the external hard object and the inferior aspect of the symphysis pubis and cause direct injury (tear or stricture) to the bulbous urethra, often even in the absence of a pelvic fracture.

The posterior male urethra is composed of the prostatic portion (encased in the prostate) and the membranous portion (contained within the urogenital diaphragm). Typically, injuries to the posterior urethra are associated with pelvic fractures and 5% of all men who sustain a pelvic fracture will also sustain a urethral injury. Specifically, the injuries tend to occur in the membranous portion of the posterior urethra secondary to shearing and rupturing of the puboprostatic ligaments.

Posterior urethral injuries are stratified into a three-tier classification system. Type 1, the least severe, includes stretch injuries caused by a pelvic hematoma. Type 2, moderately severe, includes rupture of the membranous urethra at the apex of the prostate, with extravasation of contrast above the urogenital diaphragm. Type 3, the most severe, is a rupture of the membranous and prostatic portions with disruption of the urogenital diaphragm and extravasation of contrast above and below the urogenital diaphragm.

Other causes of urethral injury include direct penile trauma, long-term bladder catheterization, and autodigestion by pancreatic enzymes after pancreatic transplantation and the drainage of pancreatic juices into the bladder.

Complications resulting from urethral injuries include strictures, incontinence, impotence, pelvic/perianal sinus tracts and fistulas, periurethral abscess, false passage, and stasis/infection.

Imaging

Retrograde urethrography is the gold standard modality for the initial evaluation of urethral injuries. If there is blood at the urethral meatus, or if there is any suspicion of a urethral injury, it is critical to get retrograde urethrography before any attempt is made to catheterize the bladder. In ~ 75% of patients with anterior urethral trauma, there would be blood at the meatus. However, statistics show a wide range (between 37 to 93%) of patients with posterior urethral injuries actually have blood at the meatus. Thus, one should have a high level of suspicion of this injury when dealing with GU trauma.[8]

Often, in the setting of trauma, a CT will be obtained immediately for another reason, much sooner than a retrograde urethrogram. Thus it is useful to know the CT signs that may indicate a urethral injury; typically, these signs may be associated with a posterior urethral injury. They include obscuration of the urogenital diaphragmatic fat plane, hematoma of the ischiocavernosus and obturator internus muscles, obscuration of the prostatic contour, and obscuration of the bulbocavernosus muscles.

If a subsequent urethral stricture is present, a simultaneous voiding cystogram and retrograde urethrogram are necessary. Also in a nonacute setting, MRI can be useful for assessing posttraumatic pelvic anatomy, determining position of the prostate, estimating the amount of pelvic fibrosis, and estimating the length of prostatomembranous defects. In general, US is not useful in the initial assessment of urethral injuries and we do not recommend it.

Treatment

The major considerations in the management of urethral injuries are whether there is a partial or complete disruption of the urethra, the length of strictures (short segment common in trauma, whereas long segment common in infection), and whether or not there is extension into the bladder neck or rectum in posterior injuries.

Blunt injuries resulting in partial tears of the anterior urethra can be conservatively managed with a suprapubic catheter or urethral catheterization. Short segment strictures are managed with optical urethrotomy or urethral dilatation. If the stricture is very dense, a surgical urethroplasty may be required. If this is necessary and the stricture is less than 1 cm long, surgical end-to-end anastomosis should be delayed. Longer strictures and complete disruptions of the urethra warrant a flap urethroplasty, though at the time of operation this procedure should be abandoned if a primary anastomosis cannot be successfully completed. End-to-end anastomosis ought to be avoided to prevent the complication of chordee. Most female urethral injuries can be sutured primarily.

Urethral stents are an option, but are not adequate as they are painful during erection, the fibrotic tissue tends to grow into the lumen of the stent, and there is always a risk of migration.

20.1.5 Penis

There are multiple causes of penile trauma including penetrating trauma, blunt force, continence- or sexual-pleasure-enhancing devices, and mutilation. Such trauma can result in penile fracture, amputation, penetrating injuries, soft tissue injuries, and priapism. Penile amputations can be complete or partial and are most often associated with an acute psychotic episode. Penetrating trauma is usually secondary to bullets, shrapnel, or stabbings.

Penile fracture is an uncommon urologic emergency. It results from the traumatic rupture of the corpora cavernosa. One or both corpus cavernosa can be involved, although it should be noted that there is a high association with urethral injuries when both are involved. Typically, it is secondary to sudden blunt trauma or abrupt lateral bending of the penis while erect. This most commonly occurs when having sexual intercourse in the female dominant position. The diagnosis is made by history (patient reports classic "popping" or "cracking" sound) and physical exam (characteristic "eggplant deformity"). An important distinction between a subcutaneous hematoma and a frank fracture is made by the history. If no sudden detumescence was present, which always occurs with a fracture, there is no need for an emergent surgical intervention.

Soft tissue injuries, by definition, do not involve the corpora and have similar etiology to soft tissue injuries of the scrotum. They are typically secondary to bites (human or animal, often dogs) and degloving injuries that involve machinery. The latter happens when the penile skin gets entrapped within clothing that then gets caught on machinery (usually farm equipment) or in motorcycle accidents. Other nontraumatic causes of soft tissue injuries include infection (such as Fournier gangrene) and burns (such as podophyllin, used in the treatment of genital warts). These will not be addressed in this chapter on GU trauma.

Priapism is classified into a low-flow state and a high-flow state. Both can result from trauma, though more commonly low-flow states are associated with veno-occlusive disease, particularly sickle cell disease. Low-flow priapism is caused by ischemia and it may occur in young men with blunt perineal or pelvic trauma that results in focal stenosis or occlusion of the common penile or cavernosal artery. High-flow priapism results from a fistulous formation between the cavernosal artery and the corpus cavernosum.

Imaging

For most of the aforementioned injuries, a good history and physical exam is sufficient to render a diagnosis. In equivocal cases, imaging may be helpful. For example, if it is unclear if a patient has a penile fracture, one can obtain a diagnostic cavernosography or an MRI to clarify.

In other cases, imaging is critical, particularly in cases of traumatic priapism. Duplex US is the most sensitive study for determining if a patient has a low-flow or a high-flow state and is considered a screening tool prior to intervention. For low-flow states, the mean systolic velocity (MSV) is the most sensitive parameter for identifying arterial insufficiency. An MSV between 35 to 60 mL/s is considered normal. In moderate arterial insufficiency, the MSV drops to 25 to 35 mL/s. A severe arterial insufficiency is less than 25 mL/s. Internal pudendal arteriography can be performed to confirm occlusive disease and plan for surgical reconstruction. High-quality selective bilateral penile pharmacoarteriography is purely anatomical and not functional, but is essential to determine the type and frequency of anatomical variance, site of obstruction, and potential collateral routes.[12]

Lastly, we must remember that in penile trauma, the urethra is often injured. As mentioned above, the best imaging technique to assess urethral injuries is the retrograde urethrography and it should be "gingerly" obtained if there is any suspicion, even without hematuria or blood at the urethral meatus.

Treatment

The goals for the treatment of all penile injuries are the same: restore normal flow to the penis and maintain erectile function, preserve penile length, and maintain the ability to void while standing. Most penile injuries, including penile fracture, amputation, and penetrating injuries, require emergent surgical exploration and reconstruction.

Historically, penile fractures were managed conservatively using cold compresses, pressure dressings, splinting, anti-inflammatory medications, fibrinolytics, and suprapubic diversion. However, it is now preferable to bring the patients immediately to the operating room to avoid possible complications such as missed urethral injury, abscess, nodule formation at the site of rupture, permanent penile curvature, painful erection, painful coitus, fibrotic plaques, and arteriovenous or arteriocalyceal fistulization.

A consideration to make in cases of penile amputation is the patient's past medical record. The literature suggests that the vast majority of patients who self-amputate their penis in an acute psychotic episode will desire penile preservation when their underlying mental illness has been treated. The exception is the patient who has repeatedly attempted amputation. Therefore, prior to repeated surgery, the risk of future self-mutilation must be weighed against the effects of replacement surgery.[13]

One instance when the interventional radiologist can provide the most therapeutic assistance is in high-flow priapism. With internal pudendal angiography, there usually is an abnormal rapid antegrade flow through the internal pudendal and penile arteries, often with pooling of contrast material in the corpus cavernosum from a ruptured cavernosal artery. A cavernosal artery-corpora cavernosal fistula may even be evident as an intense contrast blush at the base of the penis associated with early filling of venous channels in the late arterial phase. This can be corrected at the time of angiography with superselective transcatheter embolization of the internal pudendal artery and its branches with Gelfoam N-butyl-cyanoacrylate, particulate material, or platinum microcoils. Alternatively, the patient can be brought to the operating room to receive intracavernous vasoconstrictive agents, to shunt the blood away from the corpus cavernosum to the corpus spongiosum, or to ligate the internal pudendal branch arteries.[12]

20.1.6 Testicles/Scrotum

Testicular/scrotal trauma is relatively common and often occurs while playing sports or in motor vehicle crashes. Sports that are prone to testicular injuries and should raise suspicion are off-road bicycling/motor biking, in-line hockey, and rugby. Less often, the testicles can be injured by penetrating trauma or degloving accidents. Typically blunt trauma causes unilateral injuries, whereas penetrating trauma causes bilateral injuries.

Testicular injuries are testicular rupture, dislocation, torsion, or hematoma. Dislocation occurs in motor vehicle crashes or when a pedestrian is run over by a car. In 25% of cases, dislocations are bilateral.[8] If the tunica albuginea is torn/shattered, blood leaks from the site of injury and stretches the elastic scrotum until it is tense, potentially leading to infection and/or infertility.

Extratesticular injuries include hematoma, hematocele, epididymal fracture, and epididymitis and are often associated with testicular injuries. Hematoceles are collections of blood within the tunica vaginalis and can be secondary to orchiectomy, inguinal herniorrhaphy, or testicular rupture. Scrotal wall hematomas are common after blunt trauma. Epididymitis is typically seen in nontraumatic settings, but can also be a sequela of trauma.

Imaging

Ultrasound is useful in acute trauma because the degree of ecchymosis and hematoma do not accurately correlate with the severity of the testicular injury in blunt trauma. A normal parenchyma echo pattern with normal blood flow safely excludes significant injury. Ultrasound is also useful for assessing the severity of an injury by judging the echogenicity of the blood: Acute bleeding/contusion is hyperechoic; old blood is hypoechoic.

Ultrasound findings in testicular rupture include a heterogeneous echotexture of the testis with contour abnormality due to extrusion of the testes through the tunical defect, and disruption of the tunica albuginea. The most specific finding of rupture is a discrete fracture plane, but this is only seen in 17% of cases.[13]

Scrotal wall hematomas present as echogenic focal wall thickening or as complex fluid collections within the scrotal wall (depending on how much time has elapsed prior to the examination).

Doppler flow imaging helps to elucidate certain findings. Normal blood flow to the testes indicates an intact vascular pedicle. The absence of normal blood flow suggests testicular torsion (with loss of venous flow initially, and both arterial and venous flow later) or a devascularizing injury involving the spermatic cord.

Doppler flow is also useful to evaluate hematomas. The key US finding in a hematoma is lack of internal vascularity, which is particularly helpful because otherwise its appearance varies dramatically as the hematoma evolves. A hematoma superior to the testis may represent a spermatic cord hematoma in the appropriate setting (recent inguinal herniorrhaphy with iatrogenic injury, extension of retroperitoneal hemorrhage, or rarely varicocele rupture with blunt trauma).[14,15]

Doppler flow helps to differentiate epididymal pathology as well. An enlarged, ill-defined, heterogeneous epididymis may be an epididymal fracture or epididymitis. However, in a fracture there is absence of blood flow, whereas in epididymitis there is increased blood flow. Contrast-enhancement US may increase the contrast resolution and better characterize pathology. In equivocal cases, MRI or nuclear scintigraphy can provide additional information.

Treatment

The diagnostic radiologist has a role in the setting of testicular trauma. The interventional radiologist has a limited, if any, role. All scrotal traumas are treated either conservatively or with surgical exploration. If there is pain but no physical injury detected on history and physical exam, conservative management with pain medication and an athletic supporter is sufficient. Likewise, if there is pain, but only an intratesticular hematoma on US, but no fracture planes or disruption of the tunica albuginea, a conservative management is indicated. It is important to monitor all testicular hematomas to ensure they resolve completely and do not get secondarily infected, which may eventually necessitate orchiectomy. The interventional radiologist has a minimal participation in these events.

However, if a testicular rupture, dislocation refractory to manual reduction, torsion, or expanding hematoma is suspected, an emergent surgical exploration is mandatory. In fact, the salvage rate for testicular torsion decreases rapidly with almost 100% success if the patient is taken to the operating room within 6 hours of onset, a drop to 50% if taken within 6 to 12 hours, a further drop to 20% if within 12 to 24 hours, and almost unsalvageable, if presenting over 24 hours after onset.[14]

20.1.7 Female Genitalia

Trauma to the female genitalia results from many causes. The most common is childbirth, which may result in hematomas, lacerations, postpartum hemorrhage and, rarely, uterine arteriovenous fistulas (arteriovenous malformation [AVM]; AVF). Other causes are female genital mutilation (FGM), abusive assault, blunt trauma from sports (i.e., biking, snowboarding), and penetrating trauma from gunshots or stabbings.

Postpartum hemorrhage is one of the leading causes of maternal death worldwide and in the United States.[16] Hematomas and lacerations result from blunt trauma during delivery and are self-limiting. Uterine AVM and AVF are rare phenomena that can occur as a congenital anomaly (AVM) or can be acquired (AVF) after childbirth, cesarean, uterine curettage, gestational trophoblastic neoplasia, or endometrial cancer.

Female genital mutilation is any procedure that intentionally alters or causes injury to the female genital organs for nonmedical

reasons. This cruel practice considered by the international community to be a violation of human rights of girls and women, currently affects ~ 140 million women worldwide. It is divided into four subtypes: (1) clitoridectomy, (2) excision of the clitoris and labia minora, (3) Infibulation (narrowing of the vaginal opening by creating a covering seal), and (4) all other harmful procedures. There are many tragic consequences from such cruel procedures. In the immediate period, hemorrhage and infection are the major concerns. In the United States, the prevalence is low, but is increasing with the increasing number of emigrants from sub-Saharan Africa. Delayed consequences include repeat infections, infertility, painful cyst formation, vesicovaginal fistulas, dyspareunia, voiding difficulties, and psychosocial disorders.[17,18]

Imaging/Workup

Prior to any management, two important situations require immediate attention. If there is any suspicion of abusive assault, vaginal smears must be obtained for detection of spermatozoa prior to any other intervention. The other situation is if blood is present at the vaginal introitus. These women require a complete speculum exam of the vulva and vagina, preferably under sedation or general anesthesia. Careful documentation is mandatory.

For FGM, there is no workup or imaging required; a history and physical exam is sufficient.

Postpartum hemorrhage is characteristically worked up with clinical assessment in the direct postpartum period, analyzing blood loss and tracking Hb, Hct, and vital signs. If the bleeding does not stop quickly with surgical packing and suture techniques, the patient should be brought to angiography for IR management, without other imaging studies to prevent consumptive coagulopathy (▶ Fig. 20.12).[16]

Even though uterine AVM and AVF are rare, they have the potential for occurrence of significant blood loss; therefore, an accurate diagnosis is needed. Arteriovenous malformations can be detected by Doppler US, CT, MRI, and angiography.

Vulvar injuries, such as hematomas or lacerations, can be ideally studied with pelvic CT. The main goal of imaging is not to assess the vulva (which can be examined clinically), but rather to search for other related injuries. Cystography may be needed if there is suggestion of other associated pelvic injuries and there is concern.[8]

Management

Most vulvar injuries caused by blunt trauma are treated conservatively with nonsteroidal anti-inflammatory drugs and cold packs. Surgery is not warranted; however, if there is an extended vulvar hematoma, there are other abdominal or pelvic findings, or if the patient is hemodynamically unstable, surgical exploration is warranted. In cases of vulvar laceration, realignment after conservative debridement is indicated. Antibiotics must be administered.[8]

Female genital mutilation is a difficult and complicated subject steeped in psychosocial and cultural issues that must be carefully addressed in an attempt to be sensitive to the patient's desires. For delayed sequela, corrective surgery can be arranged. That is beyond the scope of this chapter.[17]

The interventional radiologist has a major role in puerperal injuries. Pelvic arteriography is needed in puerperal hematomas, postpartum hemorrhage, and uterine AVF/AVM and

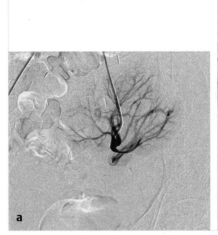
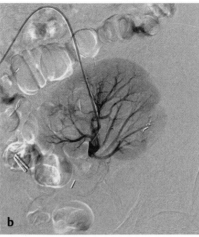

Fig. 20.12 Renal biopsy of a transplanted kidney was done resulting in macroscopic hematuria. (a) Renal arteriography shows small arterial venous fistulaat the biopsy site. (b) After superselective embolization with platinum microcoils the arterial venous fistula is no longer identified. Minimal amount of tissue was devascularized.

arterial or venous embolization can be performed. A great advantage of embolization in postpartum hemorrhage is that it preserves fertility, is easier, much safer, and more effective than surgery. The faster the hemorrhage is stopped, the better the chances for survival without risk of end organ failure. The surgical alternative is ligation of the internal iliac arteries, a technically difficult and less-effective procedure. Hysterectomy is another alternative and not ideal if fertility is desired.[16,19]

20.2 Conclusion

Trauma to the GU system in men and women is a serious cause of morbidity and mortality. A team approach with general physicians, obstetrician/gynecologists, urologists, and interventional radiologists is encouraged. Interventional radiology plays a very important role in the diagnosis and management of GU trauma injuries.

References

[1] Blair M. Overview of genitourinary trauma. Urol Nurs 2011; 31: 139–145, quiz 146

[2] Kandarpa K, Machan L. Handbook of Interventional Radiologic Procedures. 4th ed. Philadelphia, PA: Lippincott, Williams & Wilkins; 2011

[3] Kawashima A, Sandler CM, Corl FM et al. Imaging of renal trauma: a comprehensive review. Radiographics 2001; 21: 557–574

[4] Moore EE, Shackford SR, Pachter HL et al. Organ injury scaling: spleen, liver, and kidney. J Trauma 1989; 29: 1664–1666

[5] Ramchandani P, Buckler PM. Imaging of genitourinary trauma. AJR Am J Roentgenol 2009; 192: 1514–1523 Review

[6] Sagalowsky AI, McConnell JD, Peters PC. Renal trauma requiring surgery: an analysis of 185 cases. J Trauma 1983; 23: 128–131

[7] Federle MP, Brown TR, McAninch JW. Penetrating renal trauma: CT evaluation. J Comput Assist Tomogr 1987; 11: 1026–1030

[8] Lynch TH, Martínez-Piñeiro L, Plas E et al. European Association of Urology. EAU guidelines on urological trauma. Eur Urol 2005; 47: 1–15 Review

[9] American Urological Foundation. Bladder Trauma 2011. Available at: http://www.urologyhealth.org/urology/index.cfm?article=99. Accessed March 21, 2012

[10] Brant WE, Helms CA. Fundamentals of Diagnostic Radiology. 3rd ed. Philadelphia, PA: Lippincott, Williams & Wilkins; 2006

[11] Goldstein I, Cho SI, Olsson CA. Nephrostomy drainage for renal transplant complications. J Urol 1981; 126: 159–163

[12] Bakal CW, Silberzweig J, Cynamon J, et al. Vascular and Interventional Radiology: Principles and Practice. New York, NY: Thieme; 2002

[13] Santucci RA, Broghammer JA. Penile Fracture and Trauma. EMedicine; 2011. Available at: http://emedicine.medscape.com/article/456305-overview. Accessed March 22, 2012

[14] Bhatt S, Dogra VS. Role of US in testicular and scrotal trauma. Radiographics 2008; 28: 1617–1629

[15] Terlecki RP, Santucci RA. Testicular Trauma. EMedicine; 2011. Available at: http://emedicine.medscape.com/article/441362-overview. Accessed March 22, 2012

[16] Josephs SC. Obstetric and gynecologic emergencies: a review of indications and interventional techniques. Semin Intervent Radiol 2008; 25: 337–346

[17] World Health Organization. Female Genital Mutilation; 2012. Available at: http://www.who.int/mediacentre/factsheets/fs241/en/. Accessed March 22, 2012

[18] Laube DW. Evaluation and treatment of female genital mutilation Journal Watch Women's Health.; 2001: 22Accessed March 22, 2012

[19] Wang Z, Chen J, Shi H et al. Efficacy and safety of embolization in iatrogenic traumatic uterine vascular malformations. Clin Radiol 2012; 67: 541–545

21 Interventional Radiology in Extremity Vascular Trauma

Mark M. Levy, Jaime Tisnado, Malcolm K. Sydnor, and Rao R. Ivatury

21.1 Introduction

The role of digital subtraction angiography (DSA) in the evaluation and management of extremity trauma has evolved dramatically over the past decade and continues to do so. Significant improvements in noninvasive imaging such as computed tomography angiography (CTA), now widely available on an emergent basis, have altered the algorithm for diagnosing peripheral vascular injuries. Likewise, the availability of high-quality intraoperative DSA imaging diminishes the time between the diagnosis and treatment of peripheral vascular injuries. At this time, magnetic resonance imaging (MRI) is being used in certain institutions to add or replace some information as well. Most importantly, with the continuous developments of catheter and guidewire technology, the advent of covered and uncovered stents, stent grafts, and significant improvements in embolization techniques, therapeutic intervention can be provided at the time of diagnostic DSA, either in the interventional radiology (IR) suite or in the operating room (OR).

In this chapter, we present an overview of the current role of diagnostic and interventional DSA, as it relates to patients with traumatic vascular injuries of the upper and lower extremities. We provide a limited historical perspective, and try to clarify the contemporary role of IR in the current context of primary imaging modalities.

21.2 Evolution of the Role of DSA in Extremity Vascular Trauma

Although a limited number of arterial repairs were accomplished by German surgeons during World War I,[1] ligation of injured arteries remained the standard practice for arterial trauma through World War II.[2] Until the time of the Korean War, most extremity arterial injuries were managed with arterial ligation, which often required limb amputation. Arterial reconstructions were done with increased frequency in different vascular territories during the Korean War. An important work by Hughes et al documented decreased amputation rates from 49% to 13% over the WWII era.[3] Furthermore, the Vietnam war period witnessed important improvements in the rapid transport of injured soldiers to military hospitals, resulting in significantly decreased time between suffering an arterial injury and its subsequent surgical repair. Despite the fact that much more care of associated soft tissue injury resulting from high-velocity missiles were seen in the Vietnam war, limb salvage rates remained similar following arterial trauma, very likely due to a stable hospital environment and a rapid patient evacuation.[1]

Through the time of the Vietnam conflict, virtually all lower extremity injuries were managed with prompt surgical exploration of the injured vessels. Direct arterial reconstructions were then performed using autogenous conduits. There was then, little if any pragmatic role for extremity DSA, mainly due to limited availability, and the need to proceed immediately to operative repair due to tissue ischemia, given that no time for a diagnostic arteriogram was available.

Today, most modern civilian extremity vascular injuries can be localized by a clinical assessment of the injured limb. By analyzing the associated fractures and/or dislocations in the context of blunt injuries, examining bullet holes and knife wounds and reviewing plain film missile locations, accurate conclusions can be made regarding the most likely location of an arterial injury. This clinical analysis can usually localize the segment of arterial injury, particularly if only a single arterial traumatic lesion is likely.

Given the surgeon's ability to identify the likely vascular injury location without the need of DSA in many cases, what then is the role of diagnostic DSA in the evaluation of peripheral vascular traumatic injuries in the modern era? The answers are in three clinical contexts: (1) state-of-the-art current diagnostic DSA may, in some instances, rule out a surgically relevant arterial lesion, perhaps identifying arterial vasospasm, which can be treated with vasodilators; (2) a therapeutic endovascular intervention can be performed in many instances obviating the need for conventional surgical exploration and repair; (3) DSA may provide unanticipated important information regarding the true location of the arterial injuries (especially if more than one are present) and venous injuries as well.

21.3 Factors Determining the Role of DSA in Extremity Vascular Trauma

Summarizing the process of surgical decision making in extremity arterial injuries is beyond the scope of this chapter. However, a clarification of some surgical concerns is warranted because it plays a role in the decision for diagnostic imaging.

21.3.1 Severity of Limb Ischemia

Arterial injuries of the extremities may result in mild, moderate, severe, or critical ischemia. On occasion, no ischemia may be present. The degree of ischemia is assessed by the presence and character of palpable pulses, ankle-to-brachial index (or wrist-to-brachial index in the upper extremity), examination of capillary refill, and sensory and motor examination. If ischemia is severe or critical, the time for therapeutic revascularization is very limited. Therefore, no diagnostic DSA in the IR suite is required, given the patient must be taken immediately to the OR for surgical repair. When the degree of extremity ischemia is only mild to moderate, emergency revascularization is not necessary; therefore, a prompt DSA may more pragmatically proceed to subsequent surgical repair (or IR repair, if possible).

21.3.2 Isolated Vascular Injury Versus the Injured Extremity Artery in Polytrauma

The management of patients with isolated extremity vascular injuries differs from that of patients with life-threatening injuries associated with extremity vascular injuries. The simultaneous presence of intracranial, intrathoracic, and/or intra-abdominal injuries often changes, and must change the role of IR in extremity trauma management for two reasons: (1) The delay required to address the life-threatening head and/or truncal injuries may obligate a more immediate revascularization as soon as the limb injuries can be addressed. (2) Systemic heparinization indicated for peripheral vascular trauma is usually contraindicated in the context of polytrauma. For example, patients with intracranial injuries (e.g., subdural or subarachnoid hemorrhage) may require lifesaving emergent craniotomy, therefore delaying full assessment and repair of associated extremity vascular injuries.

In contrast to patients with polytrauma, patients with isolated extremity vascular injuries proceed directly to arterial evaluation and repair, with administration of systemic heparinization when indicated. Although time to presentation may still create delays prior to repair, there is usually enough time to proceed with emergent diagnostic DSA before the repair, if indicated. When one is determining whether or not conventional DSA is indicated in a trauma patient, the potential diagnostic and therapeutic benefits of DSA must be weighed against the risks associated with the study (e.g., time delay in revascularization, contrast allergies, nephrotoxicity, and/or arterial puncture site complications). In instances when the risks of diagnostic DSA are increased (e.g., acute renal failure), DSA with alternative contrast agents (e.g., CO_2) may be employed, or alternative noninvasive imaging techniques utilized (e.g., CT or duplex Doppler ultrasound (US) arterial imaging).

21.3.3 Alternative Diagnostic Imaging of Extremity Vascular Trauma

Currently, DSA is the gold standard for imaging of upper and lower extremity vascular injuries, against which other non-invasive imaging modalities—CTA, magnetic resonance angiography (MRA), duplex US, Doppler US—are compared. Furthermore at this time, CTA is being developed and used as a primary imaging method in special cases and situations. We believe that eventually it may or will replace DSA for trauma patient evaluation.

Over recent years, the alternative noninvasive imaging modalities, including duplex US, CTA, and MRA, provide other methods for the imaging of both upper and lower extremity management. In the trauma setting, those imaging methods must be considered as alternatives to conventional DSA.

Duplex Ultrasound

Duplex US provides real-time imaging of the upper extremity arterial tree from the level of the axillary artery to the radial and ulnar arteries in the wrist. The subclavian arteries can be imaged with duplex US, but the midportions of the arteries are often difficult to image adequately because of the overlying clavicles. Furthermore, in acute upper extremity trauma, duplex US imaging may be limited by the presence of hematomas and surgical wounds. If deformities or hematomas are small or absent, duplex US imaging can provide real-time information of both arterial and venous anatomy, as well as quantify flow through the upper extremity arterial tree. In the lower extremity, duplex US imaging provides real-time imaging of the

arterial tree from the common femoral artery to the popliteal artery. Imaging distal to the popliteal artery is inconsistent; although imaging of the mid-to-distal posterior and anterior tibial arteries is feasible. Also in trauma, duplex US imaging of the lower extremity may be limited by hematomas and surgical wounds. Hence, for diagnostic purposes when soft tissue abnormalities or hematomas are small or absent, duplex US imaging provides real-time information about arterial and venous anatomy and flow. The utility of duplex US imaging in penetrating extremity injuries has been examined by Knudson et al, who demonstrated a high sensitivity for detecting clinically relevant arterial injuries.[4] Unfortunately, the 24/7 availability of arterial duplex US imaging may be limited in some institutions. Whether it is not available in-house, or one must await the arrival of the on-call technologist from outside, precious time is wasted that could be critical in some severely traumatized patients. The utility and limitations of duplex US imaging in the assessment of acute arterial vascular trauma is well known.[5] Its most useful role is in surveillance and follow-up of minor vascular injuries, chronologically. (▶ Fig. 21.1)

Computed Tomography Angiography

Recent improvements in CT technology including 64-row multidetector (and more; i.e., 256), dual source scanners, and three-dimensional (3D) arterial reformats allow CT scanning in the emergent evaluation of extremity acute traumatic arterial injury.[6,7,8] During the routine CT scans in the emergency room (ER), in the evaluation of the head, chest, and abdomen of trauma patients, the arterial evaluation is much more convenient. Currently, most institutions have a multidetector array CT (MDCT) scanner in the ER which is used in the triage of patients as discussed in other chapters.

For diagnostic purposes, CTA is similar to DSA in costs, and time to complete the study. In a recent comparison of diagnostic modalities by Seamon et al, CTA had a 100% sensitivity and specificity for clinically relevant arterial abnormalities among a small cohort of 21 patients with extremity trauma and either hard signs of arterial trauma or decreased ankle or wrist pressure indices. They concluded that due to its availability, lower cost, great sensitivity and noninvasiveness, CTA will be the screening diagnostic modality of choice in vascular trauma to the extremities.[9]

Magnetic Resonance Angiography

Despite its well-established role in the diagnosis of arterial occlusive and aneurysmal disease, the use of MRA in the trauma setting is limited to neurovascular evaluation.[10,11] Moreover, many trauma patients, especially those with penetrating injuries may have metallic objects (e.g., bullets, pellets, shrapnel), contraindicating MRA. Furthermore, MRA is, in most places not routinely available, and quality imaging requires special technological expertise. Therefore, the current role of MRA in the acute evaluation of extremity arterial trauma is limited.

21.4 Blunt and Penetrating Upper Extremity Vascular Injury

Patients with blunt trauma to the upper extremity arteries due to crush, shearing, or stretching forces, usually present with no

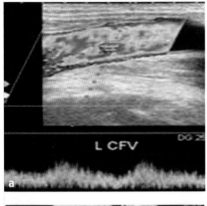
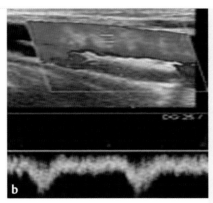

Fig. 21.1 Iatrogenic arterial venous fistula between the common femoral artery and vein. (a,b) Color Doppler ultrasound study the left groin shows the characteristic findings of an AVF. (c) The pelvic arteriogram confirms findings.

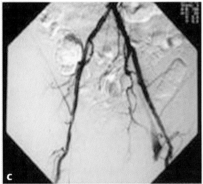

palpable radial or ulnar pulses. The initial assessment includes an accurate examination of the pulses, sensory and motor function, and capillary refill; the wrist pressure is "indexed" to the systemic pressure with a wrist-to-brachial index, using the ipsilateral brachial pressure if the injury is distal to the brachial pressure, or the contralateral brachial pressure if the injury is proximal to the ipsilateral brachial pulse. When fractures are present, the plain films often suggest the likely location of an associated vascular injury. Examining the extremity and reviewing the plain films helps in the diagnosis of an arterial injury. Blunt arterial injuries may require a DSA to better define the location, extent, and nature of the arterial injury.

Penetrating vascular injuries are assessed in a similar fashion as blunt vascular injuries. The degree of arterial insufficiency is assessed at the level of the end organ (wrist and hand, wrist-to-brachial index). The clinical assessment of an arterial injury location is frequently, but not always obvious and it is easy to define the nature of the lesion: partial or complete arterial disruption or transection. Consequently, a DSA may not be necessary and immediate surgical exploration is often indicated.

It is useful to classify upper extremity arterial injuries into proximal (subclavian and axillary) and distal (brachial and forearm). Endovascular repair of proximal injuries offers several well-documented advantages over conventional surgical repair. The endovascular repair obviates the need for a more morbid intrathoracic or supraclavicular surgical exposure, and utilizes prosthetic devices appropriate for 5- to 10-mm vessels. Some authors suggest that the majority of these injuries be managed with endovascular techniques.[12] Most main truncal injuries require management with covered stents. Due to technical limitations during stenting, the risks of sacrifice of critical branch

vessels (e.g., vertebral artery), must be weighed against the risks of surgical repair.

Hemorrhage from the more distal axillosubclavian arterial branch injuries are effectively treated with embolization. More precarious and controversial at this time is the management of radiographically diagnosed traumatic occlusions of the axillary and subclavian arteries. Such occlusions are, indeed, true transections, particularly following penetrating trauma, given that angiography cannot differentiate between a true transection and a thrombotic occlusion. Following the initial hemorrhage, the two ends of a transected vessel thrombose and retract due to physiologic vasospasm and tamponade by the hematoma and surrounding soft tissue. In this clinical setting, attempts at "probing" of the transection with a guidewire may dislodge the thrombus and resume severe hemorrhage. Hence, the risk-to-benefit ratio in these circumstances must be assessed by both the interventional radiologist and trauma vascular surgeon. In special circumstances, the placement of a proximal occlusion balloon by the IR team in the subclavian or axillary arteries may permit a safer and easier surgical exploration of the artery in question with a more desirable proximal control.[10,12,13,14,15]

In a meta-analysis[15] of the use of endovascular stenting for the treatment of subclavian (150) or axillary (10) artery injuries, this treatment was noted in penetrating injury (56.3%; 29 gunshot wounds; 61 Stab Wound), blunt trauma (21.3%), iatrogenic catheter-related injury (21.8%), and surgical injury (0.6%). These included pseudoaneurysm (77), arteriovenous fistula (AVF; 27), occlusion (16), transection (8), perforation (22), and dissection (6). Endovascular stent placement was successful in 96.9% of patients. On follow-up ranging from discharge to 70 months, patency rate was 84.4%. There were no mortalities

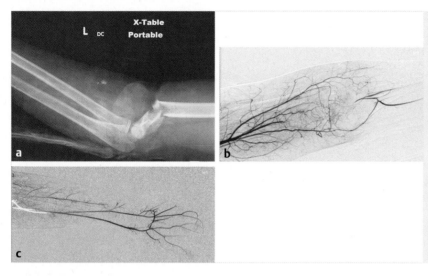

Fig. 21.2 Extensive comminuted fracture of distal humerus and radioulnar joint in a child who had a serious fall. The forearm was cold, pale, pulseless. (a–c) Arteriogram shows occlusion of the brachial artery and the three arteries of the forearm. No endovascular management is indicated. Orthopedic and vascular surgical combined approach is needed, especially in children.

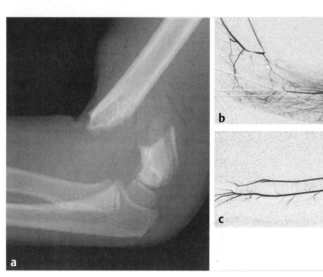

Fig. 21.3 An 8-year-old boy suffered an open supracondylar fracture of the right humerus after a fall onto an outstretched hand. (a) Increasing duskiness and loss of pulses were noted in the hand after open reduction and internal fixation. (b) Emergent angiograms demonstrated a long segment distal brachial artery disruption with reconstitution of the radial and ulnar arteries. (c) He underwent successful open thrombectomy and reconstruction with saphenous vein graft and was eventually discharged home on daily aspirin without deficit.

related to endovascular intervention and only one patient developed new neurologic deficits after its use.

The spectrum of vascular injuries to the more distal upper extremity arterial tree includes AVFs, pseudoaneurysms, arterial transections (total or partial), and thromboses. Even though endovascular repair of distal brachial or forearm arteries is feasible, vessel caliber is smaller, procedural times are likely longer, and durability of the repair remains unknown. Considering the excellent (acceptable) durability and morbidity of surgical repair, diagnostic DSA is obtained if the diagnosis of arterial injury is in doubt. If the patient has a pulseless upper extremity and a localizable obvious distal arterial injury, DSA is unnecessary prior to surgical repair. Rather, a surgical exploration and intraoperative DSA is more practical, easier, and more beneficial.

In an analysis of experience with 5 to 6 years, 135 patients and 159 upper extremity arterial injuries, Franz et al[16] noted 116 penetrating (73.0%) and 43 blunt (27.0%) injuries. Arterial distribution involved was as follows: 13 axillary (8.2%), 40 brachial (25.2%), 52 radial (32.7%), 51 ulnar (32.1%), and 3 other (1.9%). The majority of injuries (96.8%) receiving vascular management underwent surgical intervention–76 primary repair (49.7%), 41 ligation (26.8%), and 31 bypass (20.3%). Only five had endovascular (3.3%) procedures with good results (▶ Fig. 21.2, ▶ Fig. 21.3, ▶ Fig. 21.4, ▶ Fig. 21.5).

21.5 Blunt and Penetrating Lower Extremity Vascular Injury[17,18,19,20,21]

Patients with blunt lower extremity arterial trauma usually present with a pulseless extremity and/or diminished ankle-to-brachial index. The lower extremity assessment includes examination of pulses, preservation of the sensorimotor function and capillary refill and measurement of ankle-to-brachial indices. The injury location can often be estimated based upon the examination of the pulses and review of the plain film for fracture(s) and also examining the bullet holes or fragments. The injuries are rarely proximal aortoiliac (i.e., no palpable femoral pulse), or more commonly, distal (infrainguinal), (i.e., femoral pulse palpable, but more distal pulses absent).

The clinical evaluation of penetrating trauma to the arterial tree is similar to that for blunt trauma; however, with a high

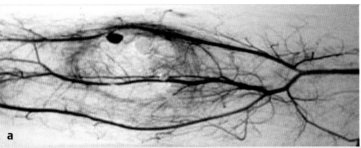
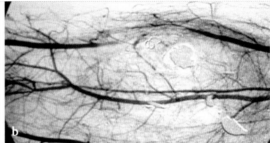

Fig. 21.4 (a) A young man received a bullet injury in the forearm. Massive swelling and destruction of tissues was evident. (b) Arteriogram showed a small pseudoaneurysm of the ulnar artery that was readily embolized.

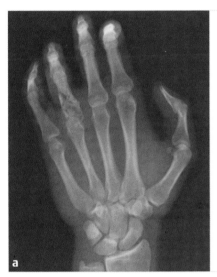
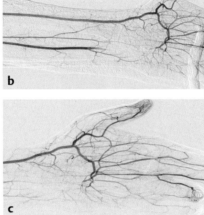

Fig. 21.5 A 17-year-old boy was shot in the left fourth phalanx during a robbery attempt with the bullet exiting the volar aspect of the wrist. (a) At exam he had an absent left ulnar pulse as well as third to fifth digit numbness and paresthesias. (b, c) Left Upper Extremity (LUE) angiogram demonstrated a traumatic occlusion of the left ulnar artery at the wrist with retrograde filling of the palmar and digital arteries via the radial artery. He underwent operative repair of the ulnar artery and was discharged into police custody in 4 days.

index of suspicion that a main artery may have been partially or completely transected. Patients with penetrating injuries to the iliac vessels are usually hemodynamically unstable, and are immediately taken to the operating room for laparotomy and vascular exploration. On the other hand, those with penetrating injuries to the infrainguinal vessels are usually hemodynamically stable. Traditionally, these patients were explored for immediate surgical repair. With improvements in endovascular and IR technology, small injuries (partial transections, intimal flaps) in stable patients are manageable with the insertion of covered or uncovered stents.

Although the durability and patency of stenting in traumatic settings is yet to be determined, endovascular therapy at least obviates the need for emergent surgery in a limb with hematomas, distorted tissue planes, and possible contamination. At this time, at least in part, the current role of DSA in these isolated cases is to accurately assess the feasibility of an endovascular repair, or provide mapping for a definitive surgical repair.

Penetrating injuries to the infrapopliteal vessels mandate surgical repair if all three leg arteries are occluded or transected. The role of DSA is to evaluate which arteries are injured. Injuries to the superficial femoral artery (SFA) and/or popliteal arteries mandate surgical vascular repair for acute severe or critical limb ischemia. However, there is a degree of redundancy

with the three leg arteries (i.e., injury to one or two of the three arteries does not necessarily mandate surgical repair, if one of the three arteries remains patent). In many instances, patency of an uninjured single leg vessel cannot be adequately determined by physical examination alone and usually is better assisted with DSA. Therefore, one of the more important roles for DSA in trauma is the assessment of patency or injury to the leg arteries.

In a 5-year period, 65 patients with 75 lower extremity arterial injuries were admitted to an institution. The majority of patients (78.4%) suffered concomitant lower extremity injuries, most frequently bony or venous injuries, whereas 35.4% experienced associated injuries to other body regions. The most common injury mechanism was a gunshot wound (46.7%). Arterial injuries were penetrating in 56% and 44% from blunt injury. Superficial femoral (32.0%), popliteal (21.3%), and tibial (36.0%) were the most frequently involved arteries. A majority of the injuries were transections (30.7%). Orthopedic surgeons performed amputations as primary procedures in three patients (4.6%). The majority (76.8%) of injuries receiving vascular management underwent surgical intervention. Only 7.5% (four patients) had endovascular procedures (▶ Fig. 21.6, ▶ Fig. 21.7, ▶ Fig. 21.8, ▶ Fig. 21.9, ▶ Fig. 21.10, ▶ Fig. 21.11).

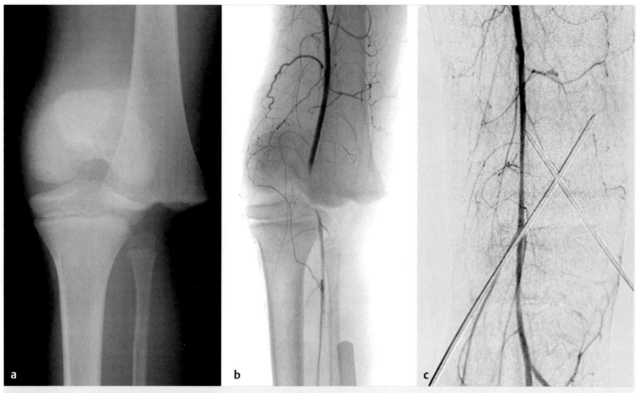

Fig. 21.6 An 11-year-old boy suffered a Salter 1 fracture through the distal femoral epiphysis with complete anterior displacement while playing tackle football. (a) Loss of pulses and worsening motor/sensory deficit after attempted reduction prompted an arteriogram. (b) This demonstrated a focal popliteal artery occlusion at the knee with reconstitution below the joint. (c) Pulses returned after open reduction and internal fixation and a repeat angiogram showed restoration of flow in the superficial femoral, popliteal, and leg arteries. He was discharged home in stable condition on daily aspirin.

21.6 Summary of the Spectrum of Traumatic Extremity Arterial Lesions

21.6.1 Vessel Occlusion

An arteriographically demonstrated arterial occlusion may represent a true complete thrombotic occlusion, as a consequence of shear or blast forces, creating an intimal or medial (or both) injury and subsequent thrombosis. The mechanisms of injury can involve deceleration associated with vessel torque and bone fractures, a blast from missiles or crush mechanisms, or penetrating injuries from bullets and knives. These often result in partial or complete transection of an artery or vein. Hemorrhage ensues and if it ceases, the injury may masquerade as a segmental arterial occlusion. Our inability to fully differentiate between a de novo arterial occlusion from an arterial transection with subsequent thrombosis has contributed to a delayed progress in the endovascular management of vascular thromboses.

Upper extremity arterial occlusions may be proximal: subclavian and axillary or distal: brachial, radial, ulnar, and interosseous. These occlusions have management algorithms that are slightly different.

Occlusions of the axillosubclavian arteries may be more conveniently managed by IR at the time of injury, with DSA, and endovascular approach if feasible because those arteries are more difficult to access with surgery. This repair is feasible in approximately half of events.[19] Lately this approach is preferred if feasible. Otherwise, surgery is needed. Placement of an occlusion balloon in the subclavian artery may be very helpful, particularly if the subclavian artery is already catherized.[20] Despite ample literature available regarding the endovascular management of axillosubclavian traumatic injuries, there is poor documentation of success in traversing occlusions owing to major difficulties in differentiating complete occlusions without a transection from a transection with thrombosis. Thrombolytic therapy, the choice therapy in occlusions or obstructions of the thoracic outlet vessels in nontraumatic pathology, is contraindicated in most, if not all, acute traumatic vascular injuries.

Traumatic occlusions of the brachial arteries are managed with open surgical reconstruction, and direct arterial repair or interposition vein grafting. The brachial artery is surgically exposed with relative ease so the advantages of traversing a "functional" (not organic) occlusion are minimal. Moreover, if a catheter has already been inserted in the brachial artery for diagnostic DSA, then a wire can be advanced easily across the occlusion. Rapid revascularization can be done with endovascular methods. Although endovascular repairs are documented to be effective in a short-term follow-up, they likely will have poor long-term durability.[12] We think this must be considered temporizing only in those patients with acute ischemia of several hours.

Single occlusions of the more distal radial and/or ulnar arteries are tolerated well and managed conservatively, unless

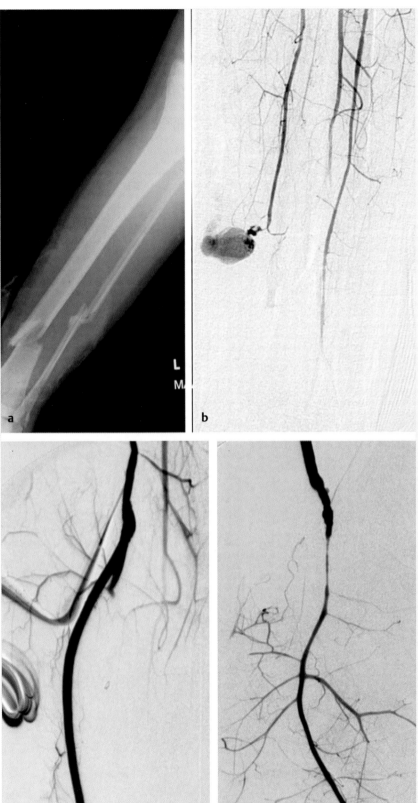

Fig. 21.7 (a) A 15-year-old boy with open left tibial and fibular fractures after a motorcycle accident, arrived in the emergency room with absent pedal pulses and no Doppler signals in his foot. (b,c) Emergency arteriography demonstrated a pseudoaneurysm and an arterial venous fistula from a transected posterior tibial artery. (d) The boy underwent repair of fractures and revascularization with proximal to distal posterior tibial artery bypass using reversed saphenous vein graft. He was discharged home in good condition in 2 weeks.

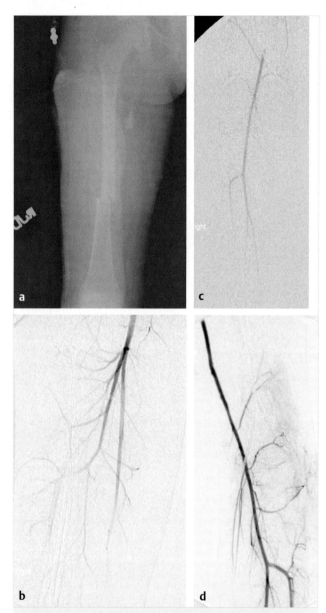

Fig. 21.8 A 7-year-old girl was struck by a car and arrived in the emergency room unstable hemodynamically with bilateral femur fractures. (a) She was resuscitated in the emergency room and underwent open repair of a right femoral fracture with loss of distal pulses noted on postoperative day 3. (b,c) Arteriogram showed a right superficial femoral artery (SFA) transection with distal reconstitution of the popliteal artery. (d) She underwent right femoral to popliteal artery bypass with reversed saphenous vein graft followed by fasciotomy for compartment syndrome.

multiple arterial occlusions render the limb ischemic. Otherwise, simultaneous radial and ulnar traumatic thromboses are managed operatively, as thrombolytic therapy is contraindicated most of the time.

Traumatic occlusions of the arteries of the lower extremities are rather common. Both blunt and/or penetrating trauma may result in arterial thrombosis. At this time, the IR management of atherosclerotic arterial occlusions includes percutaneous transluminal angioplasty (PTA) and/or stenting, but the

endovascular management of traumatic arterial thromboses has been developing slowly given that there is a lack of documentation of long-term patency with this method of therapy. Interestingly, recanalization of tibial artery thrombosis due to blunt trauma has been reported using a combination of low-profile angioplasty balloons and placement of coronary stents.

21.6.2 Vessel Transection/ Pseudoaneurysm

The demonstration of extravascular contrast material at DSA is the sine qua non of arterial disruption. The spectrum of arterial disruption severity ranges from partial and contained disruption (pseudoaneurysm) to complete transection with uncontrolled external or internal hemorrhage. Arteriography in both will show extravasation of contrast material, therefore, we cannot usually determine if there is a partial or total transection or a pseudoaneurysm, or both. Three IR techniques to effectively manage these potentially life- or limb-threatening injuries are (1) temporary balloon occlusion, (2) embolization, and (3) stenting. These methods are discussed in other chapters.

With the exception of the hemodynamically unstable patient with active hemorrhage that usually goes directly to the OR, there are well-documented applications of endovascular grafting for partial disruption of the axillosubclavian arteries.[10,15] For many years, surgeons and interventional radiologists have employed covered stent grafts successfully resulting in decreased blood loss and length of hospital stay among non-randomized patient cohorts.

Therapeutic embolization is also well documented as an effective method for treating leg artery pseudoaneurysms both at the time of the injury, as well as later in a subacute or chronic presentation.[16,17] Lopera et al recently described eight consecutive patients with penetrating trauma, with arterial transections, or pseudoaneurysms.[18] Six of eight patients had associated AVF, and all were successfully treated with embolization with coils, thrombin, and/or *N*-butyl cyanoacrylate (▶ Fig. 21.12).

21.6.3 Branch Vessel Transection Pseudoaneurysm

Active arterial hemorrhage from branches (e.g., circumflex femoral, circumflex humeral, or profunda femoris) branches, can result in external hemorrhage and/or contained hematoma. Selective catheterization of the bleeding branch permits embolization, preferably proximal and distal to the pseudoaneurysm —the so-called sandwich technique. (▶ Fig. 21.12)

21.6.4 Vasospasm

Concentric narrowing of the caliber is a nonspecific, reversible arteriographic finding that can result from arterial vasospasm secondary to trauma. In younger patients, severe vasospasm may simulate frank arterial occlusion. Arterial vasospasm can be confirmed with intra-arterial administration of vasodilators. We prefer 200 to 500 microgram boluses of nitroglycerin. If the spasm is relieved, we rule out extrinsic compression or intravascular thrombosis. In addition, vasodilatation may help to delineate an associated intimal or transmural arterial injury.

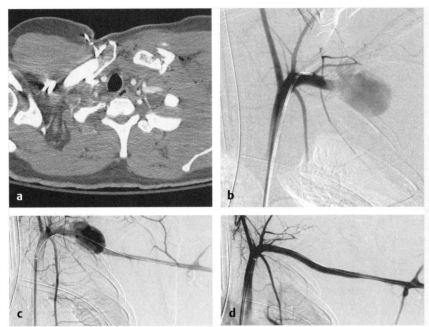

Fig. 21.9 A young boy received a stab wound in the left shoulder. (a) CT scan after the injury. (b) Emergency arteriogram shows complete occlusion of the left subclavian artery and a huge pseudoaneurysm. (b) The occluded subclavian artery was easily crossed with a glide wire using a coaxial system with a 7-French (F) sheath, a 5-F catheter, and the wire. (c) Arteriogram shows patency and relatively "normal" flow in left brachial artery. The large pseudoaneurysm remained unchanged in size. (d) After easy insertion of a 6-mm balloon-expandable covered stent. Complete patency of the subclavian artery and all branches is shown in the final arteriogram. The procedure was done in a short time. The patient recovered and went home.

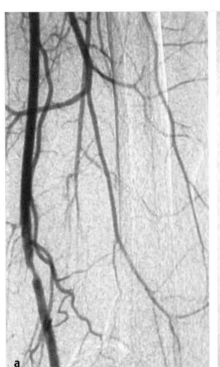
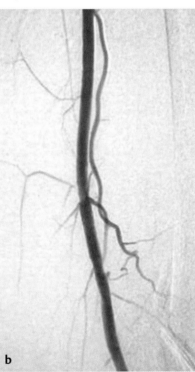

Fig. 21.10 A young man received a bullet wound in the thigh. Significant diminution of distal pulses was noted prompting an arteriogram. (a) Superficial femoral arteriogram shown localized stenosis of lumen of artery. (b) After placement of covered stent the lesion is no longer seen.

However, on occasion, vasodilators do not alter the appearance of the vessel. So, the diagnosis could still be in doubt. A high degree of suspicion and repeated clinical evaluation is needed here. (▶ Fig. 21.2, ▶ Fig. 21.3, ▶ Fig. 21.6, ▶ Fig. 21.7, ▶ Fig. 21.10)

21.6.5 Arteriovenous Fistula

Acute traumatic AVFs are common occurrences in the upper and lower extremities. The usual mechanism is penetrating trauma with simultaneous injury to an artery and adjacent vein. Physical examination may demonstrate a bruit or a thrill over the site. There may be associated limb ischemia, however, most times, the distal arterial perfusion is maintained. Sometimes the exact site of a large AVF communication can be difficult to localize due to the very rapid, near-simultaneous filling of arteries and veins. Increasing the frame rate of filming (7–15 × second), a superselective catheterization, filming in different obliquities, and increasing the amount of contrast material will help.

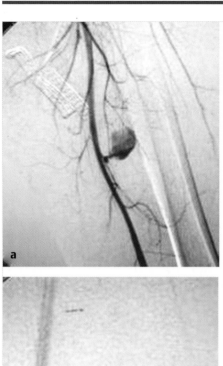

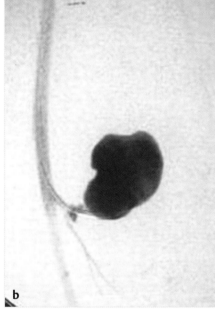

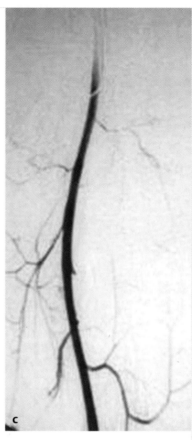

Fig. 21.11 Left superficial femoral arteriogram after a stabbing in the midthigh. Swelling and extensive bleeding ensued. (a,b) A small pseudoaneurysm is noted at the site of stabbing. (c) The lesion can be managed endovascularly by stenting and/or embolization. A selective 5-French catheter was advanced into the neck of the pseudoaneurysm and embolized. No need for stenting of this lesion. It is much simpler and certainly much less expensive. Stent here is "overkill."

Extremity AVFs are managed with different techniques, depending on the location of the lesion, and the need to maintain antegrade arterial flow. Management of these upper and lower extremity vascular lesions in the axillosubclavian, superficial femoral arteries with placement of covered stents will often suffice. However, if a significant hematoma and/or venous laceration is also present, placement of covered stents in the artery and the vein is done. Smaller caliber or branch vessels with AVF can be effectively treated with coil embolization of the arterial branch supply, preferably proximally and distally to the AVF (▶ Fig. 21.13, ▶ Fig. 21.14, ▶ Fig. 21.15, ▶ Fig. 21.16, ▶ Fig. 21.17).

21.6.6 Intimal Injury and Dissection

Intimal arterial injury spans the spectrum from subtle intimal abnormalities to severe flow-limiting dissections. Intimal flaps appear as well-defined linear filling defects that may occur proximal or distal to an arterial injury. Minor intimal injuries may be managed conservatively with observation and surveillance, follow-up clinical and US exams. These injuries can also be repaired with a balloon angioplasty to "tack" the flap, or with covered or uncovered stents.

21.6.7 Venous Injuries

Venous injuries of the extremities rarely require intervention or surgery, except in cases of external exsanguination or large hematomas. Venous hemorrhages constrained by intact skin usually tamponades, with cessation of hemorrhage. The likely outcome of venous wall distruption, without treatment, is deep venous thrombosis. Endovenous stents have been utilized in rare instances of large venous wall disruptions. The long-term patency of venous stents is poor; therefore, stents should be inserted only in rare special cases with major indications, rather than routinely in venous injuries.

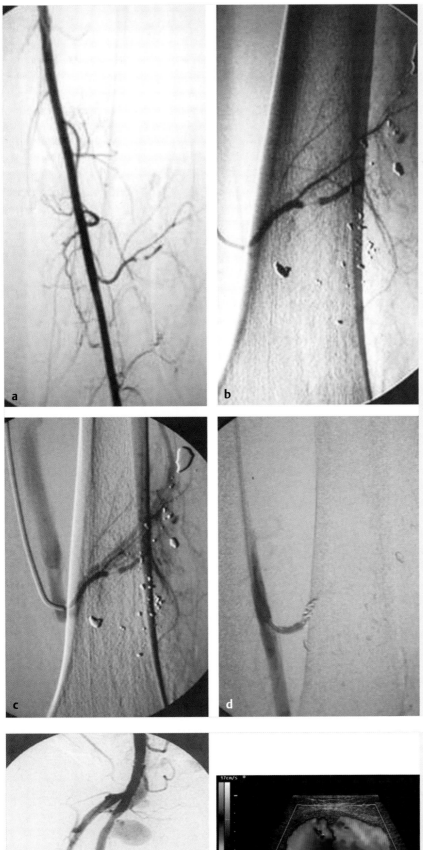

Fig. 21.12 A young man received a bullet wound in the distal left femur. (a) Selective superficial femoral arteriogram showed a small arterial venous fistula (AVF) in the distal thigh. The AVF was selectively catheterized. (b,c) Successful embolization of branch feeding the lesion with stainless steel coils. (d) Final arteriogram is normal and the AVF is no longer seen.

Fig. 21.13 A right common femoral arteriogram in a middle-aged patient after repeated attempts at femoral arterial catheterization. (a) The patient developed a large hematoma in the right groin and thigh. The arteriogram shows a large pseudoaneurysm in the proximal superficial femoral artery, with an arterial venous fistula (AVF) with the common femoral vein. (b) The color Doppler ultrasound (US) shows the large pseudoaneurysm of iatrogenic origin. There are different ways to manage this lesion, such as open surgical repair, endovascular with a covered stent, US-guided compression and also per-cutaneous thrombin injection. The easier and more effective way in this case was stenting with a covered stent.

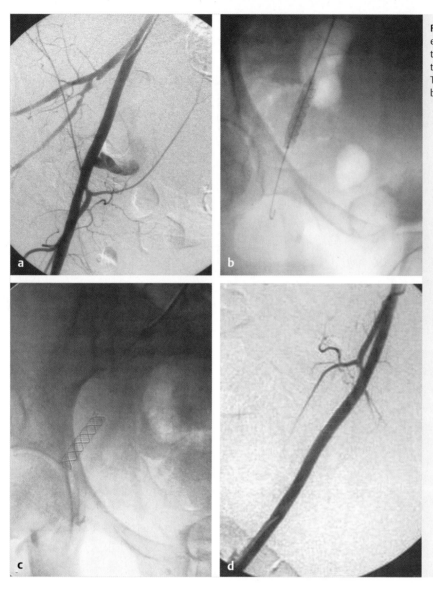

Fig. 21.14 (a) An iatrogenic injury to the right external iliac artery during cardiac catheterization. (b–d) A large pseudoaneurysm is noted in the midportion of the right external iliac artery. This was readily managed by placement of a balloon-expandable covered stent.

21.6.8 Filling Defects: Thrombus, Embolus

Current IR technology includes the potential recanalization of occluded arteries using many of the techniques for endovascular salvage of nontraumatic peripheral occlusions. In acute trauma, thrombolytic therapy is usually contraindicated, but has been used in selected instances when no other alternatives exist. Therefore, if an occlusion can be safely crossed with a guidewire, mechanical rheolytic devices (e.g., Possis Angiojet, Ekos, suction catheters, etc.) can be used to decompress a segmental arterial occlusion. Follow-up arteriography usually demonstrates thromboembolic and residual intimal disease, most often requiring stent placement (▶ Fig. 21.5, ▶ Fig. 21.8).

21.7 Upper Versus Lower Extremity Vascular Injury

In an analysis of the National Trauma Data Bank (NTDB) of 8,311 cases of extremity arterial trauma, 37% involved the lower

extremity. This cohort had higher blunt injury (56.2% vs. 37.4%; $p < 0.0001$), required more fasciotomies (23.6% vs. 6.7%; $p < 0.0001$) and had higher complications, amputations (7.8% vs. 1.3%; $p < 0.0001$) and mortality rate (7.7% vs. 2.2%, $p < 0.0001$. In multivariate analysis, lower extremity arterial trauma was associated with increased mortality (odds ratio [OR] = 2.2) and amputation (OR = 4.3) confirming that lower extremity arterial trauma is much more complex.[22]

The evolution of endovascular therapy for vascular injury is well illustrated by an analysis of 12,732 arterial injuries (1994–2003) from the NTDB[23] 7,286 open arterial repairs and 281 endovascular repairs were recorded for an overall utilization rate for endovascular procedures of 3.7%. The yearly number of endovascular procedures increased 27-fold, from 4 in 1997 to 107 in 2003. Use of stents substantially increased from 12 in 2000 to 30 in 2003; endograft use increased from one in 2000. Using multivariable regression to control for differences in injury severity score and associated injuries, mortality was significantly lower for patients undergoing endovascular procedures (OR = 0.18; $p = 0.029$) including those with an arterial injury of the torso or head and neck (OR = 0.51, $p = 0.007$). Total

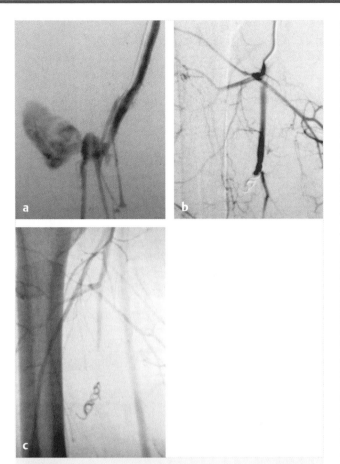

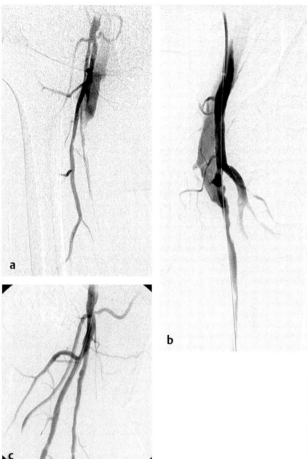

Fig. 21.15 A 15-year-old girl was stabbed in the right thigh and a pulsatile mass was noted on exam. (a) Angiography demonstrated a large pseudoaneurysm originating from the profunda femoris artery with rapid filling of the deep femoral vein, indicating a large arterial venous fistula. (b,c) The lesion was embolized with multiple 3 mm × 10 mm stainless steel coils. She had an uneventful recovery and was discharged home on hospital day 3.

Fig. 21.16 An arterial venous fistula (AVF) secondary to repeated punctures of the right groin for diagnostic and interventional cardiology procedures. (a,b) A small AVF communicating the right superficial femoral artery. (c) After placement of a covered stent, the AVF is no longer identified.

Fig. 21.17 (a,b) A small arterial venous fistula in the right groin after many punctures for cardiac catheterization was easily embolized with Gelfoam particles and coils.

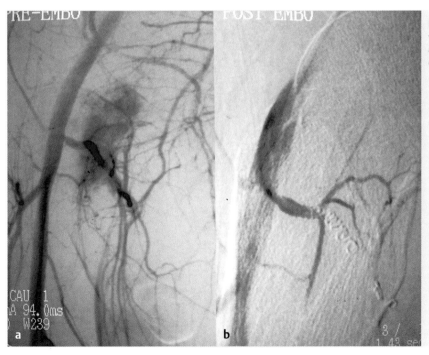

length of hospital stay also tended to be lower for patients undergoing endovascular procedures by 18% ($p = 0.064$).

21.8 Conclusion

It is apparent that, as embolic materials, catheters, microcatheters, microwires, stents, and stent grafts have developed, IR can now expand its role from a diagnostic to a therapeutic point of view, both in nonexsanguinating hemorrhage and contained vascular extravasation. A team approach including interventional radiologists and vascular surgeons will significantly improve the outcome of patients with peripheral vascular trauma to the extremities.

References

[1] Norman M. Rich. Historical and military aspects of vascular trauma (with lifetime reflections of Doctor Norman Rich). In Rich NM, Mattox KL, Hirschberg A, eds. Vascular Trauma. 2nd ed. Philadelphia, PA: Elsevier Saunders; 2004: 3–72

[2] DeBakey ME, Simeone FA. Battle injuries of the arteries in World War II: an analysis of 2,471 cases. Ann Surg 1946; 123: 534–579

[3] Hughes CW. Arterial repair during the Korean war. Ann Surg 1958; 147: 555–561

[4] Knudson MM, Lewis FR, Atkinson K, Neuhaus A. The role of duplex ultrasound arterial imaging in patients with penetrating extremity trauma. Arch Surg 1993; 128: 1033–1037, discussion 1037–1038

[5] Gaitini D, Razi NB, Ghersin E, Ofer A, Soudack M. Sonographic evaluation of vascular injuries. J Ultrasound Med 2008; 27: 95–107

[6] Soto JA, Múnera F, Cardoso N, Guarín O, Medina S. Diagnostic performance of helical CT angiography in trauma to large arteries of the extremities. J Comput Assist Tomogr 1999; 23: 188–196

[7] Foster BR, Anderson SW, Soto JA. CT angiography of extremity trauma. Tech Vasc Interv Radiol 2006; 9: 156–166

[8] Fishman EK, Horton KM, Johnson PT. Multidetector CT and three-dimensional CT angiography for suspected vascular trauma of the extremities. Radiographics 2008; 28: 653–665, discussion 665–666

[9] Seamon MJ, Smoger D, Torres DM et al. A prospective validation of a current practice: the detection of extremity vascular injury with CT angiography. J Trauma 2009; 67: 238–243, discussion 243–244

[10] Levey DS, Teitelbaum GP, Finck EJ, Pentecost MJ. Safety and efficacy of transcatheter embolization of axillary and shoulder arterial injuries. J Vasc Interv Radiol 1991; 2: 99–104

[11] DuBose JJ, Rajani R, Gilani R et alEndovascular Skills for Trauma and Resuscitative Surgery Working Group. Endovascular management of axillosubclavian arterial injury: a review of published experience. Injury 2012; 43: 1785–1792

[12] Bakhritdinov FSh, Zufarov MM, Babadzhanov SA. [The use of balloon occlusion of subclavian artery defect in patients with traumatic injuries] Angiol Sosud Khir 2003; 9: 41–42

[13] Danetz JS, Cassano AD, Stoner MC, Ivatury RR, Levy MM. Feasibility of endovascular repair in penetrating axillosubclavian injuries: a retrospective review. J Vasc Surg 2005; 41: 246–254

[14] Castelli P, Caronno R, Piffaretti G et al. Endovascular repair of traumatic injuries of the subclavian and axillary arteries. Injury 2005; 36: 778–782

[15] Xenos ES, Freeman M, Stevens S, Cassada D, Pacanowski J, Goldman M. Covered stents for injuries of subclavian and axillary arteries. J Vasc Surg 2003; 38: 451–454

[16] Franz RW, Goodwin RB, Hartman JF, Wright ML. Management of upper extremity arterial injuries at an urban level I trauma center. Ann Vasc Surg 2009; 23: 8–16

[17] Alvarez-Tostado J, Tulsyan N, Butler B, Rizzo A. Endovascular management of acute critical ischemia secondary to blunt tibial artery injury. J Vasc Surg 2006; 44: 1101–1103

[18] Piffaretti G, Tozzi M, Lomazzi C et al. Endovascular treatment for traumatic injuries of the peripheral arteries following blunt trauma. Injury 2007; 38: 1091–1097

[19] Rosa P, O'Donnell SD, Goff JM, Gillespie DL, Starnes B. Endovascular management of a peroneal artery injury due to a military fragment wound. Ann Vasc Surg 2003; 17: 678–681

[20] Lopera JE, Suri R, Cura M, Kroma G, El-Merhi F. Crural artery traumatic injuries: treatment with embolization. Cardiovasc Intervent Radiol 2008; 31: 550–557

[21] Franz RW, Shah KJ, Halaharvi D, Franz ET, Hartman JF, Wright ML. A 5-year review of management of lower extremity arterial injuries at an urban level I trauma center. J Vasc Surg 2011; 53: 1604–1610

[22] Tan TW, Joglar FL, Hamburg NM et al. Limb outcome and mortality in lower and upper extremity arterial injury: a comparison using the National Trauma Data Bank. Vasc Endovascular Surg 2011; 45: 592–597

[23] Reuben BC, Whitten MG, Sarfati M, Kraiss LW. Increasing use of endovascular therapy in acute arterial injuries: analysis of the National Trauma Data Bank. J Vasc Surg 2007; 46: 1222–1226

22 Interventional Radiology in Pediatric Trauma

Soroosh Mahboubi, Gordon K. McLean, and Jaime Tisnado

Trauma is the leading cause of morbidity and mortality in children older than one year. Mortality is most closely associated to concurrent traumatic brain injury. Despite the improvements in available multidisciplinary diagnostic and treatment modalities at tertiary care facilities, significant morbidity and mortality persist in contemporary practice.

Furthermore, survivors of childhood trauma may suffer lifelong disability and require long-term skilled care. For every child who dies from an injury, 40 others are hospitalized. An estimated 50,000 children acquire permanent disabilities each year, most of which are the result of closed head injuries. Thus, pediatric trauma is one of the major threats to the health of children and those who survive childhood injury with disability pose an enormous financial burdens to the society.[1–5]

Special training is required for appropriate management of injured children, and all physicians responsible for the care of a child-sized trauma patient (surgeons, department physicians, anesthesiologists, radiologists, and interventional radiologists) must be familiar with every tenet of modern trauma care.

Vascular injuries are uncommon during childhood and adolescence; however, trauma management in children is based largely on adult trauma experience, which has made considerable advancement in the diagnosis and management of vascular injuries,[6,7] as reported elsewhere in this book.

Many vascular injuries in children require early diagnosis and aggressive care to prevent serious sequelae. An injury to a major artery can result in ischemia and subsequent growth retardation of that limb, if not detected and treated in a timely manner. Under the age of 5, vascular trauma occurs more from iatrogenic causes, whereas injuries after 5 years of age have similar causes as in adults.[2,3,4,5]

Most vascular injuries are associated with orthopedic injuries, such as supracondylar or long bone fractures. Penetrating trauma is more likely than blunt trauma to result in a vascular injury.[8] Extremity injuries are equally divided between upper and lower extremities.[2] The superficial femoral artery and the brachial artery are the most frequently injured vessels in the extremities. Associated nonvascular injuries occur in 79% of patients, most of them being orthopedic. Neurologic injuries are next. The presence of pulsatile bleeding, expanding hematoma, absent distal pulses, cold limb, or new bruit/thrill mandates prompt operative exploration and repair after diagnosis by different modalities.

Doppler ultrasonography and/or computed tomography angiography (CTA) should be used to confirm the diagnosis. The benefit of noninvasive CTA compared with digital subtraction angiography (DSA) is that it is rapid, easy, and free of major complications. Multislice helical CTA is an alternative to DSA in the evaluation of vascular injuries. Computed tomography angiography is noninvasive, fast, and available everywhere. Its advantages are speed of acquisition, few artifacts from patient motion, and the scanning of the critically injured child is safer. Also CTA has the ability to evaluate nearby organs, surrounding soft tissues and bone as well as provide axial, sagittal, coronal, and three-dimensional images from a single scan, which may be invaluable in operative planning (▶ Fig. 22.1, ▶ Fig. 22.2).[9–13]

Radiation exposure and contrast–induced nephropathy (CIN) are potential risks with either CTA or DSA. The ability to control radiation exposure during multislice CTA in children is possible by controlling parameters such as speed, X-ray tube current peak voltage, pitch, angle, and gantry rotation time.[14] This is a very important consideration at this time. Low-radiation CT scanners are now being made.

The first issue consideration in pediatric vascular trauma is differentiation between thrombosis versus spasm of the injured vessel. The spasm is usually less than 3 hours. If the distal pulses continue absent for more than 6 hours, thrombosis or transection of the vessel is likely. Successful early revascularization of the injured limb leads to good short-term results in most injured children. A delay in diagnosing vascular injury can lead to a prolonged ischemia, compartment syndrome, and contractures with consequent long-term disability. Long-term follow-up of injured children must continue into adulthood because of the increased risk of vascular compromise, late graft failure, and even limb loss. Unfortunately, sometimes some of the children are lost to follow-up, particularly those in inner cities or in gangs. Furthermore, some children may be victims of lethal violence.

Fortunately, these injuries are rare, but clinically challenging injuries. The diagnosis and treatment must be as rapid as possible, but never without proper stabilization of the patient and primary attention to other life-threatening conditions. Even when physical examination shows definitive signs of vascular injuries, a threat to the life of the child is more important so no other imaging studies are necessary at this time. At other times, when there is a high level of suspicion, then imaging with CTA with its ability to evaluate the entire body in a few seconds may be performed. Blunt arterial injuries in children are also very rare, and diagnosis of these injuries is often made with CTA, which helps the surgeon select and plan for the appropriate vascular repair.[15]

22.1 Thoracic Aortic Rupture

Aortic transaction in pediatric and adolescent patients is extremely uncommon. Rupture of the thoracic aorta occurs in ~ 0.06% of children admitted with severe blunt chest trauma. Children comprise ~ 6% of all patients with acute rupture of the thoracic aorta. Operative repair with autologous arterial tissue has been the standard management, but when autologous tissue is unavailable or otherwise contraindicated, endovascular techniques have shown promising results.[16,17,18] However, pseudocoarctation must be kept in mind as the child grows. No complete data about this problem exist as of today.

Older children with high injury severity scores and major vascular injury are at a small but known risk for venous thromboembolism—a finding in 0.1% of children less than 16 years of age who were admitted to a level I pediatric trauma center over an 8-year period.[19,20,21] Insertion of removable (optional) filters is a topic of interest now. In selected cases, we advocate temporary filter placement if indicated.

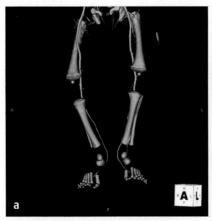

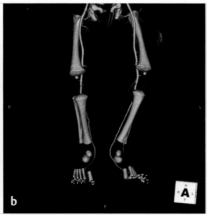

Fig. 22.1 A 9-hour newborn with right lower extremity ischemia postdelivery. Anteroposterior (a) and three-dimensional reconstruction (b) computed tomography angiography scan demonstrate a patent right superficial femoral artery, but signal loss in the distal right anterior tibial artery.

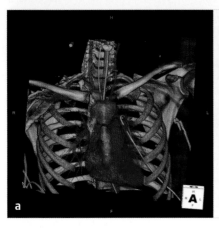

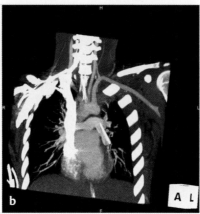

Fig. 22.2 A 16-year-old girl with a gunshot wound to the left upper chest. Computed tomography angiography (a) and scan (b) demonstrates no evidence of injury to the aorta and branches, or the carotid, subclavian, and vertebral arteries. Both internal mammary arteries are intact.

22.2 Pediatric Vascular Trauma

Usually in children with trauma, a vascular disruption producing uncontrollable hemorrhage is considered in the dominant injury. Following stabilization of the child and attention to life-threatening conditions, bleeding must be controlled before turning attention to other organ systems. On the other hand, if the vascular injury is not critical, its treatment may be delayed until the more critical neurological, visceral, or musculoskeletal injuries are addressed first. We must remember that there may be a close interrelation between organ system in children (i.e., reduction of a fracture may initiate or exacerbate a vascular injury and resulting hemorrhage may require immediate diagnosis and therapy). This is a general principle in trauma care, but relatively more important in children.

Although emergent CTA is not necessary in the majority of pediatric trauma, it should be performed if there is a question of vascular injury. Computed tomography angiography, even in the absence of signs or symptoms, is directly attributable to the vascular system. Obvious signs and symptoms of vascular injury dictate emergent CTA, so that appropriate therapy may be initiated to prevent exsanguinations of loss of limbs, as already mentioned earlier.

The demands of performing emergent interventional procedures in infants and small children are different from those in adults. The support of competent anesthesiologists, specialized nurses, and clinical care physicians is mandatory to provide the appropriate type and depth of anesthesia. Documentation of a precise angiographic diagnosis and implementation of an effective definitive therapy requires a level of patient cooperation that an acutely traumatized child (or most children) may not provide.

22.3 Pelvic Trauma

Hemorrhage is one of the leading causes of death in children with pelvic fractures.[2] Death may result from primary exsanguination or secondary infection of a hematoma. Surgical treatment is often difficult because most pelvic bleeding secondary to trauma is not caused by disruption of a single major vessel, but rather damage to multiple small pelvic branches, veins, and arteries. Additionally, the clinical diagnosis of active intrapelvic bleeding may be difficult, particularly in a patient with multiple bleeding sites. Computed tomography angiography is indicated in most children with major pelvic fractures and clinical signs of bleeding.

Venous bleeding is usually self-limited because the hematoma effectively tamponades the bleeding veins. In general, venous hemorrhages are not amenable to transcatheter embolization therapy. On occasion, major venous injuries can be managed with placement of stents. When sites of arterial extravasations are identified, transcatheter embolization therapy is extremely effective and life-saving procedure.

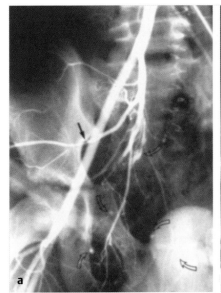
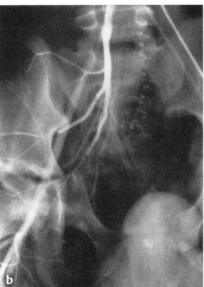
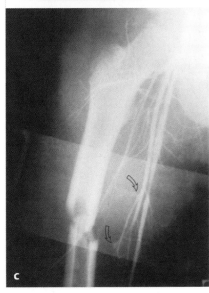

Fig. 22.3 (a) Arterial trauma following pelvic fracture successfully treated by transcatheter embolization in an 11-year-old boy struck by a car. Despite therapy with military antishock trousers, he had continuing transfusion requirements. Pelvic arteriography revealed multiple bleeding points (curved arrows) throughout the right pelvis. Note also an intimal tear of the superior gluteal artery as it passes through the sciatic notch (straight arrow). (b) An arteriogram following Gelfoam embolization shows abrupt cutoff of the treated vessels. There is no further evidence of bleeding. At this point, the catheter was placed selectively in the left internal iliac artery to rule out additional bleeding sites on the left side or collateral opacification of bleeding sites on the right. (c) Following the successful pelvic embolization, the catheter was advanced in the right common femoral artery, and arteriogram performed because of hematoma on the right thigh associated with a femoral fracture. Here, two bleeding points are identified arising from the descending branch of the profunda femoris artery (curved arrows). The catheter was placed in this branch and Gelfoam pledgets injected to control the hemorrhage. The child recovered uneventfully.

The pelvic arterial embolization procedure is performed, basically, as follows:

An aortic midstream arteriogram is obtained first to give an overview of the lower abdominal aorta and pelvis, and is a "roadmap" to guide subsequent selective catheterization. The amount and rate of injections of contrast material should be proportional to the arterial size and amount of blood flow. Rapid sequence DSA is performed for at least 10 seconds. Prolonged filming allows not only the identification of acute sources of bleeding, but finding of late contrast extravasation and may allow a subtle arterial or even a venous source to be identified.

Selective catheterization of the internal iliac arteries is then undertaken. A Shepard crook or other catheter is exchanged for the initial pigtail catheter and advanced selectively into both proximal internal iliac arteries or further into bleeding branches. Usually, with extensive pelvic fractures, multiple areas of extravasation are identified (▶ Fig. 22.3a).

Once the sites of extravasation are identified, subselective catheterization is ideally performed. Although this may be accomplished with the initial diagnostic catheter, a microcatheter is used more commonly. These catheters are less than 1 mm in diameter and can be advanced into small vessels, as selectively as possible into the affected branch for embolization to be performed. Several embolic agents are available and range from microcoils of platinum and Dacron, particulate agents such as 1 to 3 mm pledgets of Gelfoam (Pfizer, New York, NY) to intravascular adhesives such as N-butyl cyanoacrylate (NBCA) and Onyx. Polyvinyl alcohol particles can be used as well, but we must take into consideration that many agents are permanent. Therefore, temporary agents (i.e., Gelfoam pledgets) are preferred. Avitene (Bard Davol, Warwick, RI) and Oxicell (Apex Energetics, Irvine, CA) are rarely used.

Following embolization, a controlled arteriogram ensures that all sites of extravasation have been occluded (▶ Fig. 22.3b). The above steps are repeated until there is no further angiographic evidence of bleeding.

The selective catheter is then placed in the contralateral internal iliac artery. Even if no bleeding sites are identified on

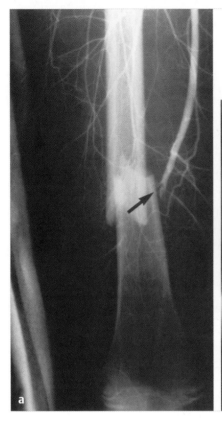

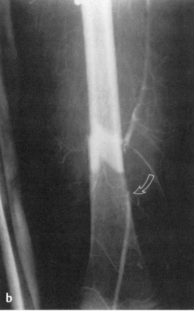

Fig. 22.4 (a) Traumatic occlusion of the superficial femoral artery in an 11-year-old girl with a fracture of the mid femur in a motor vehicle accident. Over 24 hours, pulses in the leg were reported as a "variable." An initial attempt to reduce the fracture was unsuccessful, and the child was taken to Interventional Radiology. The superficial femoral artery is occluded just at the fracture site with intraluminal thrombus (arrow). (b) There is reconstitution of the distal superficial femoral artery (arrow), which then continues in a normal popliteal artery. At surgery, the superficial femoral artery showed intimal dissection with intraluminal thrombosis, but was not transected.

the contralateral side, it is extremely important to embolize both sides. The extensive anastomotic network normally present in the pelvis in children allows rapid resupply of bleeding sites from the contralateral branches.

If the bleeding is diffuse and involves most or all of the major branches, the internal iliac circulation may be interrupted proximally with stainless steel coils (detachable occlusion balloon or other larger vessel occlusion devices) can be used: Amplatzer plugs, large coils, etc.

In the majority of cases, pelvic bleeding should be controlled. Surgery is rarely necessary unless the presence of a large hematoma and the threat of subsequent infection prompts operative removal. Surgical evacuation, if needed, should be performed once the patient is hemodynamically stable.

Complications associated with pelvic embolization are uncommon. An ischemic neurapraxic of the sciatic or femoral nerves may result if the embolization is with fine particulate matter (e.g., powdered Gelfoam) or liquid agents (e.g., NBCA). Other areas of ischemic necrosis may result from inadvertent embolization of nontarget areas (e.g., perineal or vulvar necrosis resulting from embolization of the internal pudendal artery). Profound focal ischemia is not a risk when large pledgets of Gelfoam, stainless steel coils, or detachable intravascular balloons are used. Flow interruption of the gluteal arteries may result in buttock claudication. This is always self-limited in children. With careful techniques, experience in children, and contemporary microcatheter techniques, complications should be minimal or absent.

When pelvic trauma is sufficient to cause pelvic vascular disruption, associated lower extremity vascular injury should be considered. Since the catheter is already in place, DSA of any fractured extremity may be of significant diagnostic benefit (▶ Fig. 22.3c).

22.4 Peripheral Vascular Trauma

Blunt and penetrating trauma can result in peripheral vascular damage. Injury to a peripheral artery is usually produced by fracture or dislocation. The CTA or angiographic findings may include vessel disruption (▶ Fig. 22.1, ▶ Fig. 22.4), intimal injury, and bleeding with or without a pseudoaneurysm (▶ Fig. 22.5). The clinical presentation is often that of an ischemic extremity with poor or absent pulses distal to the site of injury. If the blood loss can be controlled, a CTA or arteriography offers significant information to direct the vascular reconstruction.

In questionable cases, arteriography may be necessary to determine whether there is intrinsic arterial injury (▶ Fig. 22.6), an extravascular hematoma (causing extrinsic compression), or spasm producing distal diminished pulses. An unreduced fracture may cause extrinsic pressure without necessarily an intrinsic arterial damage. Contrast DSA or CT venography may be important when a major venous injury is suspected because venous repair may be required to prevent limb loss.

In evaluating the patient with an apparently negative imaging workup, it must be kept in mind that DSA, CT, and any imaging examination, can produce a false–negative result. A negative imaging study should never be unequivocally accepted in the face of strongly positive clinical examination when evaluating the child with a suspected vascular injury.

Penetrating trauma, such as a gunshot and stabbings, may produce occlusion of the vessel by an intimal flap, thrombosis,

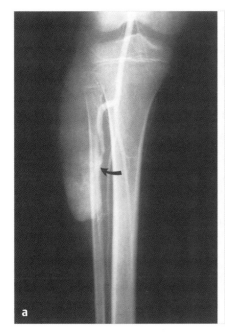

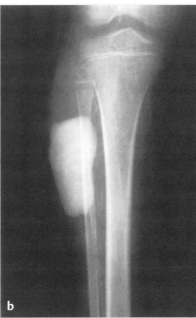

Fig. 22.5 (a) A large false aneurysm in this child struck by an automobile who presented with marked swelling of the right leg. Plain films showed no fracture. The arteriogram shows obvious extravasation or contrast material from the anterior tibial artery (arrow) into a huge false aneurysm. (b) Large false aneurysm unassociated with fracture. On later films, filling of the false aneurysm is more apparent.

disruption with overt bleeding, pseudoaneurysm (▶ Fig. 22.5), or an arteriovenous fistula (AVF).

The CTA imaging should include the entire trajectory or tissue path of the bullet from its point of entry to its resting place or point of exit (▶ Fig. 22.2). Furthermore, the site of injury may not be at or near the entry, but anywhere along the course of the bullet (permanent cavity) or even far away. In cases of high-velocity gunshot injuries, the shock wave may result in vascular disruption at some distance from the actual path of the bullet. This is due to the so-called temporary cavity, which can be 10 to 20 times larger than the permanent one. Computed tomography angiography in these patients can obviate the need for exposure of long segments of extremities and surrounding tissues reducing operative time and morbidity, and eventual permanent limb damage.

A limited number of therapeutic options are available to the interventional radiologist examining a child with acute extremity trauma. Many injuries will occur in major vessels, which are supplying or draining a significant tissue volume (e.g., the superficial femoral artery and the popliteal vein). In adults, fabric-covered stents may be used to bridge the area of focal disruption. Blood vessels in children, however, are not fixed in size, but will grow in both diameter and length as the child grows. An endovascular stent will provide only a short-term solution and will have to be eventually replaced. If the hemorrhage is from a small rather than a major artery, embolization can be safely and easily accomplished because sacrifice of one or even several of these vessels rarely produces any sequelae. Otherwise, the child eventually will develop a pseudocoarctation when older.

If transcatheter embolization is contemplated, the diagnostic catheter should be advanced into the contralateral artery. As the catheter enters the affected limb in an antegrade fashion, selection of target vessels for embolization is easy (▶ Fig. 22.3c).

22.5 Abdominal Trauma

22.5.1 Liver and Spleen

Blunt or penetrating trauma to the abdomen in the pediatric age group may result in extensive damage to the liver and spleen parenchyma, usually prompting emergent CTA. Most cases with extensive hepatic trauma, multisystem injuries, and hemodynamically stable can have an initial radiological evaluation, such as CTA scanning, which may show an acute hematoma or replacement/displacement of normal parenchyma by intrahepatic or intrasplenic subcapsular hematomas. If lesions appear to be amendable to transcatheter therapy, the procedure is as follows:

An abdominal aortogram is performed first with a pigtail or other multisided holes catheter to delineate visceral perfusion and a vascular "overview" of the abdomen. Multiple sources or arterial supply to the liver and spleen are common and must be defined for accurate diagnosis and effective therapy.

Selective celiac arteriography is then performed. The possibility of spasm or traumatic disruption of the branches should be explored prior to any attempts to subselectively catheterize the vessel or any of its branches.

Once patency of the main arteries has been documented the catheter may then be advanced subselectively progressively through the common hepatic, proper hepatic or right, left, or middle hepatic arteries (▶ Fig. 22.7). In the spleen into the hilar or, polar branches, the hepatic and splenic arteries are particularly prone to spasm, which may be the result of the primary trauma or the instrumentation with catheters and guidewires. Although the combination of general anesthesia and local antispasmodics (e.g., nitroglycerine) are helpful in reducing vessel reactivity, spasm remains a risk and care must be exercised to avoid adding catheter induced dissection and subsequent vessel

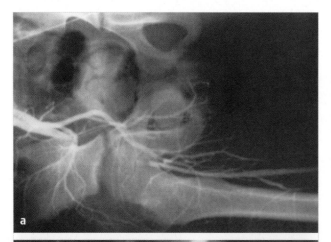

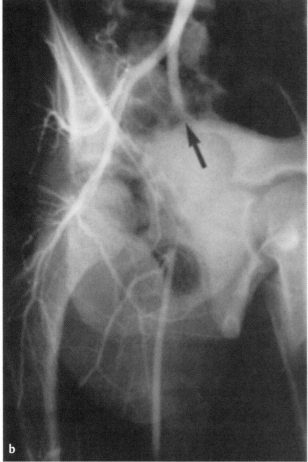

Fig. 22.6 (a) Traumatic occlusion of the right common femoral artery without fracture or dislocation in a 10-year-old boy struck by a car while riding his bicycle. Right pedal pulses were decreased, and a Doppler study showed the pedal pressures of 60 mm Hg compared with a normal reading of 120 mm Hg on the left. A right leg arteriogram performed via left femoral puncture shows complete occlusion of the common femoral artery. Reconstitution of the profunda femoris and superficial femoral artery is via collateral branches derived from the superior and inferior gluteal arteries. (b) An oblique view better demonstrates the absence of blood flow in the distal external iliac artery (arrow). There is reconstitution of the superficial femoral and proximal portion of the profunda femoris arteries. At surgery, a large intimal flap was found and repaired in the common femoral artery.

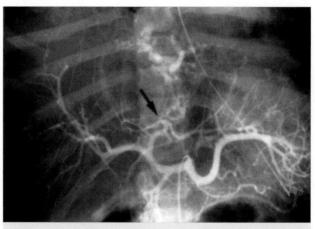

Fig. 22.7 A intrahepatic hemorrhage following blunt trauma in an 8-year-old child involved in a motor vehicle accident. Computed tomography scan showed laceration of the liver with active bleeding and extravasation. Here, arteriogram shows bleeding arising from the left hepatic artery (arrow). Contrast is seen flowing into the large area of laceration in the midportion of the liver with displacement of normal arterial branches in both hepatic lobes. Following the diagnostic arteriogram the catheter was advanced selectively into the left hepatic artery, which was then embolized with Gelfoam® pledgets.

occlusion to the existing traumatic injury making, perhaps, the situation worse. Therefore, special "soft touch" is recommend.

The presence of extravasation, pseudoaneurysms, or vessel "cutoff" will direct the therapy. The catheter should be advanced as far as possible into the relevant arterial branch to maximize effectiveness of therapy and limit the amount of damage suffered by the adjacent normal, nontraumatized liver.

In dealing with the spleen, there are two types of embolization and the choice depends on the particular case. If a small area of spleen is damaged and a localized pseudoaneurysm is found, or an AVF or extravasation localized in a small area in the spleen, then "peripheral" embolization is done with particles of Gelfoam or PVA, or coils or microcoils. On the other hand, if the entire spleen is damaged, then central embolization with coils is preferred. The general results of both techniques are similar; the outcome is similar. However, much less radiation is needed in the child with the central embolization. In both cases, the appropriate embolization agent is selected then injected until the contrast extravasation is controlled, the pseudoaneurysm occluded or the transected vessel safely occluded, or the AVF is no longer opacified.

22.5.2 Kidney

Hematuria post trauma in children is rarely an indication for emergency DSA. However, if the child has a persistent gross hematuria or signs of hemodynamic instability, the possibility of laceration of a major renal vessel or avulsion of the renal vascular pedicle must be considered (▶ Fig. 22.8). Prompt CTA or DSA diagnosis and therapy are mandatory (▶ Fig. 22.9). The procedures are performed as follows:

Because of the frequency of multiple renal arteries, a midstream aortogram should always precede any attempt at selective catheterization. This aortogram may demonstrate spasm, thrombosis, or complete avulsion of the renal pedicle.

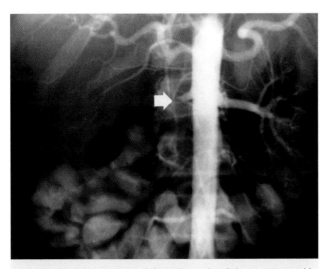

Fig. 22.8 Traumatic avulsion of the right renal pedicle in a 15-year-old boy who presented with gross hematuria and severe right flank pain following a sledding accident. A renal flow scan showed no uptake in the right kidney. The aortogram demonstrates avulsion of the right renal artery. The artery is in spasm and terminates abruptly (arrow). Because there was no extravasation, and the child was hemodynamically stable, no attempts at transcatheter therapy embolization were done. However, on occasion, to make sure no bleeding is going to occur after the artery is recanalized by the normal lytic mechanism of the child, a coil can be deposited in the arterial stump.

If the renal arteries are patent, they can be selectively catheterized. Injection rates are according to size and flow of the artery in children, generally 2 to 8 mL at a rate of 1 to 4 mL/s. Very rapid filming is necessary.

Magnification techniques are extremely helpful, and angled views should be obtained as necessary.

If contrast material extravasation is identified, the catheter is advanced subselectively into the bleeding branch. Embolization is then performed in standard fashion with Gelfoam pledgets (▶ Fig. 22.9).

22.6 Conclusion

This chapter has introduced an overview of imaging and intervention in pediatric trauma. The role of computed CTA and catheter angiography (CA) in injured pediatric patients was discussed in pelvic fractures, peripheral vascular trauma, and solid abdominal organ injury.

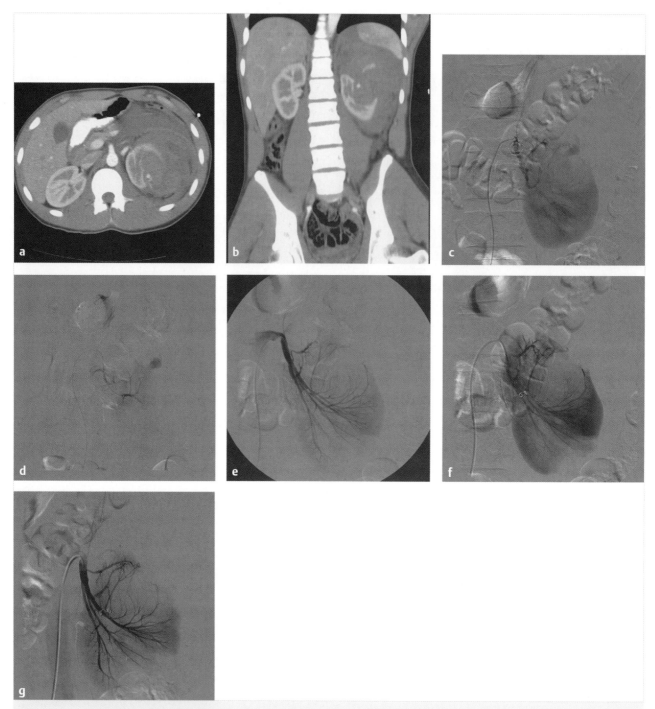

Fig. 22.9 A 17-year-old boy was hit in the abdomen with a football helmet during a football game. (a,b) Computed tomography in axial and coronal reconstruction images demonstrates lacerations of the upper pole of left kidney with active bleeding and perinephric and intrarenal hematomas. (c,d) Selective left renal angiogram shows an upper pole branch bleeding with contrast extravasation. A 3-French Renegade microcatheter was advanced into the bleeding branch and embolized with 2 mm × 2 cm platinum microcoil. (e-g) Postembolization digital subtraction angiography demonstrates cessation of bleeding and the embolized arterial branch. The child recovered from his renal injuries.

a

References

[1] Krug SE, Tuggle DW American Academy of Pediatrics Section on OrthopaedicsAmerican Academy of Pediatrics Committee on Pediatric Emergency MedicineAmerican Academy of Pediatrics Section on Critical CareAmerican Academy of Pediatrics Section on SurgeryAmerican Academy of Pediatrics Section on Transport MedicineAmerican Academy of Pediatrics Committee on Pediatric Emergency MedicinePediatric Orthopaedic Society of North America. Management of pediatric trauma. Pediatrics 2008; 121: 849–854

[2] Harris LM, Hordines J. Major vascular injuries in the pediatric population. Ann Vasc Surg 2003; 17: 266–269

[3] Reichard KW, Reyes HM. Vascular trauma and reconstructive approaches. Semin Pediatr Surg 1994; 3: 124–132

[4] Klinkner DB, Arca MJ, Lewis BD, Oldham KT, Sato TT. Pediatric vascular injuries: patterns of injury, morbidity, and mortality. J Pediatr Surg 2007; 42: 178–182, discussion 182–183

[5] de Virgilio C, Mercado PD, Arnell T, Donayre C, Bongard F, White R. Noniatrogenic pediatric vascular trauma: a ten-year experience at a level I trauma center. Am Surg 1997; 63: 781–784

[6] Rozycki GS, Tremblay L, Feliciano DV et al. A prospective study for the detection of vascular injury in adult and pediatric patients with cervicothoracic seat belt signs. J Trauma 2002; 52: 618–623, discussion 623–624

[7] Woo K, Magner DP, Wilson MT, Margulies DR. CT angiography in penetrating neck trauma reduces the need for operative neck exploration. Am Surg 2005; 71: 754–758

[8] Cox CS, Black CT, Duke JH et al. Operative treatment of truncal vascular injuries in children and adolescents. J Pediatr Surg 1998; 33: 462–467

[9] Peclet MH, Newman KD, Eichelberger MR et al. Patterns of injury in children. J Pediatr Surg 1990; 25: 85–90, discussion 90–91

[10] Lineen EB, Faresi M, Ferrari M, Neville HL, Thompson WR, Sola JE. Computed tomographic angiography in pediatric blunt traumatic vascular injury. J Pediatr Surg 2008; 43: 549–554

[11] Puapong D, Brown CV, Katz M et al. Angiography and the pediatric trauma patient: a 10-year review. J Pediatr Surg 2006; 41: 1859–1863

[12] Busquéts AR, Acosta JA, Colón E, Alejandro KV, Rodríguez P. Helical computed tomographic angiography for the diagnosis of traumatic arterial injuries of the extremities. J Trauma 2004; 56: 625–628

[13] Inaba K, Potzman J, Munera F et al. Multi-slice CT angiography for arterial evaluation in the injured lower extremity. J Trauma 2006; 60: 502–506, discussion 506–507

[14] Chan FP, Rubin GD. MDCT angiography of pediatric vascular diseases of the abdomen, pelvis, and extremities. Pediatr Radiol 2005; 35: 40–53

[15] Milas ZL, Dodson TF, Ricketts RR. Pediatric blunt trauma resulting in major arterial injuries. Am Surg 2004; 70: 443–447

[16] Milas ZL, Milner R, Chaikoff E, Wulkan M, Ricketts R. Endograft stenting in the adolescent population for traumatic aortic injuries. J Pediatr Surg 2006; 41: e27–e30

[17] Rousseau H, Soula P, Perreault P et al. Delayed treatment of traumatic rupture of the thoracic aorta with endoluminal covered stent. Circulation 1999; 99: 498–504

[18] Trachiotis GD, Sell JE, Pearson GD, Martin GR, Midgley FM. Traumatic thoracic aortic rupture in the pediatric patient. Ann Thorac Surg 1996; 62: 724–731, discussion 731–732

[19] Vavilala MS, Nathens AB, Jurkovich GJ, Mackenzie E, Rivara FP. Risk factors for venous thromboembolism in pediatric trauma. J Trauma 2002; 52: 922–927

[20] Rohrer MJ, Cutler BS, MacDougall E, Herrmann JB, Anderson FA, Wheeler HB. A prospective study of the incidence of deep venous thrombosis in hospitalized children. J Vasc Surg 1996; 24: 46–49, discussion 50

[21] Grandas OH, Klar M, Goldman MH, Filston HC. Deep venous thrombosis in the pediatric trauma population: an unusual event: report of three cases. Am Surg 2000; 66: 273–276

23 Interventional Radiology in Thromboembolic Disease in Trauma

Timothy P. Maroney and Charles A. Bruno, Jr.

Thromboembolic disease, which encompasses both deep venous thrombosis (DVT) and pulmonary embolism (PE), constitutes a major health care burden and is the third most common cardiovascular disease after ischemic heart disease and stroke.[1,2] The incidence of first-time venous thromboembolism is estimated to be 1.92 per 1,000 persons in the United States. Rates are higher in men than women, and the incidence of thromboembolic events increases with age. African Americans and Asian Americans may have slightly higher and lower rates of thromboembolism, respectively.[3,4,5] Among hospitalized patients the incidence is 100 times greater and PE is thought to be associated with 5 to 10% of deaths for that cohort of patients. Acute PE, arguably the most severe manifestation of venous thromboembolic disease, is diagnosed in 350,000 patients and results in as many as 240,000 deaths per year.[6,7,8] Additionally, postphlebitic syndrome affects more than 50% of patients with DVT. Untreated or inadequately treated patients suffering from thromboembolic disease have a 47% chance of recurrent venous thromboembolism within 3 months, and a mortality rate up to 26%, thus necessitating the need for quick, accurate diagnosis and treatment.[8,9,10] Patients suffering from trauma are at even higher risk for developing thromboembolic disease and have much higher rates of morbidity and mortality when compared with the general population. Our understanding of thromboembolic disease in trauma, including its epidemiology and pathophysiology has markedly improved over the past 10 years; as a result, prevention and treatment of this terrible disease has improved.

23.1 Trauma and Thromboembolic Disease: Historical Perspectives, Epidemiology, and Risk Factors

The relationship between trauma and thromboembolic disease has been well known for nearly a century. In a 1934 paper, Homans wrote, "It was the fatal experience of this patient which led Dr. Channing Frothingham to refer to me a woman of forty-four who, after a trifling injury to her foot, developed evidence of a similar local thrombosis."[11] That same year J.S. McCartney suggested that there was an association between trauma and death from pulmonary emboli. He reported the incidence of PE to be 1.46 times greater in patients who died of trauma than those who died of nontraumatic causes.[12] He also recognized that the association between trauma and pulmonary emboli was particularly strong in patients suffering from lower extremity fractures.[12] In 1961, S. Sevitt and N. Gallagher reported that among trauma patients the incidence of DVT and PE was 65% and 20%, respectively. They went on to conclude PE was the cause of death in a large number of these patients.[13,14] A few years later, Fitts analyzed the records of 950 fatally injured patients from Philadelphia hospitals, and found that in patients who died after hip fractures, PE was the reported cause of death in 38% of those who received autopsies. Interestingly,

PE was reported as the cause of death in only 2% of patients who had hip fractures and did not receive autopsies. Fitts concluded that the use of prophylactic anticoagulation might have decreased mortality in these patients and that such therapy "should be considered."[15] The work of Fitts and coworkers reconfirmed the magnitude of thromboembolic disease after trauma and promoted the fact that PE was rarely diagnosed premortem.

These preliminary studies stimulated the work of Freeark and others who in 1967 demonstrated roentgenographic evidence of venous thrombosis in 35% of patients with fractures. Freeark found that signs or symptoms suggesting venous thromboembolism were elicited in fewer than 25% of their patients.[16] Additionally, DVT involved both the injured and the uninjured extremity, or frequently both. Thrombus formation was observed within 24 hours after injury, a finding that was seen by Salzman a year earlier.[16,17] Freeark concluded, however, that more data were needed before routine anticoagulant prophylaxis could be recommended and strongly advocated for future study.[16]

Today we know that thromboembolic disease is a potentially preventable cause of morbidity and mortality after trauma and some form of prophylaxis is routinely used in all major trauma centers; yet these patients still have one of the highest incidences of deep venous thrombosis and PE among those hospitalized.[18,19,20] The reported incidence of thromboembolic disease after trauma varies from 7 to 58% depending on the population being studied, the nature of their injuries, the methods used to detect DVT and PE, and the type of prophylaxis being used.[18,21,22,23] The most comprehensive study on the incidence of thromboembolic disease following trauma was reported by Geerts and colleagues in 1994.[18] They prospectively studied 349 high-risk trauma patients using venography. None of the 349 patients received any form of thromboembolic prophylaxis. Deep venous thrombosis was found in 58% of those studied; the incidence of DVT involving the popliteal or more proximal veins was 18%. Seven patients (2%) had confirmed pulmonary emboli, and three died of pulmonary emboli. Only 1.5% of patients with deep vein thrombosis had signs or symptoms of thrombosis before the diagnosis was made by venography.[18] In studies using serial duplex scanning for surveillance, Knudson found proximal clot in 10% of patients despite the fact that 50% of the subjects were receiving either mechanical or pharmacologic prophylaxis.[22-26] Other reports using color-flow duplex scanning have reported the incidence of silent, asymptomatic DVT between 10 to 85% in patients with multiple injuries.[27,28]

The incidence of symptomatic PE in patients experiencing major trauma varies from 0.5 to 2%.[19,27,29] Among those who develop PE, the mortality rate is as high as 50%. Six percent of trauma patients develop PE within the first day of admission and PE is the third most common cause of death in trauma patients who survive longer than 24 hours after injury.[18,24,30] However, the true incidence of PE in high-risk trauma patients is likely much higher as a substantial number of these patients suffer from silent pulmonary emboli, and a practical screening modality does not exist. In 2004, Schultz and colleagues[31] reported that 24% of moderately to severely injured patients undergoing surveillance computed tomography pulmonary angiography (CTPA) were found to have asymptomatic PE. Four had major clot burden, including one patient with a saddle embolus, and 30% of patients receiving pharmacologic prophylaxis had a PE.[31] Some argue that Schultz's study may actually underestimate the magnitude of asymptomatic PE following trauma because of the intrinsic weakness' of CTPA. A recent study comparing CTPA to catheter pulmonary angiography for the diagnosis of PE in critically ill surgical patients (28 trauma patients were included) demonstrated poor correlation. Computed tomography pulmonary angiography resulted in nine false-negatives and two false-positives, and the sensitivity and specificity of CTPA was found to be 40% and 91% for PE, respectively.[32]

Large population-based studies, however, would suggest that the incidence of thromboembolic disease in trauma patients is in fact much lower.[23,33] Analysis of all patients contained in the National Trauma Data Bank from 1994 to 2001 showed the incidence of thromboembolism to be only 0.36%.[23] However, this study did not stratify patients by the nature and severity of their injuries and only 7% of the 450,000 patients suffered severe trauma, while 69% had minor injuries.[23] Additionally, the quality of data are questionable given that it was derived from a large database and no information regarding prophylaxis was available. It is also likely that a large number of DVTs were likely missed because the number of reported PEs was 522 and only 988 DVTs were detected; assuming that 18 cases of DVT will result in one PE.[23] Finally, the results of this study may simply speak to the suboptimal way in which DVT and PE is diagnosed and reported in trauma patients.

The identification of trauma patients at risk for the development of thromboembolic disease remains difficult. Traditionally, patients with spinal fractures, with or without paralysis, pelvic fractures, long bone fractures, head injury, and severe burns have been considered high risk for developing thromboembolic disease.[21,34] Deep-vein thrombosis rates as high as 81% in patients with spinal cord injuries, 61% in those with pelvic fractures, 80% in those with femoral fractures, 77% in those with tibial fractures, and 74% in those with ankle fractures have been reported.[18] In addition, reduced mobility, prolonged hospital stay, and a Glasgow Coma Scale of less than 8 are believed to place patients at relatively higher risk for DVT and PE.[18] Knudson[23] identified nine risk factors felt to be significant in the development of thromboembolic disease. Ninety percent of patients with clinically significant thromboembolic disease in the National Trauma Data Bank from 1994 to 2001 had at least one of those risk factors. In 2002, The Eastern Association for the Surgery of Trauma[35] reported a meta-analysis that included 73 articles reporting risk factors for thromboembolic disease. Interestingly, they discovered that the only risk factors found to place the patient at higher risk for development of DVT were spinal fractures and spinal cord injury.

23.2 Pathophysiology

Microthrombi, tiny aggregates of red cells, platelets, and fibrin, are formed and lysed continually within the venous circulatory system. This dynamic process, made up of two distinct but interlocking systems—platelets and the coagulation proteins—ensures local hemostasis without permitting uncontrolled propagation of clot.[36] When there is a breakdown of this process, microthrombi grow, propagate, and ultimately embolize. Pulmonary embolism occurs when these propagating clots break loose and block pulmonary blood vessels.[37] Rudolf Virchow was the first to recognize that blood clots in the pulmonary arteries originated as venous thrombi in the deep veins of the legs: "The detachment of larger or smaller fragments from the end of the softening thrombus which are carried along by the current of blood and driven into remote vessels. This gives rise to the very frequent process on which I have bestowed the name Embolia."[38,39]

In addition to recognizing the association between venous thrombosis and pulmonary emboli, Virchow also postulated its underlying pathophysiology. To this day Virchow's model of hypercoagulability, venostasis, and endothelial damage remains accurate, and all three components of the "triad," to some extent, have a role in the pathogenesis of the posttraumatic prothrombotic state.[37,40] Systemic hypercoagulability that ensues following trauma, venous stasis, resulting from immobilization secondary to paralytics, neurologic injury or skeletal fixation, and venous injury from the initial trauma or iatrogenic causes all contribute to the high incidence of thromboembolic disease in trauma patients.

A systemic hypercoagulable disorder secondary to excessive activation of coagulation, a reduction in coagulation inhibitors and increased fibrinolytic inhibition underlies most episodes of deep vein thrombosis and PE.[41,42] Multiple studies have shown that virtually all seriously injured patients have increased thrombin generation and increased intravascular fibrin formation.[40,43] Engelman and colleagues demonstrated laboratory evidence of hypercoagulability in 85% of seriously injured trauma patients.[42] Furthermore, this hypercoagulable state is induced almost immediately following injury and has been shown to persist for at least a month after injury.[40]

However, hypercoagulability, although necessary, is not sufficient in and of itself to produce thrombus. Venous endothelial injury leading to conversion of the normally antithrombotic endothelium into a pro-thrombotic state, followed by platelet adhesion to the venous endothelial cell junctions or exposed subendothelial matrix is also needed in the pathogenesis of venous thrombosis.[44] The third component of Virchows' triad, venous stasis, is likely a permissive factor, localizing activated coagulation at sites prone to thrombosis.

The prevailing component that underlies venous thrombosis following trauma is likely the hypercoagulable state. Thus, one should consider venous thromboembolic disease in the trauma patient as a systemic coagulation disorder that manifests locally in areas of endothelial damage and venous stasis.[40] The works of Sevitt and others helps to support this premise in several ways. Sevitt showed that in patients with lower extremity fractures, thrombosis was confined to the injured extremity in only 12% of cases and that the uninjured extremity demonstrated thrombosis almost as often as the injured extremity.[13,14] Similarly, Geerts found an unexpectedly high frequency of deep vein thrombosis in patients whose only major injuries involved the face, chest, or abdomen. Sevitt also failed to demonstrate evidence of venous wall injury in the vicinity of 49 of 50 venous thrombi in the lower extremities of 41 patients during autopsy.[45] Microscopic examination of these clots showed that they consisted of two regions; one that was composed predominantly of fibrin and trapped erythrocytes and another that was composed mainly of aggregated platelets. He referred to these as red thrombi and white thrombi, respectively. He showed that the red thrombi were found to be adjacent to the vessel wall, while the platelet-rich region localized further from the site of attachment.[45] These findings suggest that activation of the coagulation system precedes platelet activation and aggregation during the formation of venous thrombi. Additionally, it explains the limited efficacy of antiplatelet drugs in preventing and treating venous thrombosis.

23.3 Prophylaxis of Thromboembolic Disease in Trauma

Trauma patients are a heterogeneous group with marked variation in the extent and distribution of their injuries. As a result, prophylaxis of thromboembolic disease in trauma patients is a complex issue and the optimal mode of prophylaxis has yet to be determined.[46] No single agent has been shown to be effective and applicable in all injured patients and some forms of prophylaxis are contraindicated, or simply not feasible, in patients with certain types of injuries. The literature on venous thromboprophylaxis in trauma patients with multiple injuries is inconsistent and confusing, and definitive randomized controlled studies do not exist.[46,47] This has resulted in underutilization of prophylaxis and marked variation in the timing and modality of prophylaxis used.[48] Nevertheless, the literature is filled with numerous, smaller prospective studies, some of which are randomized, which can be used to help guide prophylaxis decisions.[46,47]

There are two major groups of venous thromboembolic disease prophylaxis, pharmacological and mechanical. Pharmacological prophylaxis is based on the use of unfractionated low-dose heparin (ULDH) and low-molecular weight heparin (LMWHs). Mechanical prophylaxis includes intermittent pneumatic compression devices (PCDs) and arteriovenous foot pumps (AVFPs). A third mechanical prophylactic measure used to battle thromboembolic disease in trauma patients is interruption of the inferior vena cava (IVC). The use of IVC filters will be discussed in detail later in this chapter. For now, more "traditional" methods of prophylaxis will be discussed.

Mechanical devices are an attractive means of prophylaxing against thromboembolic disease in trauma patients because of their relative safety.[49,50] External pneumatic compression devices were first described by Calnan in 1970 and have been in use since that time.[51] Although the exact mechanism by which PCDs work is not entirely understood, it is known that they increase mean and peak femoral venous blood flow, and thus decrease venous stasis.[52,53] Additionally, it is believed that intermittent pneumatic compression activates the fibrinolytic system, presumably through the production and release of pro-fibrinolytic factors by the vascular endothelium; although this has never been conclusively proven.[54–59] This concept was introduced by Knight and Dawson who showed that application of a pneumatic compression device to the upper extremity resulted in significant enhancement of fibrinolysis (as measured by euglobulin clot lysis times in blood that had been drawn from the antecubital vein of the arm) and a decreased incidence of lower extremity DVT.[54] More recent reports have shown that there is an incremental decrease in fibrinolytic activity in sites remote from the area of placement of PCDs.[60] Additionally, it has been shown that alterations in fibrinolysis are short-lived, decaying within minutes of discontinuing PCDs.[60] These observations reinforce the need for continuous use of these devices and question the ability of PCDs worn in remote sites (i.e., upper extremities) to prevent DVT in the legs.

The literature regarding PCDs in patients undergoing elective surgery has shown them to be effective in reducing postoperative thromboembolic disease.[61] Although a few smaller studies have shown PCDs to be effective in preventing thromboembolic disease in patients with multiple injuries,[25,62] the majority of the literature fails to demonstrate any benefit over no prophylaxis,[52,63,64] including a meta-analysis of randomized and nonrandomized studies by Velmahos.[65] In a 1994 prospective randomized study, Knudson found no benefit from PCDs over no prophylaxis, except in a subgroup of patients suffering from neurotrauma in which PCDs offered slightly more protection against thromboembolism than those in the control group.[25] A study by Gersin in 1994 failed to redemonstrate this benefit in that subgroup of patients.[64] One reason for PCDs lack of efficacy is poor patient compliance and improper use, given that these devices are typically uncomfortable for patients and cumbersome for nursing staff.[66,67,68]Additionally, approximately one-third of trauma patients are unable to use PCDs due to lower extremity fractures, casts, or dressings.[20,21]

Another type of mechanical device is the AVFP. In the early 1980s, Garder and Fox described a venous pump on the sole of the foot that fills by gravity and empties with weightbearing, thus increasing venous blood flow without muscular assistance.[69] The AVFP is designed to simulate the normal physiologic pumping mechanism produced by weightbearing. In contrast to PCDs, this device only requires access to the foot, and thus is suitable for patients with bulky lower extremity dressings, external fixation devices or casts.[35] The literature regarding the efficacy of AVFPs in trauma patients is very limited and not encouraging. In her 1996 study,[26] Knudson showed that patients with AVFPs had a higher incidence of DVT then those receiving LMWH or PCDs. Although the difference was not statistically significant, 8 of 53 patients wearing the foot pumps developed severe skin changes. Geerts showed that the rate of venographically proven DVT in 100 trauma patients was 57%, despite prophylaxis with bilateral AVFPs.[70] Much like pneumatic compression devices, improper application and functioning occurs in over 40% of patients with AVFPs.[71]

Based on the current data available, mechanical compression devices should not be used as first-line thromboembolic prophylaxis in trauma patients.[20,35,72] Pneumatic compression devices may be beneficial in patients with a contraindication to anticoagulation due to active bleeding or a high risk for hemorrhage.[20] Arteriovenous foot pumps may be used as a substitute for PCDs in patients who cannot wear PCDs and cannot be anticoagulated.[35]

Heparin is the most widely studied method of thromboembolic disease prophylaxis. Discovered in 1918 by Howell and

Holt,[73,74] it was the first anticoagulant to be identified. It is a naturally occurring polysaccharide that augments the activity of antithrombin 3 resulting in the interruption of both the intrinsic and extrinsic pathways.[26,35,74] In 1930, Howell and McDonald recommended intravenous (IV) heparin in the treatment of venous thrombosis.[74] Later in that decade, several studies demonstrated the efficacy of heparin in preventing postoperative thromboembolic disease, and its use was quickly adopted in that setting.[74] In the 1970s the landmark studies by Kakkar and colleagues[75,76,77] demonstrated that low-dose unfractionated heparin decreased the incidence of DVT and PE in surgical patients. Importantly, however, patients undergoing emergency surgery were excluded from his studies, including those suffering from trauma.[47] Subsequent literature regarding the use LDUH in patients suffering from multiple injuries fails to demonstrate its efficacy.

In several studies by Knudson and colleagues,[25,26] LDUH failed to demonstrate any benefit over no prophylaxis. In another study, Upchurch and colleagues[78] found no significant difference in the rate of thromboembolic disease between those receiving LDUH and no prophylaxis. As part of their study, they also performed a meta-analysis on the use of LDUH in over 1,000 trauma patients. They found that LDUH did not offer any benefit over no prophylaxis. Velmahos also performed a meta-analysis and found that the incidence of DVT between patients receiving LDUH was no different than those receiving no prophylaxis.[65] Multiple other nonrandomized studies have also failed to demonstrate any benefit from LDUH.[28,55,79] Based on the currently available literature LDUH should not be used as a sole agent for the prophylaxis of thromboembolic disease in the trauma patient at high risk for VTE.[35,72]

In contrast to unfractionated low-dose heparin, LMWHs are smaller molecules ranging in size from 2,000 to 9,000 Daltons.[35] The LMWHs have greater bioavailability than unfractionated heparin and seem to have less bleeding for equivalent antithrombotic doses.[26,35] The LMWHs work via binding to antithrombin 3 and have less activity against thrombin and platelets.[26,30,35] The first report demonstrating the efficacy of LMWH for thromboembolic prophylaxis in surgical patients was by Kakkar in 1982.[80] Since then, numerous studies showing its efficacy have been performed, including many on trauma patients. Most believe that LMWH is the most effective means of preventing thromboembolic disease in moderate and high-risk trauma patients,[20,72,81] and it received a level 2 recommendation from the Eastern Association for the Surgery of Trauma for certain groups of patients.[35]

In a landmark 1996 study, Geerts randomized 344 trauma patients to receive either LDUH or LMWH.[82] Those randomized to LMWH had a significantly lower incidence of overall DVT, 31% versus 44% (proven via venography). Additionally, the incidence of proximal DVT was significantly lower in the LMWH group, 15% versus 6%. Although there was no control group, the authors estimated that the risk reduction for LMWH was 30% for DVT and 58% for proximal DVT. The incidence of bleeding in those receiving LMWH was 2.9% versus 0.8% in the LDUH group. Although the difference was not statistically significant, it should be noted that the single LDUH patient who bled, suffered epistaxis, while the LMWH patients bled in the chest, abdomen, head, and retroperitoneum. In a 1996 study, Knudson demonstrated that the incidence of DVT was lower in patients

treated with LMWH than via mechanical methods.[26] The results were not statistically significant and one patient receiving heparin had a major bleeding complication. In a similar study, Ginzburg[83] also found LMWH to be more effective than Sequential Compression Devices (SCDs) in preventing DVT. Again, the results were not statistically significant. In a 2003 publication, the Spinal Cord Injury Thromboprophylaxis Investigators[84] compared LDUH and SCDs to LMWH. The rates of venography proven DVT were 63.3% and 65.5% in the LDUH and SCD group and the LMWH group, respectively. More importantly, however, the rate of PE was significantly lower in patients receiving LMWH, 5.2% versus 18.4%.[84] Several other prospective, noncontrolled and retrospective studies have shown LMWH to be effective in reducing thromboembolism in trauma patients.[85,86,87] However, not all reports on LMWH are as favorable, including a meta-analysis that showed no difference in PE rates between LMWH and LDUH.[65]

The paradox of thromboembolic disease prophylaxis with anticoagulation is the potential to induce or worsen bleeding in injured tissue.[30] Uncontrolled bleeding directly contributes to nearly 40% of trauma-related deaths and worsens central nervous system and organ failure.[30,88,89] Unlike other surgical cohorts, the extent and severity of injuries in trauma patients may not be apparent at the time of presentation. As a result of these uncertainties, initiation of anticoagulation is often delayed or withheld resulting in potentially devastating consequences.[90,91,92,93] Currently accepted contraindications to LMWH prophylaxis include intracranial bleeding, uncontrolled bleeding, an uncorrected major coagulopathy, and incomplete spinal cord injury with suspected or proven paraspinal hematoma.[20,72]

The routine use of thromboprophylaxis in trauma patients is standard of care. However, the type of prophylaxis, mechanical versus pharmacological, or combined mechanical and pharmacological treatment,[94] and when and for how long[95] it should be used is still a matter of debate. Additionally, mechanical and/or pharmacological prophylaxis is frequently contraindicated in many injured patients. As a result, a third method of prophylaxis should be considered, namely interruption of the IVC via filtration.

23.4 Treatment of Thromboembolic Disease

Although pharmacological therapy for thromboembolic disease is typically not suitable for trauma patients, it would be remiss not to discuss it given that it remains the primary means of treating thromboembolic disease. The use of either unfractionated or LMWH followed by 6 months of oral anticoagulation in patients with proximal DVT is over 90% effective in preventing PE or recurrent DVT.[96] Unfractionated heparin is usually administered by continuous IV infusion, although twice daily subcutaneous administration can be employed. The starting IV dose is either a bolus dose of 5,000 units, followed by a continuous infusion of at least 30,000 units for the first 24 hours or a weight-adjusted nomogram.[97,98,99] Levels are titrated to achieve an activated partial thromboplastin time ratio of 1.5 to 2.5 times control.[100,101] In a 1992 meta-analysis, Hommes and colleagues showed that subcutaneous unfractionated heparin administered twice daily appeared to be more effective and at least as safe as IV heparin.[102]

Alternatively, LMWH can be utilized via the subcutaneous route. Due to the more predictable pharmacokinetics of LMWH, it can be administered subcutaneously once or twice daily without laboratory monitoring in the majority of patients.[103, 104,105] Multiple studies have shown that LMWH is at least as effective as unfractionated heparin.[104,105] Additionally, serious potential complications of unfractionated heparin, such as heparin-induced thrombocytopenia and osteoporosis, seem less common with LMWH; although a recent meta-analysis showed no statistically significant difference in heparin-induced thrombocytopenia between the two agents.[106]

Thrombolytic agents have been used in the treatment of venous thromboembolic disease for over 30 years, yet their role is still debated.[107] Although thrombolytics result in earlier clot resolution than heparin and possibly a reduction in residual vein stenosis and valve damage, mortality and other meaningful outcome parameters have not been demonstrated.[108] Additionally, there are significantly more major hemorrhagic complications associated with thrombolytic therapy, including intracranial hemorrhage. Dalen showed that the incidence of intracranial hemorrhage among 559 patients treated with recombinant tissue-type plasminogen activator was 2.1%, and the incidence of fatal intracranial hemorrhage was 1.6%.[109] Other reports have shown the incidence of intracranial hemorrhage to be as high as 3.0%.[110] This issue is obviously very concerning in trauma patients who may be bleeding or who are at high risk for hemorrhage. The data supporting the use of thrombolytics in patients with signs of massive PE and hemodynamic shock are scarce and inconclusive.[111] Additionally, the optimal thrombolytic agent and administration methods are uncertain.[112] The Seventh ACCP Conference on Antithrombotic and Thrombolytic Therapy concluded that clinicians should not use systemic thrombolytic therapy for most patients with PE and that patients who are hemodynamically unstable and have a low risk of bleeding are the most appropriate candidates.[113] Other possible indications for thrombolytics include hemodynamically stable patients with echocardiographic evidence of right ventricular dysfunction and those with massive ileofemoral DVT who are at risk of limb gangrene secondary to venous occlusion.

23.5 History of Venous Interruption/Inferior Vena Cava Filters

Inferior vena cava interruption to prevent PE has undergone significant evolution over the last 80 years. Recognizing that most pulmonary emboli originate in the deep veins of the lower extremities, Homans recommended and first performed interruption of the lower extremity veins via surgical ligation in 1934—although John Hunter performed such interventions as far back as 1793.[11,114] Vein ligations were often performed at the level of the femoral vein, although ligation of the iliac veins was performed if thrombus was identified in the common femoral vein.[115] In 1955, Byrne advocated bilateral femoral vein ligation as multiple reports supported its benefit.[116] Femoral

vein ligation was abandoned, however, because of lack of efficacy and the high incidence of lower extremity morbidity,[117] including swelling, varicose veins, and venous ulcers.

Surgical interruption of the IVC to prevent pulmonary embolization was first suggested by Trousseau in 1868 and subsequently performed by Bottini in 1893.[118,119] However, it was not until the 1940s that the concept of IVC ligation fell into favor.[118] The procedure was performed until the late 1960s with variable success and felt by many to be far superior to femoral vein ligation in protecting against recurrent pulmonary emboli.[119,120,121] Critical evaluation of the efficacy of this procedure, however, demonstrated recurrent PE in up to 50% of patients. Additionally, IVC ligation had significant morbidity and mortality, particularly in patients with heart failure who could not tolerate the sudden drop in venous return that resulted from the procedure.[117,122,123] Mortality rates following IVC ligation were reported to be as high as 39%.[124] Severe, debilitating lower limb stasis and thrombophlebitis occurred in up to half of treated patients.[125,126]

In an attempt to avoid some of these complications, a variety of surgical procedures and devices were developed to partially interrupt IVC flow.[117,127] The idea was to convert a single large vessel, the vena cava, into multiple smaller parallel vessels, or simply narrow its diameter to preserve flow while "trapping" potentially harmful thrombi.[128,129,130] Plication with sutures was suggested by Spencer and DeWeese while plication with staples was done by Ravitch.[131,132] The Moretz clip, introduced in 1959, narrowed the lumen of the IVC to 3.5 mm, whereas the Miles and Admas-Deweese clips compartmentalized the IVC into multiple, small channels.[133,134] Clips and suture plication were associated with 30 to 40% caval occlusion. Additionally, these techniques carried the inherent risks of general anesthesia and laporotomy.[135,136]

In the early 1970s, the Hunter-Sessions balloon was introduced as an alternative to surgical ligation or plication of the IVC.[137,138] The balloon was designed to fully occlude the vena cava and insertion was via the transjugular approach in the awake patient given local anesthesia.[137,138,139,140] The Hunters-Sessions balloon, like the Mobin-Uddin umbrella, which will be discussed shortly, eliminated the morbidity and mortality associated with the above-mentioned surgical procedures. The device consisted of a 75-cm long catheter with a balloon attached to the tip. An inflation needle traversed the inside of the catheter and was attached to an inflating syringe at the proximal end. The smooth intracaval surface of the device prevented caval wall penetration and allowed for full-dose anticoagulation. Additionally, the balloon had the potential to be removed when it was felt that the patient no longer needed it; a concept that was revisited in the late 1990s. The filter was relatively well tolerated and efficacious in preventing PE.[137,139,140]

In 1967 another transjugular device for caval interruption, the Mobin-Uddin umbrella, was introduced.[141] It was hailed as the "umbrella of life" in the October 20, 1969 edition of Newsweek magazine. The device was released for general clinical use in 1970 and was placed via a catheter system through the right internal jugular vein after surgical exposure. The umbrella was designed as an adjunct to anticoagulation. Two types of umbrellas were designed, an imperforate type intended to cause immediate caval occlusion and a sieve type intended to allow for gradual caval occlusion.[141,142] Both types had six stainless

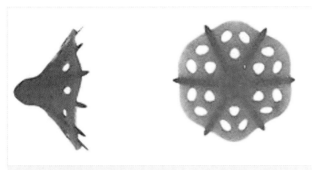

Fig. 23.1 Deployed Mobin-Uddin filter. (Palestrant AM, Prince M, Simon M. Comparative in vitro evaluation of the nitinol inferior vena cava filter. Radiology 1982;145(2):351–355. Reprinted with permission.)

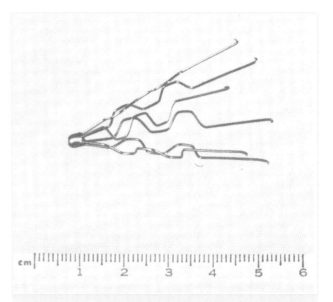

Fig. 23.2 Deployed Greenfield filter. (Greenfield LJ, McCurdy JR, Brown PP, Elkins RC. A new intracaval filter permitting continued flow and resolution of emboli. Surgery 1973;73(4):599–606. Reprinted with permission.)

steel spokes radiating from a central hub and connected with a silicone membrane (▶ Fig. 23.1). The second-generation umbrella was 28 mm in diameter because the smaller original version (23 mm) had an unacceptably high rate of migration.[141,142] Interestingly, about one-third of patients with the Mobin-Uddin umbrella maintained patency of their IVCs with no increase in the incidence of PE, which was reported to be as low as 3.6%. Ultimately, a heparin bonding was applied to the silicon membrane to aid in maintaining caval patency.[142] The Mobin-Uddin umbrella demonstrated a negligible procedure-related mortality, secondary to its transvenous placement and a lower rate of lower extremity morbidity when compared with traditional surgical procedures.[141,142,143,144] The Mobin-Uddin umbrella was removed from the market in 1986 because of an unacceptably high prevalence of caval thrombosis.[145] However, it set the stage for the development of multiple endovascular devices intended to maintain caval patency while trapping thrombi.

The next great advance in the evolution of IVC interruption came in 1973 with the introduction of the Kimray-Greenfield filter (KGF).[146] The original KGF was made of six stainless steel, radiating struts fitted at an angle of 35 degrees to an apical hub. It was 46 mm long and 30 mm wide at the base.[146,147] Each strut had several alternating bends to maximize the filtration area, and terminal hooks intended to fix the filter to the vena cava wall without penetrating it (▶ Fig. 23.2). The cone apex was positioned cephalad, as opposed to the Mobin-Uddin umbrella, which was positioned with cone apex toward the patient's feet.[146,147] The conical design of the device allowed for 80% of the depth of the filter to be filled with thrombus without the development of a pressure gradient across the filter, thus reducing the risk of venous stasis.[146,148] The design also allowed for flow around trapped thrombus, permitting endogenous thrombolysis, and in many cases resolution of clot.[146] The original KGF was inserted through a 29.5-French outer diameter sheath after surgical exposure of either the internal jugular vein or femoral vein. Percutaneous placement was first reported in 1984.[149] Clinical trials and more than 20 years of clinical experience with the KGF have shown a 4% rate of PE and a 96% patency rate.[148,150] Dr. Lazar Greenfield's goal was to design a device that permitted effective filtration of emboli, remained patent after capturing a thrombus, showed no tendency to propagate thrombus and could be inserted under local anesthesia.[146] The KGF satisfied these criteria and, although the original design is no

longer commercially available, remains the device by which other filters are compared. Today there are numerous IVC filters available, most of which are low profile and inserted percutaneously.

23.6 Available Permanent Filters

The titanium version of the Greenfield filter (Boston Scientific, Natick, MA) was introduced in 1988 and approved by the Food and Drug Administration (FDA) one year later (▶ Fig. 23.3).[151] The filter was specifically designed for percutaneous placement via a low profile (12-French [F]) delivery system; half the size of the original stainless steel filter delivery system (SSGF).[151,152,153] It was designed for either internal jugular or femoral vein insertion through a 14-F outer sheath. Although it shared the conical design of the SSGF, the original titanium Greenfield filter (TGF) had significant structural and mechanical differences.[151] The TGF was more flexible and about half the weight of the stainless steel version, 0.25 g versus 0.56 g.[151,152] It was slightly longer than the SSGF, 47 mm versus 44 mm, and had a broader base, 38 mm versus 30 mm. The TGF also had a different hook angle than the SSGF (41 degrees compared with 23.5 degrees on the SSGF) and a smaller apical cap. The design modifications allowed the TGF to be placed via a 12-F delivery system (14-F outer sheath), facilitated entry and positioning, eliminated bleeding during percutaneous insertion and markedly reduced the incidence of insertion site thrombosis (3% vs. up to 41% with a 26-F outer sheath).[151] However, in preliminary clinical studies, it had an unacceptable rate of filter migration, angulation, and caval wall penetration.[151,154] The filter was subsequently removed from the market and reintroduced after modification of the hook.[152,153,154] The currently available titanium Greenfield filter, the modified-hook titanium Greenfield filter (M-HTGF), has a hook angle of 80 degrees; a design that

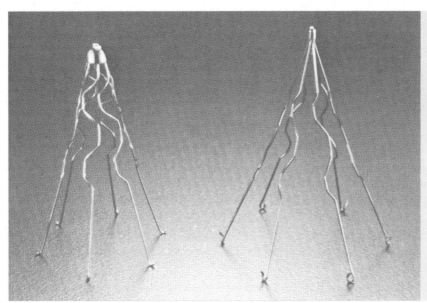

Fig. 23.3 Stainless steel and titanium Greenfield filters. (Greenfield LJ, Cho KJ, Proctor M, Bonn J, Bookstein JJ, Castaneda-Zuniga WR, Cutler B, Ferris EJ, Keller F, McCowan T, et al. Results of a multicenter study of the modified hook-titanium Greenfield filter. J Vasc Surg 1991;14(3):253–257. Reprinted with permission.)

showed a low incidence of caval penetration and filter migration in animal and human studies.[152,155,156] Preliminary results with the M-HTGF demonstrated decreased filter migration (11% vs. 27%), and lower rates of suspected and confirmed caval penetration when compared with the original TGF.[152] In contrast to the SSGF, the struts on the M-HTGF come to a point, which precludes filter deployment over a guide wire.[151,152,157] Without this centering feature, the carrier system may contact the wall of the vena cava at the time of filter discharge, resulting in clustering or asymmetric distribution of the limbs.[157] The clinical significance of strut clustering and asymmetry is debated[155,157,158] and various techniques have been employed to correct it.[157] The M-HTGF has a high caval patency rate (up to 99%) and provides equal protection against PE when compared with the SSGF.[155] The filter is designed for IVC up to 28 mm and is compatible with magnetic resonance imaging (MRI).[159]

The next improvement in the Greenfield filter came in 1994 with the introduction of the percutaneous stainless steel Greenfield filter (PSSGF), or the over-the-wire alternating hook Greenfield filter.[160] The PSSGF, which was FDA approved in 1995,[160] is a hybrid of previous Greenfield designs.[161] The small opening in the hub allows the PSSGF to be inserted and deployed over a guide wire like the original SSGF. This facilitates centering of the filter and decreases the incidence of filter tilting and asymmetry; a problem frequently encountered with the MHTGF.[160,161] The over-the-wire insertion feature also provides support for the passage of the carrier system through the relatively tortuous iliac veins and facilitates insertion from the left femoral vein.[160,161] It has an alternating hook design, to achieve optimal stabilization.[162] Separate femoral and jugular insertion systems are available that differ only in the orientation of the filter apex with respect to the introducer.[160,161] The PSSGF has similar rates of caval patency (98% vs. 93%) and recurrent PE (2.6% vs. 3.2%) as the MHTGF.[163] The filter is MRI compatible. but causes a significant amount of artifact.[159]

The Gianturco-Roehm Bird's Nest filter (BNF; Cook, Bloomington, IN) was introduced in 1982[164] and approved for clinical use by the FDA in 1989.[165] It has a unique design composed of four stainless steel wires measuring 25 cm in length and 0.18 mm in diameter.[159,166,167] The wires are preshaped with numerous random bends of varying size and attached to two V-shaped struts that have small barbs at the ends designed to engage the wall of the IVC. There are small wire loops located just proximal to the hooks that help prevent caval perforation.[166] The original version had flexible, 0.25 mm struts and came preloaded in an 8-F catheter.[166,167] However, due to the high rate of filter migration, the struts were redesigned.[166] In 1986 a new model with broader, more rigid struts measuring 0.46 mm was introduced.[159,166,167] The first step in the deployment process of the BNF is to secure one set of struts to the vena cava wall, with the apex directed caudally. This is followed by careful deployment of the wires, and then engagement of the second set of struts into the caval wall. The second set of struts should be positioned so that the apex, or junction point of the legs, is directed cephalad. The two sets of struts should overlap ~ 2 cm. The result is a maze of 100 cm of wire averaging 7 cm in the cranial caudal dimension (► Fig. 23.4).[166] Occasionally, the wires will prolapse above the cephalad struts. However, this does not affect the clot trapping ability of the filter.[168] One unique quality of the BNF is its ability to be used in vena cava larger than 28 mm in diameter because of its wide strut span (60 mm). Several studies have shown that the BNF can be used in oversized vena cava measuring up to 42 mm in diameter without insertion difficulties, or increased incidence of migration, caval thrombosis, or PE.[169,170] The manufacturer cautions against the use in vena cava larger than 40 mm. One drawback of the BNF is the extensive magnetic resonance imaging artifact that it generates (particularly abdominal imaging) because of its high degree of ferromagnetism. However, field strengths of up to 1.5 Tesla do not induce filter migration or decrease the efficacy of the BNF, and thus it is considered MRI safe.[171]

The Simon nitinol IVC filter (SNF) was introduced in 1988 and received FDA approval in 1990.[172] It is made from nitinol, an alloy of nickel and titanium that has thermal memory.[172,173] At room temperature, the SNF is pliable and can be straightened to conform to a low-profile carrier system (9-F). When

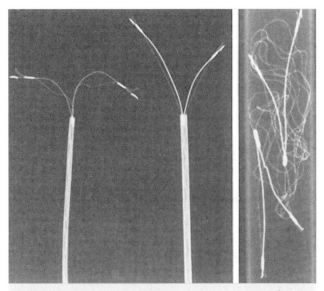

Fig. 23.4 Bird's Nest filter. (Roehm JO Jr, Johnsrude IS, Barth MH, Gianturco C. The Bird's Nest inferior vena cava filter: progress report. Radiology 1988;168(3):745–9. Reprinted with permission.)

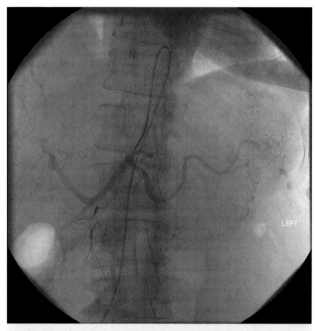

Fig. 23.5 Simon nitinol inferior vena cava filter—formed.

introduced into the body, the SNF instantly transforms into its "preformed" shape (► Fig. 23.5).[172] Nitinol is stronger than stainless steel, resists corrosion, is well tolerated in humans, and is not thrombogenic.[173] The SNF has a unique design with two levels of filtration.[172] The anchoring part of the filter is composed of six struts arranged in a conical configuration. Each strut has a small terminal hook that engages the caval wall for a depth of 1 mm.[172] In addition to anchoring the filter, the legs serve as a coarse filter.[172] The dome of the SNF consists of seven overlapping nitinol wire loops fused together at two points to form a filter daisy wheel.[159] The dome forms a fine filter designed to trap large, as well as smaller emboli.[68] The SNF is 38 mm long and the diameter of the dome in 28 mm.[68] The filter comes preloaded in a 9-F outer diameter delivery system and can be inserted via the femoral or jugular approach. Femoral and jugular delivery systems differ only in length and orientation of the filter (the jugular system is longer and the filter is delivered feet first).[68] External jugular vein[172,174] and antecubital vein[175] insertion is possible because of the flexibility and small size of the delivery system. When using the antecubital approach, a peripherally inserted central catheter (PICC) can be inserted through the same access site after removal of the delivery system.[176] The SNF can be used in vena cava up to 28 mm in diameter. The rate of recurrent PE after placement of a SNF is reported to be between 3%[177] and 4.4%.[178] The incidence of IVC occlusion is reported to be between 3.7%[177] and 11%,[172] although one smaller series reported symptomatic caval occlusion in 21% of 24 patients.[179] In smaller vena cava, tilting of the filter petals in relation to the long axis of the vena cava occurs up to 64% of the time.[172,178] However, filters positioned off-axis have been shown to be as effective in filtering emboli as well-centered filters. Migration of the SNF is uncommon, although several cases of migration to the heart and pulmonary arteries have been reported.[180] Inferior vena cava perforation is frequently seen with the SNF, but does not seem to have clinical

consequences.[177,178] The SNF is MRI compatible and causes minimal MRI artifact.[159]

The Vena Tech-LGM filter (VT-LGM; B. Braun Interventional Systems, Bethlehem, PA) has been used in Europe since 1985 and received FDA approval in 1989.[181] The filter is manufactured from phynox, a metal alloy composed of cobalt, chromium, iron, nickel, and molybdenum. It is biocompatible and nonferromagnetic.[182] The VT-LGM has a six strut conical design. Each strut has a longitudinal side rail attached at its base. The side rails are designed to run parallel to the wall of the vena cava, providing transverse stability and centering. Small hooks, which emanate from each side rail, provide longitudinal stability and minimize filter migration.[182] The original VT-LGM filter had side rails measuring 34 mm and legs measuring 45 mm. However, this design resulted in a high rate (up to 41% of filters)[183] of incomplete filter opening[182] when placed via the jugular approach. It was postulated that this complication was secondary to crossing of the relatively shorter side rails with the struts during deployment.[182] The filter was redesigned with side rails and struts that are nearly equal in length. The currently available VT-LGM filter is 38 mm in height and its base diameter is 30 mm. The filter can be used in IVCs up to 28 mm in diameter. It is placed through a 12-F introducer sheath (14.6-F outer diameter). Thrombus formation within the IVC has been reported to occur in up to 37%[182] of patients; cephalad extension of thrombus above the filter occurred in 20% of patients in one series.[182] Inferior vena cava patency rates have been shown to progressively decrease over time with the VT-LGM filter. Crochet and colleagues[187] reported a 66.8% IVC patency rate at 9-year follow-up in over 200 patients. Insertion site thrombosis, filter migration, and filter angulation have been reported in up to 23%,[182] 18%,[186] and 4.5%[188] of patients, respectively.

In 2001, an elaborated low profile version of the VT-LGM filter was approved by the FDA (► Fig. 23.6).[189] Similar to the VT-LGM, the Vena Tech LP (VT-LP) is made from a chromium-cobalt based

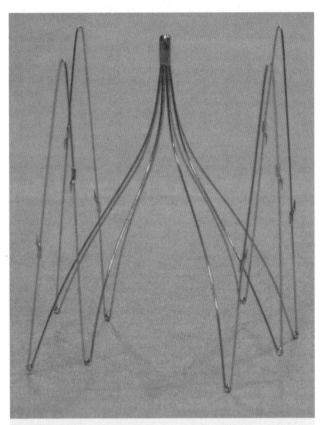

Fig. 23.6 Vena Tech™ low-profile inferior vena cava filter.

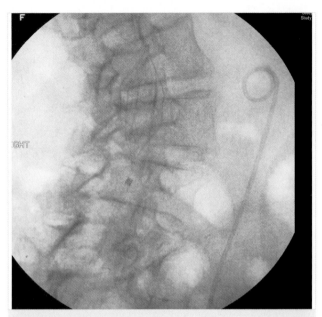

Fig. 23.7 TrapEase inferior vena cava filter.

alloy and thus, MRI-compatible.[189] The VT-LP is composed of eight phynox wires shaped in a conical configuration. The wires fuse caudally in pairs which form side rails that aid in caval centering and stabilization. Each side rail has a superiorly or inferiorly oriented fixation hook arranged in an alternating fashion. The unexpanded filter has a height of 48 mm.[189] When deployed, the VT-LP is 43 mm in height and the base diameter is 40 mm. It is FDA approved for use in IVCs up to 28 mm in diameter, but is safely used in IVCs of up to 35 mm in diameter in Europe.[189] Brachial implantation has been shown to improve patient comfort during insertion.[190] In a recently published series[189] examining the safety and effectiveness of the VT-LP filter, 106 patients were followed over a 3-month period with planned follow-up visits at days 2 to 5, day 30 ± 5, and day 90 ± 15. No clinical evidence of new PE was detected throughout the study.[189] New lower extremity DVT was detected via ultrasound (US) in 13.9% of cases at days 2 to 5, 10.7% of cases at day 30 ± 5, and 8.4% of cases at day 90 ± 15. Filters were inserted via the femoral (right side $n = 63$; left side $n = 9$), jugular ($n = 22$), brachial (right side $n = 9$; left side $n = 1$) and subclavian ($n = 1$) routes without any major complication. Filter migration was not detected on abdominal radiograph throughout the follow-up period. Filter tilting of 10 to 45 degrees was seen in up to 4.3% of cases, but was felt to be clinically insignificant.[189]

The TrapEase vena cava filter (Cordis, Miami Lakes, FL) (▶ Fig. 23.7) has a unique, symmetric, trapezoidal double-basket design. It is laser cut from a single tube of nitinol without welding.[191] Each basket is formed by six diamond or trapezoid-shaped wire polygons joined at one end to form the superior

and inferior apices. The baskets are connected to one another via six side struts that have proximal and distal hooks to provide filter anchoring. The superior basket is oriented in the conventional manner (apex is cephalad), while the inferior basket is oriented with the apex facing down. The double-basket arrangement is designed to offer dual-layer filtration and has been shown to have higher filtration efficiency in vitro when compared with conically designed filters.[192] The side struts minimize filter tilt and migration. The filter is 65 mm in length before deployment. After deployment, it ranges in size from 50 mm to 60 mm depending on the filter's expanded diameter, which is a function of the IVC diameter. The filter can expand to a maximum diameter of 35 mm. The TrapEase was approved by the FDA in 2000 for permanent deployment in IVCs up to 30 mm in diameter. The filter is inserted through an 8-F outer diameter sheath via the femoral, jugular, or antecubital veins. A 90-cm introducer sheath is suitable for the antecubital approach[193] (the jugular and femoral sheaths are 55 cm). Insertion through the subclavian veins has been found to be safe, and is valuable in patients with limited central access.[194] In 2001, Rousseau et al[191] reported their experience with the TrapEase in a multicenter, prospective study. The study included 65 patients from 12 centers in Europe and Canada. At 6 months there were no cases of symptomatic PE, filter migration, filter fracture, or IVC perforation. Two cases of filter thrombosis were reported. Liu and colleagues[195] prospectively evaluated the TrapEase IVC filter in 42 patients. Follow-up evaluations (mean: 15.4 months) were performed at 6- and 12-month intervals. No cases of symptomatic PE, filter migration, filter fracture, or IVC perforation were detected. There was one case of symptomatic filter thrombosis. Schutzer[196] reported one symptomatic PE in 189 patients with a TrapEase filter. Kalva[197] reported clinical and imaging data on 751 patients with the TrapEase filter. During a mean 295-day clinical follow-up, 7.5% of patients developed symptoms of PE, and one death was attributed to PE. Chest CT performed at a mean 192 days showed PE in 6.8% of patients; one-third were asymptomatic. Filter fracture occurred in 3.0% of patients and no cases of filter migration were reported. Twenty five percent of patients had thrombus in their filters and less than 1% of patients had IVC occlusion at a mean follow-up of 189 days. Intracardiac migration[93] and perforation of the superior vena cava (SVC) leading to cardiac tamponade[198] has been described with the TrapEase IVC filter. The authors of the second report caution against using the TrapEase filter in the SVC because of its rigid structure.[199]

23.7 Nonpermanent (Temporary, Optional, Retrievable) Filters

The concept of a nonpermanent device for caval filtration is not new. In 1967, Eichelter and Schenk[200] described an umbrella-like device that was introduced under local anesthesia into the femoral vein of dogs to filter emboli. The Eichelter–Schenk device was constructed by making longitudinal incisions circumferentially around a segment of a polyethylene tube, placing a tube of smaller diameter inside the larger tube and flaring the end protruding beyond the linear incisions. Light traction of the inner tube while holding the outer tube stable produced an umbrella-like structure. The small catheter was then secured to the femoral vein with a suture for removal of the sieve at a later time. After several weeks, the device was collapsed and removed through a small incision. The embolization of trapped or attached emboli upon removal of the Eichelter–Schenk device precluded use of this device in humans.[201,202] However, the concept laid the groundwork for future devices.

Today, numerous nonpermanent caval filtration devices are available worldwide.[203] These devices are being used more frequently and will occupy a larger proportion of the total market as interventionalists and surgeons gain experience and confidence in these products. Nonpermanent filters are classified as either temporary or optional.[204] Temporary filters[205] are devices that are not designed for permanent placement. These filters typically do not have barbs or hooks for fixation to the wall of the IVC. Instead they are attached to tethers that stabilize the filter and aid in their removal. The tethers are usually externalized or buried subcutaneously at a venous access site. Removal of the device is required, typically within 4 to 6 weeks, before the filter and/or tether becomes attached to the wall of the IVC by endothelial overgrowth.[206] If permanent filtration is required, the temporary filter must be removed and replaced by another filter device. There are no temporary filters available in the United States.

Optional filters come in two varieties, retrievable and convertible filters. Convertible devices are permanent filters that can be physically altered via a second percutaneous endovascular procedure to no longer function as filters.[203] Unlike temporary filters, these devices usually maintain their position in the IVC with hooks, barbs, or pressure. After conversion, some or all of the filter remains in the patient's IVC, but not in a configuration that provides protection from PE. If not converted, these devices are designed to function as permanent filters.[203] One such device in development is based on the B. Braun Vena Tech filter. Currently, however, we are aware of no FDA-approved conversion filters.

Retrievable filters are devices that are designed to be removed percutaneously during device-specific time windows.[203,204] They

are independent devices that affix to the wall of the IVC usually by means of hooks, barbs, or pressure. These devices can be placed with or without the intent to be retrieved, giving the physician the option of permanent filtration if needed. Currently there are three optional IVC filters that are FDA-approved for placement and retrieval: the Gunther Tulip (Cook Inc., Bloomington, IN) the OptEase (Cordis, Miami, FL), and the Celect (Cook Inc.).

Nonpermanent filters, in theory, provide protection from PE in the short-term, yet limit or eliminate the long-term complications associated with permanent filters. Although retrievable filters have been widely adopted into clinical use since their introduction there is still much debate concerning when and in whom optional filters should be used given there is a lack of long-term data supporting their safety and efficacy. The decision to use an optional filter should be based on the estimated duration of protection required against clinically significant PE and/or risk of traditional (pharmacological) therapy; although it is frequently difficult to determine the duration and reversibility of the contraindication for anticoagulation at the time of filter placement.[203] Recent studies estimate that retrievable filters are retrieved between 11.5% and 89% of the time, with a mean removal rate of only 36%.[207] The primary reason for this staggering statistic is because of persistence of contraindications to anticoagulation, the presence of significant intrafilter thrombus, and poor patient follow-up (particularly among trauma patients). We expect that in the coming years we will see multiple prospective, randomized studies comparing permanent and retrievable filters, as well as individual filters within each group.

23.8 Available Nonpermanent Filters

The Recovery nitinol filter (RNF) was approved by the FDA for use as a permanent IVC filter in 2002. One year later it gained FDA approval for retrieval, becoming the first FDA-approved optional filter. The RNF is composed of 12, 0.13-inch nitinol wires that are joined at the apex with a nitinol sleeve.[208] The two-tier cone design provides dual-level filtration via six arms forming the upper cone, and six legs forming the lower cone (▶ Fig. 23.12). The RNF was modeled after the dual-level structure of the Simon nitinol filter. Fixation hooks are only found on the struts of the lower cone. The RNF has a base diameter of 32 mm and is 40 mm in height. The filter is designed for placement in vena cava of 28 mm or less. It is delivered through a 9-F outer-diameter sheath via the femoral approach.[208] The RNF is retrieved with a device-specific retrieval cone that consists of nine metal claws covered by urethane. The open diameter of the cone is 15 mm. The cone is inserted via the jugular vein through a 10-F catheter (outer diameter 12 F).[208] In 2002, preliminary clinical experience with the RNF was reported after successful filter placement in 32 patients.[208] Twenty-four filters were successfully retrieved with a mean implantation time of 53 days (5–134 days). Trapped thrombus was seen within the filter of seven patients. Cephalad filter migration (4 cm) in one patient with a large trapped thrombus was reported. The filter and clot were successfully retrieved through a 20-F sheath. No episodes of PE or insertion-site thrombosis were reported. Grande et al[209] reported their experience with 106 patients

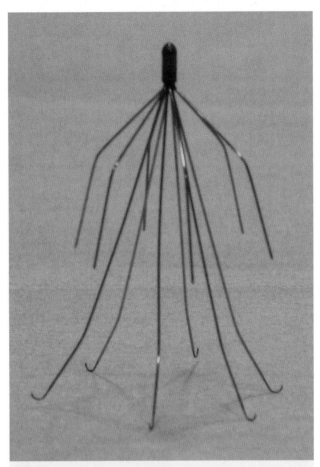

Fig. 23.8 G2 inferior vena cava filter.

In 2003, it received FDA approval as a retrievable device. The GTF is made from elgiloy and is MRI compatible. The filter has four main struts measuring 0.45 mm in diameter.[213] Each strut has a wire loop wrapped around it several millimeters from its distal end to form a tulip-petal conical-shaped structure (▶ Fig. 23.10). The loop ends are fixed to the filter apex. There is a small hook that arises from the filters apex which is used for retrieval (▶ Fig. 23.11). The GTF is 30 mm in diameter and 45 mm in height. The filter is inserted through an 8.5-F sheath via the jugular or femoral veins. The jugular introducer sheath is 45 cm and the femoral sheath is 80 cm. Retrieval is performed via the jugular approach with a wire loop device. The manufacturer recommends filter retrieval within the first 12 days after placement.[213] However, there are numerous reports of successful retrieval at 30 days[213] or longer.[214] One series reported the uneventful removal of 31 GTFs after a mean indwell time of 262 days (range 182–403 days).[215] Additionally, percutaneous repositioning of the device within the IVC via a jugular approach has been employed to "reset" the clock, and thus prolong implantation time.[216] Failed retrievals are typically secondary to strut adherence to the IVC wall, extreme filter tilt, and extensive thrombus within the filter. A venacavogram must be performed prior to retrieval to assess the volume of trapped clot within the filter. The presence of thrombus larger than 25% of the caval diameter at the level of the filter is typically regarded as contraindication to removal.[217] If permanent filtration is needed, the filter can be left in place without adjustment.

The OptEase filter is cut from a single tube of nitinol and has a similar symmetric, trapezoidal double basket design as the permanent TrapEase filter. These design modifications allow retrievability from the femoral approach, which is unique to the OptEase filter. The filter can be inserted via the femoral or jugular vein through an 8-F outer diameter sheath. The retrieval system is 10 F. The OptEase received FDA approval in 2002 for retrieval up to 23 days. Rosenthal and colleagues[218] reported their experience with 40 patients after implantation of the OptEase filter. All 40 patients underwent uncomplicated filter retrieval after a mean indwell time of 16 days (range 3–48 days). Eleven patients underwent successful filter repositioning to extend implantation time. There were no reported cases of symptomatic PE, IVC injury, filter fracture, or filter migration. Oliva et al[219] reported on 27 patients after placement of an OptEase filter. Twenty-one patients had their filters successfully retrieved without complications with a mean indwell time of 11 days. Retrieval was not performed in the remaining patients because of ongoing contraindication to anticoagulation ($n = 3$), large trapped thrombi within the filter ($n = 2$), and poor patient prognosis ($n = 1$). No symptomatic PE, vena cava wall injury, filter fracture, or filter migration was observed. Nineteen of the 21 patients had no device-related adverse events or symptomatic PE at 1-month postretrieval follow-up. In a more recent report, Keller et al[217] reported removal of 58 of 83 OptEase filters with a mean indwell time of 14 days.

The newest optional filter to receive FDA approval (2008) is the Celect filter (▶ Fig. 23.12). The Celect closely resembles the GTF and is made of the same material, elgiloy. The Celect filter has four anchoring struts that have a single fixation hook at the inferior end. Additionally, there are eight curved, secondary struts intended to improve self-centering and clot-trapping. A small retrieval hook arises from the apex of the filter similar to

with RNFs. Three patients (2.8%) were reported to have symptomatic PE after filter placement. No caval thromboses were detected. Filter removal was attempted in 15 of 106 patients at a mean of 150 days after placement. The recovery filter was successfully retrieved in 14 of 15 patients. The GNF is no longer commercially available and has been replaced by the G2 filter that is discussed next.

The G2 filter (▶ Fig. 23.13) is a modification of the RNF.[207] It was approved by the FDA in 2005 as a permanent filter. The G2 filter has not received FDA approval for retrieval, although it is used as an optional filter outside the United States. The G2 filter has longer arm processes than the RNF, a wider leg span and thicker fixation hooks.[207] It has better centering and enhanced fracture resistance. It is designed for IVCs up to 28 mm in diameter.[207] The G2 can be inserted via the femoral or jugular veins. The femoral approach uses a 7-F (inner diameter) introducer whereas the jugular kit utilizes a 10-F sheath. The filter is 42 mm in height when deployed. Oliva and colleagues[210] reported successful removal of 51 G2 filters in 51 patients with a mean implantation time of 53.4 days (7–242 days). They concluded that retrieval of the G2 filter is safe and can be performed successfully in patients who no longer need IVC filtration (▶ Fig. 23.9).[210] Two reports[211,212] of intracardiac G2 migration have been published. Both filters were retrieved endovascularly.

The Gunther Tulip filter (GTF) has been used in Europe since 1992 and was approved by the FDA in 2001 for permanent use.

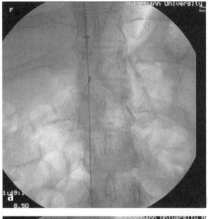
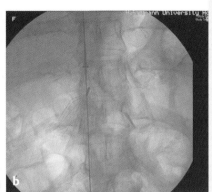
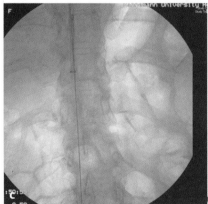

Fig. 23.9 (a) G2 inferior vena cava (IVC) filter removal-1. (b) G2 IVC filter removal-2. (c) Removal of G2 IVC filter-removal-3.

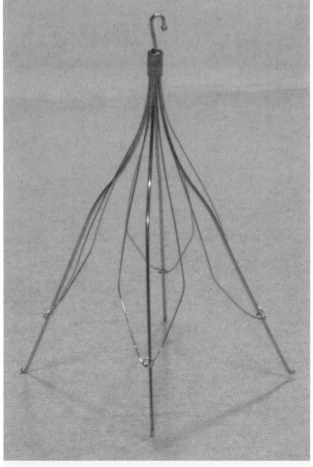

Fig. 23.10 Gunther Tulip inferior vena cava filter.

the GTF. The filter is inserted through an 8.5-F sheath via the jugular or femoral veins and retrieved via the jugular approach with a wire-loop device. Initial studies suggest that the Celect filter may have longer indwell times than other currently available optional filters.[220] Transmural penetration of the IVC within 9 days of its placement has been reported (▶ Fig. 23.13).[220]

23.9 Indications for IVC Filter Placement

Although the incidence of thromboembolic disease has remained fairly stable and the accepted standard of care for patients with venous thromboembolism remains anticoagulant therapy,[221] the use of IVC filters over the last two decades has markedly increased,[145,222,223] and future growth is projected to be as high as 16% per year.[224] Between 1979 and 1999 the number of IVC filters placed in the United States increased almost 25-fold, from an estimated 2,000 in 1979 to an estimated 49,000 in 1999.[223] This rapid increase is likely a consequence of multiple factors including improved filter technology, increasing comfort with nonpermanent filters, bedside insertion techniques with US guidance and expanded indications for insertion,[221] including prophylactic placement.[222]

Before discussing the indications for IVC filter placement it should be stated, although obvious, that the sole function of IVC filters is to prevent clinically significant pulmonary emboli. Inferior vena cava filters do not prevent the formation of DVT[225] and may actually promote DVT formation.[226] Additionally, they have no beneficial effect on the prevention of DVT extension, recurrence, or postthrombotic syndrome.[227]

227

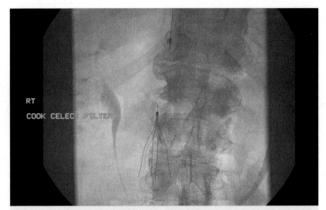

Fig. 23.12   Celect inferior vena cava filter.

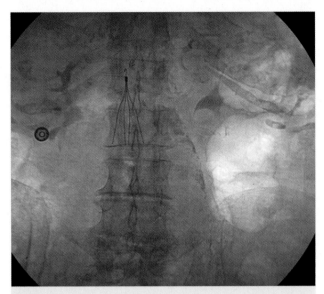

Fig. 23.11   Gunther Tulip inferior vena cava filter; arrow points to retrieval hook.

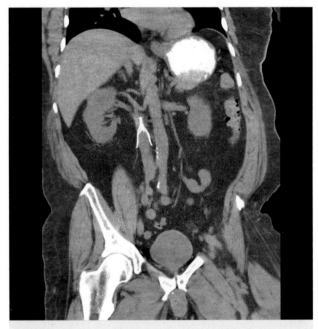

Fig. 23.13   A computed tomography scan of a Celect inferior vena cava filter with perforating struts.

The indications for IVC filter placement have evolved and significantly expanded since the introduction of the Kimray–Greenfield filter nearly 40 years ago. Currently, they can be divided into two broad categories, preventive and prophylactic.[117,224,228] Preventive indications include patients with DVT, as well as, those with a documented PE. The goal in this cohort of patients is to prevent an initial PE or recurrent PE.[117] Preventive indications can be further divided into absolute and relative indications.[117,159,224,229] Prophylactic indications refer to vena cava filter placement in patients who do not have thromboembolic disease, but are in a high risk clinical situation for the development of clini-

cally significant PE.[117] The goal in this cohort of patients is to prevent clinically significant PE if DVT develop.[159,222]

Although the last 10 years has shown an increase in the prophylactic placement of vena cava filters,[222] the majority of filters are still placed in patients with documented thromboembolic disease[222] for absolute indications (57%),[222] including contraindications to anticoagulation, anticoagulation failure or complications of heparin, including heparin induced thrombocytopenia-thrombosis syndrome.[117,159,222,224,229,230,231] Absolute contraindications to anticoagulation include recent major trauma, active internal bleeding, hemorrhagic stroke, intracranial neoplasm, and heparin-induced thrombocytopenia. Relative contraindications include hematuria, occult blood in stool, peptic ulcer disease, and "unstable" gait. Pregnancy presents a unique therapeutic dilemma because oral anticoagulation cannot be used given that it crosses the placenta and causes congenital anomalies.

About one-third of all IVC filters are placed for relative indications.[222] These include patients who are deemed poor candidates for anticoagulation, including the elderly, epileptics, noncompliant patients, and those with neoplasms with propensity to bleed, such as gastrointestinal or genitourinary cancer. Additional relative indications include patients with massive PE[232] in which recurrent emboli would potentially be fatal, after surgical embolectomy,[233] during DVT thrombolysis,[234] and in patients with free floating ileo-femoral thrombus who have a significantly greater risk of PE (50%), even with adequate anticoagulation (27%)[235,236,237,238]; although some reports fail to demonstrate an increased risk of PE in this cohort of patients.[239,240] The use of vena cava filters for these relative indications is controversial and certainly not accepted as the standard of care.

Prophylactic use of IVC filters is a relatively new concept that has recently gained popularity for certain clinical situations. Term refers to the insertion of an IVC filter in someone without DVT or PE, but who is felt to be at high risk for developing a clinically significant PE and cannot receive anticoagulation. The percentage of total filters inserted for prophylactic indications increased from 2.6% to 8% over a 10-year period in one study[222]; 58.6% of the filters were inserted in trauma patients.[222] Clinical situations where the use of prophylactic IVC filtration has been used include high-risk trauma patients, patients with repaired iliofemoral venous injuries,[241] cancer patients,[231] patients with poor pulmonary reserve with a cardiac index less than

1.5 L/min and patients undergoing complex spine, brain, total knee replacement, or bariatric surgery.[167] Additionally, some have advocated the use of prophylactic filters in surgical oncology patients. Similar to the above-mentioned relative indications, prophylactic indications are not universally accepted, and with the exception of prophylactic IVC filter use in trauma, data evaluating this practice is weak. Prospective, randomized studies are needed to clarify what role, if any, IVC filters play in the prophylactic management of thromboembolic disease in different clinical situations.

There are only a few absolute and relative contraindications to IVC filter placement. Absolute contraindications include the inability to gain access to the vena cava and complete thrombosis of the IVC.[159,230] Some relative contraindications to filter placement include severe coagulopathy and patients with septic emboli or positive blood cultures. Additionally, filters should be used with caution in pediatric patients due to the lack of long-term follow-up data on currently available devices.[159,230]

23.10 Methods of Placement of IVC Filters

Inferior vena cava filter placement techniques, imaging guidance modalities, the physical setting where filter placement is performed (operating room, angiography suite, bedside), and the personnel who place them, has undergone significant evolution over the last 30 years.[117] The first IVC filters, including the Mobin-Uddin umbrella filter and Greenfield filter,[242] were placed in the operating room under fluoroscopic guidance after internal jugular or femoral vein surgical cutdown. Percutaneous placement of the Greenfield filter was first described by Tadavarthy[149] in 1984. Following percutaneous internal jugular or common femoral vein puncture, Tadavarthy used serial coaxial dilators over a guide wire to accommodate the large sheath required for filter insertion (24 F).[149] His technique was quickly adopted because it was found that percutaneous placement was safer, easier and less costly[243,244,245,246] than previous surgical methods. Today, most, if not all, IVC filters are placed percutaneously.[247] Newer, low-profile IVC filters do not require serial dilation or balloon angioplasty[248] prior to placement.

Percutaneous placement of IVC filters is typically achieved after gaining access to either the internal jugular vein or common femoral vein.[117,159] Both approaches are similarly effective and associated with potential risks and benefits. Proponents of the internal jugular vein approach argue that there is less tendency for filter tilting during insertion because there is essentially a straight line from the point of venous puncture to the point of filter deployment[246]; in contrast to the curved route in the femoral approach. The femoral approach also carries a higher risk of access site thrombosis[246,249] and associated morbidity than the internal jugular approach, although this is encountered much less frequently with the newer, low profile devices.[250] On the other hand, accessing the femoral vein eliminates the risk of pneumothorax, air embolism, and inadvertent puncture of the carotid artery.[246] Additionally, the effects of a serious bleeding complication in the neck are potentially more dangerous than in the groin.[246,250] The femoral approach gives the operator more room to work (the wires and catheters can be placed over the sterile field formed by the patient's lower body), and is less threatening to the patient.[246] Other access sites that have been used with smaller delivery systems include the subclavian veins,[194] antecubital veins,[176,251] and the external jugular veins.[182] In our institution the approach is determined by the constraints of the patient and personal preference of the interventionalist.

Prior to filter placement, high-quality imaging of the vena cava is needed to determine renal vein location, measure IVC diameter, and confirm patency of the vena cava and iliac veins.[252,253] Preplacement imaging allows the interventionalist to plan their approach and aids in filter selection.[254] The gold standard and most frequently used method of imaging the vena cava is iodinated contrast venography. Cavography should be performed with a 5- to 7-F pigtail catheter positioned at the confluence of the iliac veins followed by injection of 20 mL of contrast for 2 seconds. Filming should be done at 3 to 6 frames per second during suspended respiration in the anteroposterior plane.[254] If variant anatomy is suspected, selective renal venography should be performed.[254,255] Some have recommended selective venography be performed in most patients because it detects significantly more abnormal and aberrant findings, most of which require major changes in filter position.[256] The importance of preplacement cavography cannot be understated, given that up to 15% of cavograms show abnormalities that significantly affect filter placement.[252,253]

Alternative contrast agents that have been employed for cavography include carbon dioxide (CO_2)[257] and gadolinium.[258] Carbon dioxide venography has been advocated in critically ill trauma patients[257] and patients with renal failure because of the low incidence of nephrotoxicity associated with its use. It is also useful in patients who have had a reaction to iodinated contrast material.[117,257] Although CO_2 venography has been shown to be safe[257,259] and well tolerated, the literature contains conflicting data on its ability to accurately estimate caval diameter and identify the renal veins.[257,259-263] Some reports have shown that carbon dioxide venography underestimates caval diameter[259,260] and it has been recommended to consider iodinated contrast-enhanced cavography when the diameter of the IVC is greater than 25 mm at carbon dioxide cavography.[260] Other studies have shown carbon dioxide cavography to be extremely accurate (within 1 mm when compared with iodinated contrast venography)[257] in determining caval diameters.[262,263] Some authors have gone so far as to recommend CO_2 as the first-line contrast agent for all critically ill patients requiring cavography for vena cava filter placement.[263] Carbon dioxide cavography has been shown to be less accurate then iodinated contrast venography in identifying the renal veins.[259] Gadolinium[258] should not be used in patients with renal disease because its use in this population has been linked to nephrogenic systemic fibrosis[264,265]—a disease characterized by scleroderma-like thickening of the skin, subcutaneous edema and joint contractures, as well as involvement of internal organs.[264,265,266] Alternative imaging methods for IVC filter placement include transabdominal and intravascular US as well as CT.[267]

Although the majority of IVC filters are placed percutaneously in the interventional suite or operating room under fluoroscopic guidance, bedside placement is becoming much more common, particularly in multiply injured trauma and critically-ill intensive care unit patients.[262,263,268-275] Furthermore, IVC filter placement eliminates the risks associated with transporting critically ill patients, including hypothermia, catheter dislodgement, and hemodynamic instability.[276,277] Additionally, it avoids potential treatment delays while waiting for an interventional suite or operating room to become available.[278,279] Also, IVC filter placement has been shown to be cost effective[268, 270,271,272,280] and is more convenient for patients, nursing staff, and managing physicians.[281]

The first descriptions of bedside IVC filter placement utilized cavography with either iodinated contrast or carbon dioxide.[262, 263,268,269] This technique requires portable fluoroscopy units, rooms large enough to accommodate the equipment and fluoroscopy-compatible beds.[262,268] Additionally, specialized rooms or shielding equipment are needed to reduce radiation exposure to medical personnel and surrounding patients.[262,268,270, 279] More recent reports have described US-guided and IVUS IVC filter placement, including transabdominal and intravascular approaches. In addition to the benefit of being able to perform filter placement at the bedside, these techniques eliminate the use of contrast and radiation, and are cost effective.[279,280,281,282] Ultrasound-guided IVC filter placement has gained popularity, particularly among trauma physicians who have taken an active role in refining these techniques.[279,280,281]

Although recent reports have shown transabdominal duplex US to be a safe and effective imaging modality for placing IVC filters at the bedside,[280,281,283,284,285] there are several limitations associated with this technique. Inadequate visualization of the relevant landmarks required for accurate filter placement[280,281,283,286] secondary to obesity,[287] abdominal wounds, or excessive bowel gas, occurs in up to 14% of patients evaluated for the procedure.[278,280] Additionally, transabdominal duplex US is relatively poor at identifying IVC and renal vein anomalies,[280,281] which, if not detected, could result in filter malpositioning and inadequate protection from PE.[288] These weaknesses are likely responsible for the lower technical success rates that have been reported with transabdominal duplex US as compared with venography.[280]

An alternative bedside technique that has gained popularity in recent years is intravascular US. This innovative approach was first described in 1999 using a single femoral vein puncture.[275,289] After gaining access to the right femoral vein, an intravascular US catheter is advanced over a super stiff guide wire to the level of the right atrium. Using the pullback technique, the renal and iliac veins are localized and external markers at the level of the renal veins and iliac vein confluence are placed on the patient. After the anatomical landmarks are verified, the intravascular US catheter is exchanged over the wire for the IVC filter catheter.[275,278,289] The IVC filter catheter is subsequently passed blindly over the wire and, using the external markers on the patient for reference, deployed.[275,278,289] Several other approaches have been reported, including a double-puncture technique that allows for real-time imaging during filter deployment,[282] and refined single-puncture techniques that have reported technical success rates of 100%.[290,291] Intravascular US has been shown to be safe[278] and very accurate in characterizing the IVC and locating the necessary anatomical landmarks needed for accurate filter placement.[289,292] In fact, one study showed IVUS to be more accurate at localizing the renal veins and measuring vena cava diameter than contrast venography.[293] Additionally, this technique is ideally suited for obese patients in whom transabdominal US guidance and

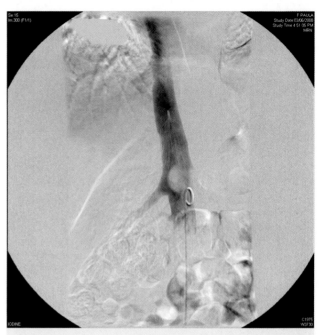

Fig. 23.14 Suprarenal placement of G2 inferior vena cava (IVC) filter for IVC thrombus.

fluoroscopic guidance are not feasible because of poor IVC visualization or weight limitations of the fluoroscopy unit.[287,294] One limitation of intravascular US is the relative inability to detect venous anomalies, including duplication of the IVC, IVC transposition, and anomalous renal veins.[278,282] Contrast venography is recommended if a significant size differential is detected between the suprarenal and infrarenal IVC, if large branches below the renal veins are seen, or if the IVC is smaller than expected.[278,282]

Traditionally, IVC filters have been placed within the infrarenal segment of the IVC with the apex of the filter positioned at the level of the lowest renal vein ostium. Additionally, positioning the filter apex slightly above the origins of the renal veins in order that renal vein inflow may help prevent filter thrombosis or thrombus propagation has also been practiced.[295] Today, infrarenal placement is still the preferred position because of the potential complications associated with suprarenal placement.[296,297,298] In comparison to the infrarenal IVC, the suprarenal IVC has a larger diameter, is shorter, and not visualized as well with venography. Additionally, the suprarenal IVC is subject to mechanical forces produced by the diaphragm and liver as well as cyclical variation in size with respiration and transmitted pulsations from the heart.[296,297,299,300] These anatomical and physiological attributes may be responsible for the higher rates of filter migration,[296,298] filter fracture,[296] and filter penetration[297] that have been reported with suprarenal placement. Another reason infrarenal positioning is favored is because of the theoretical risk of renal vein thrombosis and subsequent renal dysfunction in the event of filter / IVC thrombosis associated with placement above the renal veins.[301] There are, however, several circumstances in which infrarenal placement cannot or should not be done.[302] The most common indication for suprarenal placement is thrombosis of the IVC at or above the level of the renal veins (▶ Fig. 23.14). Other indications include renal vein thrombosis, ovarian vein thrombosis, pregnancy, or the intention to become pregnant. Additional indications include thrombus propagating proximal to an infrarenal filter and anatomical anomalies including duplication of the IVC and circumaortic left renal vein.[295] Although there are theoretical risks involved with suprarenal placement of vena cava filters (described above), many large studies have shown suprarenal IVC filters to be safe and effective.[303] Suprarenal placement does not carry any more risk than the infrarenal placement in terms of permanent renal dysfunction, increased rate of recurrent PE, and IVC occlusion and should be considered in patients in whom infrarenal placement is not feasible.

23.11 Upper Extremity Venous Thrombosis / Superior Vena Cava Filters

Most (85–95%) pulmonary emboli develop within the deep veins of the lower extremities. The remainder develop in the pelvic veins, vena cava, right atrium, or upper extremities.[115,304] Over the last several decades the concept of upper extremity thrombosis in regards to etiology, propensity to propagate and cause PE, and treatment has undergone significant evolution. Although relatively rare, thrombosis in the subclavian, axillary, or brachial veins is more common than previously reported and accounts for 4 to 10% of all venous thromboses.[305] The relatively lower incidence of upper extremity DVT (UEDVT) compared with lower extremity DVT (LEDVT) is believed to be secondary to lower gravitational stress, fewer venous valves and less stasis in the upper extremities.[305] Upper extremity DVT is divided into two groups, primary and secondary thromboses. Primary UEDVT, which accounts for 30% of all UEDVT, includes thromboses secondary to thoracic outlet syndrome[306,307] (60% of primary UEDVT),[305] Paget-Schroetter syndrome,[308,309] and idiopathic causes.[305] Secondary UEDVT includes thromboses secondary to central venous catheters[310] (most common cause), malignancy, coagulation abnormalities, oral contraceptive use, and pregnancy.[305] The rise in UEDVT over the last several decades has been attributed to the increased use of central lines, peripherally inserted central venous catheters, and pacemakers.[311] The most serious complication of UEDVT, PE, occurs in 12 to 16% of patients.[312,313,314] One series reported a PE rate of 36%[315] in patients with UEDVT, and there have been several reports of fatal PE from UEDVT.[311,316] Catheter-related thrombosis is more likely to embolize and cause PE than primary causes of thrombosis.[311,317] The data regarding UEDVT in trauma patients is extremely limited and the relationship between UEDVT and subsequent PE in this cohort of patients is not known.[314]

Therapy for UEDVT is controversial and the optimal mode of treatment is debated.[305] The first line, and most common treatment is anticoagulation with low molecular weight heparin (LMWH) and vitamin K antagonists[316]; identical to lower extremity DVT treatment.[305] In patients with mechanical causes of UEDVT (Paget-Schroetter syndrome and thoracic outlet syndrome), thrombolysis, and surgery have been advocated.[316,318,319] A third treatment option is mechanical interruption of the SVC. Superior vena cava filter placement is an attractive option for patients in whom anticoagulation is contraindicated, or who suffer a second PE despite adequate anticoagulation. Superior vena cava filtration has been used in a small number of patients with good success.[316]

Prior to use in humans, Langham and Greenfield described placement of the Greenfield filter in the SVC of 11 dogs.[311,320] Harvested thrombus was subsequently embolized into the filters. At 3-month follow-up, all filters were patent and no pulmonary emboli were detected in any animal at autopsy.[320] Superior vena cava perforation did not occur and only minimal increases in central venous pressure was noted.[321] Since then, a small number of case reports[198,322–332] and several small series regarding SVC filter placement in humans have been reported.[311,333,334] In 1996, Ascer[333] reported the use of the titanium Greenfield filter in six patients with UEDVT in whom anticoagulation was either contraindicated or ineffective in preventing recurrent PE. There were no complications related to filter insertion and no clinical evidence of PE at 4 to 14 months after filter insertion.[333]

In 1999, Spence and colleagues[311] reported on 41 patients with acute UEDVT who underwent percutaneous SVC filter placement. All patients had documented thrombus (US and/or venography proven) and failure of or contraindication to anticoagulation. Thirty-three patients received a Greenfield filter, five received a Simon nitinol filter, and two received a Vena Tech filter. The remaining patient had a Gianturco-Roehm BNF inserted. There were no complications related to filter insertion, and at a median follow up of 3 months there was no evidence of filter migration or fracture. There was no clinical evidence of SVC occlusion at 15 weeks, and only 1 PE was reported; the PE occurred 44 months after filter placement and was believed to be secondary to acute LEDVT.

In 2000, Ascher and colleagues[334] reported the largest series of SVC filter placements. Seventy-two Greenfield filters were inserted into the SVCs of 72 patients with acute UEDVT. The indication for filter placement was contraindication to full-dose anticoagulation ($n = 67$), or failure of full-dose anticoagulation to prevent recurrent PE or extension of thrombus ($n = 5$).[334]

All of the above case reports and series employed the use of permanent filters.[311,334] More recently, nonpermanent filters have been used for temporary SVC interruption. The first temporary SVC filter was placed in 2001 in a young patient with an upper extremity thrombus and PE.[335] After thrombectomy, the temporary filter was successfully removed. In 2002, Nadkarni[336] reported the first case of SVC interruption with an optional filter, the GTF. The filter was successfully placed and retrieved in the SVC of a 56-year-old woman with bilateral subclavian and internal jugular venous thromboses.

Reported complications associated with SVC filters include SVC occlusion,[325,326] erosion into the ascending aorta,[329] penetration of the right lung with subsequent tension pnemothorax,[330] perforation of SVC and cardiac tamponade.[198] Although filter dislodgment following blind central line placement has been reported,[334] right heart cannulation following SVC filter placement has been performed safely.

Superior vena cava filters are inserted percutaneously via the femoral, jugular, or subclavian veins.[316] Prior to insertion, a superior venacavogram must be performed to determine the diameter of the SVC, exclude anatomical variations (double SVC occurs in 0.3% of the population) and ensure patency of the SVC.[311,316,323,334] Superior vena cava thrombosis is a contraindication to

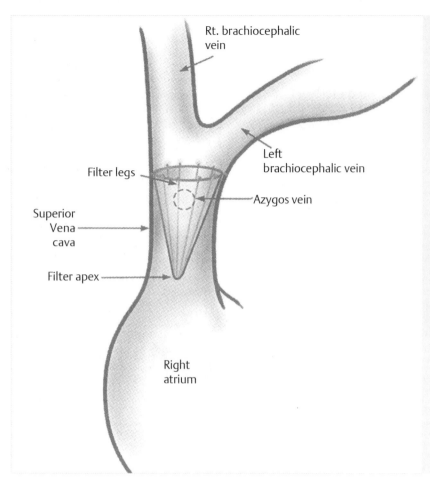

Rt. brachiocephalic vein

Left brachiocephalic vein

Filter legs

Azygos vein

Superior Vena cava

Filter apex

Right atrium

Fig. 23.15 Schematic of superior vena cava filter placement. (Spence LD, Gironta MG, Malde HM, Mickolick CT, Geisinger MA, Dolmatch BL. Acute upper extremity deep venous thrombosis: safety and effectiveness of superior vena caval filters. Radiology 1999;210(1):53–58. Reprinted with permission.)

filter placement.[316] Additionally, central venous stenosis may act as an "auto filter" and thus eliminate the need for iatrogenic filtration.[311] Ideally, SVC filters should be positioned just inferior to the confluence of the brachiocephalic veins to avoid azygous vein occlusion in the event of filter thrombosis, and above the cavoatrial junction (▶ Fig. 23.15). If the filter is released too low, migration into the heart could occur. Placement too high could result in migration into the brachiocephalic or internal jugular veins.[323] The relatively short target area for deployment makes SVC filter insertion technically more challenging than IVC filter insertion.[311,316,334] Additionally, cardiac pulsations can further complicate insertion.[316] For femoral approaches, a jugular insertion kit must be used so that proper filter orientation is achieved; the apex of the filter should face toward the heart.[311,316,334] A femoral kit must be used if a jugular approach is performed. Central lines must be removed or retracted prior to SVC filter insertion. Following deployment a superior venacavogram and chest radiograph should be obtained to document placement and exclude immediate complications.

Although SVC filter placement is technically feasible, and the majority of literature suggests that they are safe and effective, the total number of reported patients is very small and duration of follow-up is relatively short. Prospective, randomized studies using objective measures to detect asymptomatic complications and longer follow-up are needed before intelligent recommendations regarding when and in whom SVC filters should be used.

23.12 Prophylactic Use of IVC Filters in Trauma Patients

The use of prophylactic IVC filters in high-risk trauma patients has increased from 3 to 57% over the past 15 years.[337] Contraindications to traditional thromboembolic prophylaxis and the relative ineffectiveness of low-dose heparin or external mechanical devices[47,338] to prevent thrombotic complications, as well as the introduction and availability of optional filters has fueled this enthusiasm. A 1997 practitioner survey administered to over 600 U.S. trauma surgeons found that potential removability of IVC filters would significantly increase prophylactic placement from 29 to 53% in patients with multiple lower-extremity fractures.[339]

Over the last quarter century many authors have examined the effectiveness and safety of prophylactic IVC filter use in high-risk trauma patients.[338,340–353] However, it is extremely difficult to develop definitive recommendations based on this data for several reasons. First, patient demographics and what is considered "high risk" varies considerably between studies. In addition, the indications for placement of prophylactic filters are inconsistent. Additionally, the types of filters used vary from study to study; more recent literature has examined the use of optional filters. Other variables that complicate the data include insertion methods, pre- and postimaging standards, length of follow up, as well as differences in who performs the procedures—surgeons, interventional radiologists, interventional cardiologists. Finally, these studies lack adequate control groups for comparison, with most series using historical data for comparison. Nevertheless, there is a considerable amount of data available that cannot be ignored.

In 1998, Rogers and colleagues[341] reported on 132 trauma patients who received prophylactic IVC filters over a 6-year period. The study provided 5 years of follow-up data. Seventy percent of the patients received titanium Greenfield filters. The remaining patients received stainless-steel Greenfield filters, Vena Tech filters, and BNFs. The authors demonstrated a low rate of insertion-related thrombosis (3%), a low rate of PE (2%), and a 97% caval patency rate. The three pulmonary emboli, one of which was fatal, were believed to be related to strut malposition and /or significant filter tilt. They recommended careful assessment of postplacement filter position, and transcatheter manipulation or placement of a second filter if improper placement was seen.

In 1994, Leach and colleagues[342] reported on 200 trauma patients following the institution of a protocol for prophylactic IVC filtration for trauma patients at high risk for PE. They found no mortality and no patient with a Greenfield filter sustained a fatal PE. In the year prior to the initiation of prophylactic IVC filter use, 11 deaths from PE occurred. In 1996 Rodriguez et al[348] prospectively placed vena cava filters in 40 high-risk trauma patients prophylactically and compared them with 80 matched historic controls. They found a significant reduction in the frequency of PE, 2.5% versus 17%, as well as, PE-related mortality. In 2002, Carlin retrospectively reported on 78 trauma patients in whom IVC filters were place prophylactically. None of these patients developed PE. Rosenthal et al[343] reported no PE in 29 high-risk trauma patients who had received prophylactic IVC filtration. Additionally, 84% of the surviving patients (21 of 25) maintained patency of their vena cava at a mean follow-up of 33 months. Khansarinia et al[346] demonstrated a significant reduction in PE and PE-related deaths with the use of prophylactic IVC filters in select high-risk trauma patients. None of the 108 patients who received a prophylactic IVC filter developed a PE, whereas 13 of the matched historic control patients developed PE; nine of which were fatal. These differences were statistically significant for both PE and PE-related death. Carlin[338] reported a decreased incidence of PE in high-risk trauma patients from 0.29% to 0.15% after the increased use of prophylactic filtration. In 2000, Velmahos et al[349] reported a meta-analysis of several observation uncontrolled studies and found that patients with prophylactic vena cava filtration had a lower incidence of PE (0.2%) compared with those without filters (1.5%) and historical controls (5.8%). Giannoudis and colleagues examined over 25 studies containing 3,404 trauma patients who had received prophylactic IVC filters and found that the overall complication rate in this population was 13%. Recurrent PE occurred in less than 1% of this cohort. Inferior vena cava thrombosis and insertion site thrombosis occurred in 2% of patients while filter migration, misplacement and/or tilt occurred in 1%.

More recent literature on prophylactic filter use in trauma patients has focused on optional filters. In 2005 Allen et al[351] reported on 51 high-risk trauma patients who had received IVC filtration. Thirty-two filters were placed prophylactically, whereas 21 were placed for demonstrated thromboembolic disease. Retrieval was successful in 24 of 25 attempts and no complications of device migration or thrombosis, or PE were reported. In 2004 Rosenthal[282] reported on 94 patients with multiple injuries who underwent prophylactic IVCF placement using the OptEase vena cava filter. The filters were inserted at the bedside under real-time intravascular US. Thirty-one patients underwent uneventful filter retrieval. One PE was reported after filter retrieval. Hoff[352] reported equally positive results in 35 trauma patients with contraindications to LMWH.

In contrast, some investigators have experienced less favorable results with prophylactic vena cava filter placement. In 1999, McMurtry and colleagues[353] retrospectively evaluated 299 trauma patients who had received IVC filters over an 8-year period. The review failed to demonstrate a decrease in PE rate in patients who received a prophylactic IVC filter.

Although the data presented suggests that there is a clear advantage to placing prophylactic vena cava filters in trauma patients, their use is still highly debated and should not be used as first-line prophylaxis. The use of prophylactic IVC filters can be considered in patients who are at high risk for thromboembolic disease and cannot be anticoagulated. Additionally, careful examination of the patient's comorbidities, life expectancy, and overall prognosis must be considered.

References

[1] Giuntini C, Di Ricco G, Marini C, Melillo E, Palla A. Pulmonary embolism: epidemiology. Chest 1995; 107 Suppl: 3S–9S

[2] Monreal M, Barba R, Tolosa C, Tiberio G, Todolí J, Samperiz AL RIETE Investigators. Deep vein thrombosis and pulmonary embolism: the same disease? Pathophysiol Haemost Thromb 2006; 35: 133–135

[3] Heit JA. The epidemiology of venous thromboembolism in the community: implications for prevention and management. J Thromb Thrombolysis 2006; 21: 23–29

[4] Silverstein MD, Heit JA, Mohr DN, Petterson TM, O'Fallon WM, Melton LJ. Trends in the incidence of deep vein thrombosis and pulmonary embolism: a 25-year population-based study. Arch Intern Med 1998; 158: 585–593

[5] Stein PD, Henry JW. Prevalence of acute pulmonary embolism among patients in a general hospital and at autopsy. Chest 1995; 108: 978–981

[6] Francis CW. Clinical practice. Prophylaxis for thromboembolism in hospitalized medical patients. N Engl J Med 2007; 356: 1438–1444

[7] Tapson VF. Acute pulmonary embolism. N Engl J Med 2008; 358: 1037–1052

[8] Streiff MB. Vena caval filters: a comprehensive review. Blood 2000; 95: 3669–3677

[9] Prandoni P, Lensing AW, Cogo A et al. The long-term clinical course of acute deep venous thrombosis. Ann Intern Med 1996; 125: 1–7

[10] Douketis JD, Kearon C, Bates S, Duku EK, Ginsberg JS. Risk of fatal pulmonary embolism in patients with treated venous thromboembolism. JAMA 1998; 279: 458–462

[11] Homans J. Thrombosis of the deep veins of the lower leg, causing pulmonary embolism. N Engl J Med 1934; 211: 993–997

[12] McCartney JS. Pulmonary embolism following trauma. Am J Pathol 1934; 10: 709–710

[13] Sevitt S, Gallagher NG. Prevention of venous thrombosis and pulmonary embolism in injured patients. A trial of anticoagulant prophylaxis with phenindione in middle-aged and elderly patients with fractured necks of femur. Lancet 1959; 2: 981–989

[14] Sevitt S, Gallagher N. Venous thrombosis and pulmonary embolism. A clinico-pathological study in injured and burned patients. Br J Surg 1961; 48: 475–489

[15] Fitts WT, Lehr HB, Bitner RL, Spelman JW. An analysis of 950 fatal injuries. Surgery 1964; 56: 663–668

[16] Freeark RJ, Boswick J, Fardin R. Posttraumatic venous thrombosis. Arch Surg 1967; 95: 567–575

[17] Salzman EW, Harris WH, DeSanctis RW. Anticoagulation for prevention of thromboembolism following fractures of the hip. N Engl J Med 1966; 275: 122–130

[18] Geerts WH, Code KI, Jay RM, Chen E, Szalai JP. A prospective study of venous thromboembolism after major trauma. N Engl J Med 1994; 331: 1601–1606

[19] Sharma OP, Oswanski MF, Joseph RJ et al. Venous thromboembolism in trauma patients. Am Surg 2007; 73: 1173–1180

[20] Geerts WH, Pineo GF, Heit JA et al. Prevention of venous thromboembolism: the Seventh ACCP Conference on Antithrombotic and Thrombolytic Therapy. Chest 2004; 126 Suppl: 338S–400S

[21] Shackford SR, Davis JW, Hollingsworth-Fridlund P, Brewer NS, Hoyt DB, Mackersie RC. Venous thromboembolism in patients with major trauma. Am J Surg 1990; 159: 365–369

[22] Knudson MM, Collins JA, Goodman SB, McCrory DW. Thromboembolism following multiple trauma. J Trauma 1992; 32: 2–11

[23] Knudson MM, Ikossi DG, Khaw L, Morabito D, Speetzen LS. Thromboembolism after trauma: an analysis of 1602 episodes from the American College of Surgeons National Trauma Data Bank. Ann Surg 2004; 240: 490–496, discussion 496–498

[24] Knudson MM, Ikossi DG. Venous thromboembolism after trauma. Curr Opin Crit Care 2004; 10: 539–548

[25] Knudson MM, Lewis FR, Clinton A, Atkinson K, Megerman J. Prevention of venous thromboembolism in trauma patients. J Trauma 1994; 37: 480–487

[26] Knudson MM, Morabito D, Paiement GD, Shackleford S. Use of low molecular weight heparin in preventing thromboembolism in trauma patients. J Trauma 1996; 41: 446–459

[27] Piotrowski JJ, Alexander JJ, Brandt CP, McHenry CR, Yuhas JP, Jacobs D. Is deep vein thrombosis surveillance warranted in high-risk trauma patients? Am J Surg 1996; 172: 210–213

[28] Napolitano LM, Garlapati VS, Heard SO et al. Asymptomatic deep venous thrombosis in the trauma patient: is an aggressive screening protocol justified? J Trauma 1995; 39: 651–657, discussion 657–659

[29] Schuerer DJ, Whinney RR, Freeman BD et al. Evaluation of the applicability, efficacy, and safety of a thromboembolic event prophylaxis guideline designed for quality improvement of the traumatically injured patient. J Trauma 2005; 58: 731–739

[30] Latronico N, Berardino M. Thromboembolic prophylaxis in head trauma and multiple-trauma patients. Minerva Anestesiol 2008; 74: 1–5

[31] Schultz DJ, Brasel KJ, Washington L et al. Incidence of asymptomatic pulmonary embolism in moderately to severely injured trauma patients. J Trauma 2004; 56: 727–731, discussion 731–733

[32] Velmahos GC, Toutouzas KG, Vassiliu P et al. Can we rely on computed tomographic scanning to diagnose pulmonary embolism in critically ill surgical patients? J Trauma 2004; 56: 518–525, discussion 525–526

[33] Stawicki SP, Grossman MD, Cipolla J et al. Deep venous thrombosis and pulmonary embolism in trauma patients: an overstatement of the problem? Am Surg 2005; 71: 387–391

[34] Abelseth G, Buckley RE, Pineo GE, Hull R, Rose MS. Incidence of deep-vein thrombosis in patients with fractures of the lower extremity distal to the hip. J Orthop Trauma 1996; 10: 230–235

[35] Rogers FB, Cipolle MD, Velmahos G, Rozycki G, Luchette FA. Practice management guidelines for the prevention of venous thromboembolism in trauma patients: the EAST practice management guidelines work group. J Trauma 2002; 53: 142–164

[36] López JA, Kearon C, Lee AY. Deep venous thrombosis. Hematology (Am Soc Hematol Educ Program) 2004: 439–456

[37] Merli GJ. Pathophysiology of venous thrombosis and the diagnosis of deep vein thrombosis-pulmonary embolism in the elderly. Cardiol Clin 2008; 26: 203–219, vi

[38] Dalen JE. Pulmonary embolism: what have we learned since Virchow? Natural history, pathophysiology, and diagnosis. Chest 2002; 122: 1440–1456

[39] Virchow RLK. Cellular Pathology. 1859 special ed. London, UK: John Churchill; 1978: 204–207

[40] Meissner MH, Chandler WL, Elliott JS. Venous thromboembolism in trauma: a local manifestation of systemic hypercoagulability? J Trauma 2003; 54: 224–231

[41] Boldt J, Papsdorf M, Rothe A, Kumle B, Piper S. Changes of the hemostatic network in critically ill patients—is there a difference between sepsis, trauma, and neurosurgery patients? Crit Care Med 2000; 28: 445–450

[42] Engelman DT, Gabram SG, Allen L, Ens GE, Jacobs LM. Hypercoagulability following multiple trauma. World J Surg 1996; 20: 5–10

[43] Shackford SR, Davis JW, Hollingsworth-Fridlund P, Brewer NS, Hoyt DB, Mackersie RC. Venous thromboembolism in patients with major trauma. Am J Surg 1990; 159: 365–369

[44] Samuels PB, Webster DR. The role of venous endothelium in the inception of thrombosis. Ann Surg 1952; 136: 422–438

[45] Sevitt S. The structure and growth of valve-pocket thrombi in femoral veins. J Clin Pathol 1974; 27: 517–528

[46] Knudson MM, Ikossi DG. Venous thromboembolism after trauma. Curr Opin Crit Care 2004; 10: 539–548

[47] Velmahos GC. The current status of thromboprophylaxis after trauma: a story of confusion and uncertainty. Am Surg 2006; 72: 757–763

[48] Imberti D, Ageno W. A survey of thromboprophylaxis management in patients with major trauma. Pathophysiol Haemost Thromb 2005; 34: 249–254

[49] Parra RO, Farber R, Feigl A. Pressure necrosis from intermittent-pneumatic-compression stockings. N Engl J Med 1989; 321: 1615

[50] Lachmann EA, Rook JL, Tunkel R, Nagler W. Complications associated with intermittent pneumatic compression. Arch Phys Med Rehabil 1992; 73: 482–485

[51] Calnan JS, Pflug JJ, Mills CJ. Pneumatic intermittent-compression legging simulating calf-muscle pump. Lancet 1970; 2: 502–503

[52] Griffin M, Kakkos SK, Geroulakos G, Nicolaides AN. Comparison of three intermittent pneumatic compression systems in patients with varicose veins: a hemodynamic study. Int Angiol 2007; 26: 158–164

[53] Keith SL, McLaughlin DJ, Anderson FA et al. Do graduated compression stockings and pneumatic boots have an additive effect on the peak velocity of venous blood flow? Arch Surg 1992; 127: 727–730

[54] Knight MT, Dawson R. Effect of intermittent compression of the arms on deep venous thrombosis in the legs. Lancet 1976; 2: 1265–1268

[55] Inada K, Koike S, Shirai N, Matsumoto K, Hirose M. Effects of intermittent pneumatic leg compression for prevention of postoperative deep venous thrombosis with special reference to fibrinolytic activity. Am J Surg 1988; 155: 602–605

[56] Killewich LA, Cahan MA, Hanna DJ et al. The effect of external pneumatic compression on regional fibrinolysis in a prospective randomized trial. J Vasc Surg 2002; 36: 953–958

[57] Macaulay W, Westrich G, Sharrock N et al. Effect of pneumatic compression on fibrinolysis after total hip arthroplasty. Clin Orthop Relat Res 2002; 399: 168–176

[58] Cahan MA, Hanna DJ, Wiley LA, Cox DK, Killewich LA. External pneumatic compression and fibrinolysis in abdominal surgery. J Vasc Surg 2000; 32: 537–543

[59] Christen Y, Wütschert R, Weimer D, de Moerloose P, Kruithof EK, Bounameaux H. Effects of intermittent pneumatic compression on venous haemodynamics and fibrinolytic activity. Blood Coagul Fibrinolysis 1997; 8: 185–190

[60] Jacobs DG, Piotrowski JJ, Hoppensteadt DA, Salvator AE, Fareed J. Hemodynamic and fibrinolytic consequences of intermittent pneumatic compression: preliminary results. J Trauma 1996; 40: 710–716, discussion 716–717

[61] Weinmann EE, Salzman EW. Deep-vein thrombosis. N Engl J Med 1994; 331: 1630–1641

[62] Elliott CG, Dudney TM, Egger M et al. Calf-thigh sequential pneumatic compression compared with plantar venous pneumatic compression to prevent deep-vein thrombosis after non-lower extremity trauma. J Trauma 1999; 47: 25–32

[63] Fisher CG, Blachut PA, Salvian AJ, Meek RN, O'Brien PJ. Effectiveness of pneumatic leg compression devices for the prevention of thromboembolic disease in orthopaedic trauma patients: a prospective, randomized study of compression alone versus no prophylaxis. J Orthop Trauma 1995; 9: 1–7

[64] Gersin K, Grindlinger GA, Lee V, Dennis RC, Wedel SK, Cachecho R. The efficacy of sequential compression devices in multiple trauma patients with severe head injury. J Trauma 1994; 37: 205–208

[65] Velmahos GC, Kern J, Chan LS, Oder D, Murray JA, Shekelle P. Prevention of venous thromboembolism after injury: an evidence-based report—part I: analysis of risk factors and evaluation of the role of vena caval filters. J Trauma 2000; 49: 132–138, discussion 139

[66] Macatangay C, Todd SR, Tyroch AH. Thromboembolic prophylaxis with intermittent pneumatic compression devices in trauma patients: a false sense of security? J Trauma Nurs 2008; 15: 12–15

[67] Comerota AJ, Katz ML, White JV. Why does prophylaxis with external pneumatic compression for deep vein thrombosis fail? Am J Surg 1992; 164: 265–268

[68] Cornwell EE, Chang D, Velmahos G et al. Compliance with sequential compression device prophylaxis in at-risk trauma patients: a prospective analysis. Am Surg 2002; 68: 470–473

[69] Gardner AM, Fox RH. The venous pump of the human foot—preliminary report. Bristol Med Chir J 1983; 98: 109–112

[70] Geerts WH, Jay R, Code K et al. Venous foot pump as thromboprophylaxis in major trauma. Thromb Haemost 1999; 82 suppl: 650–651

[71] Anglen JO, Goss K, Edwards J, Huckfeldt RE. Foot pump prophylaxis for deep venous thrombosis: the rate of effective usage in trauma patients. Am J Orthop 1998; 27: 580–582

[72] Geerts WH, Bergqvist D, Pineo GF et al. Prevention of venous thromboembolism: the Eighth ACCP Conference on Antithrombotic and Thrombolytic Therapy. Chest 2008; 133 suppl: 381S–453S

[73] Howell WH, Holt E. Two new factors in blood coagulation-heparin and proantithrombin. Am J Physiol 1918; 47: 328–333

[74] Dalen JE. Pulmonary embolism: what have we learned since Virchow?: treatment and prevention. Chest 2002; 122: 1801–1817

[75] Kakkar VV, Corrigan T, Spindler J et al. Efficacy of low doses of heparin in prevention of deep-vein thrombosis after major surgery. A double-blind, randomised trial. Lancet 1972; 2: 101–106

[76] Fossard DP, Corrigan T, Spindler JJ, Kakkar VV. Low doses of heparin in the prevention of postoperative D.V.T.—a double-blind trial. Br J Surg 1972; 59: 914

[77] Fossard DP, Corrigan T, Fossard DP et al. Prevention of fatal postoperative pulmonary embolism by low doses of heparin. An international multicentre trial. Lancet 1975; 2: 45–51

[78] Upchurch GR, Demling RH, Davies J, Gates JD, Knox JB. Efficacy of subcutaneous heparin in prevention of venous thromboembolic events in trauma patients. Am Surg 1995; 61: 749–755

[79] Dennis JW, Menawat S, Von Thron J et al. Efficacy of deep venous thrombosis prophylaxis in trauma patients and identification of high-risk groups. J Trauma 1993; 35: 132–138, discussion 138–139

[80] Kakkar VV, Djazaeri B, Fok J, Fletcher M, Scully MF, Westwick J. Low-molecular-weight heparin and prevention of postoperative deep vein thrombosis. Br Med J (Clin Res Ed) 1982; 284: 375–379

[81] Cothren CC, Smith WR, Moore EE, Morgan SJ. Utility of once-daily dose of low-molecular-weight heparin to prevent venous thromboembolism in multisystem trauma patients. World J Surg 2007; 31: 98–104

[82] Geerts WH, Jay RM, Code KI et al. A comparison of low-dose heparin with low-molecular-weight heparin as prophylaxis against venous thromboembolism after major trauma. N Engl J Med 1996; 335: 701–707

[83] Ginzburg E, Cohn SM, Lopez J, Jackowski J, Brown M, Hameed SM Miami Deep Vein Thrombosis Study Group. Randomized clinical trial of intermittent pneumatic compression and low molecular weight heparin in trauma. Br J Surg 2003; 90: 1338–1344

[84] Cord S Spinal Cord Injury Thromboprophylaxis Investigators. Prevention of venous thromboembolism in the acute treatment phase after spinal cord injury: a randomized, multicenter trial comparing low-dose heparin plus intermittent pneumatic compression with enoxaparin. J Trauma 2003; 54: 1116–1124, discussion 1125–1126

[85] Spinal Cord Injury Thromboprophylaxis Investigators. Prevention of venous thromboembolism in the rehabilitation phase after spinal cord injury: prophylaxis with low-dose heparin or enoxaparin. J Trauma 2003; 54: 1111–1115

[86] Britt LD, Zolfaghari D, Kennedy E, Pagel KJ, Minghini A. Incidence and prophylaxis of deep vein thrombosis in a high risk trauma population. Am J Surg 1996; 172: 13–14

[87] Schwarcz TH, Quick RC, Minion DJ, Kearney PA, Kwolek CJ, Endean ED. Enoxaparin treatment in high-risk trauma patients limits the utility of surveillance venous duplex scanning. J Vasc Surg 2001; 34: 447–452

[88] Chiara O, Cimbanassi S, Brioschi PR, Bucci L, Terzi V, Vesconi S. Treatment of critical bleeding in trauma patients. Minerva Anestesiol 2006; 72: 383–387

[89] Sauaia A, Moore FA, Moore EE et al. Epidemiology of trauma deaths: a reassessment. J Trauma 1995; 38: 185–193

[90] Cothren CC, Smith WR, Moore EE, Morgan SJ. Utility of once-daily dose of low-molecular-weight heparin to prevent venous thromboembolism in multisystem trauma patients. World J Surg 2007; 31: 98–104

[91] Alejandro KV, Acosta JA, Rodríguez PA. Bleeding manifestations after early use of low-molecular-weight heparins in blunt splenic injuries. Am Surg 2003; 69: 1006–1009

[92] Kakkar AK, Davidson BL, Haas SK Investigators Against Thromboembolism (INATE) Core Group. Compliance with recommended prophylaxis for venous thromboembolism: improving the use and rate of uptake of clinical practice guidelines. J Thromb Haemost 2004; 2: 221–227

[93] Nathens AB, McMurray MK, Cuschieri J et al. The practice of venous thromboembolism prophylaxis in the major trauma patient. J Trauma 2007; 62: 557–562, discussion 562–563

[94] Stannard JP, Lopez-Ben RR, Volgas DA et al. Prophylaxis against deep-vein thrombosis following trauma: a prospective, randomized comparison of mechanical and pharmacologic prophylaxis. J Bone Joint Surg Am 2006; 88: 261–266

[95] Bridges GG, Lee MD, Jenkins JK, Stephens MA, Croce MA, Fabian TC. Expedited discharge in trauma patients requiring anticoagulation for deep venous thrombosis prophylaxis: the LEAP Program. J Trauma 2003; 54: 232–235

[96] Schulman S, Rhedin AS, Lindmarker P et al. Duration of Anticoagulation Trial Study Group. A comparison of six weeks with six months of oral anticoagulant therapy after a first episode of venous thromboembolism. N Engl J Med 1995; 332: 1661–1665

[97] Hull RD, Raskob GE, Rosenbloom D et al. Optimal therapeutic level of heparin therapy in patients with venous thrombosis. Arch Intern Med 1992; 152: 1589–1595

[98] Raschke RA, Reilly BM, Guidry JR, Fontana JR, Srinivas S. The weight-based heparin dosing nomogram compared with a "standard care" nomogram. A randomized controlled trial. Ann Intern Med 1993; 119: 874–881

[99] Hyers TM, Agnelli G, Hull RD et al. Antithrombotic therapy for venous thromboembolic disease. Chest 2002; 121: 1378–1379

[100] Brill-Edwards P, Ginsberg JS, Johnston M. Establishing a therapeutic range for heparin therapy. Ann Intern Med 1993; 119: 104–109

[101] Levine MN, Hirsh J, Gent M et al. A randomized trial comparing activated thromboplastin time with heparin assay in patients with acute venous thromboembolism requiring large daily doses of heparin. Arch Intern Med 1994; 154: 49–56

[102] Hommes DW, Bura A, Mazzolai L, Büller HR, ten Cate JW. Subcutaneous heparin compared with continuous intravenous heparin administration in the initial treatment of deep vein thrombosis. A meta-analysis. Ann Intern Med 1992; 116: 279–284

[103] Verstraete M. Pharmacotherapeutic aspects of unfractionated and low molecular weight heparins. Drugs 1990; 40: 498–530

[104] Merli G, Spiro TE, Olsson CG et al. Enoxaparin Clinical Trial Group. Subcutaneous enoxaparin once or twice daily compared with intravenous unfractionated heparin for treatment of venous thromboembolic disease. Ann Intern Med 2001; 134: 191–202

[105] Gray E, Mulloy B, Barrowcliffe TW. Heparin and low-molecular-weight heparin. Thromb Haemost 2008; 99: 807–818

[106] Morris TA, Castrejon S, Devendra G, Gamst AC. No difference in risk for thrombocytopenia during treatment of pulmonary embolism and deep venous thrombosis with either low-molecular-weight heparin or unfractionated heparin: a metaanalysis. Chest 2007; 132: 1108–1110

[107] Browse NL, Brist MD, James DC. Streptokinase and pulmonary embolism. Lancet 1964; 1: 1039–1043

[108] Anderson DR, Levine MN. Thrombolytic therapy for the treatment of acute pulmonary embolism. CMAJ 1992; 146: 1317–1324

[109] Dalen JE, Alpert JS, Hirsh J. Thrombolytic therapy for pulmonary embolism: is it effective? Is it safe? When is it indicated? Arch Intern Med 1997; 157: 2550–2556

[110] Goldhaber SZ, Visani L, De Rosa M. Acute pulmonary embolism: clinical outcomes in the International Cooperative Pulmonary Embolism Registry (ICOPER) Lancet 1999; 353: 1386–1389

[111] Douma RA, Kamphuisen PW. Thrombolysis for pulmonary embolism and venous thrombosis: is it worthwhile? Semin Thromb Hemost 2007; 33: 821–828

[112] Capstick T, Henry MT. Efficacy of thrombolytic agents in the treatment of pulmonary embolism. Eur Respir J 2005; 26: 864–874

[113] Büller HR, Agnelli G, Hull RD, Hyers TM, Prins MH, Raskob GE. Antithrombotic therapy for venous thromboembolic disease: the Seventh ACCP Conference on Antithrombotic and Thrombolytic Therapy. Chest 2004; 126 Suppl: 401S–428S

[114] Moretz WH, Still JM, Griffin LH, Jennings WD, Wray CH. Partial occlusion of the inferior vena cava with a smooth Teflon clip: analysis of long-term results. Surgery 1972; 71: 710–719

[115] Homans J. Deep quiet venous thrombosis in the lower limb: preferred levels for interruption of veins, iliac sector or location. Surg Gynecol Obstet 1994; 79: 70–82

[116] Byrne JJ. Phlebitis; a study of 748 cases at the Boston City Hospital. N Engl J Med 1955; 253: 579–586

[117] Martin MJ, Salim A. Vena cava filters in surgery and trauma. Surg Clin North Am 2007; 87: 1229–1252, xi–xiixi–xii

[118] Kempczinski RF. Surgical prophylaxis of pulmonary embolism. Chest 1986; 89 Suppl: 384S–388S

[119] Mozes M, Adar R, Bogokowsky H, Agmon M. Vein ligation in the treatment of pulmonary embolism. Surgery 1964; 55: 621–629

[120] Hann CL, Streiff MB. The role of vena caval filters in the management of venous thromboembolism. Blood Rev 2005; 19: 179–202

[121] Amador E, Li TK, Crane C. Ligation of inferior vena cava for thromboembolism. Clinical and autopsy correlations in 119 cases. JAMA 1968; 206: 1758–1760

[122] Maraan BM, Taber RE. The effects of inferior vena caval ligation on cardiac output: an experimental study. Surgery 1968; 63: 966–969

[123] Alberts WM, Tonner JA, Goldman AL. Echocardiography in planned interruption of the inferior vena cava. South Med J 1989; 82: 772–774

[124] Amador E, Li TK, Crane C. Ligation of inferior vena cava for thromboembolism. Clinical and autopsy correlations in 119 cases. JAMA 1968; 206: 1758–1760

[125] Piccone VA, Vidal E, Yarnoz M, Glass P, LeVeen HH. The late results of caval ligation. Surgery 1970; 68: 980–998

[126] Shea PS, Robertson RL. Late sequelae of inferior vena cava ligation. Surg Gynecol Obstet 1951; 93: 153–158

[127] Goldhaber SZ, Buring JE, Lipnick RJ, Stubblefield F, Hennekens CH. Interruption of the inferior vena cava by clip or filter. Am J Med 1984; 76: 512–516

[128] Spencer FC, Quattlebaum JK, Quattlebaum JK, Sharp EH, Jude JR. Plication of the inferior vena cava for pulmonary embolism: a report of 20 cases. Ann Surg 1962; 155: 827–837

[129] Moretz WH, Naisbitt PF, Stevenson GP. Experimental studies on temporary occlusion of the inferior vena cava. Surgery 1954; 36: 384–398

[130] Taber RE, Zikria E, Hershey EA, Lam CR. Prevention of pulmonary emboli with a vena caval clip. JAMA 1966; 195: 889–894

[131] Spencer FC. An experimental evaluation of partitioning of the inferior vena cava to prevent pulmonary embolism. Surg Forum 1960; 10: 680–684

[132] Ravitch MM, Snodgrass E, McEnany T, Rivarola A. Compartmentation of the vena cava with the mechanical stapler. Surg Gynecol Obstet 1966; 122: 561–566

[133] Moretz WH, Rhode CM, Shepherd MH. Prevention of pulmonary emboli by partial occlusion of the inferior vena cava. Am Surg 1959; 25: 617–626

[134] Miles RM, Chappell F, Renner O. A partially occluding vena caval clip for prevention of pulmonary embolism. Am Surg 1964; 30: 40–47

[135] Leather RP, Clark WR, Powers SR, Parker FB, Bernard HR, Eckert C. Five-year experience with the Moretz vena caval clip in 62 patients. Arch Surg 1968; 97: 357–364

[136] Hendricks GL Jr Barnes WT. Experiences with the Moretz clip: 100 cases. Am Surg 1971; 37: 558–562

[137] Hunter JA, Sessions R, Buenger R. Experimental balloon obstruction of the inferior vena cava. Ann Surg 1970; 171: 315–320

[138] Mansour M, Chang AE, Sindelar WF. Interruption of the inferior vena cava for the prevention of recurrent pulmonary embolism. Am Surg 1985; 51: 375–380

[139] Hunter JA, DeLaria GA, Goldin MD et al. Inferior vena cava interruption with the Hunter-Sessions balloon: eighteen years' experience in 191 cases. J Vasc Surg 1989; 10: 450–456

[140] Hunter JA, Dye WS, Javid H, Najafi H, Goldin MD, Serry C. Permanent transvenous balloon occlusion of the inferior vena cava: experience with 60 patients. Ann Surg 1977; 186: 491–499

[141] Mobin-Uddin K, McLean R, Bolooki H, Jude JR. Caval interruption for prevention of pulmonary embolism. Long-term results of a new method. Arch Surg 1969; 99: 711–715

[142] Mobin-Uddin K, Utley JR, Bryant LR. The inferior vena cava umbrella filter. Prog Cardiovasc Dis 1975; 17: 391–399

[143] Gomez GA, Cutler BS, Wheeler HB. Transvenous interruption of the inferior vena cava. Surgery 1983; 93: 612–619

[144] Menzoian JO, LoGerfo FW, Weitzman AF, Ezpeleta M, Sequeira JC. Clinical experience with the Mobin-Uddin vena cava umbrella filter. Arch Surg 1980; 115: 1179–1181

[145] Athanasoulis CA, Kaufman JA, Halpern EF, Waltman AC, Geller SC, Fan CM. Inferior vena caval filters: review of a 26-year single-center clinical experience. Radiology 2000; 216: 54–66

[146] Greenfield LJ, McCurdy JR, Brown PP, Elkins RC. A new intracaval filter permitting continued flow and resolution of emboli. Surgery 1973; 73: 599–606

[147] Greenfield LJ, Zocco J, Wilk J, Schroeder TM, Elkins RC. Clinical experience with the Kim-Ray Greenfield vena caval filter. Ann Surg 1977; 185: 692–698

[148] Greenfield LJ, Michna BA. Twelve-year clinical experience with the Greenfield vena caval filter. Surgery 1988; 104: 706–712

[149] Tadavarthy SM, Castaneda-Zuniga W, Salomonowitz E et al. Kimray-Greenfield vena cava filter: percutaneous introduction. Radiology 1984; 151: 525–526

[150] Greenfield LJ, Proctor MC. Twenty-year clinical experience with the Greenfield filter. Cardiovasc Surg 1995; 3: 199–205

[151] Greenfield LJ, Cho KJ, Pais SO, Van Aman M. Preliminary clinical experience with the titanium Greenfield vena caval filter. Arch Surg 1989; 124: 657–659

[152] Greenfield LJ, Cho KJ, Proctor M et al. Results of a multicenter study of the modified hook-titanium Greenfield filter. J Vasc Surg 1991; 14: 253–257

[153] Ramchandani P, Koolpe HA, Zeit RM. Splaying of titanium Greenfield inferior vena caval filter. AJR Am J Roentgenol 1990; 155: 1103–1104

[154] Teitelbaum GP, Jones DL, van Breda A et al. Vena caval filter splaying: potential complication of use of the titanium Greenfield filter. Radiology 1989; 173: 809–814

[155] Greenfield LJ, Proctor MC, Cho KJ et al. Extended evaluation of the titanium Greenfield vena caval filter. J Vasc Surg 1994; 20: 458–464, discussion 464–465

[156] Greenfield LJ, Cho KJ, Tauscher JR. Evolution of hook design for fixation of the titanium Greenfield filter. J Vasc Surg 1990; 12: 345–353

[157] Greenfield LJ, Proctor MC, Cho KJ, Wakefield TW. Limb asymmetry in titanium Greenfield filters: clinically significant? J Vasc Surg 1997; 26: 770–775

[158] Greenfield LJ, Proctor MC. Experimental embolic capture by asymmetric Greenfield filters. J Vasc Surg 1992; 16: 436–443, discussion 443–444

[159] Kinney TB. Update on inferior vena cava filters. J Vasc Interv Radiol 2003; 14: 425–440

[160] Cho KJ, Greenfield LJ, Proctor MC et al. Evaluation of a new percutaneous stainless steel Greenfield filter. J Vasc Interv Radiol 1997; 8: 181–187

[161] Johnson SP, Raiken DP, Grebe PJ, Diffin DC, Leyendecker JR. Single institution prospective evaluation of the over-the-wire Greenfield vena caval filter. J Vasc Interv Radiol 1998; 9: 766–773

[162] Greenfield LJ, Proctor MC, Roberts KR. An improved process for development and testing of vena caval filters: the percutaneous steel Greenfield filter. Surgery 1997; 121: 50–57

[163] Greenfield LJ, Proctor MC. The percutaneous greenfield filter: outcomes and practice patterns. J Vasc Surg 2000; 32: 888–893

[164] Roehm JO Jr Gianturco C, Barth MH, Wright KC. Percutaneous transcatheter filter for the inferior vena cava. A new device for treatment of patients with pulmonary embolism. Radiology 1984; 150: 255–257

[165] Rogoff PA, Hilgenberg AD, Miller SL, Stephan SM. Cephalic migration of the bird's nest inferior vena caval filter: report of two cases. Radiology 1992; 184: 819–822

[166] Roehm JO Jr Johnsrude IS, Barth MH, Gianturco C. The bird's nest inferior vena cava filter: progress report. Radiology 1988; 168: 745–749

[167] Hann CL, Streiff MB. The role of vena caval filters in the management of venous thromboembolism. Blood Rev 2005; 19: 179–202

[168] Katsamouris AA, Waltman AC, Delichatsios MA, Athanasoulis CA. Inferior vena cava filters: in vitro comparison of clot trapping and flow dynamics. Radiology 1988; 166: 361–366

[169] Reed RA, Teitelbaum GP, Taylor FC, Pentecost MJ, Roehm JO. Use of the bird's nest filter in oversized inferior venae cavae. J Vasc Interv Radiol 1991; 2: 447–450

[170] Korbin CD, Reed RA, Taylor FC, Pentecost MJ, Teitelbaum GP. Comparison of filters in an oversized vena caval phantom: intracaval placement of a bird's nest filter versus biiliac placement of Greenfield, Vena Tech-LGM, and Simon nitinol filters. J Vasc Interv Radiol 1992; 3: 559–564

[171] Watanabe AT, Teitelbaum GP, Gomes AS, Roehm JO. MR imaging of the bird's nest filter. Radiology 1990; 177: 578–579

[172] Simon M, Athanasoulis CA, Kim D et al. Simon nitinol inferior vena cava filter: initial clinical experience. Work in progress. Radiology 1989; 172: 99–103

[173] Palestrant AM, Prince M, Simon M. Comparative in vitro evaluation of the nitinol inferior vena cava filter. Radiology 1982; 145: 351–355

[174] McCowan TC, Ferris EJ, Carver DK, Harshfield DL. Use of external jugular vein as a route for percutaneous inferior vena caval filter placement. Radiology 1990; 176: 527–530

[175] Kim D, Schlam BW, Porter DH, Simon M. Insertion of the Simon nitinol caval filter: value of the antecubital vein approach. AJR Am J Roentgenol 1991; 157: 521–522

[176] Engmann E, Asch MR. Clinical experience with the antecubital Simon nitinol IVC filter. J Vasc Interv Radiol 1998; 9: 774–778

[177] Athanasoulis CA, Kaufman JA, Halpern EF, Waltman AC, Geller SC, Fan CM. Inferior vena caval filters: review of a 26-year single-center clinical experience. Radiology 2000; 216: 54–66

[178] Poletti PA, Becker CD, Prina L et al. Long-term results of the Simon nitinol inferior vena cava filter. Eur Radiol 1998; 8: 289–294

[179] Grassi CJ, Matsumoto AH, Teitelbaum GP. Vena caval occlusion after Simon nitinol filter placement: identification with MR imaging in patients with malignancy. J Vasc Interv Radiol 1992; 3: 535–539

[180] LaPlante JS, Contractor FM, Kiproff PM, Khoury MB. Migration of the Simon nitinol vena cava filter to the chest. AJR Am J Roentgenol 1993; 160: 385–386

[181] Ricco JB, Crochet D, Sebilotte P et al. Percutaneous transvenous caval interruption with the "LGM" filter: early results of a multicenter trial. Ann Vasc Surg 1988; 2: 242–247

[182] Murphy TP, Dorfman GS, Yedlicka JW et al. LGM vena cava filter: objective evaluation of early results. J Vasc Interv Radiol 1991; 2: 107–115

[183] Reed RA, Teitelbaum GP, Taylor FC et al. Incomplete opening of LGM (Vena Tech) filters inserted via the transjugular approach. J Vasc Interv Radiol 1991; 2: 441–445

[184] Taylor FC, Awh MH, Kahn CE, Lu CT. Vena Tech vena cava filter: experience and early follow-up. J Vasc Interv Radiol 1991; 2: 435–440

[185] Millward SF, Marsh JI, Peterson RA et al. LGM (Vena Tech) vena cava filter: clinical experience in 64 patients. J Vasc Interv Radiol 1991; 2: 429–433

[186] Crochet DP, Stora O, Ferry D et al. Vena Tech-LGM filter: long-term results of a prospective study. Radiology 1993; 188: 857–860

[187] Crochet DP, Brunel P, Trogrlic S, Grossetête R, Auget JL, Dary C. Long-term follow-up of Vena Tech-LGM filter: predictors and frequency of caval occlusion. J Vasc Interv Radiol 1999; 10: 137–142

[188] Ricco JB, Dubreuil F, Reynaud P et al. The LGM Vena-Tech caval filter: results of a multicenter study. Ann Vasc Surg 1995; 9 Suppl: S89–S100

[189] Le Blanche AF, Benazzouz A, Reynaud P et al. European VenaTech LP Vena Cava Filter Study Group. The VenaTech LP permanent caval filter: effectiveness and safety in the prevention of pulmonary embolism—a European multicenter study. J Vasc Interv Radiol 2008; 19: 509–515

[190] Le Blanche AF, Pautas E, Gouin I, Bagüés A, Piette F, Chaibi P. Placement of the VenaTech LP caval filter in the elderly: feasibility and clinical benefits of insertion via the arm. Cardiovasc Intervent Radiol 2005; 28: 813–817

[191] Rousseau H, Perreault P, Otal P et al. The 6-F nitinol TrapEase inferior vena cava filter: results of a prospective multicenter trial. J Vasc Interv Radiol 2001; 12: 299–304

[192] Lorch H, Dallmann A, Zwaan M, Weiss HD. Efficacy of permanent and retrievable vena cava filters: experimental studies and evaluation of a new device. Cardiovasc Intervent Radiol 2002; 25: 193–199

[193] Davison BD, Grassi CJ. TrapEase inferior vena cava filter placed via the basilic arm vein: a new antecubital access. J Vasc Interv Radiol 2002; 13: 107–109

[194] Stone PA, Aburahma AF, Hass SM et al. TrapEase inferior vena cava filter placement: use of the subclavian vein. Vasc Endovascular Surg 2004; 38: 505–509

[195] Liu WC, Do YS, Choo SW et al. The mid-term efficacy and safety of a permanent nitinol IVC filter(TrapEase). Korean J Radiol 2005; 6: 110–116

[196] Schutzer R, Ascher E, Hingorani A, Jacob T, Kallakuri S. Preliminary results of the new 6F TrapEase inferior vena cava filter. Ann Vasc Surg 2003; 17: 103–106

[197] Kalva SP, Wicky S, Waltman AC, Athanasoulis CA. TrapEase vena cava filter: experience in 751 patients. J Endovasc Ther 2006; 13: 365–372

[198] Hussain SM, McLafferty RB, Schmittling ZC et al. Superior vena cava perforation and cardiac tamponade after filter placement in the superior vena cava—a case report. Vasc Endovascular Surg 2005; 39: 367–370

[199] Porcellini M, Stassano P, Musumeci A, Bracale G. Intracardiac migration of nitinol TrapEase vena cava filter and paradoxical embolism. Eur J Cardiothorac Surg 2002; 22: 460–461

[200] Eichelter P, Schenk WG. Prophylaxis of pulmonary embolism. A new experimental appraoch with initial results. Arch Surg 1968; 97: 348–356

[201] Williams RW, Schenk WG. A removable intracaval filter for prevention of pulmonary embolism: early experience with the use of the Eichelter catheter in patients. Surgery 1970; 68: 999–1008

[202] Major WK Jr Williams RW, Schenk WG. The Eichelter catheter. Further experience. Arch Surg 1974; 109: 278–282

[203] Kaufman JA, Kinney TB, Streiff MB et al. Guidelines for the use of retrievable and convertible vena cava filters: report from the Society of Interventional Radiology multidisciplinary consensus conference. J Vasc Interv Radiol 2006; 17: 449–459

[204] Millward SF. Temporary and retrievable inferior vena cava filters: current status. J Vasc Interv Radiol 1998; 9: 381–387

[205] Darcy MD, Smith TP, Hunter DW, Castaneda-Zuniga W, Lund G, Amplatz K. Short-term prophylaxis of pulmonary embolism by using a retrievable vena cava filter. AJR Am J Roentgenol 1986; 147: 836–838

[206] Lorch H, Welger D, Wagner V et al. Current practice of temporary vena cava filter insertion: a multicenter registry. J Vasc Interv Radiol 2000; 11: 83–88

[207] Kim HS, Young MJ, Narayan AK, Hong K, Liddell RP, Streiff MB. A comparison of clinical outcomes with retrievable and permanent inferior vena cava filters. J Vasc Interv Radiol 2008; 19: 393–399

[208] Asch MR. Initial experience in humans with a new retrievable inferior vena cava filter. Radiology 2002; 225: 835–844

[209] Grande WJ, Trerotola SO, Reilly PM et al. Experience with the recovery filter as a retrievable inferior vena cava filter. J Vasc Interv Radiol 2005; 16: 1189–1193

[210] Oliva VL, Perreault P, Giroux MF, Bouchard L, Therasse E, Soulez G. Recovery G2 inferior vena cava filter: technical success and safety of retrieval. J Vasc Interv Radiol 2008; 19: 884–889

[211] Kuo WT, Loh CT, Sze DY. Emergency retrieval of a G2 filter after complete migration into the right ventricle. J Vasc Interv Radiol 2007; 18: 1177–1182

[212] Bui JT, West DL, Pinto C, Gramling-Babb P, Owens CA. Right ventricular migration and endovascular removal of an inferior vena cava filter. J Vasc Interv Radiol 2008; 19: 141–144

[213] De Gregorio MA, Gamboa P, Bonilla DL et al. Retrieval of Gunther Tulip optional vena cava filters 30 days after implantation: a prospective clinical study. J Vasc Interv Radiol 2006; 17: 1781–1789

[214] Looby S, Given MF, Geoghegan T, McErlean A, Lee MJ. Gunther Tulip retrievable inferior vena caval filters: indications, efficacy, retrieval, and complications. Cardiovasc Intervent Radiol 2007; 30: 59–65

[215] Rosenthal D, Wellons ED, Hancock SM, Burkett AB. Retrievability of the Günther Tulip vena cava filter after dwell times longer than 180 days in patients with multiple trauma. J Endovasc Ther 2007; 14: 406–410

[216] de Gregorio MA, Gamboa P, Gimeno MJ et al. The Günther Tulip retrievable filter: prolonged temporary filtration by repositioning within the inferior vena cava. J Vasc Interv Radiol 2003; 14: 1259–1265

[217] Keller IS, Meier C, Pfiffner R, Keller E, Pfammatter T. Clinical comparison of two optional vena cava filters. J Vasc Interv Radiol 2007; 18: 505–511

[218] Rosenthal D, Swischuk JL, Cohen SA, Wellons ED. OptEase retrievable inferior vena cava filter: initial multicenter experience. Vascular 2005; 13: 286–289

[219] Oliva VL, Szatmari F, Giroux MF, Flemming BK, Cohen SA, Soulez G. The Jonas study: evaluation of the retrievability of the Cordis OptEase inferior vena cava filter. J Vasc Interv Radiol 2005; 16: 1439–1445, quiz 1445

[220] Sadaf A, Rasuli P, Olivier A et al. Significant caval penetration by the celect inferior vena cava filter: attributable to filter design? J Vasc Interv Radiol 2007; 18: 1447–1450

[221] Crowther MA. Inferior vena cava filters in the management of venous thromboembolism. Am J Med 2007; 120 Suppl 2: S13–S17

[222] Yunus TE, Tariq N, Callahan RE et al. Changes in inferior vena cava filter placement over the past decade at a large community-based academic health center. J Vasc Surg 2008; 47: 157–165

[223] Stein PD, Kayali F, Olson RE. Twenty-one-year trends in the use of inferior vena cava filters. Arch Intern Med 2004; 164: 1541–1545

[224] Rutherford RB. Prophylactic indications for vena cava filters: critical appraisal. Semin Vasc Surg 2005; 18: 158–165

[225] Kaufman JA, Kinney TB, Streiff MB et al. Guidelines for the use of retrievable and convertible vena cava filters: report from the Society of Interventional Radiology multidisciplinary consensus conference. J Vasc Interv Radiol 2006; 17: 449–459

[226] Decousus H, Leizorovicz A, Parent F et al. A clinical trial of vena caval filters in the prevention of pulmonary embolism in patients with proximal deep-vein thrombosis. Prévention du Risque d'Embolie Pulmonaire par Interruption Cave Study Group. N Engl J Med 1998; 338: 409–415

[227] Girard P, Stern JB, Parent F. Medical literature and vena cava filters: so far so weak. Chest 2002; 122: 963–967

[228] Proctor MC. Indications for filter placement. Semin Vasc Surg 2000; 13: 194–198

[229] Büller HR, Agnelli G, Hull RD, Hyers TM, Prins MH, Raskob GE. Antithrombotic therapy for venous thromboembolic disease: the Seventh ACCP Conference on Antithrombotic and Thrombolytic Therapy Chest 2004; 126 (3 Suppl): 401S–428S

[230] Giannoudis PV, Pountos I, Pape HC, Patel JV. Safety and efficacy of vena cava filters in trauma patients. Injury 2007; 38: 7–18

[231] Quirke TE, Ritota PC, Swan KG. Inferior vena caval filter use in U.S. trauma centers: a practitioner survey. J Trauma 1997; 43: 333–337

[232] Kucher N, Rossi E, De Rosa M, Goldhaber SZ. Massive pulmonary embolism. Circulation 2006; 113: 577–582

[233] Mo M, Kapelanski DP, Mitruka SN et al. Reoperative pulmonary thromboendarterectomy. Ann Thorac Surg 1999; 68: 1770–1776, discussion 1776–1777

[234] Thery C, Asseman P, Amrouni N et al. Use of a new removable vena cava filter in order to prevent pulmonary embolism in patients submitted to thrombolysis. Eur Heart J 1990; 11: 334–341

[235] Radomski JS, Jarrell BE, Carabasi RA, Yang SL, Koolpe H. Risk of pulmonary embolus with inferior vena cava thrombosis. Am Surg 1987; 53: 97–101

[236] Norris CS, Greenfield LJ, Herrmann JB. Free-floating iliofemoral thrombus. A risk of pulmonary embolism. Arch Surg 1985; 120: 806–808

[237] Monreal M, Ruiz J, Salvador R, Morera J, Arias A. Recurrent pulmonary embolism. A prospective study. Chest 1989; 95: 976–979

[238] Berry RE, George JE, Shaver WA. Free-floating deep venous thrombosis. A retrospective analysis. Ann Surg 1990; 211: 719–2, discussion 722–723

[239] Baldridge ED, Martin MA, Welling RE. Clinical significance of free-floating venous thrombi. J Vasc Surg 1990; 11: 62–67, discussion 68–69

[240] Pacouret G, Alison D, Pottier JM, Bertrand P, Charbonnier B. Free-floating thrombus and embolic risk in patients with angiographically confirmed proximal deep venous thrombosis. A prospective study. Arch Intern Med 1997; 157: 305–308

[241] Sue LP, Davis JW, Parks SN. Iliofemoral venous injuries: an indication for prophylactic caval filter placement. J Trauma 1995; 39: 693–695

[242] Greenfield LJ, McCurdy JR, Brown PP, Elkins RC. A new intracaval filter permitting continued flow and resolution of emboli. Surgery 1973; 73: 599–606

[243] Hye RJ, Mitchell AT, Dory CE, Freischlag JA, Roberts AC. Analysis of the transition to percutaneous placement of Greenfield filters. Arch Surg 1990; 125: 1550–1553

[244] Pais SO, Tobin KD, Austin CB, Queral L. Percutaneous insertion of the Greenfield inferior vena cava filter: experience with ninety-six patients. J Vasc Surg 1988; 8: 460–464

[245] Rose BS, Simon DC, Hess ML, Van Aman ME. Percutaneous transfemoral placement of the Kimray-Greenfield vena cava filter. Radiology 1987; 165: 373–376

[246] Pais SO, Mirvis SE, De Orchis DF. Percutaneous insertion of the Kimray-Greenfield filter: technical considerations and problems. Radiology 1987; 165: 377–381

[247] Crystal KS, Kase DJ, Scher LA, Shapiro MA, Naidich JB. Utilization patterns with inferior vena cava filters: surgical versus percutaneous placement. J Vasc Interv Radiol 1995; 6: 443–448

[248] Shetty PC, Bok LR, Burke MW, Sharma RP. Balloon dilation of the femoral vein expediting percutaneous Greenfield vena caval filter placement. Radiology 1986; 161: 275

[249] Kantor A, Glanz S, Gordon DH, Sclafani SJ. Percutaneous insertion of the Kimray-Greenfield filter: incidence of femoral vein thrombosis. AJR Am J Roentgenol 1987; 149: 1065–1066

[250] Molgaard CP, Yucel EK, Geller SC, Knox TA, Waltman AC. Access-site thrombosis after placement of inferior vena cava filters with 12–14-F delivery sheaths. Radiology 1992; 185: 257–261

[251] Stavropoulos SW, Clark T, Jacobs D et al. Placement of a vena cava filter with an antecubital approach. Acad Radiol 2002; 9: 478–481

[252] Martin KD, Kempczinski RF, Fowl RJ. Are routine inferior vena cavograms necessary before Greenfield filter placement? Surgery 1989; 106: 647–650, discussion 650–651

[253] Mejia EA, Saroyan RM, Balkin PW, Kerstein MD. Analysis of inferior venacavography before Greenfield filter placement. Ann Vasc Surg 1989; 3: 232–235

[254] Kaufman JA, Geller SC, Rivitz SM, Waltman AC. Operator errors during percutaneous placement of vena cava filters. AJR Am J Roentgenol 1995; 165: 1281–1287

[255] Hicks ME, Malden ES, Vesely TM, Picus D, Darcy MD. Prospective anatomic study of the inferior vena cava and renal veins: comparison of selective renal venography with cavography and relevance in filter placement. J Vasc Interv Radiol 1995; 6: 721–729

[256] Danetz JS, McLafferty RB, Ayerdi J, Gruneiro LA, Ramsey DE, Hodgson KJ. Selective venography versus nonselective venography before vena cava filter placement: evidence for more, not less. J Vasc Surg 2003; 38: 928–934

[257] Holtzman RB, Lottenberg L, Bass T, Saridakis A, Bennett VJ, Carrillo EH. Comparison of carbon dioxide and iodinated contrast for cavography prior to inferior vena cava filter placement. Am J Surg 2003; 185: 364–368

[258] Kaufman JA, Geller SC, Bazari H, Waltman AC. Gadolinium-based contrast agents as an alternative at vena cavography in patients with renal insufficiency—early experience. Radiology 1999; 212: 280–284

[259] Boyd-Kranis R, Sullivan KL, Eschelman DJ, Bonn J, Gardiner GA. Accuracy and safety of carbon dioxide inferior vena cavography. J Vasc Interv Radiol 1999; 10: 1183–1189

[260] Dewald CL, Jensen CC, Park YH et al. Vena cavography with CO(2) versus with iodinated contrast material for inferior vena cava filter placement: a prospective evaluation. Radiology 2000; 216: 752–757

[261] Brown DB, Pappas JA, Vedantham S, Pilgram TK, Olsen RV, Duncan JR. Gadolinium, carbon dioxide, and iodinated contrast material for planning inferior vena cava filter placement: a prospective trial. J Vasc Interv Radiol 2003; 14: 1017–1022

[262] Sing RF, Stackhouse DJ, Jacobs DG, Heniford BT. Safety and accuracy of bedside carbon dioxide cavography for insertion of inferior vena cava filters in the intensive care unit. J Am Coll Surg 2001; 192: 168–171

[263] Schmelzer TM, Christmas AB, Jacobs DG, Heniford BT, Sing RF. Imaging of the vena cava in the intensive care unit prior to vena cava filter insertion: carbon dioxide as an alternative to iodinated contrast. Am Surg 2008; 74: 141–145

[264] Canavese C, Mereu MC, Aime S et al. Gadolinium-associated nephrogenic systemic fibrosis: the need for nephrologists' awareness. J Nephrol 2008; 21: 324–336

[265] Stratta P, Canavese C, Aime S. Gadolinium-enhanced magnetic resonance imaging, renal failure and nephrogenic systemic fibrosis/nephrogenic fibrosing dermopathy. Curr Med Chem 2008; 15: 1229–1235

[266] Samtleben W. [Nephrogenic systemic fibrosis] Radiologe 2007; 47: 778–784

[267] Vesco PA, Falimirski ME, Williams HK, Rodriguez A, Young J. Abdominal computed tomography and the placement of inferior vena caval filters. J Trauma 2006; 60: 1197–1201, discussion 1202–1203

[268] Sing RF, Smith CH, Miles WS, Messick WJ. Preliminary results of bedside inferior vena cava filter placement: safe and cost-effective. Chest 1998; 114: 315–316

[269] Sing RF, Jacobs DG, Heniford BT. Bedside insertion of inferior vena cava filters in the intensive care unit. J Am Coll Surg 2001; 192: 570–575, discussion 575–576

[270] Tola JC, Holtzman R, Lottenberg L. Bedside placement of inferior vena cava filters in the intensive care unit. Am Surg 1999; 65: 833–837, discussion 837–838

[271] Paton BL, Jacobs DG, Heniford BT, Kercher KW, Zerey M, Sing RF. Nine-year experience with insertion of vena cava filters in the intensive care unit. Am J Surg 2006; 192: 795–800

[272] Van Natta TL, Morris JA, Eddy VA et al. Elective bedside surgery in critically injured patients is safe and cost-effective. Ann Surg 1998; 227: 618–624, discussion 624–626

[273] Uppal B, Flinn WR, Benjamin ME. The bedside insertion of inferior vena cava filters using ultrasound guidance. Perspect Vasc Surg Endovasc Ther 2007; 19: 78–84

[274] Benjamin ME, Sandager GP, Cohn EJ et al. Duplex ultrasound insertion of inferior vena cava filters in multitrauma patients. Am J Surg 1999; 178: 92–97

[275] Bonn J, Liu JB, Eschelman DJ, Sullivan KL, Pinheiro LW, Gardiner GA. Intravascular ultrasound as an alternative to positive-contrast vena cavography prior to filter placement. J Vasc Interv Radiol 1999; 10: 843–849

[276] Lahner D, Nikolic A, Marhofer P et al. Incidence of complications in intrahospital transport of critically ill patients—experience in an Austrian university hospital. Wien Klin Wochenschr 2007; 119: 412–416

[277] Smith I, Fleming S, Cernaianu A. Mishaps during transport from the intensive care unit. Crit Care Med 1990; 18: 278–281

[278] Ebaugh JL, Chiou AC, Morasch MD, Matsumura JS, Pearce WH. Bedside vena cava filter placement guided with intravascular ultrasound. J Vasc Surg 2001; 34: 21–26

[279] Spaniolas K, Velmahos GC, Kwolek C, Gervasini A, De Moya M, Alam HB. Bedside placement of removable vena cava filters guided by intravascular ultrasound in the critically injured. World J Surg 2008; 32: 1438–1443

[280] Corriere MA, Passman MA, Guzman RJ, Dattilo JB, Naslund TC. Comparison of bedside transabdominal duplex ultrasound versus contrast venography for inferior vena cava filter placement: what is the best imaging modality? Ann Vasc Surg 2005; 19: 229–234

[281] Benjamin ME, Sandager GP, Cohn EJ et al. Duplex ultrasound insertion of inferior vena cava filters in multitrauma patients. Am J Surg 1999; 178: 92–97

[282] Rosenthal D, Wellons ED, Levitt AB, Shuler FW, O'Conner RE, Henderson VJ. Role of prophylactic temporary inferior vena cava filters placed at the ICU bedside under intravascular ultrasound guidance in patients with multiple trauma. J Vasc Surg 2004; 40: 958–964

[283] Conners MS III Becker S, Guzman RJ et al. Duplex scan-directed placement of inferior vena cava filters: a five-year institutional experience. J Vasc Surg 2002; 35: 286–291

[284] Matsumura JS, Morasch MD. Filter placement by ultrasound technique at the bedside. Semin Vasc Surg 2000; 13: 199–203

[285] Nunn CR, Neuzil D, Naslund T et al. Cost-effective method for bedside insertion of vena caval filters in trauma patients. J Trauma 1997; 43: 752–758

[286] Sato DT, Robinson KD, Gregory RT et al. Duplex directed caval filter insertion in multi-trauma and critically ill patients. Ann Vasc Surg 1999; 13: 365–371

[287] Kardys CM, Stoner MC, Manwaring ML et al. Safety and efficacy of intravascular ultrasound-guided inferior vena cava filter in super obese bariatric patients. Surg Obes Relat Dis 2008; 4: 50–54

[288] Trigaux JP, Vandroogenbroek S, De Wispelaere JF, Lacrosse M, Jamart J. Congenital anomalies of the inferior vena cava and left renal vein: evaluation with spiral CT. J Vasc Interv Radiol 1998; 9: 339–345

[289] Oppat WF, Chiou AC, Matsumura JS. Intravascular ultrasound-guided vena cava filter placement. J Endovasc Surg 1999; 6: 285–287

[290] Jacobs DL, Motaganahalli RL, Peterson BG. Bedside vena cava filter placement with intravascular ultrasound: a simple, accurate, single venous access method. J Vasc Surg 2007; 46: 1284–1286

[291] Chiou AC. Intravascular ultrasound-guided bedside placement of inferior vena cava filters. Semin Vasc Surg 2006; 19: 150–154

[292] Ashley DW, Gamblin TC, McCampbell BL, Kitchens DM, Dalton ML, Solis MM. Bedside insertion of vena cava filters in the intensive care unit using intravascular ultrasound to locate renal veins. J Trauma 2004; 57: 26–31

[293] Ashley DW, Gamblin TC, Burch ST, Solis MM. Accurate deployment of vena cava filters: comparison of intravascular ultrasound and contrast venography. J Trauma 2001; 50: 975–981

[294] Wellons ED, Rosenthal D, Shuler FW, Levitt AB, Matsuura J, Henderson VJ. Real-time intravascular ultrasound-guided placement of a removable inferior vena cava filter. J Trauma 2004; 57: 20–23, discussion 23–25

[295] Kalva SP, Chlapoutaki C, Wicky S, Greenfield AJ, Waltman AC, Athanasoulis CA. Suprarenal inferior vena cava filters: a 20-year single-center experience. J Vasc Interv Radiol 2008; 19: 1041–1047

[296] Ganguli S, Tham JC, Komlos F, Rabkin DJ. Fracture and migration of a suprarenal inferior vena cava filter in a pregnant patient. J Vasc Interv Radiol 2006; 17: 1707–1711

[297] Kim D, Porter DH, Siegel JB, Simon M. Perforation of the inferior vena cava with aortic and vertebral penetration by a suprarenal Greenfield filter. Radiology 1989; 172: 721–723

[298] Matchett WJ, Jones MP, McFarland DR, Ferris EJ. Suprarenal vena caval filter placement: follow-up of four filter types in 22 patients. J Vasc Interv Radiol 1998; 9: 588–593

[299] Lemmon GW, Litscher LJ. Incomplete caval protection following suprarenal caval filter placement—a case report. Angiology 2000; 51: 155–159

[300] Chen L, Kim Y, Santucci KA. Use of ultrasound measurement of the inferior vena cava diameter as an objective tool in the assessment of children with clinical dehydration. Acad Emerg Med 2007; 14: 841–845

[301] Marcy PY, Magné N, Frenay M, Bruneton JN. Renal failure secondary to thrombotic complications of suprarenal inferior vena cava filter in cancer patients. Cardiovasc Intervent Radiol 2001; 24: 257–259

[302] Greenfield LJ, Peyton R, Crute S, Barnes R. Greenfield vena caval filter experience: late results in 156 patients. Arch Surg 1981; 116: 1451–1456

[303] Greenfield LJ, Proctor MC. Suprarenal filter placement. J Vasc Surg 1998; 28: 432–438, discussion 438

[304] Horattas MC, Wright DJ, Fenton AH et al. Changing concepts of deep venous thrombosis of the upper extremity—report of a series and review of the literature. Surgery 1988; 104: 561–567

[305] Flinterman LE, Van Der Meer FJ, Rosendaal FR, Doggen CJ. Current perspective of venous thrombosis in the upper extremity. J Thromb Haemost 2008; 6: 1262–1266

[306] Jamieson WG, Chinnick B. Thoracic outlet syndrome: fact or fancy? A review of 409 consecutive patients who underwent operation. Can J Surg 1996; 39: 321–326

[307] Jamieson CW. Venous complications of the thoracic outlet syndrome. Eur J Vasc Surg 1987; 1: 1–3

[308] Liang HW, Su TC, Hwang BS, Hung MH. Effort thrombosis of the upper extremities related to an arm stretching exercise. J Formos Med Assoc 2006; 105: 182–186

[309] van Stralen KJ, Blom JW, Doggen CJ, Rosendaal FR. Strenuous sport activities involving the upper extremities increase the risk of venous thrombosis of the arm. J Thromb Haemost 2005; 3: 2110–2111

[310] Abdullah BJ, Mohammad N, Sangkar JV et al. Incidence of upper limb venous thrombosis associated with peripherally inserted central catheters (PICC). Br J Radiol 2005; 78: 596–600

[311] Spence LD, Gironta MG, Malde HM, Mickolick CT, Geisinger MA, Dolmatch BL. Acute upper extremity deep venous thrombosis: safety and effectiveness of superior vena caval filters. Radiology 1999; 210: 53–58

[312] Horattas MC, Wright DJ, Fenton AH et al. Changing concepts of deep venous thrombosis of the upper extremity—report of a series and review of the literature. Surgery 1988; 104: 561–567

[313] Hingorani A, Ascher E, Marks N et al. Morbidity and mortality associated with brachial vein thrombosis. Ann Vasc Surg 2006; 20: 297–300

[314] Spaniolas K, Velmahos GC, Wicky S et al. Is upper extremity deep venous thrombosis underdiagnosed in trauma patients? Am Surg 2008; 74: 124–128

[315] Prandoni P, Polistena P, Bernardi E et al. Upper-extremity deep vein thrombosis. Risk factors, diagnosis, and complications. Arch Intern Med 1997; 157: 57–62

[316] Mir MA. Superior vena cava filters: hindsight, insight and foresight. J Thromb Thrombolysis 2008; 26: 257–261

[317] Ascher E, Hingorani A, Mazzariol F, Jacob T, Yorkovich W, Gade P. Clinical experience with superior vena caval Greenfield filters. J Endovasc Surg 1999; 6: 365–369

[318] Molina JE, Hunter DW, Dietz CA. Paget-Schroetter syndrome treated with thrombolytics and immediate surgery. J Vasc Surg 2007; 45: 328–334

[319] Machleder HI. Evaluation of a new treatment strategy for Paget-Schroetter syndrome: spontaneous thrombosis of the axillary-subclavian vein. J Vasc Surg 1993; 17: 305–315, discussion 316–317

[320] Langham MR, Etheridge JC, Crute SL, Greenfield LJ. Experimental superior vena caval placement of the Greenfield filter. J Vasc Surg 1985; 2: 794–798

[321] Murphy KD. Superior vena cava filters. Tech Vasc Interv Radiol 2004; 7: 105–109

[322] Hoffman MJ, Greenfield LJ. Central venous septic thrombosis managed by superior vena cava Greenfield filter and venous thrombectomy: a case report. J Vasc Surg 1986; 4: 606–611

[323] Pais SO, De Orchis DF, Mirvis SE. Superior vena caval placement of a Kimray-Greenfield filter. Radiology 1987; 165: 385–386

[324] Owen EW, Schoettle GP, Harrington OB. Placement of a Greenfield filter in the superior vena cava. Ann Thorac Surg 1992; 53: 896–897

[325] Lidagoster MI, Widmann WD, Chevinsky AH. Superior vena cava occlusion after filter insertion. J Vasc Surg 1994; 20: 158–159

[326] Black MD, French GJ, Rasuli P, Bouchard AC. Upper extremity deep venous thrombosis. Underdiagnosed and potentially lethal. Chest 1993; 103: 1887–1890

[327] Rajan DK, Sniderman KW, Rubin BB. Retrieval of the Bard recovery filter from the superior vena cava. J Vasc Interv Radiol 2004; 15: 1169–1171

[328] Nadkarni S, Macdonald S, Cleveland TJ, Gaines PA. Placement of a retrievable Günther Tulip filter in the superior vena cava for upper extremity deep venous thrombosis. Cardiovasc Intervent Radiol 2002; 25: 524–526

[329] Cousins GR, DeAnda A. Images in cardiothoracic surgery. Superior vena cava filter erosion into the ascending aorta. Ann Thorac Surg 2006; 81: 1907

[330] Bhatt SP, Nanda S, Turki MA. Tension pneumothorax: a complication of superior vena cava filter insertion. Ann Thorac Surg 2008; 85: 1813

[331] Hirano Y, Kasashima F, Abe Y et al. The use of a Greenfield filter to treat a pregnant woman for internal jugular venous thrombosis: report of a case. Surg Today 2002; 32: 635–637

[332] Kanda Y, Yamamoto R, Chizuka A et al. Treatment of deep vein thrombosis using temporary vena caval filters after allogeneic bone marrow transplantation. Leuk Lymphoma 2000; 38: 429–433

[333] Ascer E, Gennaro M, Lorensen E, Pollina RM. Superior vena caval Greenfield filters: indications, techniques, and results. J Vasc Surg 1996; 23: 498–503

[334] Ascher E, Hingorani A, Tsemekhin B, Yorkovich W, Gunduz Y. Lessons learned from a 6-year clinical experience with superior vena cava Greenfield filters. J Vasc Surg 2000; 32: 881–887

[335] Watanabe S, Shimokawa S, Shibuya H, Iguro Y, Moriyama Y, Taira A. Superior vena caval placement of a temporary filter: a case report. Vasc Surg 2001; 35: 59–62

[336] Nadkarni S, Macdonald S, Cleveland TJ, Gaines PA. Placement of a retrievable Günther Tulip filter in the superior vena cava for upper extremity deep venous thrombosis. Cardiovasc Intervent Radiol 2002; 25: 524–526

[337] Shackford SR, Cook A, Rogers FB, Littenberg B, Osler T. The increasing use of vena cava filters in adult trauma victims: data from the American College of Surgeons National Trauma Data Bank. J Trauma 2007; 63: 764–769

[338] Carlin AM, Tyburski JG, Wilson RF, Steffes C. Prophylactic and therapeutic inferior vena cava filters to prevent pulmonary emboli in trauma patients. Arch Surg 2002; 137: 521–525, discussion 525–527

[339] Quirke TE, Ritota PC, Swan KG. Inferior vena caval filter use in U.S. trauma centers: a practitioner survey. J Trauma 1997; 43: 333–337

[340] Rohrer MJ, Scheidler MG, Wheeler HB, Cutler BS. Extended indications for placement of an inferior vena cava filter. J Vasc Surg 1989; 10: 44–49, discussion 49–50

[341] Rogers FB, Strindberg G, Shackford SR et al. Five-year follow-up of prophylactic vena cava filters in high-risk trauma patients. Arch Surg 1998; 133: 406–411, discussion 412

[342] Leach TA, Pastena JA, Swan KG, Tikellis JI, Blackwood JM, Odom JW. Surgical prophylaxis for pulmonary embolism. Am Surg 1994; 60: 292–295

[343] Rosenthal D, McKinsey JF, Levy AM, Lamis PA, Clark MD. Use of the Greenfield filter in patients with major trauma. Cardiovasc Surg 1994; 2: 52–55

[344] Wilson JT, Rogers FB, Wald SL, Shackford SR, Ricci MA. Prophylactic vena cava filter insertion in patients with traumatic spinal cord injury: preliminary results. Neurosurgery 1994; 35: 234–239, discussion 239

[345] Winchell RJ, Hoyt DB, Walsh JC, Simons RK, Eastman AB. Risk factors associated with pulmonary embolism despite routine prophylaxis: implications for improved protection. J Trauma 1994; 37: 600–606

[346] Khansarinia S, Dennis JW, Veldenz HC, Butcher JL, Hartland L. Prophylactic Greenfield filter placement in selected high-risk trauma patients. J Vasc Surg 1995; 22: 231–235, discussion 235–236

[347] Rogers FB, Shackford SR, Ricci MA, Wilson JT, Parsons S. Routine prophylactic vena cava filter insertion in severely injured trauma patients decreases the incidence of pulmonary embolism. J Am Coll Surg 1995; 180: 641–647

[348] Rodriguez JL, Lopez JM, Proctor MC et al. Early placement of prophylactic vena caval filters in injured patients at high risk for pulmonary embolism. J Trauma 1996; 40: 797–802, discussion 802–804

[349] Velmahos GC, Kern J, Chan LS, Oder D, Murray JA, Shekelle P. Prevention of venous thromboembolism after injury: an evidence-based report—part II: analysis of risk factors and evaluation of the role of vena caval filters. J Trauma 2000; 49: 140–144

[350] Greenfield LJ, Proctor MC, Michaels AJ, Taheri PA. Prophylactic vena caval filters in trauma: the rest of the story. J Vasc Surg 2000; 32: 490–495, discussion 496–497

[351] Allen TL, Carter JL, Morris BJ, Harker CP, Stevens MH. Retrievable vena cava filters in trauma patients for high-risk prophylaxis and prevention of pulmonary embolism. Am J Surg 2005; 189: 656–661

[352] Hoff WS, Hoey BA, Wainwright GA et al. Early experience with retrievable inferior vena cava filters in high-risk trauma patients. J Am Coll Surg 2004; 199: 869–874

[353] McMurtry AL, Owings JT, Anderson JT, Battistella FD, Gosselin R. Increased use of prophylactic vena cava filters in trauma patients failed to decrease overall incidence of pulmonary embolism. J Am Coll Surg 1999; 189: 314–320

24 Interventional Radiologic Management of Retrievable Vena Cava Filters

Riyad Karmy-Jones

The advent of retrievable filters have stimulated an increased utilization of filters in the hopes that the incidence of fatal pulmonary embolism (PE) is reduced without the risk of long-term complications that have been attributed to permanent filters, notably venous hypertension and IVC thrombosis. Several critical questions have been raised, not all of which have been clearly answered.

1. Are all retrievable filters equivalent?
2. Do retrievable filters reduce the incidence of PE without affecting the indications for use?
3. Are they retrieved?
4. If not, are they equivalent to permanent filters?
5. Can they be removed if there is a residual deep venous thrombosis (DVT)?

24.1 Currently Available Retrievable Filters

There are three retrievable filters used commonly: The Gunther Tulip (GTF; Cook, Bloomington, IN), the Recovery (Bard Peripheral Vascular, Tempe, AZ) and the Optease (Cordis Endovascular, Miami Lakes,FL). The GTF and Recovery are conical, while the Optease is hexagonal (▶ Fig. 24.1). All can be placed via a femoral or jugular approach, but only the Optease can be removed or repositioned from a femoral approach. The Optease's configuration may permit it to more reliably trap small emboli and be associated with a lower tilt rate, but it also appears to be associated with a higher rate of caval thrombosis.[1,2] This appears to be related to two mechanisms. Thrombus trapped in the apex is exposed to large shear forces, which should aid lysis. However, downstream of the thrombus, an area of stagnation is created as the shear forces are directed laterally against the caval wall. Thrombus trapped in the inferior portion of the basket results in shear forces being directed against the contralateral IVC wall, whereas an area of stagnation extends along the ipsilateral wall. These result in firm thrombus build-up that can be resistant to attempts at lysis.[3]

Timing of retrievability varies between types as well. In general, the GTF is thought to be retrievable up to 6 weeks, although longer intervals have been described while the Recovery filter is felt to be retrievable up to 6 months from placement. Hermson noted a higher rate of tip-to-caval wall "touching" among the Recovery (43%) versus 6% with the GTF. This had an impact of retrievability because filters whose tip touched the caval wall (i.e., tilted) had a reduced rate of retrievability (50% vs. 88%).[4] The Optease appears to be associated with a vigorous inflammatory reaction, and it is recommended that removal or repositioning be performed within 2 to 3 weeks.[5,6,7,8]

In one multicenter study (albeit with limited follow-up) the Optease was associated with a significantly higher rate of inability to retrieve (72% vs. GTF and recovery combined, $p = 0.01$) and symptomatic caval thrombosis (▶ Table 24.1).[1] Although our bias has been to avoid the Optease, others have

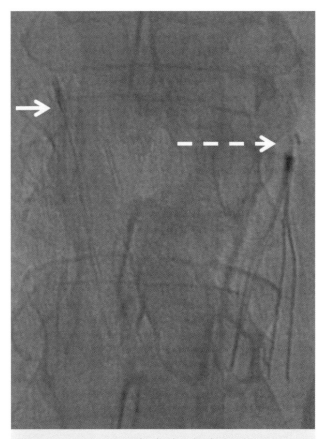

Fig. 24.1 A trauma patient who developed a deep vein thrombosis. The patient was found on initial cavogram to have dual vena cava and required two filters, a Recovery (solid arrow) and a Gunther Tulip (GTF) (stippled arrow). The choice was made simply because that was what was available. Note the GTF tip is turned so that the hook can be easily seen. Both filters were subsequently removed.

Table 24.1 Comparison of retrievable filters[1]

	Gunther Tulip N=152	Recovery N=224	Optease N=37
Attempts made to retrieve	54	50	11
Technically unable	5 (10%)	7 (14%)	3 (27%)
Residual thrombus	3 (6%)	2 (4%)	5 (46%)
Migration	0	3 (1.3%)	0
Breakthrough pulmonary embolism	1 (0.6%)	1 (0.4%)	0
Symptomatic caval occlusion	0	2 (1%)	4 (11%)

reported excellent results, which have been linked to close follow-up and early repositioning or retrieval.[8]

24.2 Do Prophylactic Retrievable Filters Reduce the Incidence of Pulmonary Embolism?

It is clear that patients who have a documented DVT that extends to or above the popliteal veins, and who cannot be adequately treated with anticoagulation or who fail anticoagulation, are candidates for vena cava filters.[9,10,11] To what extent the utility of prophylactic retrievable filters have in reducing the incidence of PE is less clear. Certainly, certain populations are at increased risk of DVT and subsequent PE, and in these groups the majority of studies present data that supports the notion that the incidence of symptomatic (but perhaps not fatal) PE can be reduced by using prophylactic filters (whether permanent or retrievable).[12,13] One application that retrievable filters may be uniquely suited for is the patient at risk for DVT or with documented DVT who requires multiple repeat procedures in a short period which precludes adequate consistent prophylaxis or treatment. Whether retrievable filters can be demonstrated to have uniform clinical benefit across a population, particularly if specific guidelines are not followed, is less clear.[13,14,15] It does appear that the availability of retrievable filters has led to increased utilization, particularly for prophylaxis, with a decreased regard for current guidelines.[16,17] Antevil and colleagues compared the utilization of filters in their trauma population following the introduction of retrievable technology. They found a threefold increase in utilization of filters, a reduction (from 73% to 42%) among patients who underwent filter placement and who meet East criteria for high risk, but no change in the overall incidence of PE (0.2%).[18] Clearly, this mirrors the debate about the role of prophylactic filters in the pre-retrievable era, and is linked to how PE is detected and severity attributed.[12,15,19] In addition, the perceived utility of prophylactic filter placement depends upon whether or not there is adherence to practice guidelines with respect to chemical prophylaxis and surveillance.[20] It is probable that when used appropriately, following strict criteria (which may vary from institution to institution, but should be based on consensus guidelines) that retrievable filters do reduce (but do not eliminate) the risk of PE, but that loosening indications do not confer an advantage to the population as a whole while being associated with an increased risk of complications.[13,18,21,22]

24.3 Are Retrievable Filters Actually Retrieved?

In general, the majority of retrievable filters are not, in fact, retrieved. Antevil and associates noted that of 161 retrievable filters placed, an attempt at removal was made in only 43 (27%) and was successful in only 33 (21%). Kirilcuk and colleagues noted that of 23 filters placed with the intention of removing them, an attempt was made in only 10 (43%) and successful in 8 (35%). The multicenter trial performed by the American Association for the Surgery of Trauma found that of 413 filters placed, an attempt to retrieve was made in only 116 (28%) of cases and was successful in 90 (22%). The two primary reasons for lack of an attempt to retrieve was loss to follow up (31%) and prolonged immobility with perceived risk of deep venous thrombosis (30%). The primary reason for failure to retrieve filters was because of loss to follow up (31%). This was sixfold higher (6% to 44%, p=0.001) when the service placing the filters was not directly responsible for follow up.[1] This underscores the importance of establishing a firm protocol for following patients if the desire is to actually remove the filters.[21,22] Although the concern of prolonged immobility is often used as a rationale for leaving filters in, particularly in patients with vertebral or head injuries, this is not a broadly applicable indication for prophylactic filters.[11] However, if there is concern, in most cases it can be anticipated that these will be prolonged, perhaps life-long issues, and it may be more reasonable to utilize permanent filters for this indication.

24.4 Do Retrievable Filters Have Lower Complication Rates than Permanent Filters?

There is no literature that compares permanent versus retrievable filters in a prospective fashion in the trauma population. There are excellent reviews available, but in general the majority of the literature concerns cancer or nontrauma settings.[5,13] Trauma, although there is a hypercoagulable state, is transient (between 4–6 weeks) and in the absence of other hereditary coagulation deficits, is presumably not lifelong.[23] In terms of acute complications, there is no data that supports one form or type of filter in terms of reduced complications at placement. At best, one can review available reports dealing with specific populations, usually using one filter type alone. Some reports regarding complications of permanent filters can be used as a basis for comparison. Greenfield and colleagues reported a 2-year follow-up study of trauma patients, comparing those who underwent filter placement for prophylactic as opposed to therapeutic indications. This data showed no difference in terms of recurrent PE rate or caval occlusion between groups, although there was a significantly higher incidence of leg swelling and need for compressive stockings among patients who underwent intervention for therapeutic reasons (▶ Table 24.2).[24] Wojick and associates, with a mean follow-up of 29 months, found an incidence of filter migration of 0.95%, caval occlusion of 0.95%, and symptomatic leg swelling of 10%.[25] Rogers and colleagues at 5 years found an incidence of filter tilt (> 14 degrees) of 5.5% and strut malposition in 38%.[26]

Table 24.2 A 2-year follow-up of patients who underwent filter placement[24]

	Prophylactic (%)	Therapeutic (%)
New pulmonary embolism	1.5	2
Caval occlusion	3.5	2.3
Lower extremity edema	25	43
Support stockings	3.5	25

Presumably, if the filter is retrieved, a significant portion of these long-term complications should not occur. However, there is limited data regarding the efficacy of retrievable filters left in permanently. Ota and associates reported on 52 GTF left in and noted a patency rate of 93% (97% when "low intensity" anticoagulation with warfarin was used).[27] In addition, in 56% of cases the filter struts penetrated > 3 mm through the cava walls, although there were no sequelae. The AAST study described a new DVT rate of 20% (3% access site DVT) among patients who underwent filter placement, a tilt or migration rate of 1.3% among the recovery filters, and as noted, an 11% incidence of caval thrombosis after placement of an Optease filter (► Table 24.1).[1] In this same study there were no complications recorded among patients who underwent permanent filter placement, although the follow-up was extremely limited. These data suggest that there may be lower tilt/migration when permanent filters are placed compared with retrievable filters, but that there is no data that clearly show a difference in caval thrombosis between the two types. In general, conical filters appear to have a lower incidence of caval thrombosis than trapezoid, whether retrievable or permanent.

If retrievable filters offer the promise of reduced occlusive complications, assuming they are retrieved, they also have a unique complication, PE after removal. In theory, once a patient can be anticoagulated, the standard of care would be to remove the filter, even in the presence of a documented DVT. Many centers are inhibited by medicolegal concerns from doing this. In the AAST study, the overall incidence of PE following filter removal was 6% among patients who underwent filter placement for therapeutic indications, 0 among the prophylactic group. Of note, given that as many as 25% of patients who have a filter placed will develop a DVT, none of these patients had undergone duplex screening prior to filter removal.[1,28]

Thus, the primary benefit in terms of reduced filter complications with retrievable filters appears to hold true only if the filters are indeed retrieved. In terms of complications if the filters are left in place there are no data suggesting that retrievable filters have a lower complication rate than permanent filters, and there are hints that there may be a higher incidence of filter migration.

24.5 Placement Considerations

Vena cava filters can be placed in the intensive care unit or at the bedside without resorting to using the imaging suites.[29] Intravascular or transabdominal ultrasound can also be used for insertion at the bedside in critically ill patients.[30] Jugular approaches may be associated with a lower risk of infection or DVT, but there is no proof of this. Key steps include measuring the diameter of the cava relative to the choice of filter, and ensuring that there are no critical anatomical variations (► Fig. 24.1). With the Recovery or GTF, attention should be made to carefully deploying the filter so that the tip does not angle away, making recovery difficult. In the case of the GTF, it is ideal to rotate the filter so that the hook can be clearly seen, aiding later retrieval. At the time of retrieval, a cavogram should be performed to rule out significant thrombus residing in the filter or more distally prior to removal.

24.6 Conclusion

Retrievable filters probably reduce PE in patients who are defined as being at increased risk based on published criteria. In the majority of institutions, however, they are not in fact retrieved. The primary reason for this is a lack of a consistent follow-up program. No data confirm that when retrievable filters are left in permanently they are "safer" than permanent filters; indeed, there may be increased complications of tilt and/or migration. Lowering the indications for prophylactic filter placement, based on the assumption that retrievable filters are temporary, does not translate into a global reduction in PE. Not all retrievable filters are equivalent. The Optease filter is associated with an increased incidence of caval thrombosis. Prior to retrieving a filter, a repeat venous duplex should be performed to confirm that no new above-knee thrombosis has occurred that would either suggest that the filter be left or that anticoagulation be started on removal.

References

[1] Karmy-Jones R, Jurkovich GJ, Velmahos GC , et al. Practice patterns and outcomes of retrievable vena cava filters in trauma patients: an AAST multicenter study. J Trauma 2007; 62: 17–24, discussion 24–25

[2] Mahrer A, Zippel D, Garniek A , et al. Retrievable vena cava filters in major trauma patients: prevalence of thrombus within the filter. Cardiovasc Intervent Radiol 2008; 31: 785–789

[3] Leask RL, Johnston KW, Ojha M. Hemodynamic effects of clot entrapment in the TrapEase inferior vena cava filter. J Vasc Interv Radiol 2004; 15: 485–490

[4] Hermsen JL, Ibele AR, Faucher LD, Nale JK, Schurr MJ, Kudsk KA. Retrievable inferior vena cava filters in high-risk trauma and surgical patients: factors influencing successful removal. World J Surg 2008; 32: 1444–1449

[5] Kinney TB. Update on inferior vena cava filters. J Vasc Interv Radiol 2003; 14: 425–440

[6] Ashley DW, Mix JW, Christie B , et al. Removal of the OptEase retrievable vena cava filter is not feasible after extended time periods because of filter protrusion through the vena cava. J Trauma 2005; 59: 847–852

[7] Rosenthal D, Wellons ED, Lai KM, Bikk A, Henderson VJ. Retrievable inferior vena cava filters: initial clinical results. Ann Vasc Surg 2006; 20: 157–165

[8] Rosenthal D, Swischuk JL, Cohen SA, Wellons ED. OptEase retrievable inferior vena cava filter: initial multicenter experience. Vascular 2005; 13: 286–289

[9] Pasquale M, Fabian TC. Practice management guidelines for trauma from the Eastern Association for the Surgery of Trauma. J Trauma 1998; 44: 941–956, discussion 956–957

[10] Rogers FB, Cipolle MD, Velmahos G, Rozycki G, Luchette FA. Practice management guidelines for the prevention of venous thromboembolism in trauma patients: the EAST practice management guidelines work group. J Trauma 2002; 53: 142–164

[11] Proceedings of the Seventh ACCP Conference on Antithrombotic and Thrombolytic Therapy: evidence-based guidelines. Chest 2004; 126 Suppl: 172S–696S

[12] Rodriguez JL, Lopez JM, Proctor MC , et al. Early placement of prophylactic vena caval filters in injured patients at high risk for pulmonary embolism. J Trauma 1996; 40: 797–802, discussion 802–804

[13] Martin MJ, Salim A. Vena cava filters in surgery and trauma. Surg Clin North Am 2007; 87: 1229–1252, xi–xii

[14] Knudson MM, Ikossi DG, Khaw L, Morabito D, Speetzen LS. Thromboembolism after trauma: an analysis of 1602 episodes from the American College of Surgeons National Trauma Data Bank. Ann Surg 2004; 240: 490–496, discussion 496–498

[15] McMurtry AL, Owings JT, Anderson JT, Battistella FD, Gosselin R. Increased use of prophylactic vena cava filters in trauma patients failed to decrease overall incidence of pulmonary embolism. J Am Coll Surg 1999; 189: 314–320

[16] Shackford SR, Cook A, Rogers FB, Littenberg B, Osler T. The increasing use of vena cava filters in adult trauma victims: data from the American College of Surgeons National Trauma Data Bank. J Trauma 2007; 63: 764–769

[17] Spain DA, Richardson JD, Polk HC, Bergamini TM, Wilson MA, Miller FB. Venous thromboembolism in the high-risk trauma patient: do risks justify

aggressive screening and prophylaxis? J Trauma 1997; 42: 463–467, discussion 467–469

[18] Antevil JL, Sise MJ, Sack DI , et al. Retrievable vena cava filters for preventing pulmonary embolism in trauma patients: a cautionary tale. J Trauma 2006; 60: 35–40

[19] Schultz DJ, Brasel KJ, Washington L , et al. Incidence of asymptomatic pulmonary embolism in moderately to severely injured trauma patients. J Trauma 2004; 56: 727–731, discussion 731–733

[20] Nathens AB, McMurray MK, Cuschieri J , et al. The practice of venous thromboembolism prophylaxis in the major trauma patient. J Trauma 2007; 62: 557–562, discussion 562–563

[21] Offner PJ, Hawkes A, Madayag R, Seale F, Maines C. The role of temporary inferior vena cava filters in critically ill surgical patients. Arch Surg 2003; 138: 591–594, discussion 594–595

[22] Kirilcuk NN, Herget EJ, Dicker RA, Spain DA, Hellinger JC, Brundage SI. Are temporary inferior vena cava filters really temporary? Am J Surg 2005; 190: 858–863

[23] Meissner MH, Chandler WL, Elliott JS. Venous thromboembolism in trauma: a local manifestation of systemic hypercoagulability? J Trauma 2003; 54: 224–231

[24] Greenfield LJ, Proctor MC, Michaels AJ, Taheri PA. Prophylactic vena caval filters in trauma: the rest of the story. J Vasc Surg 2000; 32: 490–495, discussion 496–497

[25] Wojcik R, Cipolle MD, Fearen I, Jaffe J, Newcomb J, Pasquale MD. Long-term follow-up of trauma patients with a vena caval filter. J Trauma 2000; 49: 839–843

[26] Rogers FB, Strindberg G, Shackford SR , et al. Five-year follow-up of prophylactic vena cava filters in high-risk trauma patients. Arch Surg 1998; 133: 406–411, discussion 412

[27] Ota S, Yamada N, Tsuji A , et al. The Günther-Tulip retrievable IVC filter: clinical experience in 118 consecutive patients. Circ J 2008; 72: 287–292

[28] Duperier T, Mosenthal A, Swan KG, Kaul S. Acute complications associated with Greenfield filter insertion in high-risk trauma patients. J Trauma 2003; 54: 545–549

[29] Sing RF, Cicci CK, Smith CH, Messick WJ. Bedside insertion of inferior vena cava filters in the intensive care unit. J Trauma 1999; 47: 1104–1107

[30] Rosenthal D, Wellons ED, Levitt AB, Shuler FW, O'Conner RE, Henderson VJ. Role of prophylactic temporary inferior vena cava filters placed at the ICU bedside under intravascular ultrasound guidance in patients with multiple trauma. J Vasc Surg 2004; 40: 958–964

25 Interventional Radiology in Iatrogenic Trauma

João Pisco, Tiago Bilhim, and Marisa Duarte

Iatrogenic vascular injuries amenable to endovascular repair are becoming more frequent because they represent a potential complication of numerous medical procedures. Its incidence has been rising due to an increasing number of new interventional procedures and more accurate diagnoses. Vascular injuries are well known and feared complications of surgery and percutaneous interventions. They can occur following open or laparoscopic surgeries, biopsies, drainage procedures, percutaneous radiofrequency ablation, arterial or venous access, sclerotherapy, injection of anesthetic agents, infusions, catheterizations, and endoscopic procedures. Some of these procedures will result in iatrogenic injuries requiring treatment.

Most injuries involve the arterial system. However, veins can also involved. Some of these complications can occur near the sites of treatment or at access puncture sites. There are different complications such as arteriovenous fistulas (AVFs), arterial pseudoaneurysms, thrombosis, rupture, dissection, embolization, laceration/avulsion, hemorrhage, or embolization and rupture of intravascular devices. Clinical signs can be acute or chronic with hemodynamic instability, ischemia, and even death. Diagnosis can sometimes be very difficult and delayed, so that procedures are frequently not treated until a later stage because they may be initially overlooked.

Treatment options are conservative open surgery or endovascular management. Endovascular treatment options have developed during the last decades. There are many new techniques available making this the first-line approach in many cases. With shorter procedure times and less blood loss. There are now available microcatheters, better embolization materials, and stents that allow superselective catheterization and treatment of the lesions at the site of injury. Balloon occlusion or dilatation, embolization with coils, polyvinyl alcohol (PVA) and/or Gelfoam (Pfizer, New York, NY) particles, and stent deployment are some of the options available. Treatment must be tailored to each situation according to the organ or vessel involved, and the clinical presentation and type of lesion found at angiography.

25.1 Etiology

Iatrogenic vascular injuries are well known and have been described since the beginning of interventional radiology (IR) in the 1970s. There are reports of arterial embolization control of iatrogenic injuries in postsurgical bleeding, hemorrhage following hip arthroplasty, or after percutaneous renal biopsy.[1]

There are many different causes of iatrogenic injuries, such as biopsies, drainage procedures, open or laparoscopic surgeries, arterial or venous access, sclerotherapy, injection of anesthetic agents, intravenous (IV) infusions, catheterizations and endoscopic procedures, and following tracheostomy, percutaneous radiofrequency ablation, or neurosurgical spine surgery.

When the lesions affect only veins, the approach is usually conservative. Unfortunately, the arteries are frequently injured and require treatment by surgery or by endovascular techniques, depending on the etiology of the injury, vessel injured, type of lesion, clinical manifestation, and available resources.

There are many reports of management of arterial complications related to diagnostic angiography or heart catheterization, after puncture or cannulation for monitoring of blood gas values or blood pressure of the radial artery, gynecological operations, operations for varicose veins, or emergency resuscitation.[2] With the increasing performance of percutaneous transluminal angioplasty and insertion of intravascular devices, iatrogenic arterial complications are increasing, with a minority of these procedures requiring treatment.

Arterial rupture or dissection during balloon angioplasty/stenting and indwelling intravascular devices with arterial rupture, thrombosis, or embolization are becoming another common source of iatrogenic injury.[3] Frequent injuries are also observed in orthopedic and abdominal/laparoscopic operations, and there are increasing reports of vascular lesions following therapeutic procedures for malignancy as well.

The endovascular treatment of arterial lesions is well known and has good results. Stopping bleeding by embolization can be achieved with different techniques and methods.[4] The most frequent arterial injuries embolized are hepatic, renal, and mesenteric. Less frequent reports of injuries to the vertebral artery and the carotid cavernous sinus are available.

An alternative endovascular procedure is the placement of covered stents, as in coronary artery perforations, in axillary and subclavian arterial injuries. This is much safer and more efficient than open repair.

Some reports indicate that the endovascular management of visceral artery aneurysms and pseudoaneurysms is more effective than surgery.[5] Transarterial embolization of postoperative hemorrhage after abdominal surgery,[6] and arterial injuries to the hepatic, mesenteric, and renal arteries has been reported.[1,6,7,8,9,10,11]

25.2 Clinical Presentation

The clinical presentation is variable and depends on different factors such as the vessel injured, the type of lesion, the amount and rate of blood loss, and the type of iatrogenic procedure responsible for the complication. The symptoms can be acute (hemorrhagic or ischemic), subacute, or chronic.

In cases of hemodynamic instability, urgent angiography is mandatory to visualize arterial lesions and plan treatment options either by endovascular approach or by open surgery. If there is little blood loss, or over a long period, the clinical symptoms may be unremarkable and only become evident some days to months later thus making the diagnosis more difficult. In these cases, iatrogenic injuries are frequently not treated until a later stage because they are initially overlooked.

In the setting of orthopedic iatrogenic lesions, the most common symptoms are acute limb ischemia with loss of Doppler arterial flow/pulses, intraoperative arterial bleeding, nonhealing wounds, and limb edema. Indications for angiography include absent pulses, signs and symptoms of ischemia, a bruit, and history of a posterior knee or allow dislocation. Relative indications are decreased pulses, significant hematoma, and proximity of a fracture. The most frequent angiographic signs

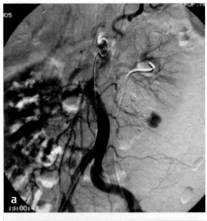
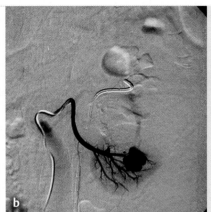
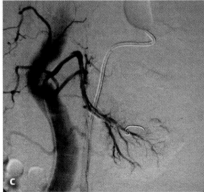

Fig. 25.1 Hematuria following left renal biopsy. (a) Abdominal aortogram shows extravasation of contrast material. (b) Selective angiography of left lower pole renal artery shows a pseudoaneurysm. (c) After embolization with a single coil, the pseudoaneurysm is no longer seen.

are thrombosis, laceration/avulsion, and pseudoaneurysm development. The most frequently involved arteries are the iliac, common femoral, profunda, superficial femoral, popliteal, or tibial. Concomitant venous injuries are sometimes present.

Vascular trauma from therapeutic procedures for malignancies can result from intra-arterial chemotherapy or by resection of tumors with local invasion.

Clinical symptoms related to complications of hepatic, biliary, and pancreatic interventions can be hemobilia, massive intra-abdominal bleeding, hematemesis and/or melena, jaundice related to strictures or compression of the common hepatic duct, nausea and vomiting, upper abdominal pain, bleeding from drainage catheters, or pancreatitis. They are usually secondary to percutaneous, surgical or laparoscopic procedures, or ablation procedure as well, can be diagnosed by digital subtraction angiography, and treated with endovascular procedures. The hepatic arteries (common, proper, right and left branches) are the most commonly affected, with the celiac axis, the splenic, left gastric, gastroduodenal, subphrenic, and superior mesenteric arteries less commonly affected.[12,13,14,15]

Iatrogenic vascular complications after renal procedures can occur after percutaneous nephrostomy, renal biopsy, biopsy-related vascular injuries in renal allografts, percutaneous nephrolithotomy, nephron-sparing surgery, percutaneous antegrade endopyelotomy, transitional cell carcinoma resection, and transurethral resection of the prostate. Clinical signs are usually gross or microscopic hematuria, azotemia, decrease of hemoglobin, and acute flank pain with perirenal hematoma. False aneurysm and contrast extravasation are the usual angiographic signs and usually involve the main renal artery or the interlobar arteries. Retroperitoneal hemorrhage due to an

iatrogenic perioperative injury of a ureteric artery has also been described. Complications resulting from renal ablations are rare but now seen with increasing frequency.

25.3 Endovascular Techniques

Selective catheterization and angiography is done with catheters selected by the vessel injured. After the source of the bleeding is identified, superselective catheterization is done placing the catheter in a more distal position using a steerable 0.035-inch guidewire. If necessary a 3-French (F) superselective coaxial microcatheter is introduced in proximity to the bleeding branch.

After identifying pseudoaneurysms, with or without extravasation of the contrast media, embolization is performed. The embolic agents frequently used are coils, and polyvinyl alcohol (PVA) and/or Gelfoam particles. Gelfoam has been used since the 1980s. It provides temporary embolization.[16] It can be used alongside coils, especially in patients with coagulopathy. Coils are the preferred embolizing agent, considered the first option for some authors (▶ Fig. 25.1). They can be placed distal and proximal to the pseudoaneurysm, providing a nidus for thrombus formation to achieve hemostasis.

Polyvinyl alcohol is a permanent embolizing agent. The particle size is generally of 150 to 1,200 µm. It can be used alone or in conjunction with coils. Care must be taken to avoid reflux of particles or occlusion of the catheter.

Although liquid adhesives or glues have been used as embolic agents for nearly three decades, experience with them outside of neurointerventional indications is generally limited. Cyanoacrylates are the main liquid adhesives used in the vascular

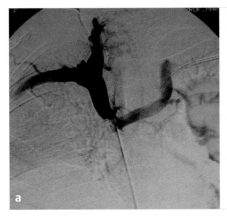
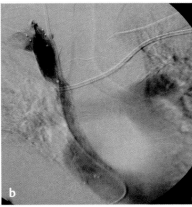

Fig. 25.2 Stent placement in superior vena cava thrombosis due to central venous catheter placements. (a) Superior vena cava occlusion. (b) Recanalization after stent placement.

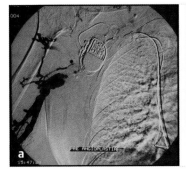
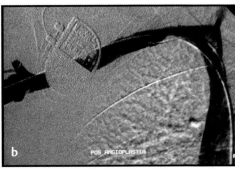

Fig. 25.3 Fibrinolysis of venous thrombosis due to pacemaker. (a) Venogram of the right axillary vein of a patient with pacemaker shows thrombosis of the right axillary and subclavian veins and superior vein cava. (b) After regional fibrinolysis, there is total recanalization of the thrombotic veins

system and have an important role in managing vascular abnormalities, especially arteriovenous malformations.[17]

Embolization of the afferent artery can be done in pseudoaneurysms that arise from a donor artery of a transplanted organ without collateral supply such as a visceral branch, whereas in the case of native visceral arteries with well-established collateral supply, the embolization of both proximal and distal branches to the pseudoaneurysm is mandatory to prevent backflow from collateral circulation.

In case of arterial rupture or laceration, prolonged (from a few minutes to hours) low-pressure balloon inflation can achieve temporary hemostasis allowing a later treatment with embolization or stent placement.

Endovascular treatment options for visceral artery pseudoaneurysms depend on lesion location and size. Exclusion methods fall into two categories—embolization and stent placement—and these procedures aim to exclude the pseudoaneurysm from the circulation, and if possible, to maintain distal blood flow. Covered stents are a feasible alternative to open repair in properly selected patients, resulting in a shorter procedure time and less blood loss.

Stents may be used in iatrogenic occlusive vascular disease such as those caused by dialysis fistulas, central venous catheters bypass anastomosis or in renal transplant artery trauma (▶ Fig. 25.2). Some iatrogenic thrombotic occlusions may be treated by regional fibrinolysis as well (▶ Fig. 25.3).

Interventional radiological procedures are effective in the management of iatrogenic lesions of most of the arterial vessels because they are minimally invasive, have a high success rate, and a low incidence of complications compared with the more complex surgical or laparoscopic options.

An iatrogenic pseudoaneurysm can be effectively treated by direct percutaneous puncture with a needle followed by insertion of the embolic agent. This technique is used in femoral artery pseudoaneurysms after angiographic procedures. It can also be used in deep abdominal lesions. Thrombin can also be injected. Thrombin is a liquid agent being increasingly used for postcatheterization pseudoaneurysms by direct puncture. It can also be used alongside with coils to promote thrombosis.

25.4 Hepatobiliary and Pancreatic Injuries

Some hepatobiliary and pancreatic procedures causing iatrogenic injuries are laparoscopic cholecystectomy for gallstones, pylorus-preserving pancreatoduodenectomy, conventional pancreatoduodenectomy, distal pancreatectomy, segmental resection of the pancreas, total pancreatectomy, bile duct resection with partial hepatectomy, hepatopancreatoduodenectomy, hemihepatectomy, and hepatic resection—with removal of the bile duct with lymphadenectomy generally for malignancies. Complications of ablative procedures are uncommon but seen with increased frequency at this time.

The hepatic, common, proper, right, and left branches are usually affected. The celiac trunk, splenic, left gastric, gastroduodenal, subphrenic, lumbar, and superior mesenteric arteries are less commonly affected (▶ Fig. 25.4).

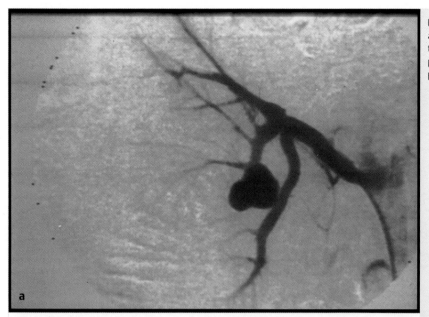

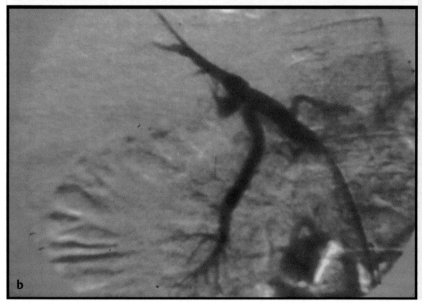

Fig. 25.4 Pseudoaneurysm of a right hepatic artery branch following percutaneous cholecystectomy. (a) Right hepatic arteriography shows a pseudoaneurysm. (b) Following embolization, the pseudoaneurysm is no longer seen.

Pseudoaneurysm, artery stumps, intact but ectatic arteries with surgical clips closely applied, arterial erosions/lacerations and arteriovenous, arterio-portal or arterio-biliary fistulas can be managed with embolization with coils with proximal and distal deployment in the injured vessel. Other embolizing agents used are polyvinyl alcohol (PVA) and/or Gelfoam particles. When indicated, covered stents are a reasonable treatment option.

25.5 Renal Injuries

Percutaneous nephrostomy, renal biopsy of native or transplanted allografts, and percutaneous nephrolithotomy are the common causes of iatrogenic lesions after renal procedures (► Fig. 25.5). Nephron-sparing surgery, percutaneous antegrade endopyelotomy, upper-tract transitional cell carcinoma resection, and transurethral resection of the prostate are less frequent causes.[18,19]

The usual findings are pseudoaneurysms, AVFs, and frank contrast extravasation (► Fig. 25.6, ► Fig. 25.7, ► Fig. 25.8). The main renal artery or one or multiple interlobar arteries are frequently injured, although ureteric arteries can also be affected.

Coils are the choice of embolizing agents with proximal and distal deployment in the injured vessel the so called "sandwich" method. Other agents are polyvinyl alcohol (PVA) and/or Gelfoam particles. Cyanoacrylate, with or without Lipiodol, can be used in special cases.

25.6 Orthopedic Injuries

Spinal operations (cervical, lumbosacral or herniated disk arthrodesis), shoulder operations (recurrent dislocation, excision of first rib), hip surgery (prosthesis, plate and screws, fractured acetabulum), and operations on the lower limbs may cause iatrogenic vascular complications (► Fig. 25.9, ► Fig. 25.10).

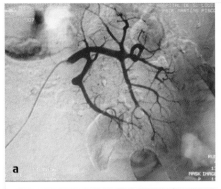

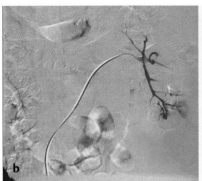

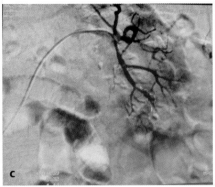

Fig. 25.5 Hematuria after left percutaneous nephrolithotomy. (a) Left renal arteriogram—extravasation of contrast from a lower pole branch. (b) Selective arteriography of the injured vessel—the extravasation better demonstrated. (c) Left renal arteriogram after embolization—the extravasation is no longer evident.

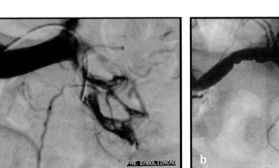

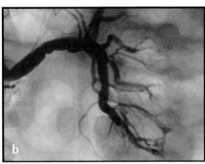

Fig. 25.6 Hematuria after left percutaneous nephrolithotomy. (a) Left renal arteriography shows an arteriovenous fistula with early renal vein opacification. (b) After embolization, the renal vein is no longer seen.

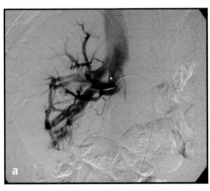

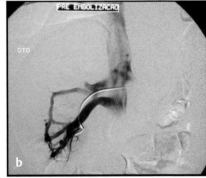

Fig. 25.7 Hematuria after right renal biopsy. (a) Right renal arteriogram shows an arteriovenous fistula (AVF) with opacification of the inferior vein cava. (b) Catheter placed selectively at the fistula level. (c) During embolization with coils. (d) After embolization, no longer AVF opacification.

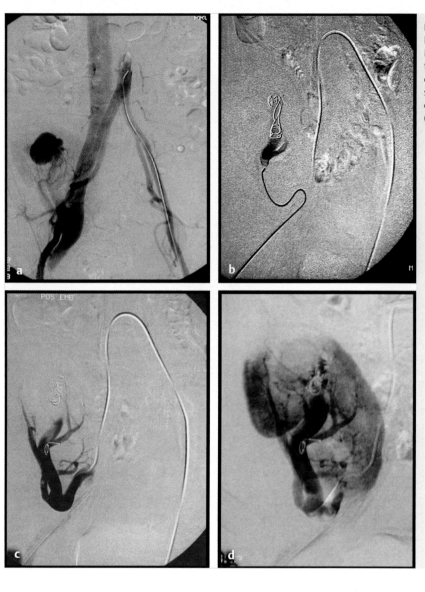

Fig. 25.8 Hematuria after biopsy of a transplant kidney. (a) Angiography of right iliac artery. There is a pseudoaneurysm with an arteriovenous fistula (AVF) and opacification of the inferior vena cava. (b) Angiography through a catheter placed selectively at the level of the fistula. (c) After embolization with coils, the AVF is not identified. (d) Late phase there is minimal parenchymal loss.

Concomitant venous injuries may be present in some cases. False aneurysms, AVF, ischemia and arterial thrombosis are the abnormalities identified. Arterial laceration/avulsion is rare.

Coils placed on the pseudoaneurysm are a viable option. Intervential radiological management is aimed at restoring blood supply. Therefore, angioplasty and stent placement are the preferred choices.

25.7 Endovascular Complications

Complications can occur after endovascular procedures. At the site of puncture, hematoma, dissection, an AVF or pseudoaneurysms can occur. The embolizing agents can migrate and cause ischemia in unwanted territories. This can be prevented with gentle injection of the embolizing agents avoiding reflux, having the emboli suspended in contrast and fluoroscopic monitoring of the injection, and having the catheter securely positioned in the target artery.

Retrieval of misplaced coils is easy with snares or detachable coils. Angioplasty and stent deployment can cause arterial lacerations or even ruptures or the stents can migrate.

Intravascular devices, such as broken guidewires or catheters with detached portions of the arterial vessel, can be treated with stent placement. Catheters and guidewires can cause arterial spasm or dissection which can be avoided with careful handling.

Hepatic infarction after arterial embolization is very rare, but possible. Filling of the distal tissue of an embolized branch through collaterals generally is well tolerated. The absence of collateral filling may be associated with liver infarction in the area corresponding to the embolized branch. Hepatic infarction is related to lack of immediate collateral flow.[20] Liver failure due to total liver necrosis has been described, but is very rare. Rupture of aneurysm during coil embolization; thrombosis extension to the right hepatic artery; delayed common bile duct stricture due to ischemia; and rupture, obstruction, or hypertension of the portal vein are other possible but uncommon complications.

Rebleeding can be successfully managed with repeat embolization. Surgical intervention can be needed because of failed re-embolization.

Abscess formation is rare and can be managed by percutaneous drainage.

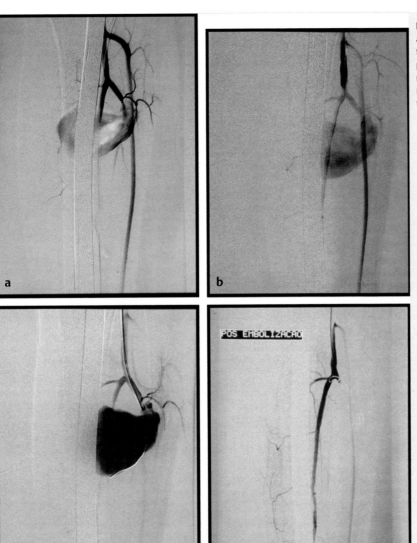

Fig. 25.9 Pseudoaneurysm of the peroneal artery after tibia osteosynthesis. (a) Arteriography of the popliteal artery shows a laceration of the peroneal artery. (b) Filing of a large pseudoaneurysm. (c) Total opacification of the pseudoaneurysm. (d) After embolization with a single coil the pseudoaneurysm is no longer opacified.

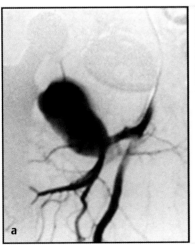
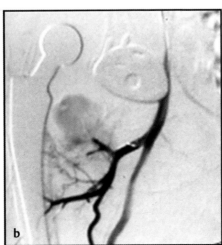

Fig. 25.10 Pseudoaneurysm after right hip arthroplasty. (a) Right femoral arteriogram shows a huge pseudoaneurysm. (b) After embolization with particles, the pseudoaneurysm is no longer opacified.

Transcatheter arterial embolization (TAE) for pelvic trauma has been associated with gluteal skin and muscle necrosis. However, the ultimate and typical signs of gluteal necrosis resulting from TAE have not been investigated.

Renal infarct after embolization is prevented with superselective embolization of the interlobar arteries with a mean postembolization parenchymal ischemic area of around 11.7% and a mean parenchymal infarcted area of 6 to 10%. Serum creatinine level may be normal one week after the procedure and at the latest follow-up. However, a progressive deterioration of renal function has been described in rare cases.

Postembolization syndrome (PES; pain, fever, nausea, and vomiting during the next few hours following the embolization), happens frequently, but it is not a complication. Arterial hypertension and migration of coils are other possible complications.

Coils or segments of wires and catheters can also be embolized. Coils can be retrieved percutaneously with developed devices.

25.8 Comments

Hepatic artery pseudoaneurysms are rare (up to 4.5% of incidence in patients with bile duct injury), but rupture is common and can occur in up to 76%, thus requiring prompt attention. The clinical presentation is with bleeding. If discovered early, the bleeding may be intermittent, but if not identified, massive hemorrhage may occur with rupture and reported mortality rate as high as 50%. Angiography with embolization of the pseudoaneurysm is safe and effective. Operative intervention should be reserved for patients for whom embolization fails, if not feasible, or for more complex injuries. Embolization offers a minimally invasive treatment in unstable patients, does not disrupt recent biliary reconstruction, allows distal as well as proximal control of the hepatic artery, and is an effective treatment for potentially life-threatening complications.

Massive arterial bleeding can occur early or late in the postoperative course of hepatobiliary pancreatic surgery with mean time between the initial intervention and diagnosis of 5.7 months (range 7 days–38 months). Early bleeding within 24 hours after the operation usually originates from vessels at the anastomotic suture line or in the intra-abdominal cavity due to inadequate hemostasis. On the other hand, delayed bleeding occurs mainly due to erosion or pseudoaneurysm of major visceral arteries and has a higher mortality rate than those with suture-line bleeding. Selective embolization of hepatic arteries is usually successful.

Pseudoaneurysms of the superior mesenteric artery should be embolized carefully because of the risk of occlusion of intestinal branches resulting in ischemia. Endovascular stenting, temporary creation of an ileocolic arterioportal shunt, or vascular reconstruction by relaparotomy, should be considered as alternatives.

During the early postoperative period after partial nephrectomy, major hemorrhage is a common complication, with an incidence of between 0 and 5%. Although serum creatinine levels can rise during the first days after renal endovascular treatment, there is generally a gradual recovery of the renal function with normalization a few days later. Superselective embolization allows permanent cessation of bleeding without significant parenchymal infarction or renal function deterioration, even when more than one feeding artery needs to be occluded. It is important to avoid occlusion of the proximal arteries to keep parenchymal loss to a minimum (10%). Therefore, embolization as distal as possible is mandatory—at least at the level of the interlobar arteries. This can be achieved using microcatheters and microcoils as embolic agents. Polyvinyl alcohol particles can be an alternative to coils, but only if the microcatheter can be placed in an interlobar artery or even distally.

Transcatheter embolization is a safe and effective technique to treat biopsy-related vascular injuries in renal transplants with immediate clinical success and significant benefit in renal function without affecting the longevity of the allograft. Major hemorrhage requiring intervention after percutaneous renal surgery is uncommon. In up to 95% of cases, angiography reveals a lesion. This supports the use of angiography for intractable bleeding in this setting. Embolization is sufficient for the treatment of vascular complications due to trauma with pseudoaneurysm or active bleeding. At some institutions, immediate surgical exploration in hemodynamically unstable patients is done. This aggressive approach is being increasingly replaced by endovascular therapy, which can achieve immediate and effective control.

Further studies are needed with larger series of patients comparing endovascular and surgical treatments, comparing the results with different embolizing agents and/or covered stents. Microcatheters and detachable coils are important agents for preventing tissue ischemia and avoiding untargeted embolization, but they are very expensive and very difficult to use.

It remains to be proven the benefits of prophylactic antibiotics to prevent bacterial seeding of infarcted tissues. Endovascular treatment must be the first line of treatment of hepatobiliary, pancreatic, and renal iatrogenic vascular injuries. The importance of embolization in other organs or territories is less well documented.

25.9 Conclusion

Although rare in the past, iatrogenic injuries are becoming more frequent with increasing radiologic diagnostic, interventional and therapeutic medical and surgical procedures. Angiography is mandatory when there is a clinical suspicion of a vascular lesion following one of these procedures. The lesions found involve the arterial system with AVF and arterial pseudoaneurysms being the most frequent. Venous injuries are less common and less important. Arterial thrombosis, rupture, dissection, embolization, laceration/avulsion, hemorrhage, and embolization of intravascular devices are less frequent complications. Management of arterial iatrogenic lesions must be individualized according to the site of bleeding, clinical presentation, and type of iatrogenic lesion. Interventional radiological procedures are effective in the management of iatrogenic lesions in most vascular territories because they are minimally invasive, have a high rate of success, and a low incidence of complications compared with the more risky open surgical or laparoscopic options.

The IR team must be available on a 24-hour basis. Embolization is less invasive than surgery and is likely to reduce morbidity and improve the chances of tissue salvage.

References

[1] Barbaric ZL, Cutcliff WB. Control of renal arterial bleeding after percutaneous biopsy. Urology 1976; 8: 108–111

[2] Lacombe M. [Iatrogenic vascular injuries] Bull Acad Natl Med 2006; 190: 1209–1222, discussion 1222–1224

[3] Lazarides MK, Tsoupanos SS, Georgopoulos SE et al. Incidence and patterns of iatrogenic arterial injuries. A decade's experience. J Cardiovasc Surg (Torino) 1998; 39: 281–285

[4] Chuang VP, Reuter SR, Schmidt RW. Control of experimental traumatic renal hemorrhage by embolization with autogenous blood clot. Radiology 1975; 117: 55–58

[5] Tulsyan N, Kashyap VS, Greenberg RK et al. The endovascular management of visceral artery aneurysms and pseudoaneurysms. J Vasc Surg 2007; 45: 276–283, discussion 283

[6] Kim J, Kim JK, Yoon W et al. Transarterial embolization for postoperative hemorrhage after abdominal surgery. J Gastrointest Surg 2005; 9: 393–399

[7] Christensen T, Matsuoka L, Heestand G et al. Iatrogenic pseudoaneurysms of the extrahepatic arterial vasculature: management and outcome. HPB (Oxford) 2006; 8: 458–464

[8] Basile A, Lupattelli T, Giulietti G et al. Interventional treatment of iatrogenic lesions and hepatic arteries. Radiol Med (Torino) 2005; 110: 88–96

[9] Tzeng WS, Wu RH, Chang JM et al. Transcatheter arterial embolization for hemorrhage caused by injury of the hepatic artery. J Gastroenterol Hepatol 2005; 20: 1062–1068

[10] Maleux G, Messiaen T, Stockx L, Vanrenterghem Y, Wilms G. Transcatheter embolization of biopsy-related vascular injuries in renal allografts. Long-term technical, clinical and biochemical results. Acta Radiol 2003; 44: 13–17

[11] Richstone L, Reggio E, Ost MC et al. First Prize (tie): Hemorrhage following percutaneous renal surgery: characterization of angiographic findings. J Endourol 2008; 22: 1129–1135

[12] Carrafiello G, Laganà D, Dizonno M, Cotta E, Ianniello A, Fugazzola C. Emergency percutaneous treatment in iatrogenic hepatic arterial injuries. Emerg Radiol 2008; 15: 249–254

[13] Tessier DJ, Fowl RJ, Stone WM et al. Iatrogenic hepatic artery pseudoaneurysms: an uncommon complication after hepatic, biliary, and pancreatic procedures. Ann Vasc Surg 2003; 17: 663–669

[14] Madanur MA, Battula N, Sethi H, Deshpande R, Heaton N, Rela M. Pseudoaneurysm following laparoscopic cholecystectomy. Hepatobiliary Pancreat Dis Int 2007; 6: 294–298

[15] Tsai CC, Chiu KC, Mo LR et al. Transcatheter arterial coil embolization of iatrogenic pseudoaneurysms after hepatobiliary and pancreatic interventions. Hepatogastroenterology 2007; 54: 41–46

[16] Kuo WT, Lee DE, Saad WEA, Patel N, Sahler LG, Waldman DL. Superselective microcoil embolization for the treatment of lower gastrointestinal hemorrhage. J Vasc Interv Radiol 2003; 14: 1503–1509

[17] Pollak JS, White RI. The use of cyanoacrylate adhesives in peripheral embolization. J Vasc Interv Radiol 2001; 12: 907–913

[18] Heye S, Maleux G, Van Poppel H, Oyen R, Wilms G. Hemorrhagic complications after nephron-sparing surgery: angiographic diagnosis and management by transcatheter embolization. AJR Am J Roentgenol 2005; 184: 1661–1664

[19] Chatziioannou A, Brountzos E, Primetis E et al. Effects of superselective embolization for renal vascular injuries on renal parenchyma and function. Eur J Vasc Endovasc Surg 2004; 28: 201–206

[20] Hashimoto M, Akabane Y, Heianna J et al. Hepatic infarction following selective hepatic artery embolization with microcoils for iatrogenic biliary hemorrhage. Hepatol Res 2004; 30: 42–50

26 Endovascular Techniques and the Hybrid Operating Room

Megan L. Brenner and Thomas M. Scalea

The use of interventional procedures in trauma has increased steadily over the past 10 years. An analysis of the National Trauma Data Bank (NTDB) reported that 8.1% of acute arterial injuries in 2003 were treated with endovascular therapy, compared with only 2.1% in 1994. Nearly an equal number of blunt (55%) and penetrating (45%) injuries were treated with endovascular therapy.[1] A more recent study, also using NTDB data, reported that 16% of traumatic vascular injuries were treated with endovascular therapy, including 20% who were hypotensive at the time of intervention. The authors report decreased mortality with the increased use of endovascular interventions.[2] With advancements in both imaging and device technology, the use of endovascular techniques has become part of the treatment algorithm for the injured patient.

Endovascular therapy in trauma involves a minimally invasive, catheter-based approach to vascular injury. Sheaths, catheters, and guidewires are the universal instruments used regardless of procedure. Devices passed over guidewires form the basis of diagnosis and treatment. This requires coordinated fluoroscopic hand-eye movements, the ability to predict guidewire-lesion interactions, navigate anatomical challenges, apply technology where appropriate and safe, and an understanding of the limits of endovascular therapy in trauma.

26.1 Endovascular 101

Guidewires are available in many different sizes, shapes, coatings, stiffness, and length (▶ Fig. 26.1). Most are coated with a Teflon or silicone coat to decrease the coefficient of friction. Furthermore, their hydrophilic covering seeks the path of liquid, helping to navigate through high-grade stenoses. The two most common guidewire diameters are 0.35 inches for larger vessels, and 0.14 inches for smaller vessels. These are advanced most safely under fluoroscopy, although the experienced interventionalist may blindly advance the guidewire up to the aortic arch in an emergent setting. Catheters also are available in many different varieties, and it is the size and tip of the catheter that determines its function (▶ Fig. 26.2). Similar to guidewires, they are advanced under fluoroscopy. Catheters are generally used to navigate difficult anatomy, guide devices, and obtain angiographic images with contrast injection. Angioplasty and occlusion balloons are tools used for dilation of high-grade lesions, for dilation of stents after deployment to prevent or treat endoleaks, or to obtain proximal control in an emergent setting. This application has many potential uses in trauma. The balloon may be advanced over a guidewire and inflated under fluoroscopy at the proximal aorta (▶ Fig. 26.3), subclavian, iliac, or femoral arteries to achieve hemorrhage control prior to endovascular or open treatment of a more distal injury. This rapid maneuver can be life-saving by dramatically reducing blood loss and delaying the onset of coagulopathy.

Technological advances in the interventional industry have significantly increased the applicability of many devices to the treatment of vascular injury. The earliest stents were bare metal stents, originally used for dilating and providing radial force to prevent restenosis (▶ Fig. 26.4). As many vascular injuries require coverage of the damaged area, these were not useful in vascular injury. However, there are now very many types of covered stents with bare metal scaffolding interlaced with polytetrafluoroethylene. These covered stents, or stent grafts, are now able to exclude lesions such as partial or full-thickness lacerations that cause or could potentially cause hemorrhage

26.2 Aortic Injury

Thoracic endovascular aortic repair (TEVAR) is currently the most studied endovascular intervention in trauma. The short-term data suggests that aortic stent grafting is comparable to

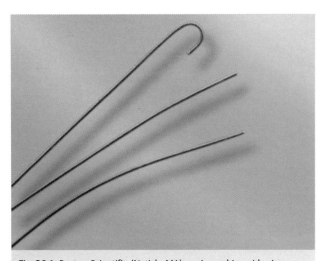

Fig. 26.1 Boston Scientific (Natick, MA) angiographic guidewires.

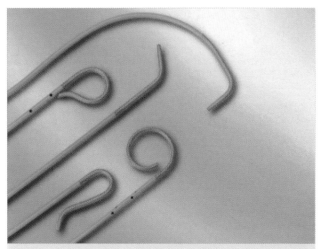

Fig. 26.2 Boston Scientific (Natick, MA) angiographic catheters.

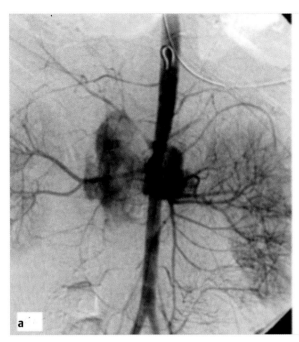

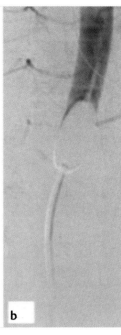

Fig. 26.3 (a) Angiogram demonstrating active extravasation at the level of the celiac axis. (b) Intra-aortic occlusive balloon technique at the proximal abdominal aorta. (Reprinted with permission from author, S. Shalhub, Thompson, C. M., Deboard, Z. M.,Maier, R. V. Revisiting the pancreaticoduodenectomy for trauma: A single institution's experience. Journal of Trauma and Acute Care Surgery 2013:Aug;75(2):225–228)

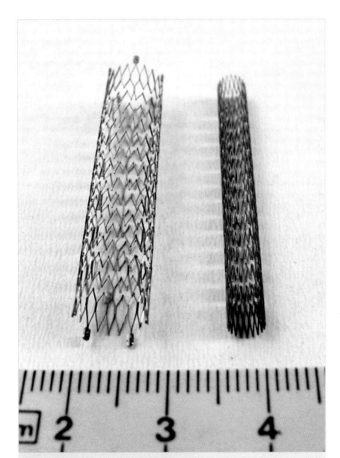

Fig. 26.4 Bare metal endovascular stents.

open repair, citing lower rates of paraplegia, blood loss, complications, and shorter hospital stays.[3,4,5] The difficulty in determining whether this is the standard of care comes from a lack of long-term data. With so many young patients receiving aortic stent grafts, the relationship of the aging stent graft to the aging aorta is unknown. Complications of TEVAR include stent collapse (▶ Fig. 26.5) and "bird beaking" (the proximal portion of the stent graft does not oppose to the aortic wall) due to size mismatching and/or a small arch radius, and may ultimately lead to the need of additional endovascular or open repair. Technology is advancing rapidly, and many industry-sponsored multi-institutional trials are currently investigating aortic devices with improved deployment systems and conformability, particularly suitable for the small arch radius aortas seen in younger patients.

Injuries to the thoracic and abdominal aorta that are within proximity to major branch vessels present a challenge when the proximal or distal landing zones for the device includes the take-off of major branch vessels. The use of standard stent grafts would cover the ostium of those vessels. In the thoracic aorta, coverage of the left subclavian artery has been routinely performed with minimal morbidity. Close observation is usually sufficient, in the event that symptoms develop and progress, a carotid-subclavian bypass is required. Other situations, such as prior cardiac surgery, may necessitate a bypass procedure prior to stent-graft placement. In the abdominal aorta, major injuries near the visceral and renal vessels would not be amenable to stent placement. Technological advancements such as fenestrated (▶ Fig. 26.6) or branched grafts are only used in the United States in trials for elective aortic surgery. These devices have been used with success in other countries, and will be available in the future for off-label use in the injured aorta. Additionally, the chimney technique, in which the branch vessels are stented along with the aorta (▶ Fig. 26.7) may be an option for select patients. Unfortunately, this technique is time

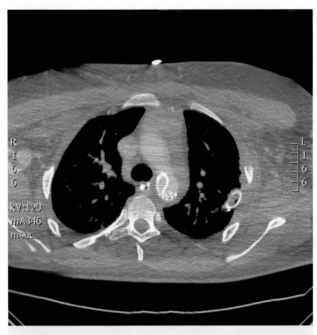

Fig. 26.5 Aortic stent graft collapse following repair of traumatic transection.

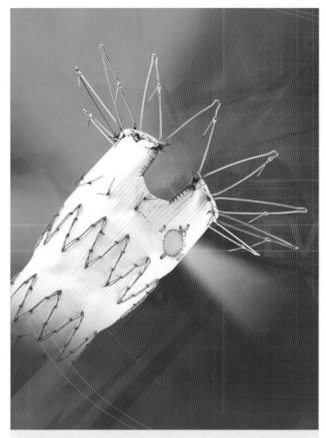

Fig. 26.6 Fenestrated aortic stent graft.

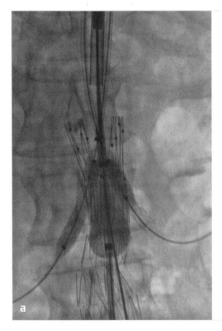

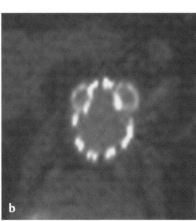

Fig. 26.7 (a) Chimney technique for perirenal lesions, treated with bilateral renal stent grafts and an aortic stent graft. (b) The axial view demonstrates patent bilateral renal stent grafts and good apposition of the renal and aortic stent grafts. (Reprinted with permission from the author W Anthony Lee, Kevin J Bruen; Robert J Feezor; Michael J Daniels; Adam W Beck. Endovascular chimney technique versus open repair of juxtarenal and suprarenal aneurysms. Journal of vascular surgery 2011;53(4):895–904; discussion 904–5.Source:

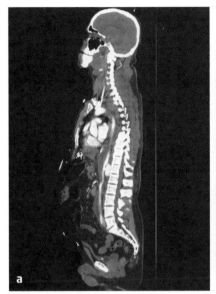
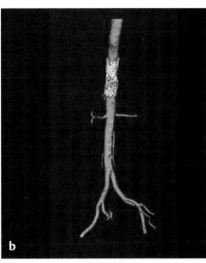

Fig. 26.8 (a) Supraceliac aortic pseudoaneurysm with hematoma 2 cm proximal to celiac origin. (b) Treated with stent graft.

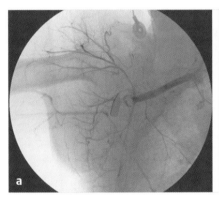
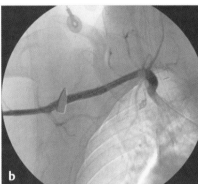

Fig. 26.9 Gunshot wound to the axillary artery (a) treated with a stent graft (b). (Reprinted with permission from the author, M. Cox, O'Brien J. P > Stents in Tents: endovascular therapy on the battlefields of the global war on terror. Surg. Radiol., 2011;2:1–27)

consuming and requires a high degree of interventional experience. Rarely, an aortic injury occurs where the proximal and distal landing zones do not place branch vessels at risk, and a stent is an excellent and minimally invasive treatment option (▶ Fig. 26.8).[6]

26.3 Injury to the Extremities

Treatment of extremity injury may be performed using endovascular techniques. As previously described, the occlusion balloon may be a life-saving measure in the event of exsanguinating hemorrhage, particularly where body habitus may impede rapid dissection and proximal control. Injuries to the distal subclavian or axillary arteries can be managed with balloon tamponade, which may prevent an upper median sternotomy incision to achieve proximal control. A stent can then be placed across the lesion to prevent further blood loss (▶ Fig. 26.9), or the balloon may stay in place while an open exploration is performed. Injury to the subclavian or axillary vein, or brachial plexus, as well as the physiological status of the patient and their body habitus, will determine whether an endovascular or a hybrid procedure is necessary.

Endovascular treatment of extremity injuries is more common, although there exists only small case series in the literature. Limb-salvage and survival rates are reported up to 100%, but no comparison between open and endovascular therapy treatment has been reported.[7] Injury to the carotid arteries is also amenable to endovascular therapy. With reported 30-day mortality and stroke rates of 5%, this therapy may be comparable to open repair.[8]

26.4 Venous System

Although injury to the venous system less commonly requires operative intervention, stent grafts have been used with success for injuries to the inferior vena cava (IVC). The more common type of lesion due to trauma occurs in the venous system in the form of deep vein thrombosis (DVT). Prevention of pulmonary embolism (PE) from DVT in many trauma patients, especially those with traumatic brain injury, cannot be achieved with anticoagulation. Inferior vena cava filters may be placed in such patients to prevent the migration of clot and subsequent PE. There are many varieties of filters ranging from temporary to long-term, and they may be placed under fluoroscopic guidance

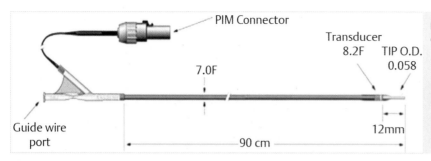

Fig. 26.10 Intravascular ultrasound transducer, catheter, and connecting system.

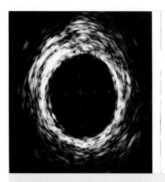 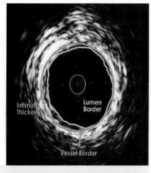

Fig. 26.11 Intravascular ultrasound 360-degree view of a vessel lumen.

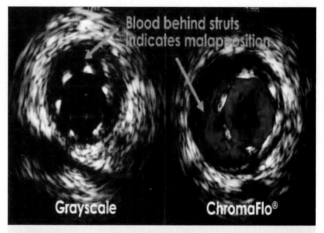

Fig. 26.12 Intravascular ultrasound color-flow mode (ChromaFlo) can visualize blood flow within the vessel lumen, and around malapposed stent grafts.

in the interventional suite or at bedside. Some interventionalists have successfully utilized intravascular ultrasound (IVUS) to place these filters when the use of contrast is contraindicated.

Endovascular techniques of thrombolysis using equipment such as the AngioJet (MEDRAD, Inc., Warrendale, PA) or Trellis (Covidien plc, Dublin, Ireland) allow dissolution of a DVT without use of anticoagulation (AngioJet), or focal use of thrombolytics as in the case of the Trellis. Additionally, catheters such as the Export catheter (Medtronic, Minneapolis, MN) may be effective by using simple suction therapy along the affected vein. There are many potential applications for endovascular therapy in the setting of venous injury, or sequelae of injury.

26.5 Diagnosing Vascular Injury

With the advent of the 64-slice helical computed tomography (CT) scan, vascular injury is being diagnosed more commonly, and smaller injuries are detected that would never have been seen decades ago. The CT angiogram (CTA) has become an established tool for diagnosing vascular injury by its ability to give three-dimensional (3D) views along with the sensitivity to detect intimal flaps, dissections, pseudoaneurysms, hematomas, and contrast extravasation through full-thickness injuries. The disadvantages include administration of intravenous (IV) contrast, radiation exposure, and travel risks. Angiograms, once thought to be the gold standard in diagnosis of vascular injury, have been replaced by the CTA in many situations. Small, partial-thickness injuries to large vessels without hematoma or extravasation on CTA can largely be observed. Equivocal traumatic lesions require a formal angiogram to examine the vessel and determine the extent of the injury. Disadvantages of angiograms include IV contrast administration, radiation exposure, travel risks, and access complications. Magnetic resonance

angiography (MRA) is useful in select situations such as contrast allergy or renal dysfunction, but its function is limited in the trauma population. Duplex ultrasound is a simple, noninvasive tool whose role in diagnosing vascular injury remains to be declared.

26.6 Looking Inside Out

Intravascular ultrasound is an endovascular imaging tool that may play a significant role in the diagnosis of vascular injury in the future. Developed in the 1960s by Born for two-dimensional (2D) imaging of coronary vessels, IVUS takes the concept of ultrasound and applies it to a "view from the inside" approach. The miniature ultrasound transducer is mounted on a catheter tip, and the ultrasound beam rotates around the axis of the catheter (▶ Fig. 26.10) to give a 360-degree axial view of the vessel (▶ Fig. 26.11). Intravascular ultrasound is the most sophisticated diagnostic tool available; it is the only modality able to visualize all three vessel layers simultaneously. It can measure lumen diameter to accurately size stent grafts, examine wall thickness, lesion shape, size, and type, as well as the position of the lesion within the vessel lumen. Intravascular ultrasound can distinguish intimal flaps, dissections, pseudoaneurysms, and transections as well as visualizing blood flow with the color-flow mode (▶ Fig. 26.12). There are no additional risks associated with IVUS if performed as part of angiography; risks of use without angiography include contrast exposure and access site complications. Several reports in the literature have

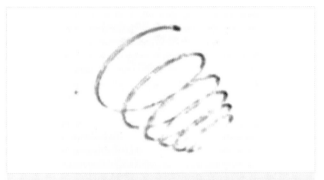

Fig. 26.13 Cook Medical (Bloomington, IN) Tornado embolization coil.

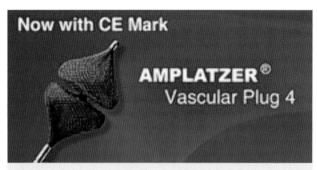

Fig. 26.14 AGA Medical (Plymouth, MN) Amplatzer vascular plug.

solidified the utility of IVUS in the diagnosis of vascular trauma by both changing the diagnosis and ruling out injuries previously equivocal on angiogram.[9] Furthermore, a comparison of CT, angiography, and IVUS studies in blunt traumatic aortic injury reported an unmatched sensitivity and specificity (100%) of the IVUS compared with all other modalities.[10] Intravascular ultrasound has been used to place IVC filters at the bedside when IV contrast and/or traveling outside the intensive care unit is unsafe.

Intravascular ultrasound can be used for diagnostic purposes because it can help to determine chronic variants from acute injuries, rule out injuries deemed indeterminate by other modalities, and determine candidates for endovascular therapy. During the treatment of a vascular injury, IVUS can give accurate measurements for sizing and placement of stent grafts as well as confirm apposition and absence of endoleak (potentially decreasing contrast exposure). Intravascular ultrasound may be used as a screening tool, for follow-up of minor injuries, or in lieu of CTA or angiogram when iondinated contrast is contraindicated.

26.7 Endovascular Damage Control

The concept of damage control can be applied to endovascular therapy in trauma. Approximately 20% of those trauma patients in a recent review who presented with hypotension were treated with endovascular therapy, thus hemodynamic instability should not itself necessitate an open operation.[2] Endovascular technology can be effectively used to provide life-saving hemorrhage control. A balloon catheter can be advanced quickly up a guidewire to the aorta or branch vessel to provide proximal vascular control (▶ Fig. 26.3). This can remain in place throughout the operation regardless of whether the repair is performed open or not. The balloon can be deflated, readjusted, and reinflated for optimal positioning, which may change throughout the procedure. This is a basic maneuver which can significantly alter the outcome of the patient.

Diagnostic angiography may also be used for diagnostic purposes, particularly in the multitrauma patient whose body habitus or hemodynamic instability prevents travel to the CT

scanner. Interventionalists have been providing endovascular control of splenic, hepatic, pelvic, carotid, and intercostal artery injuries for decades. Technology has advanced from simple coils (▶ Fig. 26.13) to Gelfoam (Pfizer, New York, NY) and plug devices (▶ Fig. 26.14), which can be used to stop hemorrhage in these locations. Angiographic embolization has gained tremendous success in the control of hemorrhage in locations such as the pelvis where direct access is problematic.

Endovascular therapy as damage control can also be used as a bridge to open repair. Stent grafts may be used temporarily or permanently to cover partial- or full-thickness injuries. In cases of major vascular injury that cannot be easily or rapidly accessed with surgical exposure, stent grafting is rapidly becoming the procedure of choice. Placing a stent across a full thickness injury may decrease blood loss and ensuing complications in a physiological devastated patient more effectively than complex open procedures.

Endovascular skills are rapidly gaining momentum in the early treatment of vascular injury. As technology improves, the applicability for endovascular techniques in trauma will only increase. A recently proposed treatment algorithm for blunt abdominal trauma outlines two specific indications for intra-aortic balloon tamponade: in hemodynamically unstable patients with a positive focused assessment with ultrasound for trauma (FAST) or diagnostic peritoneal lavage (DPL), or in hemodynamically unstable patients with a pelvic fracture and a negative FAST or DPL.[4] Furthermore, the proposed algorithm recommends an aortic or pelvic angiogram after balloon occlusion in unstable patients with a negative FAST or DPL. Damage control surgery is being redefined to include endovascular techniques such as balloon occlusion, angiography, and embolization.

26.8 Minimal Vascular Injury

For many vascular injuries, follow-up timing and modality of imaging is under investigation. Minor injuries usually require serial imaging and antiplatelet therapy if safe. No consensus exists for optimal timing or modality of follow-up. Given each patient's unique injury, presentation, recovery, and confounding medical factors, most injuries require a case-by-case approach to follow-up.

26.9 Hybrid Trauma Operating Room

The current model in a many trauma hospitals today are operating suites without full angiographic capabilities, which leads to increased risk to the patient by means of delays due to room or staff availability. Furthermore, some patients (often the most severely injured) require both multiple and urgent procedures which are available only in remote areas of the hospital. Those operating rooms (ORs) that have fluoro tables and a C-arm may be able to accommodate basic angiographic procedures; however, imaging tends to be suboptimal, and the tools and experienced staff required to complete the necessary interventions are likely unavailable.

The answer is a trauma hybrid operating and angiography suite, where the table itself is amenable to fluoroscopy, and the available equipment, devices, and experienced staff are available within minutes and are located only a few feet from the trauma admitting area. A suite that is equipped with a fluoroscopy table, C-arm, monitors, and equipment for both endovascular and open procedures is of significant benefit to the injured patient. The ability to perform multiple procedures almost simultaneously—for example, an exploratory laparotomy and an extremity angiogram—without change in location or time delay, provides more rapid assessment and care of any trauma patient.

The equipment required for a hybrid OR is profound. A fluoroscopy table, C-arm, monitors, lights, as well as anesthesia, surgical, and endovascular supplies form the basis of the hybrid trauma suite. Additional instruments such as a transesophageal echocardiography (TEE), Radiology Information Systems (RISS), IVUS, as well as bypass and dialysis pumps may be needed. Advancements in C-arm technology have led to the production of a CT/C-arm hybrid machine, the Artis Zeego by Siemens (Munich, Germany), which combines high-resolution angiography with CT fluoroscopy. This "CT" is not as sensitive as the 64-slice helical CT, but can give excellent quality 3D views to supplement 2D angiography. Advantages to this modality include obtaining CT images without travel, no additional contrast use, and acquiring sensitive information such as endoleaks, which are not seen or poorly visualized on angiography.

The technology for a hybrid OR is costly, approximately $3 to 9 million total for the room, and 1.5 to 5 million for just the fluoroscopic equipment. In addition, the experience and knowledge of the OR staff is critical to successful hybrid procedures. The circulators and especially scrub technicians need to be comfortable with the acquisition, preparation, use, and billing of devices. A competent radiation technologist is essential to help provide images critical to decision making and treatment. Radiation safety should also be practiced with vigilance.

26.10 Preparing the Trauma Patient for a Hybrid Procedure

Once the patient has been declared a candidate for open/and or endovascular repair, rapid mobilization of the staff and equipment must occur. The anesthesiologists (preferably trauma-trained) must prepare for a variety of scenarios, including blood pressure control and manipulation, rapid transfusions, need for bypass, extracorporeal membrane oxygenation, or TEE. In the absence of an innominate or right subclavian injury, it is wise to obtain arterial and venous monitoring devices on the patient's right upper extremity if possible, leaving the left upper extremity and bilateral groins available for endovascular access. The left brachial artery provides secondary access to the aorta and branch vessels if one or both groins is unavailable, or the lesion is better suited to treatment via this approach. In most cases, the patient should be prepped from chin to toes, with the left upper extremity prepped on an arm board. Certain situations may require slight modifications such as shoulder or back rolls, but the prepping should be nearly all-inclusive. In the event of a gravid patient, lead should be used where possible to minimize exposure. The preparation of the patient for multiple procedures, both endovascular and open, allows significant time to be saved, leading to shorter operative time, and ultimately better patient outcomes.

Many situations arise in the setting of trauma in which a hybrid operating room is ideal. For an unstable patient requiring an exploratory laparotomy for intra-abdominal bleeding and hemostasis of pelvic hemorrhage, the procedures may be done near-simultaneously, and certainly more quickly than if the patient travels to another area of the hospital after the exploration. During or after any open procedures, diagnostic angiograms/IVUS studies may be obtained also within a short period, with no additional travel risks. The hybrid suite is ideal for the treatment of patients with intra-abdominal bleeding and extremity trauma, which can be treated simultaneously, as well as severe traumatic brain injury patients who require emergent craniotomies and endovascular or open treatment of additional injuries.

26.11 The Future

Traditionally, catheter therapy has been limited to use in patients that are stable. Conventional wisdom still states that unstable patients are best served by open exploration and control of vascular injuries. However, this is predicated on the belief that open exposure is more rapid than catheter therapy.

Certainly, in most hospitals this is true most of the time. Interventional radiologists and the staff that runs the angiography suite generally are not in house on off hours. Even in busy trauma centers, it takes an hour to mobilize resources to begin the procedure. This added to the time it takes to do the procedure makes this a poor option in patients who are not stable.

This has placed significant restrictions on our use of catheter therapy. For instance, extraperitoneal pelvic packing has become a popular therapy for pelvic hemostasis after blunt trauma. Although this is sometimes definitive therapy, in many centers this is done as a bridge to angiographic embolization. If embolization was available more quickly, many clinicians would likely utilize it over pelvic packing.

Computed tomography angiography has essentially replaced diagnostic catheter angiography. For many patients, CTA is equal or perhaps even superior to a traditional catheter study. However, CTA is a snapshot in time. The timing of contrast determines the quality and clinical utility of images. There are times when a dynamic study is preferable such as injuries around the popliteal trifurcation. This allows a dynamic assessment of the level of injury and collateral flow around it. Computed tomography angiography cannot provide this. Yet, increasingly, interventional radiologists are more and more reluctant to perform a diagnostic study.

We believe that catheter therapy should become part of the routine armamentarium for the acute care surgeon. Acute care surgeons are in house and are immediately available. Hybrid operating rooms are becoming more common. Quicker access will reduce the time to hemostasis. In addition, acute care surgeons understand the disease of injury and blood loss. Interventional radiologists, though talented operators do not treat critically ill and/or injured patients as the majority of their practice. They may wish to persist to get a better technical result such as superselective embolization in the pelvis when a less selective approach will be equally effective and quicker.

As acute care surgeons become trained in catheter therapy, the possibilities will explode. Balloon catheter vascular control, expanded use of embolization, diagnostic angiography, and stent grafting for injuries currently being managed with open vascular repair, will be the future. It is imperative that acute care surgeons define this future and drive the conversation at a local, regional, national, and international level.

References

[1] Reuben BC, Whitten MG, Sarfati M, Kraiss LW. Increasing use of endovascular therapy in acute arterial injuries: analysis of the National Trauma Data Bank. J Vasc Surg 2007; 46: 1222–1226

[2] Avery LE, Stahlfeld KR, Corcos AC et al. Evolving role of endovascular techniques for traumatic vascular injury: a changing landscape? J Trauma Acute Care Surg 2012; 72: 41–46, discussion 46–47

[3] Demetriades D, Velmahos G, Scalea TM et al. Operative repair or endovascular stent graft in blunt traumatic thoracic aortic injuries: results of an American Association for the Surgery of Trauma Multicenter Study. J Trauma 2008; 64: 561–570

[4] Nicholls S, Karmy-Jones R. Ten-year follow-up after endovascular repair of traumatic abdominal aortic rupture. Innovations (Phila) 2011; 6: 51–53

[5] Dake M, White R, Diethrich EB et al. Report on endograft management of traumatic thoracic aortic transections at 30 days and 1 year from a multidisciplinary subcommittee of the SVS. J Vasc Surg 2011; 53: 1091–1096

[6] Willis M, Neschis D, Menaker J, Lilly M, Scalea T. Stent grafting for a distal thoracic aortic injury. Vasc Endovascular Surg 2011; 45: 187–190

[7] duToit DF, Coolen D, Lambrechts A. de V Odendaal J, Warren BL. The endovascular management of penetrating carotid injuries. Eur J Vasc Surg 2009; 38: 267–272

[8] Piffaretti G, Tozzi M, Lomazzi C et al. Endovascular treatment for traumatic injuries of the peripheral arteries following blunt trauma. Injury 2007; 38: 1091–1097

[9] Azizzadeh A, Valdes J, Miller CC III. et al. The utility of intravascular ultrasound compared to angiography in the diagnosis of blunt traumatic aortic injury. J Vasc Surg 2011; 53: 608–614

[10] Malhotra AK, Fabian TC, Croce MA, Weiman DS, Gavant ML, Pate JW. Minimal aortic injury: a lesion associated with advancing diagnostic techniques. J Trauma 2001; 51: 1042–1048

27 The Future of Interventional Radiology in Trauma

Michael J. Rohrer and Timothy C. Fabian

Although the future is impossible to predict, the recent past and the rapid evolution in the fields of interventional radiology and endovascular surgery allows one to recognize important trends in the delivery of trauma care. The drive to provide less invasive, focally directed, and more cost-effective care will certainly continue. This ensures the continued evolution of innovative technology and procedures. However, the nature of these procedures, the location where these procedures are performed, and even who is performing them is in an ongoing state of flux.

27.1 Future Techniques in Interventional Radiology

At the foundation of the application of the minimally invasive techniques of interventional radiology in trauma is the ability of accurate imaging to establish an exact diagnosis so that a targeted and minimally invasive procedure can be utilized to solve a specific clinical problem. Although the use of diagnostic ultrasound in trauma may be useful, most of the improvements in the care of trauma patients have been driven by improvements in computed tomography (CT) imaging.[1] The ability to obtain high-resolution diagnostic images in a timely fashion has changed the algorithm in the management of trauma and allows the more liberal screening for the identification of injury.[2] For example, the decision to perform an arch aortogram to define the presence of a blunt aortic injury was, in the past, based upon a clinical evaluation of the mechanism of injury combined with a critical review of the chest radiograph to identify indirect evidence of aortic injury such as widening of the mediastinum, the presence of a fractured first rib, and deviation of the trachea.[3] Now, the ease and speed with which a CT scan can be performed liberalizes the indications for screening for an aortic injury substantially, and allows for the increased recognition of this lethal problem before catastrophic symptoms lead to its discovery.[4,5] Improved image acquisition times and image quality have also allowed CT scanning to be the modality that defines the presence of cerebrovascular injury, leading to more opportunities to treat specific problems using catheter-based techniques. Similarly, the ability to define that a focal area of splenic injury is the source of hemoperitoneum permits splenic artery embolization to be performed rather than a laparotomy followed by splenectomy. Embolization of a lacerated lumbar artery is not a technical milestone, but the ability to define this lesion on a CT scan and treat it in a minimally invasive fashion is a quantum leap forward in the care of the injured patient.

Engineering accomplishments such as the development of covered stents, combined with imagination and ingenuity, will continue to drive the evolution of minimally invasive techniques in the care of trauma patients. The development of large covered stents for the treatment of abdominal and thoracic aneurysms, for example, has allowed for the "off-label" use of these devices to treat aortic and great vessel injuries, a practice that is gaining increased popularity as evidenced by the number of case reports and case series that have appeared in the literature over the past several years.[6,7,8,9]

27.2 Future Trauma Operating Rooms

Both interventional procedures and traditional operations play a large role in the contemporary management of injured patients. To date, however, it is rare to combine these two resources in a single location, which leads to frequent patient transport and the need to prioritize the sequential care of injuries. It would be advantageous to not have to move patients so frequently and to allow uninterrupted care of multiple injuries. It is clear, however, that a traditional interventional radiology suite is a poor location to perform an operation, and it is equally clear that an operating room with a portable C-arm is a poor substitute for state-of-the-art imaging equipment.[10,11,12] Many hospitals have already identified the advantages of providing operating rooms with fixed imaging equipment for the performance of endovascular procedures that combine the benefits of the availability of general anesthesia and operative exposure of access vessels with high-quality imaging. The quality of the imaging equipment, ease of use, ergonomics, and ability to perform both open and percutaneous procedures illustrate its value.[10] Future improvements will be derived from the experience of organizing the high density of equipment in a small space and optimizing the placement of overhead operating lights and imaging booms along with the placement of imaging monitors and accompanying operating equipment such as suction and electrocautery. The perfect operating table for this suite that combines the advantages of ease of patient movement, radiologic translucency, as well as ability to provide positioning such as the Trendelenburg and cradling side to side is elusive.[13]

Although the combination of the strengths of the classic operating room and the traditional interventional radiology suite is well established, the intraoperative use of other imaging modalities is in its infancy. Operating rooms have been developed incorporating intraoperative CT scanning as well as intraoperative magnetic resonance imaging (MRI) scanning capabilities.[14] Just one of the many challenges in this case includes fabricating a procedure table that is functional both for the performance of an operation as well as remaining MRI compatible.

In the future, some operating rooms will become very procedure and technology specific, as will the teams who staff those rooms.[12,15] Perhaps the future trauma operating room will be where the trauma patient can undergo an initial trauma evaluation, resuscitation, diagnostic imaging with CT scanning and angiography, and operative treatment in a single location.

27.3 Future Interventional Radiology Practitioners

The term "surgery" has been defined as "the therapeutic use of manual skills."[16] By this definition, the traditional interventional radiologist has long been a "surgeon." Similarly, the traditional vascular surgeon has become expert in vascular imaging and endovascular procedures, and has become an "interventional radiologist." This blending of clinical skills has furthered the evolution of less invasive approaches to the delivery of care. As even basic endovascular skills are acquired by other more traditionally trained surgeons such as trauma surgeons, the performance of angiographic procedures and the use of occlusion balloons placed through sheaths inserted by the Seldinger technique may become routinely incorporated into trauma-management algorithms. With this development, training programs will need fundamental revision to ensure that practitioners are competent to carry out these new procedures.[15]

27.4 Conclusion

The ability to noninvasively image traumatic injuries promptly and definitively allows the application of specific modalities in a less invasive fashion. The exploratory laparotomy will be replaced by the performance of very selectively directed procedures to repair defects that have been identified, and many of these will be minimally invasive procedures performed by the interventional radiologist. Recent applications of interventional procedures such as the use of covered stents to treat blunt thoracic aortic injuries and the use of removable vena cava filters typify the desire to minimize both the short-term and long-term impact of procedures on injured patients. Other advances will be driven by new technology such as the development of biodegradable stents, and the delivery of lysosomes containing bioactive drugs that are activated when required by using ultrasound.[1] Catheters will be used for the delivery of stem cells to areas of spinal cord injury or to deliver medications to injured brain tissue.[1] Improved communication, surgical robots, and applications of teleradiology may even challenge the concept of regionalization of care and allow expert interventions to be provided at remote locations, changing the paradigm of regionalization of care.

The ability to treat problems in a less invasive fashion will translate into a decreased systemic complication rate and decreased physiologic stress. The tradeoff, however, will be the need to identify and address access-site complications, and to be expert at identifying device-specific complications, provide long-term imaging surveillance,[4] and evaluate the long-term effect of these radiological procedures.

References

[1] Sclafani SJ. A look into the future of interventional radiology for the injured patient. Injury 2008; 39: 1304–1307

[2] Sofocleous CT, Hinrichs CR, Hubbi B, Doddakashi S, Bahramipour P, Schubert J. Embolization of isolated lumbar artery injuries in trauma patients. Cardiovasc Intervent Radiol 2005; 28: 730–735

[3] Malloy PC, Richard HM III. Thoracic angiography and intervention in trauma. Radiol Clin North Am 2006; 44: 239–249, viiiviii

[4] Hoffer EK. Endovascular intervention in thoracic arterial trauma. Injury 2008; 39: 1257–1274

[5] Arthurs ZM, Starnes BW. Blunt carotid and vertebral artery injuries. Injury 2008; 39: 1232–1241

[6] Singh MJ, Rohrer MJ, Ghaleb M, Kim D. Endoluminal stent-graft repair of a thoracic aortic transection in a trauma patient with multiple injuries: case report. J Trauma 2001; 51: 376–381

[7] McPhee JT, Asham EH, Rohrer MJ et al. The midterm results of stent graft treatment of thoracic aortic injuries. J Surg Res 2007; 138: 181–188

[8] Kasirajan K, Heffernan D, Langsfeld M. Acute thoracic aortic trauma: a comparison of endoluminal stent grafts with open repair and nonoperative management. Ann Vasc Surg 2003; 17: 589–595

[9] Amabile P, Collart F, Gariboldi V, Rollet G, Bartoli JM, Piquet P. Surgical versus endovascular treatment of traumatic thoracic aortic rupture. J Vasc Surg 2004; 40: 873–879

[10] Hudorović N, Rogan SA, Lovricević I, Zovak M, Schmidt S. The vascular hybrid room—operating room of the future. Acta Clin Croat 2010; 49: 289–298

[11] Kpodonu J. Hybrid cardiovascular suite: the operating room of the future. J Card Surg 2010; 25: 704–709

[12] Kpodonu J, Raney A. The cardiovascular hybrid room a key component for hybrid interventions and image guided surgery in the emerging specialty of cardiovascular hybrid surgery. Interact Cardiovasc Thorac Surg 2009; 9: 688–692

[13] Nollert G, Wich S. Planning a cardiovascular hybrid operating room: the technical point of view. Heart Surg Forum 2009; 12: E125–E130

[14] Matsumae M, Fukuyama H, Osada T et al. Fully functional MR-compatible flexible operating table resolves the neurosurgeon's dilemma over use of intraoperative MRI. Tokai J Exp Clin Med 2008; 33: 57–60

[15] Wickham JE. Minimally invasive surgery. Future developments. BMJ 1994; 308: 193–196

[16] Shaftan GW. How interventional radiology changed the practice of a trauma surgeon. Injury 2008; 39: 1229–1231

Index

Note: Page numbers set **bold** or *italic* indicate headings or figures, respectively.